The Global Impact of the COVID-19 Pandemic on Institutional and Community Corrections

The authors of the chapters included in this volume provide preliminary answers to questions such as:

- How extensive were COVID-19 outbreaks in prisons, jails, and community corrections systems globally? Which regions and countries reported the largest outbreaks?
- Why were prisons and jails found to be "hot spots" for the spread of COVID-19 in most countries?
- How did governments initially respond to COVID-19 outbreaks in their corrections systems?
- Did the mitigation strategies used in each country reduce the spread of the infection in the corrections system (both in prisons and jails, and in community corrections)?
- Did the corrections-focused mitigation strategies used in each country have a positive or an adverse impact on public health and public safety?
- How likely is it that the varied short-term mitigation strategies implemented by governments will result in long-term changes in corrections policies and practices?

The book includes three chapters examining the global impact of the COVID-19 outbreaks, six regional overviews, and 27 country-specific reviews, including reviews targeting 21 of the 50 largest prison systems globally. This collection will be an excellent resource for researchers, policymakers, practitioners, and the general public interested in knowing more about the nature and extent of COVID-19 outbreaks in corrections systems globally, and about the diversity of responses developed and implemented by governments from each global region.

The chapters in this book were originally published as a special issue of the journal *Victims & Offenders*.

James M. Byrne is Professor in the School of Criminology and Justice Studies at the University of Massachusetts Lowell, and Director of the Global Community Corrections Initiative (www.glob.cci.org). His edited texts include *The Social Ecology of Crime* (1986), *Smart Sentencing: The Emergence of Intermediate Sanctions* (1994), *The New Technology of Crime, Law and Social Control* (2007), and *The Culture of Prison Violence* (2008).

Don Hummer is Associate Professor in the School of Public Affairs, Penn State Harrisburg. His research focuses on corrections policy, violence, and the implications of technological advances for justice system actors. He is co-editor of *The Culture of Prison Violence* (2008) and *Handbook of Police Administration* (2008).

Sabrina S. Rapisarda is a doctoral student in the School of Criminology and Justice Studies at the University of Massachusetts Lowell. Much of Sabrina's work has been anchored in the public health framework. Her current research investigates various aspects of the criminal justice system's response to COVID-19.

The Global Impact of the COVID-19 Pandemic on Institutional and Community Corrections

Edited by
James M. Byrne, Don Hummer, and Sabrina S. Rapisarda

Routledge
Taylor & Francis Group
LONDON AND NEW YORK

First published 2022
by Routledge
2 Park Square, Milton Park, Abingdon, Oxon OX14 4RN

and by Routledge
605 Third Avenue, New York, NY 10158

Routledge is an imprint of the Taylor & Francis Group, an informa business

British Library Cataloguing in Publication Data
A catalogue record for this book is available from the British Library

ISBN: 978-1-032-01491-3 (hbk)
ISBN: 978-1-032-03896-4 (pbk)
ISBN: 978-1-003-18957-2 (ebk)

Typeset in Minion Pro
by Newgen Publishing UK

Publisher's Note
The publisher accepts responsibility for any inconsistencies that may have arisen during the conversion of this book from journal articles to book chapters, namely the inclusion of journal terminology.

Contents

Citation Information

The chapters in this book were originally published in *Victims & Offenders*, volume 15, issues 7–8 (October 2020). When citing this material, please use the original page numbering for each article, as follows:

Introduction

Introduction to Special Issue
James Byrne, Don Hummer, and Sabrina Rapisarda
Victims & Offenders, volume 15, issues 7–8 (October 2020), pp. 835–838

Chapter 1

The Global Impact of the Pandemic on Institutional and Community Corrections: Assessing Short-Term Crisis Management and Long-Term Change Strategies
Kathryn M. Nowonty and Alex R. Piquero
Victims & Offenders, volume 15, issues 7–8 (October 2020), pp. 839–847

Chapter 2

Commentary: Assessing the Global Impact of the Covid-19 Pandemic on Prison Populations
Catherine Heard
Victims & Offenders, volume 15, issues 7–8 (October 2020), pp. 848–861

Chapter 3

An Imperfect Storm: Identifying the Root Causes of COVID-19 Outbreaks in the World's Largest Corrections Systems
James Byrne, Sabrina S. Rapisarda, Don Hummer, and Kimberly R. Kras
Victims & Offenders, volume 15, issues 7–8 (October 2020), pp. 862–909

Chapter 4

An Examination of COVID-19 Outbreaks in African Prisons and Jails
Sabrina S. Rapisarda and James M. Byrne
Victims & Offenders, volume 15, issues 7–8 (October 2020), pp. 910–920

Chapter 5

The Silver Lining in the Covid-19 Cloud: An Appraisal of Accelerated Prison Decongestion in Kenya
Mercy Deche and Conrad Bosire
Victims & Offenders, volume 15, issues 7–8 (October 2020), pp. 921–932

Chapter 6

The Social and Environmental Implications of the Novel Coronavirus on Institutional and Community Corrections in South Africa
Kimberly R. Kras and Lincoln Fitz
Victims & Offenders, volume 15, issues 7–8 (October 2020), pp. 933–947

Chapter 7

An Examination of COVID-19 Outbreaks in Prisons and Jails Throughout Asia
Sabrina S. Rapisarda and James M. Byrne
Victims & Offenders, volume 15, issues 7–8 (October 2020), pp. 948–958

Chapter 8

Correctional System's Response to the Coronavirus Pandemic and Its Implications for Prison Reform in China
Spencer D. Li and Tzu-Hsuan Liu
Victims & Offenders, volume 15, issues 7–8 (October 2020), pp. 959–969

Chapter 9

Lock Unlock: The Impact of COVID-19 on Health Security in Pakistani and Indian Prisons
Jared R. Dmello and Sheetal Ranjan
Victims & Offenders, volume 15, issues 7–8 (October 2020), pp. 970–987

Chapter 10

National Responses for Persons Deprived of Liberty during the COVID-19 Pandemic in the Philippines
Michael B. Cahapay
Victims & Offenders, volume 15, issues 7–8 (October 2020), pp. 988–995

Chapter 11

South Korea's Responses regarding Mitigating the COVID-19 Crisis behind Bars
Claire Seungeun Lee
Victims & Offenders, volume 15, issues 7–8 (October 2020), pp. 996–1008

Chapter 12

An Examination of COVID-19 Outbreaks in South American Prisons and Jails
Sabrina S. Rapisarda, James M. Byrne, and Lina Marmolejo
Victims & Offenders, volume 15, issues 7–8 (October 2020), pp. 1009–1018

Chapter 13

The Brazilian Penitentiary System under the Threat of COVID-19
Ludmila Ribeiro and Alexandre M. A. Diniz
Victims & Offenders, volume 15, issues 7–8 (October 2020), pp. 1019–1043

Chapter 14

Assessing the Effects of COVID-19 in Prisons in the Northern Triangle of Central America
Wayne J. Pitts and Christopher S. Inkpen
Victims & Offenders, volume 15, issues 7–8 (October 2020), pp. 1044–1061

Chapter 15

Responding to COVID-19 in Latin American Prisons: The Cases of Argentina, Chile, Colombia, and Mexico
Lina Marmolejo, Daniela Barberi, Marcelo Bergman, Olga Espinoza, and Gustavo Fondevila
Victims & Offenders, volume 15, issues 7–8 (October 2020), pp. 1062–1085

Chapter 16

Women Providing and Men Free Riding: Work, Visits and Gender Roles in Mexican Prisons
Carolina Agoff, Sveinung Sandberg, and Gustavo Fondevila
Victims & Offenders, volume 15, issues 7–8 (October 2020), pp. 1086–1104

Chapter 17

The Impact of COVID-19 Outbreaks in the Prisons, Jails, and Community Corrections Systems Throughout Europe
Sabrina S. Rapisarda and James M. Byrne
Victims & Offenders, volume 15, issues 7–8 (October 2020), pp. 1105–1112

Chapter 18

The Impact of Covid-19 on Prisons and Penal Policy in Germany
Frieder Dünkel
Victims & Offenders, volume 15, issues 7–8 (October 2020), pp. 1113–1123

Chapter 19

Fears of COVID-19 Contagion and the Italian Prison System Response
April Pattavina and Michael J. Palmieri
Victims & Offenders, volume 15, issues 7–8 (October 2020), pp. 1124–1132

Chapter 20

An Examination of The Romanian Prison System During The COVID-19 pandemic. Are "Zero Cases" Possible?
Ioan Durnescu and Ioana Morar
Victims & Offenders, volume 15, issues 7–8 (October 2020), pp. 1133–1147

Chapter 21

The Penitentiary System of Russia during the COVID-19 Pandemic: A Global Challenge and Initial Results
Sergei Ovchinnikov
Victims & Offenders, volume 15, issues 7–8 (October 2020), pp. 1148–1155

Chapter 22

Corrections and Crime in Spain and Portugal during the Covid-19 Pandemic: Impact, Prevention and Lessons for the Future
Santiago Redondo, Rui Abrunhosa Gonçalves, Javier Nistal, Carlos Soler, José Semedo Moreira, Joana Andrade, and Antonio Andrés-Pueyo
Victims & Offenders, volume 15, issues 7–8 (October 2020), pp. 1156–1185

Chapter 23

Telematic Control and Semi-Freedom as a Response to the Pandemic: The Spanish Penitentiary System Experience
Esther Montero Perez de Tudela
Victims & Offenders, volume 15, issues 7–8 (October 2020), pp. 1186–1202

Chapter 24

Sweden's Response to the COVID-19 Outbreak
Maria Lindström, Emma Ahlstrand, and Jenny Kärrholm
Victims & Offenders, volume 15, issues 7–8 (October 2020), pp. 1203–1214

Chapter 25

Responses Taken to Mitigate COVID-19 in Prisons in England and Wales
Pauline K. Brennan
Victims & Offenders, volume 15, issues 7–8 (October 2020), pp. 1215–1233

Chapter 26

An Examination of COVID-19 Outbreaks in Prisons and Jails in North America, Central America, and the Caribbean
Sabrina S. Rapisarda, James Byrne, and Lina Marmolejo
Victims & Offenders, volume 15, issues 7–8 (October 2020), pp. 1234–1243

Chapter 27

Institutional Responses to the COVID-19 Pandemic in American Prisons
Meghan A. Novisky, Chelsey S. Narvey, and Daniel C. Semenza
Victims & Offenders, volume 15, issues 7–8 (October 2020), pp. 1244–1261

Chapter 28

United States Bureau of Prisons' Response to the COVID-19 Pandemic
Don Hummer
Victims & Offenders, volume 15, issues 7–8 (October 2020), pp. 1262–1276

Chapter 29

Adaptations to COVID-19 in Community Corrections Agencies across the United States
Jill Viglione, Lucas M. Alward, Ashley Lockwood, and Sara Bryson
Victims & Offenders, volume 15, issues 7–8 (October 2020), pp. 1277–1297

Chapter 30

The Response to the COVID19 Crisis by the Pennsylvania Department of Corrections
John E. Wetzel and Janeen M. Davis
Victims & Offenders, volume 15, issues 7–8 (October 2020), pp. 1298–1304

Chapter 31

A Case Study of the Westchester County New York's Jail Response to COVID-19: Controlling COVID while Balancing Service Needs for the Incarcerated-A National Model for Jails
Kimberly Collica-Cox and Louis Molina
Victims & Offenders, volume 15, issues 7–8 (October 2020), pp. 1305–1316

Chapter 32

British Columbia Provincial Corrections' Response to the COVID-19 Pandemic: A Case Study of Correctional Policy and Practice
Danielle J. Murdoch
Victims & Offenders, volume 15, issues 7–8 (October 2020), pp. 1317–1336

Chapter 33

Management of COVID-19 for Persons with Mental Illness in Secure Units: A Rapid International Review to Inform Practice in Québec
Ashley J. Lemieux, Audrey-Anne Dumais Michaud, Jean Damasse, Julie-Katia Morin-Major, To Nhu Nguyen, Alain Lesage, and Anne G. Crocker
Victims & Offenders, volume 15, issues 7–8 (October 2020), pp. 1337–1360

Chapter 34

An Examination of COVID-19 Outbreaks in Prisons and Jails in Oceania
Sabrina S. Rapisarda and James M. Byrne
Victims & Offenders, volume 15, issues 7–8 (October 2020), pp. 1361–1366

Chapter 35

COVID-19 and Corrections in Australia: A Summary Review of the Available Data and Literature
Jason L. Payne and Natalia Hanley
Victims & Offenders, volume 15, issues 7–8 (October 2020), pp. 1367–1384

Chapter 36

"We Must Go Hard and We Must Go Early": How New Zealand Halted Coronavirus in the Community and Corrections
Laura J. Murray and Kimberly R. Kras
Victims & Offenders, volume 15, issues 7–8 (October 2020), pp. 1385–1395

Notes on Contributors

Carolina Agoff is a senior researcher at the National Autonomous University of Mexico (UNAM) since 2004. She received her Ph.D. in Psychology at Free University of Berlin (Germany) in 2001. Her main research interest is the empirical study of gender violence in different settings such as indigenous communities and universities, among undocumented Latino workers in the USA or lower-class urban working women. Her current work focuses on prison populations in Mexico with a narrative criminological approach.

Emma Ahlstrand serves as an officer for the Security Planning Unit in the headquarters of the Swedish Prison and Probation Service (SPPS). After earning her degree in forensic psychology, she started working for the SPPS in 2016 as a correctional officer at a jail and prison; she currently teaches at the SPPS National Correctional Officer Training Program.

Lucas M. Alward is a doctoral candidate in the Department of Criminal Justice at the University of Central Florida. His primary research interests include procedural justice and legitimacy, reentry and desistance, and the implementation of effective correctional interventions. His recent research has appeared in *Journal of Criminal Justice, Criminal Justice and Behavior,* and *European Journal of Probation.*

Joana Andrade, M.S. in Applied Psychology, is a researcher in the Psychology Research Centre at the University of Minho. She is involved in several research projects, conferences and international publications in criminal psychology. Her research interests are mainly in criminality, offending behavior, and offender treatment and rehabilitation.

Antonio Andrés-Pueyo is a Professor of Violence Psychology and Criminal Psychology and Director of the Department of Clinical Psychology and Psychobiology at the University of Barcelona. His main research area is violence risk assessment in professional settings. He has published papers and reports in violence prevention, aggression, impulsivity, individual differences and personality.

Daniela Barberi is a doctoral student in the Criminology, Law and Society program at George Mason University (GMU). She holds a Master's in Criminal Justice from the Pennsylvania State University (USA) where she earned two awards (Outstanding Graduate Student and Outstanding Master's Thesis) and a Bachelor of Arts in Psychology from the Universidad de Los Andes (Bogota, Colombia). Daniela currently works with the Pan American Development Foundation (PADF) based in Bogota, Colombia. Her research interests include corrections, translational research, alternatives to incarceration, reentry programs, prisoner treatment, and minority populations.

Marcelo Bergman is a Professor of Sociology and Criminology at Universidad Tres de Febrero (UNTREF), Argentina. He is also the Director of the Center for Latin American Studies on Insecurity and Violence (CELIV). He has been an advisor to the Ministry of Justice in Argentina in prisoner reentry topics and coordinated more than 15 surveys of prisoners in Latin America and the Caribbean. His areas of expertise include public security, illegal drugs and public policy, taxation, compliance, and the rule of law in Latin America. Dr. Bergman is particularly interested in evidence-based research on criminal justice, citizen security and illegal drug policies in Latin America, with a focus on sound data collection. His two most recent books are: *More Money, More Crime* (Oxford U Press, 2018) and *Prisons and Crime in Latin America* (coauthored with Gustavo Fondevila, Cambridge U. Press, 2021).

Conrad Bosire is the Chief of Staff in the Office of the Chief Justice, and the Acting Executive Director of the National Council on the Administration of Justice (NCAJ), a statutory body that coordinates justice sector agencies to ensure coherence in the administration of justice. Dr. Bosire is an expert in law, governance, and human rights, and holds a Doctor of Philosophy (Law) from the University of the Western Cape (UWC), South Africa, and a Master of Law (LLM) from the University of Pretoria (UP).

Pauline K. Brennan is a Professor and the Ph.D. Program Director for the School of Criminology and Justice Studies at the University of Massachusetts Lowell. Her research focuses on racial and gender inequities in court processing, corrections policy, and issues related to female offenders and victims. She has been the principal investigator on projects funded by the National Institute of Corrections and the Foundation for the Carolinas and has worked closely on policy-relevant research with community practitioners in North Carolina, Nebraska, and Iowa. For over a decade, she has served as the Director of a study abroad program to London, England, through her professional contacts with English prison staff, court personnel, and police officers. Her work has appeared in *Justice Quarterly, The Journal of Quantitative Criminology*, and *Criminal Justice and Behavior.*

Sara L. Bryson, Ph.D., is an Assistant Professor in the Department of Criminal Justice at East Carolina University. Her research interests include the juvenile justice system, juvenile delinquency, and school safety. Her most recent research appears in *Youth Violence and Juvenile Justice, School Psychology Review,* and the *Journal of Interpersonal Violence.*

James M. Byrne is a Professor in the School of Criminology and Justice Studies at University of Massachusetts Lowell, and Director of the Global Community Corrections Initiative (www.glob.cci.org). His edited texts include: *The Social Ecology of Crime* (1986), *Smart Sentencing: The Emergence of Intermediate Sanctions* (1994), *The New Technology of Crime, Law and Social Control* (2007), and *The Culture of Prison Violence* (2008). Dr. Byrne currently serves as a member of the Independent Review Committee responsible for advising the U.S. Attorney General on the design and implementation of the Risk Need Assessment System that is a central component of the Congressionally mandated 2018 First Step Act, a major federal prison reform initiative. Dr. Byrne also serves as a member, Panel of Experts – Correctional Services Advisory and Accreditation Panel, Ministry of Justice, United Kingdom. He previously served as the External Inspector of Prisons, Office of the Inspector General, Queensland Correctional Services, Australia (2014), where he conducted an independent review of the prison assault problem in Queensland's prisons.

Michael B. Cahapay is an Assistant Professor at Mindanao State University, General Santos City, Philippines. He is completing his Ph.D. in Education at the University of the Philippines, Diliman. His recent research examines the vulnerable groups of society amid the COVID-19 crisis.

Kimberly Collica-Cox is a Professor in the Criminal Justice and Security Department with PACE University and the Director of the Parenting, Prison, & Pups Program. Prior to teaching, Dr. Collica-Cox worked for a women's correctional facility in NYS coordinating an HIV prison-based peer education program and for a NY jail supervising the jail-based transitional services unit. She trains professionals in HIV-related issues in the NYS Metropolitan area and is a certified ACA (American Correctional Association) and PREA (Prison Rape Elimination Act) Auditor. Her research focuses on incarcerated women, rehabilitation, reintegration, prison-based programming, and female correctional executives. She is the recipient of the prestigious National Jefferson Award for Public Service and the Ken Peak Innovation in Teaching Award from the Academy of Criminal Justice Sciences.

Anne G. Crocker is full Professor at the Department of Psychiatry & Addictions and the School of Criminology at the Université de Montréal, the Director of Research and Academics at the Philippe Pinel Institute, and President of the International Association of Forensic Mental Health Services. She sits on many national forensic mental health policy advisory committees. Her research program focuses on the interface between justice and mental health, forensic mental health services, and pathways to violence.

Jean Damasse is a member of the Rapid Evidence Assessment Team that conducted the review of COVID-19 responses in secure psychiatric settings. He has contributed to various research projects in the field of social research, and his work has appeared in *the Journal of Urban Sociology*. Since 2012, he has worked as a research professional in health technology assessment in the social services sector.

Janeen M. Davis is an RN Supervisor with over 26 years of correctional experience transitioning from line staff, Training Academy educator, Diagnostic and Classification Center RN supervisor to working with the Department's Bureau of Health Care Administration on policy development, internal management reviews, and special projects. She graduated from Penn State University with a BS in Nursing and a Master's in Health Education. Ms. Davis has been a key member of the COVID-19 medical assessment team providing critical guidance to the field and leadership.

Mercy Deche is a Lecturer at the School of Law, University of Nairobi, Mombasa Campus. She is also the current Vice Chairperson of the Judicial Service Commission. In the past, she has served as a Special Prosecutor for Sexual and Gender Based Violence cases. Her areas of specialization are access to justice, restorative justice, legal research, and gender.

Alexandre M. A. Diniz is a Professor in the Geography Department at the Pontifical Catholic University of Minas Gerais (PUC Minas). He holds a bachelor's degree in Advertising from PUC Minas; a master's degree in Geography from Kansas State University, and a Ph.D. in Geography from Arizona State University. He was a visiting scholar at McGill University, Université de Lille, Curtin University, and Texas State University. His experience is in the field of Human Geography, acting on the following subjects: Geography of Crime and Violence, Urban Geography, and Regional Geography.

Jared R. Dmello is an Assistant Professor of Criminal Justice in the Department of Social Sciences at Texas A&M International University. His research focuses on collective action, covering primarily terrorism, ethnic conflict, and criminal street gangs. Dr. Dmello is the recipient of the 2020 Ken Peak Innovations in Teaching Award from the Academy of

Criminal Justice Sciences and the Principal Investigator on a National Institute of Justice funded examination of street gang networks.

Audrey-Anne Dumais Michaud holds a Ph.D. in Sociology and is an Associate Professor of Social Work at the Université du Québec en Outaouais. Her research focuses on mental health, social problems, as well as social and penal policies. She is also a researcher at the Mental Health and Justice Hub.

Frieder Dünkel was the previous President of the European Society of Criminology (ESC, 2015–2016), a previous Dean of Law (1994–1995), and Vice-Rector (2010–2013) of the University of Greifswald in northeast Germany. He taught criminology, penology, juvenile justice, criminal procedure and criminal law at the University of Greifswald Faculty of Law and Economics, from 1992 to 2015 and has conducted many research projects, including international comparative projects on male prisons in the countries around the Baltic Sea, female imprisonment in Europe, long-term imprisonment in 10 European countries, youth violence and juvenile justice systems in Europe (covering 33 European jurisdictions). From 2011 to 2015, he coordinated a survey on the legal aspects and practice of restorative justice in 36 European jurisdictions (funded by the EU). He has published widely in these areas (by 2020, 47 books and 615 articles in criminal justice journals and books) and organized numerous international conferences on prison research, juvenile justice, and restorative justice.

Ioan Durnescu is a Professor at the University of Bucharest/Faculty of Sociology and Social Work. He worked previously in the prison and probation departments in Romania. He is currently co-editor of the *European Probation Journal*. Ioan Durnescu conducts research, delivers training and courses and offers consultancy services in Romania, Kenya and other countries on prison, probation, and deradicalization issues.

Olga Espinoza is a doctoral candidate in the Social Sciences Department at the University of Chile. She is a lecturer at the School of Public Affairs at the University of Chile, where she teaches public policy in criminal justice, prison systems, and citizen security issues. She has worked as consultant in international organizations (Ford Foundation, Interamerican Development Bank, Organization of American States, United Nations Development Program, and EU – EUROsociAL) and as a researcher in academic centers, mainly in Chile and Brazil. Her research interests include criminal justice, citizen security, female criminality, prison policies, and social reintegration processes. She is a lawyer and holds a Master of Law from the University of Sao Paulo (Brazil).

Lincoln Fitz is a Professor of Corrections Management in the School of Criminal Justice at the University of South Africa, where he teaches Fundamental Penology and Security Management. He had a prior career with the Correctional Service of South Africa and is currently an editor at the journal *Acta Criminologica*.

Gustavo Fondevila is a Professor at the Center for Economic Research and Teaching (CIDE) in Mexico City. He holds a Ph.D. in Law from the University of Buenos Aires (Argentina). He is the author of numerous papers in specialized academic publications. Author — with Marcelo Bergman — of *Prisons and Crime in Latin America*, Cambridge University Press (2020). His research focuses on empirical comparative criminology in Latin America.

Rui Abrunhosa Gonçalves is an Associate Professor with tenure in the School of Psychology at the University of Minho (Braga, Portugal). His research interests include violent and dangerous offenders (psychopaths, sexual abusers, spouse abusers) and the correctional system's response. He also works as a forensic psychologist court expert.

Natalia Hanley is a Senior Lecturer in Criminology in the School of Health and Society at the University of Wollongong. She is a qualitative researcher working on gender-based violence, practices of punishment, and wildlife crime.

Catherine Heard is a Senior Research Fellow at the Institute for Crime & Justice Policy Research (ICPR), based at Birkbeck, University of London. At ICPR, Catherine directs the World Prison Research Programme. This program of international comparative research on prisons and imprisonment builds on the work of the World Prison Brief, ICPR's online database providing details of the prison systems of over 220 independent countries and dependent territories. Catherine worked as a commercial litigation lawyer in London before moving into criminal justice policy and international human rights law, and has held positions at the Law Commission of England & Wales and the NGOs Fair Trials and the Center for Crime and Justice Studies.

Don Hummer is an Associate Professor in the School of Public Affairs, Penn State Harrisburg. His research interests are broadly focused on corrections policy, violence, and the implications of technological advances for justice system actors. He is co-editor of *The Culture of Prison Violence* (2008) and *Handbook of Police Administration* (2008). Recent peer-reviewed articles have appeared in *The Prison Journal, Federal Probation*, and *Journal of Urban Affairs*.

Christopher S. Inkpen is a Research Sociologist and Demographer in the Division for Applied Justice Research at RTI International. He studies quantitative criminology, specifically the application of machine learning techniques to social science data. His substantive research focuses on the intersection of migration and crime.

Jenny Kärrholm is the Head of the Research and Evaluation Unit within the Swedish Prison and Probation Service (SPPS). Jenny earned a Ph.D. in Rehabilitation Medicine and has many years of experience within Swedish government agencies.

Kimberly R. Kras is an Assistant Professor of Criminal Justice in the School of Public Affairs at San Diego State University. Her research considers the experiences of formerly incarcerated persons upon reentry and how the community supervision system supports this transition. Dr. Kras' work has been published in *Criminology, Justice Quarterly*, and *Criminology and Public Policy*.

Ashley J. Lemieux is a Planning, Programming and Research Officer, in the Justice, Security, and Mental Health Technology Assessment Unit at the Institut National de Psychiatrie Légale Philippe-Pinel, Quebec. Ashley's research interests include forensic psychiatry and vulnerable populations, recovery in mental illness, violence risk assessment, homelessness, justice diversion, sexual health, and intimacy.

Alain Lesage is a Professor in the Department of Psychiatry at the University of Montréal, a psychiatrist at the Montréal University Mental Health Institute (IUSMM) and a researcher at its Research Center. Through evaluative and epidemiological research, he studies the care and services needs of people with severe mental disorders. In 1997, he founded a module to evaluate the development of psychiatric services which, in autumn 2011, became the hospital-based mental health technology assessment unit of the IUSMM. Alain Lesage's research interests include schizophrenia, suicide, mood disorders, and other related disorders.

Spencer D. Li is a Professor in the Department of Sociology at University of Macau. His research interests include substance abuse, child development, corrections, and survey research. Dr. Li has served as principal investigator on many publicly and privately funded projects related to adolescent development, religion, substance abuse and criminal justice, including grants from the U.S. National Institute of Health, U.S. Administration for Children and Families, and Social Welfare Bureau of the Government of Macau. His publications have appeared in several leading criminology and penology journals.

Maria Lindström is currently working as Head of the Security Planning Unit in the headquarters of the Swedish Prison and Probation Service (SPPS). She previously served as Liaison and Policy Officer for CEP (Confederation of European Probation) and as governor of the Probation Services in the county of Stockholm. Maria has an academic background in social work and criminology. Maria has a broad range of experience from different managerial positions in prison, jail and probation offices in national and international positions. Maria has been working in different positions within the SPPS since the beginning of the twenty-first century.

Tzu-Hsuan Liu is an Assistant Professor at School of Political Science and Public Administration at Huaqiao University. Her research interests include the Chinese criminal justice system, drug policy, and juvenile delinquency. She has published several articles on the Chinese problem-solving courts, juvenile delinquency and family violence.

Ashley Lockwood is a doctoral student in the Department of Criminal Justice at the University of Central Florida. Ashley's primary research interests examine the intersections of the criminal justice system, mental health and trauma, and disadvantaged groups. Her recent research appears in the *Journal of Police* and *Criminal Psychology and Perspectives.*

Lina Marmolejo is a doctoral candidate in the Criminology, Law and Society Department at George Mason University (GMU). She holds a master's degree in Public Administration from the Institute of Political Studies (Paris, France) and a bachelor's on Finance and International Relations from Universidad Externado de Colombia (Bogota, Colombia). Her research interests include criminal justice and security sector reform, pretrial justice, community corrections, rehabilitation, and reentry programs. Prior to her studies at GMU, she worked at the Inter-American Development Bank and the Organization of American States, in the design, management and implementation of international development projects, with an emphasis on crime and violence prevention in Latin America and the Caribbean.

Louis Molina is the First Deputy Commissioner at Westchester County Department of Corrections. He is a second generation, decorated veteran of the U.S. Marine Corps, with over twenty years of experience in the public sector, namely in the criminal justice arena having worked in policing, the District Attorney's office and corrections. His current role as

First Deputy Commissioner has allowed him to operationalize sustainable criminal justice reform practices that advance the principles of social justice in an effort to break the cycle of poverty, crime, and abuse.

Esther Montero Perez de Tudela is a Penitentiary Institutions Jurist and Associate lecturer in the Criminal Law and Criminology Department at the Universidad Loyola Andalucía. She has a law degree from the University of Seville and a Ph.D. in Criminology from the University of Lausanne (Switzerland), at the School of Criminal Sciences. Since 2010, Dr. Montero has been a member of the Technical Superior Body of Penitentiary Institutions (Spanish Ministry of the Interior). She was Deputy Director of Treatment at the Huelva Penitentiary Center from 2012 to 2017 and is currently Jurist-criminologist at the Alcalá de Guadaira Penitentiary Center. She has participated as an expert in several international exchange programs on prison issues (among them several EU Twinning Projects) and has participated in a range of international research projects funded by the European Commission, all related to prison issues.

Ioana Morar is an Associate Professor at the University of Bucharest/Faculty of Sociology and Social Work. She has more than 16 years of continuous experience working in the field of corrections (e.g., treatment of persons deprived of liberty, mental health care, rehabilitation and reducing re-offending, human resources, and staff training) in Romania, Azerbaijan, Lebanon, Moldova, Montenegro, Algeria. For more than seven years, she has been the Eastern Europe Regional Representative in the European Prison Education Association.

Julie-Katia Morin-Major is currently a pediatric resident at Beaumont Hospital, Royal Oak. She holds a Master of Science in Neurosciences, which she conducted at the Center for Studies on Human Stress. She has also worked as a research professional in health technology assessment.

Danielle J. Murdoch is a Lecturer in the School of Criminology at Simon Fraser University where she obtained her Ph.D. after completing an M.Phil in Criminological Research at the University of Cambridge. Her main research interests concern correctional policy, practice and pedagogy. Dr. Murdoch is the coauthor, with Dr. Curt T. Griffiths, of an introductory corrections textbook, *Canadian Corrections*, and has recent publications in the *Journal of Crime and Justice and the Journal of Criminal Justice Education*. She is also the winner of the 2019 Lesley B. Cormack Award for Excellence in Teaching in the Faculty of Arts and Social Sciences at SFU.

Laura J. Murray is a graduate student in the Criminology and Criminal Justice Program at San Diego State University and researches reentry experiences, especially for women, and the public and correctional policies governing the transition from prison to the community.

Chelsey S. Narvey is an Assistant Professor in the College of Criminal Justice at Sam Houston State University. Her research interests include criminological theory, corrections, and developmental/life-course criminology, and she does work at the intersection of corrections and life-course theory. She has published on telemedicine and the way it can be used in correctional settings. Some of her work can be found in *the Journal of Correctional Healthcare*, as well as in *Aggression & Violent Behavior*.

To Nhu Nguyen is the Associate Director of the Office of the Academic Mission of Montreal's Mental Health University Institute (IUSMM) and of the Ultra-Specialized Mental Health Services in the Mental Health, Addictions and Homelessness Directorate of the East-Montreal Integrated University Health and Social Services Center (CIUSSS de l'Est-de-l'Île-de-Montréal). She has more than 20 years of experience in the health and social services sector.

Javier Nistal is a lawyer in the Spanish prison system, where he has held important positions, such as Director General of Criminal Enforcement and Social Reintegration. He is the author of several publications on prison issues and a regular contributor to seminars, conferences and courses for various institutions. He has also participated as an expert in several international exchange programs on prison issues.

Meghan A. Novisky is an Assistant Professor of Criminology at Cleveland State University. Her research investigates the implications of carceral contact for health and well-being, conditions of confinement, and the collateral consequences of criminal justice policy. Her work has been published in *Criminology*, *Justice Quarterly*, the *Journal of Correctional Health Care*, and the *Journal of Crime and Justice*.

Kathryn M. Nowonty is an Assistant Professor in the University of Miami Department of Sociology. Her research uses both quantitative and qualitative methods to examine the multilevel factors that create increased risk for poor health among justice-involved people. Dr. Nowotny is the cofounder of COVID Prison Project and Site-Principal Investigator of a multi-site longitudinal cohort study examining barriers to PrEP for HIV prevention among individuals under community supervision in the South (NC, FL, KY). She is also PI of a Center for HIV and Research in Mental Health (CHARM) funded project exploring the syndemic pathways to suboptimal care for justice-involved patients living with HIV, and Co-I of a binational study investigating how the migration process influences health, including experiences with immigration enforcement and confinement to detention centers.

Sergei Ovchinnikov is the Deputy Head of the Research Institute of the FSP of Russia, Moscow, RU, Ph.D. in Sociology. His research focuses on the penitentiary system of Russia, and judicial practices in the European Court of Human Rights involving the protections of conventional rights in the field of criminal justice. He is the author of more than 90 scientific papers on criminal justice and penitentiary policy.

Michael J. Palmieri is a graduate student at the University of Massachusetts Lowell in the School of Criminology and Justice Studies. Recently, he engaged in research using technology to assess the experiences of substance using probationers under community supervision. His research mostly focuses on terrorist use of the internet, cybercrime, and online radicalization through interdisciplinary theoretical approaches.

April Pattavina is a Professor in the School of Criminology and Justice Studies at the University of Massachusetts Lowell. Her research focuses on correctional reform, program evaluation, and the criminal justice system's response to violence. Her work often involves collaborative researcher practitioner partnerships with criminal justice agencies, and she has extensive experience working with large law enforcement and corrections related data sources. She has received grant funding from federal agencies such as the National Science Foundation, the National Institute of Justice, and the Office of Violence Against Women. Her most recent project includes a National Science Foundation funded project to explore ways in which emerging technologies can support people on community supervision.

Jason L. Payne is a Professor of Criminology and Social Policy in the School of Health and Society at the University of Wollongong. His research interests include quantitative crime data analysis, program evaluation, drugs and crime, and developmental and life-course criminology. Jason is formerly a Research Manager with the Australian Institute of Criminology.

Alex R. Piquero is Chair and Professor of the Department of Sociology and Arts & Sciences and Distinguished Scholar at the University of Miami and Professor of Criminology at Monash University in Melbourne Australia. He is also editor of *Justice Evaluation Journal.* His research interests include criminal careers, criminological theory, crime policy, evidence-based crime prevention, and quantitative research methods. He has received several research, teaching, and service awards, is fellow of both the American Society of Criminology and the Academy of Criminal Justice Sciences. In 2019 he received the Academy of Criminal Justice Sciences Bruce Smith, Sr. Award for outstanding contributions to criminal justice and in 2020 he was awarded the Lifetime Achievement Award from the Division of Developmental and Life Course Criminology, a division within the American Society of Criminology.

Wayne J. Pitts is a Research Criminologist in the Applied Justice Research Division at RTI International. He has conducted research and implemented projects in the Dominican Republic, Belize, Guatemala, El Salvador, and Honduras. His current research interests include international criminology, especially in Central America; transnational migration; and international corrections.

Sheetal Ranjan is a Professor in the Department of Sociology & Criminal Justice at William Paterson University, USA. Her primary focus is applied research and she has received more than one million dollars in federal funding to establish evidence-based violence prevention and intervention programs. Dr. Ranjan is a past chair of the Division on Women & Crime (DWC) of the American Society of Criminology (ASC). In her term as DWC's chair, she led its First Congressional Briefing at the Capitol Hill and its first participation in the Commission on the Status of Women CSW63 at the United Nations Headquarters in New York City. She also serves on the New Jersey Study Commission on Violence, on ASC's policy committee and the board of the Crime and Justice Research Alliance.

Sabrina S. Rapisarda is a doctoral student in the School of Criminology and Justice Studies at the University of Massachusetts Lowell. Much of Sabrina's work has been anchored in the public health framework, where she studies topics in the realm of sexual perpetration, namely campus sexual misconduct in university and college community contexts as well as sex offender supervision and treatment. She has recently embarked on research that investigates various aspects of the criminal justice system's response to COVID-19, including global correctional mitigation strategies and domestic responses to COVID-19 among vulnerable populations – individuals who are experiencing homelessness and/or engaging in chronic illicit drug use.

Santiago Redondo is Professor of Psychology and Criminology at the University of Barcelona (Spain). His research encompasses the fields of program evaluation, institutional and community treatment, and the prevention and control of criminal behavior. His recent research studies involve analyses of the link between juvenile delinquency and adult crime, and the effectiveness of treatment strategies targeting violent and sex offenders. He has published numerous books, book chapters, and papers on all of these subjects.

Ludmila Ribeiro is an Associate Professor in the Department of Sociology and a researcher in the Center for Crime and Public Safety Studies (CRISP), both at the Federal University of Minas Gerais (UFMG). She holds a bachelor's degree in Law from the Federal University of Minas Gerais, a master's and a bachelor´s degree in Public Administration from João Pinheiro Foundation, and a Ph.D. in Sociology from Rio de Janeiro Research Institute (IUPERJ). She was a visiting scholar at the University of Florida, University of Groningen, and Texas State University. During her career, she has coordinated several research projects on how the criminal justice system operates in Brazil. Nowadays, her research interests are focused on first appearance hearings, homicide trials, and management of penitentiary systems.

Sveinung Sandberg is a Professor of Criminology at the University of Oslo. He holds a Ph.D. in sociology from the University of Bergen, Norway. He has written the book *Street Capital* (2011, Policy Press with Willy Pedersen) and several journal articles on street culture and crime with a Bourdieusian approach. Sandberg is also co-founder of Narrative Criminology (e.g., Presser and Sandberg 2015) and has worked to integrate narrative and discourse analytical approaches in criminology. His research focuses on processes of marginalization, violence, illegal drugs, social movements, and political and religious extremism.

José Semedo Moreira is an anthropologist with a variety of publications about the prison system. At present, he is Director of Communication Services and External Relations at the General Directorate of Reinsertion and Prison Services in Portugal.

Daniel C. Semenza is an Assistant Professor in the Department of Sociology, Anthropology, and Criminal Justice at Rutgers University – Camden. His research interests include gun violence, victimization, and the dynamic links between health, crime, and the criminal justice system.

Claire Seungeun Lee is an Assistant Professor in the School of Criminology and Justice Studies at the University of Massachusetts Lowell. Her research interests include human, social, and big data aspects of cybercrime and cybersecurity and global and comparative perspectives on crime and deviance.

Carlos Soler is Deputy Director of Prison Services of Catalonia for Rehabilitation Programs. His work is focused on rehabilitation and treatment programs for offenders, community corrections, risk assessment and management of violent behavior, strategic planning, and project management. He also works on research and training for correctional services and offender desistance.

Jill Viglione, Ph.D., is an Assistant Professor in the Department of Criminal Justice at the University of Florida. Her research focuses on organizational change and implementation of evidence-based practices. She recently published in *Criminal Justice and Behavior, Victims & Offenders,* and *Implementation Science.*

John E. Wetzel is the Secretary of Corrections in the state of Pennsylvania, USA. He was appointed Secretary of Corrections in January 2011, following a 22-year career in county corrections. During his tenure as Secretary, not only did the Department of Corrections experience the end of a 24-year average growth of 1,500 inmates per year, but also the first population reduction in Pennsylvania in over 4 decades, with a total reduction, thus far, of over 4,200 inmates. He has served as Chair of the Justice Center's Executive Board of the Council of State Government, of which he is now a member. He also served as the recent President of the CLA (Correctional Leaders Association), formerly ASCA, and a member of Harvard's Executive Session on Community Corrections. On the federal level, he was tapped by the Obama administration to be the corrections expert on the Chuck Colson Taskforce – which was a congressionally created group tasked with assessing the Federal Bureau of Prisons and providing the Administration and Congress with recommendations on improvement. More recently, he was named by the Trump administration to the congressionally created oversight committee to the federal First Step Act. He is a graduate of Bloomsburg University and recipient of honorary Doctorate degrees from both Indiana University of Pennsylvania and Chestnut Hill College.

Introduction

James M. Byrne, Don Hummer, and Sabrina S. Rapisarda

Introduction

The following special issue of *Victims & Offenders* addresses three critical questions about the impact of the COVID-19 crisis in corrections systems:

(1) How extensive were COVID-19 outbreaks in prisons, jails, and community corrections systems globally?
(2) How did governments respond to the COVID-19 outbreaks in their corrections systems?
(3) How likely is it that the short-term mitigation strategies implemented by governments will result in long-term changes in corrections policies?

The authors of the articles included in this volume provide preliminary answers to each of these questions, but it is clear from the research presented here that there is much that we simply do not know about both the extent of the problem and the effectiveness of various front-end, in-prison, and back-end mitigation strategies designed to reduce the spread of COVID-19 within prisons and jails while protecting the health (physical, mental) of inmates and staff. The articles included here also highlight the lack of information currently available about community corrections systems globally, which made it difficult to provide an assessment on (1) the extent of COVID-19 outbreaks in the *community corrections* system globally, (2) the types of mitigation strategies employed in community corrections, and (3) the effectiveness of these mitigation strategies.

To prepare for the next phase of this pandemic and/or the inevitable *next* public health crisis, several of the authors included in this volume[1] recommend that we immediately commence an aggressive global research agenda that – when completed – will provide the research evidence that governments desperately need, focusing on two basic questions:

(1) Did the mitigation strategies used in each country reduce the spread of the infection in the corrections system (both in prisons and jails, and in community corrections)?
(2) Did the corrections-focused mitigation strategies used in each country have an adverse impact on either public health or public safety?

Without conducting the research needed to answer these two questions, it will be impossible to offer advice to governments looking to develop evidence-based policies and practices, both in the short term and the long term.

Organization of the special issue

During the initial stages of the COVID-19 outbreak, the *Victims & Offenders* editorial team followed the news reports describing the movement of virus from one global region to the next. During this same initial period, we began to hear disturbing reports by watchdog groups about major outbreaks of the virus in prisons and jails in each global region. These reports were often at odds with official statements offered by corrections officials in many of these countries, who – at least initially – either minimized the extent of the problem in their facilities or presented data to support their contention that they had the problem under control. However, the available data – provided by government leaders and corrections officials in many countries to support these statements – were often incomplete, with little information provided on testing levels, testing rates, the number of positive tests, hospitalizations, and deaths in prisons and jails.

Not surprisingly, skepticism was voiced by many observers regarding the transparency of the official reports and the narratives being presented for public consumption by governments in several countries, including those countries with the world's largest prison systems: USA, China, Brazil, Russia, and India. Over half of the global prison population is housed in these five countries. We decided initially that we needed to examine the response to COVID-19 outbreaks in these five countries in a special issue of this journal, but we quickly expanded our group of target countries to include countries with the 50 largest prison and jail systems, following a strategy that two members of the editorial team recently employed to examine the expansion of the private prison industry globally (Byrne et al., 2019). We should note here that over 90% of the global prison population resides in these top 50 countries. We also decided to solicit profiles from some of the smaller countries in each global region, to increase regional representation and assess whether "size matters" when mitigation strategies are developed and implemented.

We contacted country-level experts in each global region in mid-June, 2020, and asked them if they could provide an initial assessment of the extent of the problem in their country's corrections system, and then describe the initial mitigation strategies being used to address the problem. Our country-level experts include international corrections experts, individuals on our journal's international editorial board with expertise in their country's corrections system, members of the global community corrections initiative identified as country-level experts (www.globcci.org), and academic researchers we identified because of their knowledge of a particular country's corrections system, their access to data on both the extent of COVID-19 outbreaks in prisons, jails, and/or community corrections systems, and their knowledge of the front-end, in-prison, and back-end mitigation strategies being used to address the problem in their country. Because of the importance of providing an accurate and timely global snapshot, we set deadlines for submission aggressively (mid-August, 2020).[2]

The following special issue includes three articles examining the global impact of the COVID-19 outbreaks, six regional overviews, and twenty-seven country-specific reviews, including reviews targeting 21 of the 50 largest prison systems globally. We think you will agree that the issue is an excellent resource for those researchers, policymakers, practitioners, and the general public interested in knowing more about the nature and extent of the COVID-19 outbreaks in corrections systems globally, and about the diversity of responses developed and implemented by governments from each global region that is detailed in these country-level reviews.

One final note: we include a list of global COVID-19 corrections-focused resources below (see Table 1). These resource links provide the latest available data on the continued spread of the pandemic globally, the recommendations of major international organizations regarding best practices, and a variety of region-specific resources.

Table 1. Global resources: responding to COVID-19 in corrections.

Global Resources

- Centers for Disease Control and Prevention (CDC) – Correctional and detention facilities: Plan, prepare, and respond *(Worldwide)*
- CDC – Interim guidance on the management of Coronavirus Disease 2019 (COVID-19) in correctional and detention facilities *(Worldwide)*
- CDC – Toolkit for correctional and detention facilities *(Worldwide)*
- Global Community Corrections Initiative – Resources for the Global Community Corrections Initiative *(Worldwide)*
- Harm Reduction International – COVID-19, prisons and drug policy *(Worldwide)*
- Interagency Standing Committee (IASC) – Interim Guidance COVID-19: Focus on persons deprived of their liberty *(Worldwide)*
- International Committee of the Red Cross (ICRC) – COVID-19: Preparedness and response in detention
- International Corrections and Prisons Association (ICPA) – COVID-19 resources *(Worldwide)*
- International Drug Policy Consortium: A global network promoting objective and open debate on drug policy (IDPC) – Coronavirus disease (COVID-19): Resources and information *(Worldwide)*
- Penal Reform International (PRI) – Coronavirus: Preventing harm and human rights violations in criminal justice systems *(Worldwide)*
- The United Nations Subcommittee on Prevention of Torture (SPT) – Advice of the subcommittee on prevention of torture to states parties and national preventive mechanisms relating to the coronavirus pandemic (adopted on 25th March 2020) *(Worldwide)*
- United Nations Office on Drugs and Crime (UNODC) – Coronavirus disease (COVID-19): UNODC updates *(Worldwide)*
- World Health Organization: Regional Office for Europe – Prevention and control of COVID-19 in prisons and other places of detention *(Worldwide)*
- World Prison Brief (WPB) & Institute for Crime and Justice Policy Research (ICPR) – International news and guidance on COVID-19 and prisons *(Worldwide)*

Europe

- Center for Crime & Justice Studies: European Prison Observatory – COVID-19 in European countries: Tracking preparedness, prevention, & control *(Europe)*
- EUROPRIS: Promoting Professional Prison Practice – Prevention measures in European prisons *(Europe)*
- Innovative Prison Systems (IPS) – COVID-19 pandemic response: Fighting the invisible threat in prisons *(Europe and North America)*
- Royal Colleges of Psychiatrists – COVID-19: Secure hospital and criminal justice settings *(United Kingdom)*

North America

- American Correctional Association (ACA) – Coronavirus COVID-19 resources and information *(United States)*
- Beyond Prisons – COVID-19 resources for incarcerated people *(United States)*
- Correctional Service Canada – COVID-19 preparedness and plans *(Canada)*
- Council on Criminal Justice: The National Commission on COVID-19 and Criminal Justice – Impact report: COVID-19 and prisons (September 2, 2020) *(United States)*
- National Commission on Correctional Health Care (NCCHC) – COVID-19 Coronavirus: What you need to know in corrections *(United States)*
- NCCHC – Study of COVID-19 in correctional facilities *(United States)*
- National Conference of State Legislatures (NCSL) – COVID-19 in U.S. prisons and jails *(United States)*
- NCSL – Criminal Justice System responses to COVID-19 *(United States)*
- Prison Policy Initiative (PPI) – Five ways the criminal justice system could slow the pandemic *(United States)*
- PPI – Responses to the COVID-19 pandemic *(United States)*
- Prisonology – COVID-19 resources related to Federal Bureau of Prisons response *(United States)*
- The COVID Prison Project – The COVID Prison Project tracks data and policy across the country to monitor COVID-19 in correctional facilities *(United States + Puerto Rico)*
- The National Academies of Sciences, Engineering, & Medicine – Academies study will examine COVID-19 in correctional facilities and strategies for decarceration *(United States)*

South/Latin America

- United Nations – Policy brief: The impact of COVID-19 on Latin America and the Caribbean *(Latin America & the Caribbean)*

Africa

- Journal of Human Rights Practice (Muntingh) – Africa, prisons, and COVID-19 *(Africa)*

Asia

- International Drug Policy Consortium (IDPC) – COVID-19: Prisons and detention in Southeast Asia *(Asia)*

Oceania

- Communicable Diseases Network Australia (CDNA) – Coronavirus disease 2019 (COVID-19) outbreaks in correctional and detention facilities *(Australia)*
- Government of New South Wales (NSW) – Community corrections COVID-safe roadmap *(Australia)*

Notes

1. See, the overview articles by Nowotny and Piquero (this volume), Heard (this volume), and Byrne, et al., (this volume).
2. We had hoped to include additional countries from both the Asian and African regions, but the very short timeframe for submission, and the lack of available data needed to complete the review, made finding qualified experts a challenge. We addressed this problem by conducting our own global overview targeting the countries with the largest prison systems globally, providing region-specific overviews, and adding selected country-specific reviews where needed. These articles are authored or coauthored by the co-editors (Byrne and Hummer) and associate editor (Kras)of the journal.

Reference

Byrne, J., Kras, K., & Marmolejo, L. (2019). International perspectives on the privatization of corrections. *Criminology and Public Policy*, *18*(2), 477–503.

Global Impact Assessment

The Global Impact of the Pandemic on Institutional and Community Corrections: Assessing Short-Term Crisis Management and Long-Term Change Strategies

Kathryn M. Nowonty and Alex R. Piquero

ABSTRACT
This introduction discusses the global impact of Covid-19 on corrections.

Introduction

By many standards, the United States has more individuals under some form of correctional supervision – but especially in jails and prisons – than any other high income countries. On any given day, there are 2.3 million people behind bars (Sawyer & Wagner, 2020) and another 4.5 million under community supervision (Jones, 2018). Each year in the US, over 600,000 incarcerated people are released from American prisons (Bronson & Carson, 2019). Nearly 11 million filter in and out of local jails (Zeng, 2020); that amount of individuals is roughly the size of the daily New York City population or the entire state of Ohio. There are over 400,000 people employed as correctional officers and jailers (U.S. Bureau of Labor Statistics, 2020); this does not include administrative, medical, and service staff and other vendors. The U.S. spends billions of dollars a year locking people up. In just 45 states in 2015, the state prison systems collectively spent 43 USD billion (Mai & Subramanian, 2017), a number that does not include local county jails, or federal prisons and detention centers. The U.S. comprises about 4% of the world population, but 25% of the world's incarcerated population, and 25% of the world's COVID-19 cases. These intertwining epidemics are not surprising given that the US has among the highest levels of inequality (OECD Center for Opportunity and Equality, n.d.) and lowest levels of life expectancy (Ho & Hendi, 2018) compared to other high-income countries, as well as high levels of racial inequality, which are also apparent in the prison (The Sentencing Project, 2018) and COVID-19 epidemics (Wortham et al., 2020).

Prisons and jails are meant to detain people who have been convicted and sentenced to an incarceration term and/or are awaiting further justice system processing. In some cases, these facilities provide rehabilitation and other types of services, including mental health and substance abuse treatment, as well as reentry planning. However, prisons and jails are designed for security not public health and health care delivery. In recent years, this tension has come to the forefront as correctional facilities have become the largest mental health care providers in the U.S. (Al-Rousan et al., 2017; Torrey, 1995), and prisons have had to respond to an aging population by developing guidelines for assisted living and end of life care (McKillop & Boucher, 2018) – especially given the many long-term and mandatory sentences previously imposed.

Historically, global infectious disease outbreaks of influenza (Besney et al., 2017; Maruschak et al., 2009; Robinson et al., 2012; Young et al., 2005) tuberculosis (TB; Centers for Disease Control Prevention, 2006; Lambert et al., 2016) and H1N1 "swine flu" (Chao et al., 2017; Turner & Levy, 2010) in correctional settings have illustrated their vulnerability. Due in part to a lack of social distancing, close quarters, shared spaces, and inadequate ventilation systems, infection control in jails and prisons is nearly impossible (Bick, 2007; Dannenburg, 2007). In the U.S., it is estimated that up to a quarter of the prison population has been infected with TB (Hammett et al., 1997), with a rate of active TB infection that is 6–10 times higher than the general population (Centers for Disease Control Prevention, 2006). Thus, it is not surprising that San Quentin prison in California has been an epicenter of three epidemics: 1918 influenza and 2009 swine flu epidemics (Chaddock, 2018), and, currently, the COVID-19 pandemic (Egelko, 2020).

People incarcerated in prisons and jails are more susceptible to acquiring and experiencing complications from infectious diseases than the population in the community. This is because people who are incarcerated are more likely than people in the community to have chronic underlying health conditions, including diabetes, heart disease, chronic lung disease, chronic liver disease, and lower immune systems from HIV (Maruschak et al., 2015). Correctional settings also have dramatic effects on psychological and physical health, subjecting people to higher rates of infectious disease and medical neglect; exacerbating or causing mental health conditions; and hastening death (Brinkley-Rubinstein et al., 2019; Cloud, Bassett et al., 2020; Nowotny & Kuptsevych-Timmer, 2018; Patterson, 2013). In the era of COVID-19, this places inmates, staff members, and the outside community at a non-negligible risk of contracting and spreading the virus, which can lead to hospitalizations and death. Global agencies such as the United Nations and Human Rights Watch have warned that the conditions of confinement, such as overcrowding and lack of basic hygiene, could be catastrophic for COVID-19 (Colville, 2020; Human Rights Watch, 2020a, 2020b). For example, in Philippine jails COVID-19 cases jumped from 194 among inmates and staff to 870 over the span of three weeks (Patag, 2020), prompting the release of over 15,000 people (Aben, 2020).

A Closer Look at the U.S.

The Covid Prison Project (CPP) tracks COVID-19 testing, cases, and deaths in 53 U.S. prison systems, including 50 states, Puerto Rico, Federal Bureau of Prisons, and Immigration and Customs Enforcement (see www.covidprisonproject.com). In the first seven months of 2020, there have been 84,082 reported cases of COVID-19 among people incarcerated in prisons along with 780 COVID-related deaths. These numbers for staff working in prisons are 17,042 and 47, respectively. Using criteria developed by the Kaiser Family Foundation (2020), 21 out of 53 prison systems are currently COVID-19 "hotspots" (Hamblett, 2020), with the 10 largest single-site outbreaks occurring at correctional facilities (New York Times, 2020). CPP data indicate that COVID-19 testing strategies vary greatly by state, with some states engaging in one-time universal testing (e.g., MI, MN, TN, TX, VT, WI), and some states having prison testing rates lower than community testing rates (e.g., AL, LA, IN). Even still, a handful of states do not report any information on testing.

Therefore, it is important to keep in mind that the reported cases are likely underestimates of the true prevalence. Nevertheless, COVID-19 outcomes have been more severe in prisons. The standardized mortality ratio is 2.84 (95% confidence interval 2.64, 3.04), meaning that adjusting for age and sex the prison population has a COVID-19 mortality rate 285% higher than the general population.

Policy Recommendations

Prisons and jails are not completely isolated, as staff and venders go to and from work daily and incarcerated people are frequently transferred between facilities. Preliminary analysis from Cook County Jail, IL shows that jail cycling was associated with 15.7% of documented cases in IL, exceeding other known predictors (e.g., population density and public transit utilization) (Reinhart & Chen, 2020). A simple stochastic susceptible exposed-infected-recovered model of COVID-19 disease spread in Immigration and Customs Enforcement detention centers shows that under optimistic conditions outbreaks among a minimum of 65 ICE facilities would overwhelm ICU beds within a 10-mile radius (Irvine et al., 2020). Additional epidemiologic modeling of ICE facilities indicates potential under-reporting of cases (Siulc, 2020). Indeed, a number of recent publications have provided warning and guidance concerning COVID-19 in correctional facilities, including mitigation strategies (Barnert et al., 2020; Williams et al., 2020; Wurcel et al., 2020) and the imperative to "flatten the curve" (Akiyama et al., 2020), expanding early and compassionate release (Nowotny et al., 2020) and increasing other decarceration efforts (especially among non-violent offenders and/or soon-to-be-released inmates) (B. Williams & Bertsch, 2020), emergency discharge planning (Howell et al., 2020), and the ethical use of medical isolation (Cloud, Ahalt et al., 2020). Unfortunately, gauging the risk of this spread has remained quite difficult, as many local and state facilities do not provide asymptomatic testing (much less engage in contact tracing). And if you do not test, then you do not know the nature of the problem. Even in the absence of testing, what is known about the spread of COVID-19 within incarceration facilities is that they rank second behind nursing homes with the number of positive cases (Sears et al., 2020) and that figure is likely an undercount.

Perhaps the most effective COVID-19 mitigation strategy proposed is reducing the carceral population. Italy (Cingolani et al., 2020), Iran (Payne, 2020), Philippines (Aben, 2020), and other countries have engaged in release efforts. In the United States, more than 100,000 people were released from state and federal prisons between March and June of 2020, an overall decrease of 8% ranging from 2% in VA to 22% in CT (Sharma et al., 2020). However, the prison population overall has dropped largely because prisons have stopped accepting new transfers from county jails, not because of release of COVID-vulnerable inmates. Thus, the trend toward decarceration is likely short-term. Among jails, data from 29 large cities found that all jails reduced their population, even slightly, due to COVID-19 (ACLU Analytics, 2020). For example, Los Angeles County Jail, the largest jail in the U.S., released 25% of its population (Hamilton et al., 2020). Recent analysis finds that the reduction in jail populations across the 29 cities was functionally unrelated to crime trends in the following months (ACLU Analytics, 2020). In fact, overall crime has been decreasing (Rosenfeld & Lopez, 2020), with the exception of short-term increases in intimate partner violence (Piquero et al., 2020), which is likely unrelated to decarceration.

Most recently, Sears et al. (2020) provided guidance for correctional facilities amid the COVID-19 crisis. Because we agree with them, we reproduce them here and encourage jail and prison facilities to these strategies: (1) screen staff at entry and provide universal tests in hot spots; (2) assign staff and residents to cohorts for distancing; (3) improve sick leave policy; (4) provide and train in PPE; and (5) provide no-cost tests and evaluation for staff and inmates at regular intervals. To that, we would add other improvements to aging facilities including, for example, adequate ventilation systems, considering more time outdoors, and the provision of earlier release among nonviolent offenders/soon-to-be-released offenders to receive reentry planning and services in community-based halfway houses and/or facilities to ease correctional population. And it goes without saying that we would urge researchers to collect the necessary criminal justice data to examine both short- and long-term crime trends among those offenders released and the communities they are released too more generally.

Conclusion

The novel coronavirus has exacerbated the many social, racial/ethnic, and health inequalities and injustices found among those individuals who are under some form of correctional supervision as well as the many disadvantaged communities from which they come from and will return. A 2017 report on the state of health affairs and disparities in the United States from the National Academies of Sciences (2017) shows that, while there have been some gains in reducing health disparities by race/ethnicity, it remains the case that compared to whites, minorities exhibit worse outcomes on many physical and mental health outcomes. A 2020 report by the Center for American Progress continues to document sharp differences in physical and mental health problems (Carratala & Maxwell, 2020). For example, compared to whites, both African Americans and Hispanics are also less likely to have health insurance and to also experience chronic health conditions. There is also evidence to suggest that the morbidity burden of Black men in the United States is understated due to their systematic exclusion from national health surveys (Nowotny et al., 2017). Moreover, these disparities are not solely driven by individual-level factors, as research has continuously shown that neighborhood disadvantage is strongly related to adverse health outcomes such as asthma, infant mortality, low birthweight, etc. (Finch et al., 2008). These disadvantaged communities tend more often than not to be dense, segregated areas of major cities where access to health care, public transportation, high performing schools, gainful employment, and healthy food options are severely limited. These roadblocks, in turn, influence attitudes that favor aggression (Anderson, 1999), increase the risk of crime and victimization (Shaw & McKay, 1942), and lead to shortened life spans (Wolff et al., 2020). And, as many incarcerated people will return back to many of these marginalized communities, the chronicity of adverse health will continue to recycle over time and within families (Clear et al., 2001).

In this regard, Covid-19 has brought to the forefront the need for meaningful criminal justice reform, both within the United States and throughout the world (Nowotny et al., 2020; B.H. Williams & Piquero, 2020). There is no shortage of what these reforms could look like and the coronavirus crisis offers what may be an opportunity to re-imagine the correctional system, including community corrections. Some candidate reforms could include: increasing and resourcing community-based alternatives that offer wrap-around services to include substance abuse and mental health treatment, reducing the number of persons incarcerated – especially for longer periods of time, employing evidence-based risk assessment tools that are impartial across race/ethnicity, eliminating excessive fines and overhauling the bail system, and increasing the adoption of early-release strategies for less violent offenders to include an earlier reentry. Some of these reforms are easier to employ than others, i.e., eliminating fines and fees and overhauling the bail system, while others are likely to take a longer period of time to put into place and then see their effects.

Beyond decarceration efforts and reforms of current systems of criminal justice, the COVID-19 pandemic has reinforced the imperative to invest in other societal institutions with the explicit goal of supporting human rights, wellbeing, and equity, such as education, healthcare, employment, social security, social safety nets, and housing. Investing in these sectors will help address the root causes of "crime", namely resource deprivation and social and institutional marginalization, and improve population health, thereby decreasing the harms caused by and reducing the need for criminal justice systems. In other words, governments should think beyond prisons and policing to solve society's problems (Critical Resistance, 2020; Washington, 2018).

In the end, it is important to not let perfection be the enemy of progress. The impact of the coronavirus within the correctional system has pinpointed an opportune moment to initiate and execute meaningful criminal justice reform and policymakers should seize this moment.

Disclosure statement

No potential conflict of interest was reported by the author(s).

References

Aben, E. (2020). Philippine jails release over 15,000 inmates amid pandemic. *Arab News*. https://www.arabnews.com/node/1699156/world

ACLU Analytics. (2020). *Decarceration and crime during COVID-19*. American Civil Liberties Union. https://www.aclu.org/news/smart-justice/decarceration-and-crime-during-covid–19/

Akiyama, M. J., Spaulding, A. C., & Rich, J. D. (2020). Flattening the curve for incarcerated populations —Covid-19 in Jails and Prisons. *New England Journal of Medicine*, *382*(22), 2075–2077. https://doi.org/10.1056/NEJMp2005687.

Al-Rousan, T., Rubenstein, L., Sieleni, B., Deol, H., & Wallace, R. B. (2017). Inside the nation's largest mental health institution: A prevalence study in a state prison system. *BMC Public Health*, *17*(1), 342. https://doi.org/10.1186/s12889-017-4257-0

Anderson, E. (1999). *Code of the street: Decency, violence, and the moral life of the inner city*. W.W. Norton.

Barnert, E., Ahalt, C., & Williams, B. (2020). Prisons: Amplifiers of the COVID-19 pandemic hiding in plain sight. *American Journal of Public Health*, *110*(7), 965–966. https://doi.org/10.2105/AJPH.2020.305713

Besney, J., Moreau, D., Jacobs, A., Woods, D., Pyne, D., Joffe, A. M., & Ahmed, R. (2017). Influenza outbreak in a Canadian correctional facility. *Journal of Infection Prevention*, *18*(4), 193–198. https://doi.org/10.1017/s0950268804003243

Bick, J. A. (2007). Infection control in jails and prisons. *Clinical Infectious Diseases*, *45*(8), 1047–1055. https://doi.org/10.1086/521910

Brinkley-Rubinstein, L., Sivaraman, J., Rosen, D. L., Cloud, D. H., Junker, G., Proescholdbell, S., Shanahan, M. E., & Ranapurwala, S. I. (2019). Association of restrictive housing during incarceration with mortality after release. *JAMA Network Open*, *2*(10), e1912516. https://doi.org/10.1001/jamanetworkopen.2019.12516

Bronson, J., & Carson, E. A. (2019). *Prisoners in 2017*. U.S. Department of Justice, Bureau of Justice Statistics: NCJ 252156. https://www.bjs.gov/content/pub/pdf/p17.pdf

Carratala, S., & Maxwell, C. (2020). *Health disparities by race and ethnicity*. Center for American Progress. https://www.americanprogress.org/issues/race/reports/2020/05/07/484742/health-disparities-race-ethnicity/

Centers for Disease Control Prevention (CDC). (2006). Prevention and control of tuberculosis in correctional and detention facilities: Recommendations from CDC. *MMWR*, *55*(RR09), 1–48. https://www.cdc.gov/mmwr/preview/mmwrhtml/rr5509a1.htm

Chaddock, D. (2018). *1918 flu pandemic puts prison medical staff to test.* California Department of Corrections and Rehabilitation. https://www.cdcr.ca.gov/insidecdcr/2018/10/18/1918-flu-pandemic-puts-prison-medical-staff-to-test/

Chao, W., Liu, P., & Wu, C. (2017). Control of an H1N1 outbreak in a correctional facility in central Taiwan. *Journal of Microbiology, Immunology and Infection*, *50*(2), 175–182. https://doi.org/10.1016/j.jmii.2015.05.005

Cingolani, M., Caraceni, L., Cannovo, N., & Fedeli, P. (2020). The COVID-19 epidemic and the prison system in Italy. *Journal of Correctional Health Care*. https://journals.sagepub.com/doi/full/10.1177/1078345820929733

Clear, T. R., Rose, D. R., & Ryder, J. A. (2001). Incarceration and the community: The problem of removing and returning offenders. *Crime & Delinquency*, *47*(3), 335–351. https://doi.org/10.1177/0011128701047003003

Cloud, D. H., Ahalt, C., Augustine, D., Sears, D., & Williams, B. (2020). Medical isolation and solitary confinement: Balancing health and humanity in US jails and prisons during COVID-19. *Journal of General Internal Medicine*. https://doi.org/10.1007/s11606-020-05968-y

Cloud, D. H., Bassett, M. T., Graves, J., Fullilove, R. E., & Brinkley-Rubinstein, L. (2020). Documenting and addressing the health impacts of carceral systems. *American Journal of Public Health*, *110*(S1), S5–S5. https://doi.org/10.2105/AJPH.2019.305475

Colville, R. (2020). *Press briefing note on Americas/Prison conditions.* United Nations Human Rights Office of the High Commissioner. https://www.ohchr.org/EN/NewsEvents/Pages/DisplayNews.aspx?NewsID=25864&LangID=E

Critical Resistance. (2020). *Abolitionist tools.* Critical Resistance. http://criticalresistance.org/resources/abolitionist-tools/

Dannenburg, J. E. (2007). Prisons as incubators and spreaders of disease and illness. *Prison Legal News*. https://www.prisonlegalnews.org/news/2007/aug/15/prisons-as-incubators-and-spreaders-of-disease-and-illness.

Egelko, B. (2020). San Quentin coronavirus outbreak apparently result of missed steps by prison overseer. *San Francisco Chronicle*. https://www.sfchronicle.com/news/article/San-Quentin-coronavirus-outbreak-apparently-15421664.php

Finch, B. K., Do, D. P., Basurto-Davila, R., Bird, C., Escarce, J., & Lurie, N. (2008). Does place explain racial health disparities? Quantifying the contribution of residential context to the Black/White Health Gap in the United States. *Social Science & Medicine*, *67*(8), 1258–1268. https://doi.org/10.1016/j.socscimed.2008.06.018

Hamblett, A. (2020). *Covid-19 case watch.* Covid Prison Project. https://covidprisonproject.com/covid-19-case-watch/

Hamilton, M., Queally, J., & Tchekmedyian, A. (2020). California's prisons and jails have emptied thousands into a world changed by coronavirus. *Los Angeles Times*. https://www.latimes.com/california/story/2020-05-17/coronavirus-prison-jail-releases

Hammett, T. M., Harmon, M. P., & Rhodes, W. (1997). The burden of infectious disease among inmates of and releases from US correctional facilities. *American Journal of Public Health*, *92*, 1789–1794. https://doi.org/10.2105/ajph.92.11.1789.

Ho, J. Y., & Hendi, A. S. (2018). Recent trends in life expectancy across high income countries: Retrospective observational study. *BMJ*, *362*, k2562. https://doi.org/10.1136/bmj.k2562

Howell, B. A., Batlle, H. R., Ahalt, C., Shavit, S., Wang, E. A., Zaller, N., & Williams, B. A. (2020). Protecting decarcerated populations in the era of COVID-19: Priorities for emergency discharge planning. *Health Affairs Blog*, *13*, 2020. https://doi.org/10.1377/hblog20200406.581615

Human Rights Watch. (2020a). *DR Congo: Prisons face Covid-19 Catastrophe.* Human Rights Watch. https://www.hrw.org/news/2020/04/17/dr-congo-prisons-face-covid-19-catastrophe

Human Rights Watch. (2020b). *Latin America: Cut prison crowding to fight COVID-19.* Human Rights Watch. https://www.hrw.org/news/2020/04/02/latin-america-cut-prison-crowding-fight-covid–19

Irvine, M., Coombs, D., Skarha, J., Del Pozo, B., Rich, J., Taxman, F., & Green, T. C. (2020). Modeling COVID-19 and its impacts on U.S. immigration and custom enforcement (ICE) detention facilities. *Journal of Urban Health.*, *97*(4), 439–447. https://doi.org/10.1007/s11524-020-00441-x.

Jones, A. (2018). *Correctional control 2018: Incarceration and supervision by state.* Prison Policy Initiative. https://www.prisonpolicy.org/reports/correctionalcontrol2018.html

Kaiser Family Foundation. (2020). *State data and policy actions to address Coronavirus.* https://www.kff.org/coronavirus-covid-19/issue-brief/state-data-and-policy-actions-to-address-coronavirus/

Lambert, L. A., Armstrong, L. R., Lobato, M. N., Ho, C., France, A. M., & Haddad, M. B. (2016). Tuberculosis in jails and prisons: United States, 2002-2013. *American Journal of Public Health, 106* (12), 2231–2237. https://doi.org/10.2105/AJPH.2016.303423.

Mai, C., & Subramanian, R. (2017). *The price of prisons: Estimating state spending trends, 2010–2015.* Vera Institute of Justice. https://www.vera.org/downloads/publications/the-price-of-prisons-2015-state-spending-trends.pdf

Maruschak, L. M., Berzofsky, M., & Unangst, J. 2015. *Medical problems of state and federal prisoners and jail inmates, 2011–12.* US Department of Justice, Bureau of Justice Statistics. 2015 February Report No.: NCJ 248491.

Maruschak, L. M., Sabol, W. J., Potter, R. H., Reid, L. C., & Cramer, E. W. (2009). Pandemic influenza and jail facilities and populations. *American Journal of Public Health, 99*(Suppl 2), S339–S344. https://doi.org/10.2105/AJPH.2009.175174

McKillop, M., & Boucher, A. (2018). *Aging prison populations drive up costs.* Pew Trusts. https://www.pewtrusts.org/en/research-and-analysis/articles/2018/02/20/aging-prison-populations-drive-up-costs

National Academies of Sciences, Engineering, and Medicine; Health and Medicine Division; Board on Population Health and Public Health Practice; Committee on Community-Based Solutions to Promote Health Equity in the United States, A. Baciu, Y. Negussie, & A. Geller. (2017). *Communities in action: Pathways to health equity.* National Academies Press (US). https://www.ncbi.nlm.nih.gov/books/NBK425844/

New York Times. (2020). Coronavirus in the U.S.: Latest map and case count. https://www.nytimes.com/interactive/2020/us/coronavirus-us-cases.html#clusters

Nowotny, K. M., Bailey, Z., Omori, M., & Brinkley-Rubinstein, L. (2020). COVID-19 exposes need for progressive criminal justice reform. *American Journal of Public Health, 110*(7), 967–968. https://doi.org/10.2105/AJPH.2020.305707.

Nowotny, K. M., & Kuptsevych-Timmer, A. (2018). Health and justice: Framing incarceration as a social determinant of health for Black men in the United States. *Sociology Compass.*, *12*(3), e12566. https://doi.org/10.1111/soc4.12566

Nowotny, K. M., Rogers, R. G., & Boardman, J. D. (2017). Racial disparities in health conditions among prisoners compared with the general population. *SSM-Population Health, 3,* 487–496. https://doi.org/10.1016/j.ssmph.2017.05.011.

OECD Centre for Opportunity and Equality. (n.d.). *Inequality.* Economic Co-operation and Development (OECD). http://www.oecd.org/social/inequality.htm

Patag, K. J. (2020). *COVID-19 cases in prisons jump to 194; 161 are inmates.* PhilStar Global. https://www.philstar.com/headlines/2020/05/27/2016915/covid-19-cases-prisons-jump-194-161-are-inmates

Patterson, E. J. (2013). The dose–response of time served in prison on mortality: New York State, 1989–2003. *American Journal of Public Health, 103*(3), 523–528. https://doi.org/10.2105/AJPH.2012.301148

Payne, A. (2020). *Iran has released 85,000 prisoners in an emergency bid to stop the spread of the coronavirus.* Business Insider. https://www.businessinsider.com/coronavirus-covid-19-iran-releases-eighty-five-thousand-prisoners–2020–3

Piquero, A. R., Riddell, J. R., Bishopp, S. A., Narvey, C., Reid, J. A., & Piquero, N. L. (2020). Staying home, staying safe? A short-term analysis of COVID-19 on Dallas domestic violence. *American Journal of Criminal Justice, 45*(4), 601–635. https://doi.org/10.1007/s12103-020-09531-7

Reinhart, E., & Chen, D. (2020). Incarceration and its disseminations: COVID-19 Pandemic lessons from Chicago's Cook County Jail. *Health Affairs, 39*(8), 1412–1418. https://doi.org/10.1377/hlthaff.2020.0065

Robinson, S., Smith, P., Sears, S., Shubert, D., Reed, J., & Manning, S. E. (2012). Influenza outbreaks at two correctional facilities — Maine, March 2011. *MMWR, 61*(13), 229–232. https://www.cdc.gov/mmwr/preview/mmwrhtml/mm6113a3.htm

Rosenfeld, R., & Lopez, E. (2020). *Pandemic, social unrest, and crime in U.S. Cities*. Council on Criminal Justice.

Sawyer, W., & Wagner, P. (2020). Mass incarceration: The whole pie 2020. Prison Policy Initiative. https://www.prisonpolicy.org/reports/pie2020.html

Sears, D., Ahalt, C., Augustine, D., & Williams, B. (2020). Occupational health: A key to the control of COVID-19 in correctional facilities. *Annals of Internal Medicine*. https://doi.org/10.7326/M20-4543.

Sharma, D., Li, W., Lavoie, D., & Lauer, C. (2020). Prison populations drop by 100,000 during pandemic: But not because of COVID-19 releases. The Marshall Project. https://www.themarshallproject.org/2020/07/16/prison-populations-drop-by-100-000-during-pandemic

Shaw, C. R., & McKay, H. D. (1942). *Juvenile delinquency and urban areas*. University of Chicago Press.

Siulc, N. (2020). *Vera's new prevalence model suggests COVID-19 is spreading through ICE detention at much higher rates than publicized*. Vera Institute of Justice. https://www.vera.org/blog/covid-19-1/veras-new-prevalence-model-suggests-covid-19-is-spreading-through-ice-detention-at-much-higher-rates-than-publicized

The Sentencing Project. (2018). *Report to the United Nations on racial disparities in the U.S. criminal justice system*. https://www.sentencingproject.org/publications/un-report-on-racial-disparities/

Torrey, E. F. (1995). Jails and prisons–America's new mental hospitals. *American Journal of Public Health, 85*(12), 1611–1613. https://doi.org/10.2105/AJPH.85.12.1611

Turner, K. B., & Levy, M. H. (2010). Prison outbreak: Pandemic (H1N1) 2009 in an Australian prison. *Public Health, 124*(2), 119–121. https://doi.org/10.1086/521910

U.S. Bureau of Labor Statistics. (2020). *Occupational employment and Wages, May 2019*. https://www.bls.gov/oes/current/oes333012.htm

Washington, J. (2018). What is prison abolition? The Nation. https://www.thenation.com/article/archive/what-is-prison-abolition/#:~:text=Abolitionists%20believe%20that%20incarceration%2C%20in,harms%20instead%20of%20fixing%20them.&text=Abolitionists%20don't%20stop%20at,our%20society%20as%20a%20whole

Williams, B., Ahalt, C., Cloud, D., Augustine, D., Rorvig, L., & Sears, D. (2020). Correctional facilities in the shadow of COVID-19: Unique challenges and proposed solutions. *Health Affairs Blog, 26*, 2020. https://doi.org/10.1377/hblog20200324.784502

Williams, B., & Bertsch, L. (2020). *No excuses: Governors must pursue decarceration along with investments in reentry services*. The Justice Collaborative Institute. https://tjcinstitute.com/research/no-excuses-governors-must-pursue-decarceration-along-with-investments-in-reentry-services/

Williams, B. H., & Piquero, A. R. (2020). The coronavirus does not ignore prisoners, nor should we. *Dallas Morning News*. https://www.dallasnews.com/opinion/commentary/2020/04/18/covid-does-not-ignore-prisoners-nor-should-we/

Wolff, K. T., Intravia, J., Baglivio, M. T., & Piquero, A. R. (2020). Adherence to the street code predicts an earlier anticipated death. *Journal of Research in Crime and Delinquency, 57*(2), 139–181. https://doi.org/10.1177/0022427819868754

Wortham, J. M., Lee, J. T., Althomsons, S., Latash, J., Davidson, A., Guerra, K., Murray, K., McGibbon, E., Pichardo, C., Toro, B., Li, L., Paladini, M., Eddy, M. L., Reilly, K. H., McHugh, L., Thomas, D., Tsai, S., Ojo, M., Rolland, S., Bhat, M., & Reagan-Steiner, S. (2020). Characteristics of persons who died with COVID-19–United States, February 12-May 18, 2020. *MMWR, 69*(28), 923–929. https://dx.doi.org/10.15585/mmwr.mm6928e1external icon

Wurcel, A. G., Dauria, E., Zaller, N., Nijhawan, A., Beckwith, C., Nowotny, K. M., & Brinkley-Rubinstein, L. (2020). Spotlight on jails: COVID-19 mitigation policies needed now. *Clinical Infectious Diseases*, ciaa346. https://doi.org/10.1093/cid/ciaa346

Young, L. C., Dwyer, D. E., Harris, M., Guse, Z., Noel, V., & Levy, M. H., & Prison Influenza Outbreak Investigation Team. (2005). Summer outbreak of respiratory disease in an Australian prison due to an influenza A/Fujian/411/2002(H3N2)-like virus. *Epidemiology & Infection*, *133*(1), 107–112. https://doi.org/10.1017/s0950268804003243

Zeng, Z. (2020). *Jail inmates in 2018*. U.S. Department of Justice, Bureau of Justice Statistics.

Commentary: Assessing the Global Impact of the Covid-19 Pandemic on Prison Populations

Catherine Heard

ABSTRACT
The author directs the World Prison Research Programme at the Institute for Crime & Justice Policy Research, based at Birkbeck (University of London). The programme's research team monitors trends in world prison populations and examines the causes and the consequences of rising levels of imprisonment. A core component of the programme involves compiling and hosting the World Prison Brief, an online database providing free access to information about prison systems throughout the world. This Commentary revisits key findings from the Programme's ongoing work on prison population growth and its links to prison overcrowding and poor standards of prison healthcare. Within this context, some of the main impacts of the COVID-19 pandemic on prison systems worldwide will be discussed, with a focus on measures taken to reduce prison population sizes and restrictions put in place in prison regimes (including suspending social and other visits to prisons, home or work leave for prisoners, and related restrictions) to help control spread of the virus. Compensatory measures introduced to lessen the adverse effects of greater isolation and reduced contact with the outside world are discussed. It is argued that the pandemic has revealed an unprecedented need for a more health-informed approach to penal reform.

In June 2019, six months before the first cases of COVID-19 emerged in Wuhan, we published a report on research we had conducted on prisoner health and healthcare (Heard, 2019), research undertaken as part of our ongoing project: *Understanding and reducing the use of imprisonment in ten countries.*[1] In a blog at the time of publication, I described the public health risks of prison overcrowding as a "global time bomb".

The research that we and our partners had carried out produced disturbing evidence of the impact on prisoners' health and wellbeing of being held in cramped, under-resourced prisons. Prisoners described extreme overcrowding (for example, 60 men sharing cells built for 20 in Brazil; cells holding up to 200 people in Thailand); inadequate medical treatment, with too few doctors to deal even with routine health issues let alone serious disease outbreaks; constant hunger; lack of fresh air and exercise; shared buckets instead of toilets; insufficient fresh water or soap; and having to eat while seated on the toilet due to lack of space in a shared cell.

To quote some of the prisoners and ex-prisoners whom we and our partners interviewed about the conditions they had faced:

'It was very dirty, our children regularly got sick with diarrhoea, skin diseases, cholera, they had colds all the time.' (Kenya)

'We spend 23 hours a day in the cell. There are 30 inmates in a cell for 15 inmates. Hygiene is bad.' (South Africa)

'People died when I was there. I had fevers, I had TB. I thought I would die.' (Brazil)

'There are about 40 detainees in my cell. We lie down next to each other.' (Thailand)

When the pandemic was declared in March 2020, it was all too clear that conditions like those described by our research participants would mean high levels of risk in many countries, not only for prisoners themselves, but also for those working in prisons, and for families and wider communities. Over the weeks and months that followed, we have been monitoring countries' responses to the crisis, and collecting information on the various measures that have been introduced to contain the risks and prevent spread of the virus, and on their impacts.

Incidence of COVID-19 in prisons worldwide

It has long been known that prisons can be epicenters for infectious diseases. They offer the ideal conditions for a contagious virus to spread. Infections such as tuberculosis and even syphilis have recently been shown to spread rapidly between prisons and the local communities (Correa et al., 2017). When the pandemic was declared it was clear that many prison systems around the world would struggle to cope. During the months that followed, prisons across much of the world saw large numbers of infections, their environments being especially ill-equipped to take the social distancing and hygiene precautions urged on us by governments and public health bodies.

In late April 2020 there were around 14,000 reported cases among prisoners in 14 countries and at least 385 prisoners had died.[2] By mid-September, confirmed cases had exceeded 205,000 in 101 countries, with almost 2,200 deaths among those cases. (These figures do not include prison staff, among whom infection rates in many countries have been higher than among prisoners.) For several reasons, the reported numbers of confirmed cases and deaths will undoubtedly be significantly lower than the true figures. Prison health systems in much of the world struggle to provide even basic healthcare, so many sick prisoners and prison staff will not have been tested. Without routine and regular testing in prisons, numbers of asymptomatic inmates and staff will present a further, unseen risk to those within and beyond the confines of the prison.

Official responses and their impacts

In March 2020, days after formally declaring the disease a pandemic, the World Health Organization warned that global efforts to tackle the spread of COVID-19 would fail without proper attention to infection control inside prisons (WHO, 2020). It issued detailed guidance running to 32 pages, and warned: "The risk of rapidly increasing transmission of the disease within prisons or other places of detention is likely to have an amplifying effect on the epidemic, swiftly multiplying the number of people affected." The document called for "strong infection prevention and control measures, adequate testing, treatment and care" and provided detail on what this would mean in practice. Many other public health and human rights agencies provided a range of guidance and other materials, in a bid to prevent a catastrophic spread of the disease with the potential to overwhelm community healthcare systems.[3]

Official responses ranged across three main areas: managing prison populations (through inflow constraints and expanded release measures) to reduce overcrowding and facilitate social distancing; suspending or restricting visits from family members and others and halting temporary leave for home visits, work or other previously permitted purposes; and ensuring provision of sanitation and protective equipment, testing and treatment facilities. The focus of this commentary will be on the first and second areas of activity, beginning with the first.

Managing prison population numbers[4]

As the data we compile for our World Prison Brief database show, overcrowding currently blights the prison systems of over 60% of countries worldwide, with grave consequences for health, rehabilitation and community safety.[5] People held in overcrowded prisons are especially vulnerable to COVID-19. Reducing numbers of prisoners was therefore identified as a key weapon in governments' armories in the fight against COVID-19. The WHO recommended that "enhanced consideration should be given to resorting to non-custodial measures at all stages of the administration of criminal justice, including at the pre-trial, trial and sentencing as well as post-sentencing stages".

Similar calls for reduced prisoner numbers came from the United Nations bodies. The UN's Subcommittee on the Prevention of Torture called on governments to "reduce prison populations and other detention populations wherever possible" and to implement "schemes of early, provisional or temporary release for those detainees for whom it is safe to do so" (United Nations Office on Drugs and Crime, 2020) This was echoed by Michelle Bachelet, the UN High Commissioner for Human Rights, who said: "Now, more than ever, governments should release every person detained without sufficient legal basis, including political prisoners and others detained simply for expressing critical or dissenting views." The UNODC likewise urged consideration of release mechanisms for prisoners facing particular risks due to COVID-19, such as the elderly and pregnant women and those affected by chronic diseases. It also suggested consideration of release mechanisms for people near the end of their sentences, those sentenced for minor crimes and those whose release would not compromise public safety.

Civil society organizations throughout the world echoed the international agencies' calls. Many issued detailed recommendations for reducing numbers in (and entering) custody and for ensuring the safety of people being considered for release and those in the community who could come into contact with them.[6]

In the weeks that followed, some national governments and justice systems took bold steps to reduce their prison populations, as some of the contributions to this Special Issue will attest. Notable examples reported in late March 2020 included: Iran, where the temporary release of 85,000 prisoners was approved; India, where it was announced that the largest New Delhi prison complex would release 3,000 prisoners, half of them sentenced inmates to be released on temporary furlough or parole, and the other half pre-trial prisoners released on bail; and Ethiopia, where over 4,000 prisoners were released under an executive amnesty order. Across much of Europe, too, prisoner release measures were announced, while prison administrations sought to work with police and prosecutors to limit numbers of new receptions into prisons (EuroPris, 2020). Remands in custody and short-term custodial sentences were replaced by house arrest or electronic monitoring.

Because of significant time lags in the availability of national prison populations data for most countries, it is too soon to know what effects the various initiatives states have been taking to reduce prisoner numbers will have had on prison population sizes worldwide. In addition, it will be difficult, perhaps impossible, to distinguish the impacts of these initiatives from those of other factors attributable to the pandemic, including fewer reported crimes, arrests and prosecutions as well as the temporary closure of many courts.

Despite these challenges in understanding precisely how prison population reduction policies have impacted prisoner numbers worldwide so far in the pandemic's history, we can obtain insights from prison population data produced by countries for which data were available as at February 2020 and have been updated since. This is the case for 20 jurisdictions, eight of which had prison populations above 70,000 as at February. These eight countries are shown in Table 1, together with information on how their prison populations changed during the first 5 months of the pandemic. All these countries were reported to have announced policies aimed at reducing prison population sizes as part of their efforts to control spread of the virus (as summarized in the table).

According to current World Prison Brief occupancy data, most of these countries were running their prison systems significantly above official capacity prior to the pandemic, with particularly severe levels of overcrowding in Nigeria (147%), Thailand (145%), Indonesia (176%) and Colombia (130%).[7]

Table 1. Prison population change in eight countries since February 2020.

	Total prisoners February 2020	Total prisoners July/ August 2020	Reduction policies (reported as at end July 2020)
Nigeria	74,106	62,258 (24.8.20)	Almost 8,000 released including the elderly or sick, and those with 6 months or less to serve. More use of non-custodial orders reported.
Colombia	122,085	102,637 (31.8.20)	Around 4,000 released to temporary house arrest including the vulnerable, pregnant women, and those who had committed minor offenses.
Indonesia	269,062	232,736 (31.8.20)	Over 39,000 released early or granted parole, with a further 11,000 releases planned.
Thailand	371,461	379,274 (1.8.20)	Some sentences suspended. Some early releases. Greater focus on creating more space in prisons.
England & Wales	83,868	79,433 (28.8.20)	Early release scheme introduced for some categories of prisoner. Limited use made of scheme, with 275 released.
France*	70,651	58,695 (1.7.20)	Early releases and reduced new receptions led to fall of around 10,000.
Poland	75,664	69,375 (31.7.20)	Temporary release programme announced for up to 12,000; unclear how many released.
Russian Federation	519,618	496,791[b] (1.8.20)	Amnesty programme potentially applicable to 30,000; unclear how far implemented.
Combined totals	1,586,515	1,481,199(105,316 fewer prisoners: a 6.64% reduction)	

*The French data are for "France entière" (ie including French overseas departments and territories), as at 1 January (data for February unavailable) and 1 July 2020.

[a]Information sourced from national news reports and official policy announcements.

[b]The recent falls in Russia's prison population rate have left it at an historic low, though it is still very high by European standards, at 344 per 100,000 of the population.

As the data in Table 1 show, all the countries in this group except Thailand saw reductions in their prison populations over the period from February to July 2020. During this period there were reports of many countries (including those in the table) implementing new early or temporary release schemes, and making wider use of alternatives to custody (both pre-trial and at sentencing). In several cases, the population reduction measures were expressed to be temporary and therefore any amelioration in the countries' prison overcrowding will, likewise, be short-lived. By way of example, on 20 August, Nigeria's federal government announced that 9,900 new receptions would soon take place in prisons across the country.

With the last national figures from the USA's Bureau of Justice Statistics dating back to June 2018, it will not be possible to track the precise changes in the country's prison population during the course of the pandemic. Some analysis has been carried out by justice reform organizations such as the Prison Policy Initiative, the Marshall Project, the Vera Institute and others, in an effort to mitigate against this data lag. In their review of changes in the country's jail population, the Prison Policy Initiative reported a median drop of over 30% in jail populations between March and May 2020, which they ascribed to quick action at local government level to reduce the numbers incarcerated. However, the NGO has since reported a slowing of these reductions and even a reversal of the downward trend in some cases.[8]

The Marshall Project (in a study conducted with the Associated Press) found that between March and June 2020, US state and federal prison populations decreased by around 100,000, equating to an 8% drop nationwide.[9] (This compared to a 2.2% decrease in state and federal prison populations over the whole of 2019.) The research showed that the reduction came about largely due to prohibitions on new prisoners being transferred from local jails, parole officers sending fewer people back to prison for low-level violations, and fewer people being sentenced to prison (due to court closures).

England & Wales failed fully to implement its early release programme, heralded as capable of reducing the prison population by 4,000 when introduced. The programme was shelved in August after just 275 prisoners had been released. The Government concluded at that point that it had sufficient extra headroom to ease overcrowding and facilitate isolation of COVID-19-positive inmates, so the early release scheme would not be required. The scheme has been criticized by some penal reform experts as having been designed to make early release very difficult even where prisoners met eligibility criteria. It had so many exclusions and so many layers of decision-making, that it was described by independent monitoring boards as having "simply added to bureaucracy without any noticeable effect" (Independent Monitoring Boards, 2020).[10] As a result of considerable falls in the numbers of reported crimes, and reduced arrests and court hearings, fewer people were remanded in custody or sentenced to prison. It is these changes, rather than any deliberate strategies to reduce prisoner numbers overall, that explain the fall in the England & Wales prison population over the first 6 months of the pandemic.

In Thailand, recent reports suggest that a mass prisoner amnesty will take effect over the remainder of 2020, as part of the royal pardon process implemented in the country every few years.[11] The last such amnesty was declared in late 2016 and reportedly extended to around 30,000 prisoners including people with disabilities, chronic illnesses, and any prisoner over 60 who had served at least a third of their sentence. This will no doubt go some way to reducing prisoner overcrowding, while not assuaging the need for structural change in pre-trial and sentencing policy and practice.

Limiting prisoners' contact with the outside world

Across the world, state authorities and prison administrations moved quickly to "lock down" prisons in order to reduce risk of infection passing between communities and prisons. Regimes became even more closed and restricted than before. Measures taken typically included:

- suspending visits from family members and other loved ones;
- suspending meetings with lawyers, religious counselors, consular staff;
- curtailment of visits by prisons inspectorate staff and other monitoring bodies – a vital check on conditions and standards;
- suspension of training and work activities in prison factories and workshops;
- stopping the normal day-to-day activities involving outside volunteers, probation or social work staff, or businesses in the local community, all of which routinely provide advice, support, training, education, rehabilitation and resettlement help to prisoners;
- restricting or ending schemes for day release for purposes of work and rehabilitation programmes;
- ending furloughs and family leave schemes (including leave for attending funerals or other important family events);
- restrictions on use of gyms, libraries and other communal spaces within prisons;
- reduced movement around prison spaces, with smaller groups being moved to help facilitate distancing and maintain order;
- more time spent inside cells and longer periods of isolation.

As at August 2020, restrictions had begun to be eased in many countries, notably in many parts of Europe (EuroPris, 2020), while in others they remained in place, the picture sometimes varying considerably from prison to prison in a given country.

Reports suggest that restrictions of this nature will frequently have led to increased anxiety for both prisoners and their loved ones, and to a worrying fall in housing, healthcare and similar support for people being released from prison (whether during the pandemic or after it). In a recent report by one English prison's independent monitoring board ("IMB"), prisoners described the mental health impacts of the highly restricted regime in place between March and July 2020:

> [The prisoners'] view was that the harmful effects did not stem simply from being locked up and having nothing to do ('*we can get used to that*'). It was the reduced contact with the outside world, particularly families, that was '*doing people's heads in*'. This reinforces the critical role that family contact plays in keeping prisons stable.[12]

The joint IMBs' annual report for the whole of England reached similar conclusions, noting that many prisoners had been locked in their cells for around 23 hours a day, with all social interaction and face-to-face education and training stopped. While these policies undoubtedly helped keep infection and mortality rates lower than had been feared, the IMBs reported a damaging cumulative impact on prisoners' mental and physical health and wellbeing and their chances of progression and rehabilitation (Independent Monitoring Boards, 2020). Concerns were raised about the impact of isolation on young people in custody, about the withdrawal of rehabilitative work, and evidence of growing frustration and rising incidence of self-harm, particularly in some women's prisons. There were particular concerns about hidden levels of distress and mental ill-health, often due to difficulties in accessing treatment and medication (for problems not principally related to COVID-19).

A similar picture emerges from the Correctional Association of New York (CANY), which also performs an oversight role and enjoys access to state prisons across New York State. CANY's survey of family members of prisoners across the state found that "the lack of regular and predictable communication between incarcerated people and their loved ones, and the longstanding and well-documented inadequacy of medical services in New York prisons [had] culminated in a high level of distrust" in the prison authorities' ability to care properly for prisoners during the pandemic' (Correctional Association of New York, 2020).

Family contact

Research shows that people who receive visits and maintain relationships while in prison are 38% less likely to reoffend after release than those who do not (Ministry of Justice and Department for Business Innovation and Skills, 2014). Family visits are vital to the maintenance of prisoner–family relationships, and extended visits of a few hours to a few days can provide opportunities for prisoners to spend quality time with their families. Maintaining family ties during a prison sentence is not just important for the prisoner but also for the prisoner's children and other family members. In many countries, prisoners also rely on relatives and loved ones to bring in goods such as medicines, nutritious foods, sanitary or hygiene products and sometimes cash, which prisoners may need to purchase items from prison commissaries.

Visits and contact with the outside world are a lifeline for many of the world's prisoners. This goes some way to explaining why, in the earliest stages of the pandemic, protests, riots and disturbances took place at prisons in many countries, some of them with tragic consequences. In Italy, unrest among prisoners when visits were abruptly suspended in March eventually spread to two dozen of the country's prisons, leading to 12 prisoners' deaths and widespread injuries to prisoners and prison staff. Riots or protests also occurred in prisons across most Central and Latin American countries, many Middle Eastern countries, in Sierra Leone, South Africa and a few other African states, India, Thailand, Sri Lanka, England, Scotland, France, Luxembourg and several other countries. In many cases, lives were lost during the unrest. The suspension of visits, along with fears that prisons would fail to put in place sufficient protection measures for prisoners, were most commonly cited as catalysts for the unrest.

A less obvious but potentially equally damaging consequence of the severely restricted regimes imposed in response to the pandemic is the psychological harm they will have caused for many prisoners. Peter Clarke, the Chief Inspector of Prisons in England & Wales, presented stark findings from the "short scrutiny visits" which replaced the usual, more comprehensive inspection regime for several weeks in the early phase of the pandemic (HM Chief Inspector of Prisons, 2020). In an amalgamated report covering 35 prisons visited during eleven weeks, Mr Clarke noted that prisoners were initially willing to accept and cooperate with the suspension of social visits, limited time out of the cell, and other restrictions, because of a sense of "being in this together" with staff and the community outside during "lockdown". However, after these initial few weeks: "Our visits identified increasing levels of stress and frustration among many prisoners and evidence that prisoner well-being was being increasingly affected by the continuation of restrictions." The most commonly identified cause was the suspension of visits.

The report pointed to the particularly severe consequences for women prisoners:

> 'In the women's estate, there are some exceptionally vulnerable individuals who usually benefit from a range of specialist support services provided by external providers; their absence was extremely damaging. For these prisoners, the long hours of lock up were compounded by the sudden withdrawal of services on which they depended, and self-harm among prisoners in prisons holding women has remained consistently high throughout the lockdown period.'

The report also addressed the risk of mental illness:

> [I]n prisons, there is now a real risk of psychological decline among prisoners, which needs to be addressed urgently, so that prisoners, children and detainees do not suffer long-term damage to their mental health and well-being, and prisons can fulfil their rehabilitative goals.

In countries where many prisoners are serving exceptionally long (or indeterminate) sentences, the importance of family visits, and the potential psychological harm caused by greater isolation, are all the greater. In New York State, visiting loved ones had already been fraught with difficulty for many even before the pandemic. Traveling for several hours at great expense (cost of travel and lost earnings) was just one aspect of this, but the highly restricted visiting hours, security checks and other features of the visiting system were also seen as needlessly punitive for families. Most New York State prisons and jails were closed to visitors from March to August 2020 (and in many cases remained so beyond August). On 6 August, New York's Alliance of Families for Justice held a rally outside the Governor's office to call for visiting rights to be restored.[13] In a statement, it said:

> These restrictions deepen the pain felt by the COVID-19 pandemic by limiting visiting hours, forbidding physical contact, limiting the number of visitors to two, closing the children's play area and shuttering the Family Reunion Program.[14]

Prisoners in Thailand could receive two types of visit before the pandemic. There were standard visits several times per week over several hours each day, where prisoners would be separated from the visitors outside by both a fence and a screen (communicating by fixed phones). There were also less frequent "open visits" when the prisoner's family members would be allowed into closer physical contact with the prisoner, sitting together in the yard or admissions area of the prison; such visits would be restricted to three or four per prisoner annually before the pandemic. Prisoners interviewed for our project in 2019 described the hardship caused when their families lived in parts of the country remote from the prison location. One, a woman 6 years into a life sentence for a drug-dealing offense, said simply: "My family do not have much money. They visit me twice a year."[15] Such prisoners will benefit from the advent of video calls (introduced in 2019 in some prisons but by no means all), particularly during the pandemic when visits were suspended for two months. Calls have been made for greater investment in the required technology and infrastructure to ensure larger numbers of prisoners can have some form of contact with their families.[16]

In the largest Dutch prison, housing around 800 prisoners, the usual practice of family visits was altered, but to a fairly limited extent. Face-to-face visits in which physical contact was allowed were replaced by visits separated by a plexiglass screen. As at early September following a successful pilot, prisons were planning to revert to normal family visits but with masks having to be worn by family members (apart from children under 12 years).

Work, education, preparation for release

External work placements and internal work and training schemes in prison factories and workshops often provide a basic level of income on which prisoners rely, whether to help support their families, or to save toward a fund they can have recourse to on release. Education programmes, where available and properly supported, can also make prison life bearable and equip prisoners with the tools to transform their chances on release.

In many countries these opportunities to earn an income, receive training or education, along with the routine interaction with others which participation entails, were abruptly halted with the pandemic.

In Thailand, the country's severe prison overcrowding has been mitigated to a limited extent by regimes in which 10 hours each day would typically be spent outside the communal cells.[17] A range of activities are provided to prisoners during these hours (including using prison library and gym facilities, meditation, dance, music, viewing pre-recorded film and TV content, training and some work opportunities). Much of this activity came to a halt during the early stages of the pandemic, although restrictions began to be eased from July. Day release schemes allowing prisoners near the end of their sentence to work outside the prison were also put on hold. It is feared that the resulting lack of earnings, together with the economic hardships families themselves are experiencing due to the pandemic and associated restrictions, could result in financial difficulties for many prisoners and their families.

In England & Wales, the system of release on temporary license ("ROTL") was suspended in order to minimize the spread of COVID-19. ROTL aims to facilitate rehabilitation, by helping prisoners to prepare for resettlement in the community after release. Many prisoners who had been working in the community and beginning to build a new life were reported to have felt the loss of opportunity keenly and expressed frustration at the scheme's suspension.

Substitute work schemes were introduced in parts of the USA to enable prisoners to use workshop facilities to make protective equipment. Some reports suggested that prisoners themselves were not allowed to use masks despite being required to mass-produce them in prison workshops.[18]

The Netherlands, with its low prison population rate and occupancy levels at around 75% of available capacity, experienced very low numbers of confirmed COVID-19 cases (11 cases according to Justice Project Pakistan).[19] In one of the country's larger establishments, it was possible to keep the prison workshops open but create different working shift patterns and reduce overall time in the workshop, to ensure social distancing would be possible.[20]

In Kenya, NGOs have in recent years become increasingly involved with many aspects of prisoner release. One, the Faraja Foundation, regularly participates in prisoner resettlement and discharge committee meetings. Their staff provide support and counseling to prisoners likely to face major problems on release because of poverty, ill health, illiteracy and other challenges. Faraja also carry out important and sensitive work to prepare communities for the return of people being released from prison. This work can help ensure protection from revenge attacks and also safeguard vulnerable individuals, including children who have been incarcerated with their mothers and who would otherwise be at risk of exploitation or abuse. As late as August 2020, restrictions on prison visits were still preventing this work to a large extent, leaving many prisoners effectively "stuck" in the system who would otherwise be moving toward a successful managed release.

Compensatory measures

In some countries, compensatory measures were announced to reduce the isolation and deprivation experienced by prisoners due to restrictions on visits and similar activities. These have included introducing secure video calls for "virtual visits", prison-administered e-mail systems, and increased access to internet and telephones. Some prison services provide additional or unlimited phone credits to prisoners and some have purchased extra mobile phones and video conferencing equipment. EuroPris have reported that there have been negotiations with telecommunication providers by some prison services in European Union countries to reduce the costs of prisoners' calls, "not all of them successful" (EuroPris, 2020).

Provision of video conferencing has presented challenges for many countries where it was not yet available (or in use for family communication) in the national prison systems. For other countries, the pandemic has been a spur to faster implementation of what had already been piloted or planned. In England & Wales, for example, prisons are reported to be moving at last toward national roll-out of free family-prisoner video visits, following years of stop-start on various pilots. In Kenya, while some of the work of organizations providing mentoring, counseling and training has been made available to prisoners via large screens, more hardware and other investment will be needed for this to have any lasting positive impact.

While these various compensatory measures were welcomed, there were also concerns over the inadequacy of supplies or the poor implementation of the measures promised. In England & Wales the Government announced in March that secure phone handsets would be given to "prisoners at 55 jails" and, in May, that video calls for family contact would now be available in 26 prisons. The inadequacy of these steps to mitigate the loss of in-person visits was described as "obvious" by the NGO Prison Reform Trust, in a report noting that demand for the new provision entirely outstripped supply, resulting in a post-code lottery of available means of staying in touch with families. The compensatory measures promised were "raising hopes but leading to frustration, distress and anger". Many family members and prisoners providing information to the NGO spoke of their intense feelings of loss and hopelessness during the months in question (Prison Reform Trust, 2020).

The restrictions imposed by the Dutch prison regime appear to have been limited and short-lived in comparison with England & Wales and many other countries we have studied. Although in-person family visits were suspended for a brief period and some restrictions were placed on prisoners' movement, family and other visits – conducted through plexiglass screens – were still possible. In addition, by staggering the periods of circulation of small groups of prisoners, significant time out of the cell engaging in purposeful activity – which had long been a hallmark of Dutch prison regimes – was still being maintained in this more restricted regime.[21]

What will COVID-19 mean for penal reform?

COVID-19 has made particularly evident the permeability of prison walls, as the virus spread from prison staff to prisoners and back into communities, taking a heavier toll in areas where prisons are located.[22] Just as it was impossible for prison administrations to keep the virus out, so, too, it is futile and dangerous to expect prison walls to contain the risk of crime or keep communities safe from harm. So, can we hope for a silver lining from the COVID-19 cloud, in the shape of a health-informed approach to criminal justice reform?

As we have seen, when the pandemic was declared, some countries moved decisively to reduce prisoner numbers in order to minimize the risk that overcrowded conditions would present. For this and other reasons related to the pandemic, it is likely that prisoner numbers across the world will fall during 2020– 2021, following decades of growth.[23] If these lower levels can be maintained, the resulting savings could be reinvested in health and social interventions known to reduce crime. For the present, it is too soon to know whether falls seen in some prison populations will be maintained, and whether the lifting of pandemic restrictions will bring with it a return to criminal justice business-as-usual.

The devastating public health consequences of the pandemic should make us all wary of returning to prison population growth, or of accepting it as an inevitable facet of modern times. Overcrowded prisons mean increased prevalence of communicable and chronic diseases, mental illness, substance misuse, violence, self-harm and suicide. The risks affect prisoners, staff, the families of prisoners and staff, and wider communities. Prison populations already bear a far greater burden of mental and physical health problems than general populations. People who enter custody usually come from the poorest and most marginalized sections of society – communities that often have worse health due to socio-economic and health inequalities. People with mental health problems, drug or alcohol dependency or other vulnerabilities are also over-represented in prison populations. It is far too easy for them to be propelled into the criminal justice system and custody *because* of those problems, when their needs would be better addressed through health-led interventions. Furthermore, prison environments tend to exacerbate existing health problems and often give rise to new ones, because of poor living conditions, lack of healthcare, availability of illicit drugs, social and psychological stresses, violence and mistreatment.

The COVID-19 pandemic has revealed an unprecedented need for a health-informed approach to penal reform. What would this entail? For most countries, reducing prisoner numbers overall is an essential first step to ensuring better conditions and access to healthcare and treatment in custody. That means limiting the use of pre-trial detention, as many European countries have done in recent years (Heard & Fair, 2019; Walmsley, 2020). It means fairer, more proportionate sentencing and making smarter use of alternatives to custody. It also means reducing the numbers of people in poor health who go to prison. To achieve that, most countries need to improve healthcare provision in the community, particularly for mental health conditions and drug and alcohol problems.

Then, for those reduced numbers of prisoners for whom custody is inevitable, there must be proper access to healthcare, screening and treatment, harm reduction measures, and decent living conditions. Daily life in prison settings should be modeled to resemble life outside in as many ways as possible; deprivation of liberty should be the only detriment of a prison sentence, because it already entails the pain of separation from loved ones, friends and community. These are principles that underlie prison regimes in the Netherlands,

Finland and a few other countries. Time spent out of the cell is maximized, visits and communication with family and loved ones are encouraged and enabled, activities and interaction involving outside organizations and volunteers are promoted and supported, and the regime's focus is on resocialisation and getting the prisoner ready for life outside.

It is likely that some of the technology introduced during the pandemic to make up for lost in-person visits will be placed on a permanent footing, either to provide extra connectivity for prisoners and better linkage with the outside world, or as a cheaper, easier substitute for face-to-face visits and real-life interactions with people from outside the prison. While remote contact would help increase the frequency of contact with family, in-person contact plays a key role and its facilitation should remain a priority even after technological connectivity has been enhanced. The "new normal" as we move out of the pandemic should therefore mean that prison systems provide and promote in-person visits and real-life activities to the widest extent possible, *and* make wider use of remote technology-enabled communication and learning.

Notes

1. The countries under study in the project are: Kenya, South Africa, Brazil, the United States of America, India, Thailand, England & Wales, Hungary, the Netherlands and Australia. https://www.icpr.org.uk/theme/prisons-and-use-imprisonment/understanding-and-reducing-use-imprisonment-ten-countries.
2. Global tracking conducted by Justice Project Pakistan: at https://www.jpp.org.pk/covid19-prisoners/.
3. These materials can be found under "resources" on our World Prison Brief site at: https://www.prisonstudies.org/news/news-covid-19-and-prisons.
4. All prison population data in this Commentary are drawn from the World Prison Brief site (except where stated), and reflect the latest available figures as at 10 September 2020. World Prison Brief data are updated on the website on a monthly basis, using data largely derived from governmental or other official sources. https://www.prisonstudies.org/.
5. National occupancy levels can be found on each country page on the World Prison Brief website; in addition, the "Highest to Lowest" function can be selected to rank countries globally or regionally, by occupancy level.
6. Examples include Human Rights Watch, the International Legal Foundation, Penal Reform International, Fair Trials, the European Prisons Observatory, Center for Crime and Justice Studies, the Thailand Institute of Justice, and the Commonwealth Human Rights Initiative. For further information, see the COVID-19 news and resources page on our World Prison Brief website at: https://www.prisonstudies.org/news/news-covid-19-and-prisons.
7. Estimated occupancy levels based on latest official capacity data available can be found on the World Prison Brief website.
8. Prison Policy Initiative, 'Jails and prisons have reduced their populations in the face of the pandemic, but not enough to save lives', article, 5 August 2020, https://www.prisonpolicy.org/blog/2020/08/05/jails-vs-prisons-update-2/.
9. The Marshall Project, "Prison populations drop by 100,000 during pandemic: but not because of COVID-19 releases", article, 16 July 2020, https://www.themarshallproject.org/2020/07/16/prison-populations-drop-by-100-000-during-pandemic.
10. The independent monitoring boards are statutory bodies performing the role of the national preventive mechanism in the United Kingdom following ratification of the Optional Protocol to the United Nations Convention against Torture and Other Cruel, Inhuman or Degrading Treatment or Punishment.

11. Thailand Bail, 23 August 2020, "Thailand royal pardon 2020: many in Thai prisons receive sentence reductions". http://www.thailandbail.com/thailand-royal-pardon-2020-many-in-thai-prisons-receive-sentence-reductions/.
12. Extract from draft annual report of an English prison's Independent Monitoring Board, provided to author by a member of the board.
13. Brooklyn Daily Eagle, 6 August 2020, "Families of incarcerated people rally outside Cuomo's office to demand visitation rights." https://brooklyneagle.com/articles/2020/08/06/families-of-incarcerated-people-rally-outside-cuomos-office-to-demand-visitation-rights/.
14. The Department of Corrections and Community Supervision of New York's website states that the Family Reunion Program "provides approved incarcerated individuals and their families the opportunity to meet for a designated period of time in a private home-like setting". https://doccs.ny.gov/family-reunion-program.
15. Around one quarter of all prisoners in Thailand are serving sentences ranging between 10 and 50 years. At least 80% of the country's sentenced prisoners have been convicted of drug offenses. Thailand Institute of Justice, March 2020, *Report on the COVID-19 situation in prisons and policy recommendations for Thailand.*
16. Thailand Institute of Justice (fn 17).
17. Information drawn from interviews with serving prisoners conducted in the course of ICPR's ongoing project *Understanding and reducing the use of imprisonment in ten countries* (see fn 1).
18. Delaware News Journal, 17 April, 2020, "Delaware officials: Prisoners won't get masks or release during COVID-19 fight", https://eu.delawareonline.com/story/news/2020/04/16/delaware-officials-prisoners-wont-get-masks-release-during-coronavirus-fight/2988586001/.
19. As fn. 2 above.
20. Information obtained in early September from a deputy governor of a prison holding around 800 inmates.
21. See fn 20.
22. In the USA, several studies have demonstrated the significant capacity for community spread of COVID-19 infections in areas with jails and prisons. See for example, Ollove (2020).
23. For the most comprehensive data on prison population trends since 2000 see Walmsley (2018).

Disclosure statement

No potential conflict of interest was reported by the author(s).

References

Correa, M. E., Croda, J., Coimbra Motta de Castro, A. R., Maria do Valle Leone de Oliveira, S., Pompilio, M. A., Omizolo de Souza, R., Ferreira de Sá Queiroz, J. H., da Silva, K. E., Ko, A. I., & Simionatto, S. (2017). High prevalence of treponema pallidum infection in Brazilian prisoners. *American Journal of Tropical Medical Hygiene*, *97*(4), 1078–1084. https://doi.org/10.4269/ajtmh.17-0098

Correctional Association of New York. (2020). *He has a home to go to: Family and friends of people in prison in New York respond to CANY's COVID-19 survey*. https://static1.squarespace.com/static/5e7b9e66cf507e048ef3f08b/t/5ecf917c38a54333593b5ca8/1590661511538/CANY+COVID-19+Report+May+2020.pdf

EuroPris. (2020). *Reducing overcrowding: EuroPris COVID-19 pandemic fact sheet, updated July 2020.*

Heard, C. (2019). *Towards a health-informed approach to penal reform? Evidence from ten countries.* Institute for Crime & Justice Policy Research.

Heard, C., & Fair, H. (2019). *Pre-trial detention and its over-use: Evidence from ten countries.* Institute for Crime & Justice Policy Research.

HM Chief Inspector of Prisons. (2020). *Aggregate report on short scrutiny visits: 21 April – 7 July 2020.* https://www.justiceinspectorates.gov.uk/hmiprisons/wp-content/uploads/sites/4/2020/08/SSV-aggregate-report-web-2020.pdf

Independent Monitoring Boards. (2020). *National annual report 2019–20.* https://www.imb.org.uk/report/10718/

Ministry of Justice and Department for Business Innovation and Skills. (2014). *Parenting and relationship support programmes for offenders and their families: Executive summary.* https://policis.com/pdf/moj/MOJ_BIS_Parenting_Support_for_offenders_and_families_Executive_Summary_280114_FINAL.pdf

Ollove, M. (2020). *How COVID-19 in jails and prisons threatens nearby communities.* Stateline. https://www.pewtrusts.org/en/research-and-analysis/blogs/stateline/2020/07/01/how-covid-19-in-jails-and-prisons-threatens-nearby-communities/

Prison Reform Trust. (2020, June). *How prisons are responding to Covid-19: Briefing #1, Families and communications* (part of series in project 'CAPPTIVE: Covid-19 Action Prisons Project: Tracking Innovation, Valuing Experience'). http://www.prisonreformtrust.org.uk/Portals/0/Documents/CAPPTIVE_families_webfinal.pdf

United Nations Office on Drugs and Crime. (2020). *Position paper: COVID-19 preparedness and responses in prisons.* https://www.unodc.org/documents/justice-and-prison-reform/UNODC_Position_paper_COVID-19_in_prisons.pdf

Walmsley, R. (2018). *World prison population list* (12th ed.). Institute for Criminal Policy Research.

Walmsley, R. (2020). *World pre-trial/remand imprisonment list* (4th ed.). Institute for Criminal Policy Research.

World Health Organization. (2020). *Preparedness, prevention and control of COVID-19 in prisons and other places of detention: Interim guidance 15 March 2020.* WHO Regional Office for Europe.

An Imperfect Storm: Identifying the Root Causes of COVID-19 Outbreaks in the World's Largest Corrections Systems

James M. Byrne, Sabrina S. Rapisarda, Don Hummer, and Kimberly R. Kras

ABSTRACT

We review the nature and extent of COVID-19 outbreaks across corrections systems globally, and document the types of front-end, in-prison, and back-end mitigation strategies used to address the COVID-19 problem in the 50 countries with the largest prison systems; these countries house over 90% of the global prison population. For most countries, the reported rates of COVID-19 infections and deaths during the first phase of the pandemic are higher in prisons and jails than in the general community, but similar baseline data on the extent of outbreaks in the community corrections systems of these countries were unavailable. We find that: prison expansion has resulted in prison overcrowding in many large prison systems, making in-prison mitigation strategies harder to implement; large prison systems are characterized by inadequate prison infrastructure and health care services; and the current global prison population includes a significant number of individuals with poor physical and mental health, placing them "at risk" for infection, both in prison and in their home communities. Based on our review of the short-term impact of reforms on inmate and staff health, the size of the prison and jail population, and public safety, we recommend an aggressive three-pronged COVID-19-based corrections research agenda.

Introduction: An imperfect storm (that was not caused by global warming)

Over 33.5 million people have been infected with COVID-19 globally, and over 1 million people have died of COVID-19-related illnesses between the months of March and September 2020 (Elflein, 2020). While there are indications that the pandemic may be winding down in some countries, the World Health Organization has warned that a - new, second wave of the pandemic may be arriving soon (World Health Organization (WHO), 2020). It is with this warning in mind that we provide the following assessment of the preliminary impact of the COVID-19 crisis on corrections systems in each global region. We begin by assessing the nature and extent of COVID-19 outbreaks in prison systems globally, and then review the various mitigation strategies employed by corrections administrators. We conclude our review by (1) offering a preliminary assessment of the effectiveness of current mitigation strategies, and (2) identifying reforms that will reduce the likelihood of future outbreaks in corrections systems in each global region.

Prisons and jails in each global region have been reported to be hot spots for the spread of the virus, but there has been little attention on whether *community corrections* systems in these same global regions face similar problems. There have been conflicting reports on the infection rates in prisons, with corrections leaders in some countries downplaying the extent of the problem (e.g., China, Romania, Venezuela), and making the claim that prisons and jails are *safer* than the surrounding communities due to mitigation strategies (Li & Liu, this volume; Durnescu, this volume; Marmolejo et al., this volume). Meanwhile, corrections leaders in other countries (e.g., Germany and the USA) have been more transparent about the extent and seriousness of the outbreaks in their prison systems and have spoken publicly about the need for more resources to address the problem (Dunkel, 2020; Wetzel and Davis, 2020). So, who is correct? To answer this question, we examine the available data on the extent of COVID-19 outbreaks in prisons and jails globally, using both official and unofficial data sources.[1] We also attempted – unsuccessfully, it turns out – to document the extent of the COVID-19 outbreaks in community corrections systems.[2] Our review highlights the paucity of data on community corrections systems globally, which makes an examination of the extent of these outbreaks impossible at the current time. As we note in our conclusion, we have the data available to examine prison systems globally, thanks in large part to the efforts of the World Prison Research Programme; we are in dire need of a similar research program targeting community corrections systems globally.[3]

Our review targets the top 50 countries with the largest prison systems for a simple and pragmatic reason: over 90% of the global prison population is housed in correctional facilities in these 50 countries (World Prison Brief, 2020). In fact, over half of the world's current prison population is held in the prison systems of just five countries: USA, China, Brazil, Russia, and India (see Figure 1). After documenting the prison/jail COVID-19 infection and death rates in these "top 50" countries, we identify three likely factors that explain the high rates reported in prisons and jails, focusing on the outbreaks in the largest prison systems: (1) prison crowding due to prison upsizing, (2) inadequate prison infrastructure and heath care, and (3) the poor health status (both physical and mental health) of the current global prison population. These three pre-pandemic conditions have created what we refer to as an "imperfect storm" that has resulted in significant harm to both inmates and staff in prisons globally. Unless the conditions that led prisons and jails to become COVID-19 hot spots in the first wave of the pandemic are addressed, additional waves of infections are likely inevitable in prison systems within and across global regions.[4]

After documenting the nature and extent of the outbreak of COVID-19 in prisons within and across global regions, we then examine the types of front-end, within-prison, and back-end mitigation strategies employed in these countries and assess the intended and unintended consequences of these strategies for inmates, workers, and the community. We conclude this review by offering an assessment of the known effect of various mitigation strategies in the short-term (in terms of public safety and reducing physical and mental health risks). Building on this assessment, we consider the likely longer-term impact of the COVID-19 crisis on sentencing and corrections reform within and across global regions.

There is a common theme that emerges from discussions by reformers of every ilk when a country or region is faced with either a serious political crisis or a "natural" disaster: never let a good (or serious) crisis go to waste.[5] In this instance, there is nothing good about this crisis in the short-term. However, it is certainly possible to speculate – perhaps naively, but that will not deter us – that the harm caused by the pandemic will force policymakers to

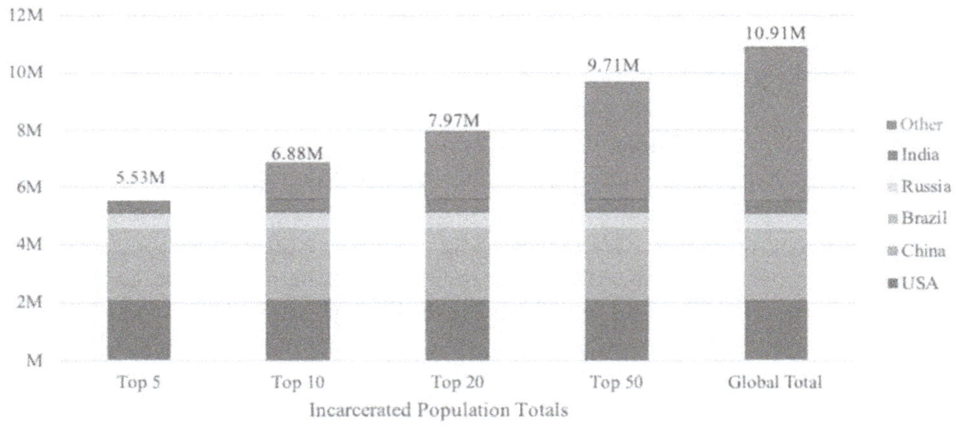

Figure 1. Cumulative global incarcerated population totals (milions). ***Note**: "Other" indicates the remaining prison systems (excluding the USA, China, Brazil, Russia, and India) within the top 10, top 20, top 50, and global total (cumulatively). The top 5 prison systems comprise nearly 51% of the cumulative global prison population total (N = 10,911,380), while the top 10 make up 63%, the top 20 comprise over 73%, and the top 50 (out of 223 prison systems worldwide) account for 89% of the world's cumulative prison population total. Taking a closer look at the world's 50 largest prison systems, the top 5 prison systems comprise nearly 55% of the world's top 50 prison systems (N = 5,534,665), while the top 10 prison systems (the USA, China, Brazil, Russia, India, Thailand, Turkey, Iran, Indonesia, and Philippines) account for approximately 71% of the top 50 prison systems' cumulative prison population total. All data were extracted from the World Prison Brief database (World Prison Brief, 2020).

move aggressively to downsize prisons, improve prison health care and infrastructure, and to address the myriad of health-related problems found in the (poverty pocket, high crime) communities where most inmates reside before and after their time in prison.

Lies, damn lies, and statistics: Whom do you trust?

A quote that has been alternately (and, it appears, inaccurately) attributed to both Benjamin Disraeli and Mark Twain is an appropriate way to start our assessment of available data documenting the extent of COVID-19 outbreaks in both prisons and the general community: *There are three kinds of lies: Lies, damn lies, and statistics.*[6] The community and prison COVID-19 data that we examine in this section of our review should be viewed with a healthy dose of skepticism, given the stakes involved for corrections administrators and political leaders within and across global regions. Several authors of articles included in this special issue have observed that in the countries they profiled, corrections administrators faced loss of their jobs if the full extent of the crisis was shared with either the central government or the general public.[7] Other authors observed that political leaders in their countries argued – without providing supporting evidence – that prisons were safer places during the pandemic than the general community.[8] To support this contention, it is certainly possible that leaders in these countries have suppressed the release of these data, and/or not tested inmates or the community at levels that would allow for us to assess these conflicting claims. For this reason, the data presented here should be viewed cautiously.

Out of sight, but in danger: Documenting and tracking outbreaks in prisons globally

We begin our review by looking at the data on the COVID-19 outbreak in the community and in the prison systems of the 50 countries with the largest prison systems (see Table 1). Taken collectively, over 90% of the world's prison population is housed in these 50 countries. In terms of regional representation, this top 50 list includes 17 countries from Asia, 10 from Africa, 10 from Europe, 3 from North America, 7 from South America, 3 from Central America/Caribbean and 1 from Oceania (World Prison Brief, 2020). Looking at individual countries, we see that the top 5 largest prison systems – USA, China, Brazil, Russia, and India – house slightly over 50% of the world's total prison population (see Figure 1). Any serious discussion of global prison downsizing needs to begin with an examination of the drivers of incarceration in these 5 countries (Byrne et al., 2015).

Table 2 presents the current data (as of September 29, 2020) on the extent of the *community-level* COVID-19 outbreaks in countries with the largest prison systems, including the number of reported infections, the rate of infections, and the number (and rate) of deaths attributed to COVID-19. According to Worldometer (2020), the cumulative global COVID-19 case count as of September 29, 2020, was 33,773,629. The 50 countries housing the largest prison systems in the world account for 30,333,348, or 90%, of the global case count total. Worldwide, there have been 1,010,510 reported COVID-19-related deaths, of which 928,392 of those cases, or 92%, of the global cumulative death count occurred within the countries with the top 50 prison systems (as of September 29, 2020).

No global region can be described as "COVID-free," but there is variation across regions that is important to consider. In terms of the number of known and officially reported cases, countries with large prison systems in both North America (USA, Mexico) and South America (Brazil, Chile, Argentina) have the largest *reported* community-level COVID-19 outbreaks. Not surprisingly, prison systems in each of these countries also have high numbers of reported infections. Is this an artifact of higher testing rates in both the general community and in prisons by these countries? Unfortunately, we do not have access to the global testing rate data for prison and the general community that would allow us to answer this question.

Based on the official data on the number of reported COVID-19 cases (Worldometer, 2020), China has significantly lower reported community-level COVID-19 infection rates (and death rates) than other countries with large prison systems; they also report the lowest prison infection rates (and death rates) among these top 5 countries (see Table 3). We are skeptical of these data, but absent of alternative data sources and alternative estimates, we do not have an answer to the question: Are China's official reports accurate or prima facia evidence of a cover-up? However, it is worth noting that the review of China's response to the COVID-19 crisis by Li and Liu (2020) includes a discussion of why local government leaders and corrections administrators were initially reluctant to report community-level or prison-level infection and death data to the central government: fear of retaliation and job loss.

One question that we *can* answer with the available data for the five countries with the largest prison populations (representing just over 50% of the global prison population) is whether prisons are safer to reside during the pandemic than the general community, as some leaders have suggested. Table 3 provides an answer: the rate of infections in prison is

Table 1. Top 50 countries by global region and prison population totals (*updated 9/30/20).

Rank	Country	Global Region	Prison Population Total	Year	Source
1	USA	North America	2,094,000	2018	U.S. Bureau of Justice Statistics/World Prison Brief
2	China	Eastern Asia	1,710,000	2018	National Prison Administration/World Prison Brief
3	Brazil	South America	755,274	December 2019	National Prison Administration/World Prison Brief
4	Russian Federation	Europe/Asia	496,791	August 1, 2020	National Prison Administration/World Prison Brief
5	India	Southern Asia	478,600	December 31, 2019	World Prison Brief
6	Thailand	South-Eastern Asia	379,274	August 1, 2020	National Prison administration/World Prison Brief
7	Turkey	Europe/Asia	281,094	July 2020	Ministry of Justice
8	Iran	Southern Asia	240,000	2018	World Prison Brief
9	Indonesia	South-Eastern Asia	232,736	August 31, 2020	National Prison Administration/World Prison Brief
10	Philippines	South-Eastern Asia	215,000	November 2018	Health Secretary/World Prison Brief
11	Mexico	North America	198,384	April 2019	Animal Politico/World Prison Brief
12	South Africa	Southern Africa	154,437	April 1, 2020	National Prison Administration/World Prison Brief
13	Vietnam	South-Eastern Asia	123,697	2019	Thai Criminology/World Prison Brief
14	Ethiopia	Eastern Africa	113,727	2013–14	National Prison Administration/World Prison Brief
15	Egypt	Northern Africa	106,000	August 2016	National Prison Administration/World Prison Brief
16	Argentina	South America	103,209	December 31, 2018	Ministry of Justice/World Prison Brief
17	Colombia	South America	102,637	August 31, 2020	National Prison Administration/World Prison Brief
18	Peru	South America	96,440	April 30, 2020	Ministry of Justice/World Prison Brief
19	Myanmar (formerly Burma)	South-Eastern Asia	92,000	2018	National Prison Administration/World Prison Brief
20	Bangladesh	Southern Asia	88,084	February 2020	Ministry of Home Affairs/World Prison Brief
21	Morocco	Northern Africa	85,767	September 2019	National Prison Administration/World Prison Brief
22	United Kingdom: England & Wales	Northern Europe	79,433	August 28, 2020	Ministry of Justice
23	Pakistan	Southern Asia	77,275	September 30, 2019	Federal Ombudsman/World Prison Brief
24	Poland	Central/Eastern Europe	69,375	July 31, 2020	National Prison Administration/World Prison Brief
25	Malaysia	South-Eastern Asia	68,603	August 2020	Ministry of Home Affairs/World Prison Brief
26	Rwanda	Eastern Africa	65,000	October 2019	National Human Rights Commission/World Prison Brief
26	Algeria	Northern Africa	65,000	2019	U.S. State Department Human Rights Report/World Prison Brief
28	Nigeria	Western Africa	62,258	August 24, 2020	National Prison Administration/World Prison Brief
29	Saudi Arabia	Western Asia	61,000	June 2017	Informed sources in Al-Watan/World Prison Brief
30	Taiwan	Eastern Asia	60,956	December 31, 2019	Ministry of Justice/World Prison Brief
31	France	Western Europe	58,695	July 1, 2020	National Prison Administration/World Prison Brief
32	Spain	Southern Europe	58,642	February 14, 2020	National Prison Administration/World Prison Brief
33	Germany	Western Europe	57,600	June 30, 2020	Federal Statistical Office/World Prison Brief
34	Cuba	Caribbean	57,337	May 2012	El Diario Oficial Granma/World Prison Brief
35	Venezuela	South America	57,096	2017	Observatorio Venezolano de Prisiones/World Prison Brief
36	Uganda	Eastern Africa	55,229	2019	Ministry of Internal Affairs/World Prison Brief
37	Republic of (South) Korea	Eastern Asia	53,920	June 30, 2020	National Prison Administration/World Prison Brief
38	Italy	Southern Europe	53,619	July 31, 2020	Ministry of Justice/World Prison Brief

(Continued)

Table 1. (Continued).

Rank	Country	Global Region	Prison Population Total	Year	Source
39	Kenya	Eastern Africa	53,348	2019	National Prison Administration/World Prison Brief
40	Ukraine	Central/Eastern Europe	52,609	April 1, 2020	National Prison Administration/World Prison Brief
41	Japan	Eastern Asia	48,802	October 31, 2019	National Prison Administration/World Prison Brief
42	Iraq	Western Asia	45,000	2015	U.N. Human Rights Committee/World Prison Brief
43	Australia	Oceania	44,358	March 2020	Australian Bureau of Statistics/World Prison Brief
44	Canada	North America	M = 39,579	March 31, 2018	Statistics Canada/World Prison Brief
45	Chile	South America	39,284	July 31, 2020	National Prison Administration/World Prison Brief
46	Ecuador	South America	39,251	January 1, 2020	National Prison Administration/World Prison Brief
47	El Salvador	Central America	36,693	August 17, 2020	National Prison Administration/World Prison Brief
48	Cambodia	South-Eastern Asia	36,600	November 2019	National Prison Administration/World Prison Brief
50	Tanzania	Eastern Africa	35,803	December 2019	Home Ministry/World Prison Brief
50	Belarus	Central/Eastern Europe	32,500	October 1, 2018	Ministry of Internal Affairs/World Prison Brief

Table 2. Community COVID-19 case and death prevalence in countries housing the top 50 largest prison systems (*updated 9/29/20).

Rank	Country	Total Case Count	Case Rate/1 million persons	Total Death Count	Death Rate/1 million persons
1	USA	7,394,635	22,308	210,571	635
2	China	85,384	59	4,634	3
3	Brazil	4,753,410	22,324	142,280	668
4	Russian Federation	1,167,805	8,001	20,545	141
5	India	6,223,519	4,499	97,529	71
6	Thailand	3,559	51	59	0.8
7	Turkey	317,272	3,752	8,130	96
8	Iran	453,637	5,384	25,986	308
9	Indonesia	282,724	1,031	10,601	39
10	Philippines	309,303	2,814	5,448	50
11	Mexico	733,717	5,676	76,603	593
12	South Africa	672,572	11,306	16,667	280
13	Vietnam	1,094	11	35	0.4
14	Ethiopia	74,584	645	1,191	10
15	Egypt	103,079	1,003	5,914	58
16	Argentina	723,132	15,964	16,113	356
17	Colombia	824,042	16,153	25,828	506
18	Peru	808,714	24,445	32,324	977
19	Myanmar (formerly Burma)	12,425	228	284	5
20	Bangladesh	362,043	2,193	5,219	32
21	Morocco	121,183	3,274	2,152	58
22	United Kingdom: England & Wales	446,156	6,564	42,072	619
23	Pakistan	311,516	1,404	6,474	29
24	Poland	89,962	2,378	2,483	66
25	Malaysia	11,135	343	134	4
26	Rwanda	4,836	321	29	2
26	Algeria	51,368	1,166	1,726	39
28	Nigeria	58,647	283	1,111	5
29	Saudi Arabia	334,187	9,563	4,739	136
30	Taiwan	513	22	7	0.3
31	France	550,690	8,432	31,893	488
32	Spain	758,172	16,214	31,614	676
33	Germany	290,466	3,464	9,556	114
34	Cuba	5,531	488	122	11
35	Venezuela	73,528	2,588	614	22
36	Uganda	8,017	174	75	2
37	Republic of (South) Korea	23,699	462	407	8
38	Italy	313,011	5,179	35,875	594
39	Kenya	38,378	710	707	13
40	Ukraine	204,932	4,693	4,065	93
41	Japan	82,494	653	1,557	12
42	Iraq	358,290	8,860	9,122	226
43	Australia	27,055	1,058	882	34
44	Canada	156,856	4,147	9,290	246
45	Chile	461,300	24,081	12,725	664
46	Ecuador	135,749	7,666	11,312	639
47	El Salvador	29,981	4,463	839	129
48	Cambodia	277	17	0	0
50	Tanzania	509	8	21	0.3
50	Belarus	78,260	8,283	828	88

Countrywide cumulative COVID-19 count and rate data from Worldometer retrieved on September 29, 2020.

consistently higher in prison than in the community for 4 out of the 5 countries with the largest prison systems (USA, China, Brazil, and India), but lower in Russia. Russia reports that their infection rates are 5 times lower in prisons than in the community. In China, the rate of infection in its prisons is reported to be approximately 8.5 times higher than in the

Table 3. Comparison of COVID-19 case and death counts & rates in communities and prison systems of countries housing the top 50 largest prison systems.

Rank	Country	Prison Population Total [a]	Total Community Case Count [b]	Community Case Rate per 10,000 persons [b]	Total Prison Case Count*	Prison Case Rate per 10,000 persons*	Total Community Death Count [b]	Community Death Rate per 10,000 persons [b]	Total Prison Death Count*	Prison Death Rate per 10,000 persons*
1	USA	2,094,000	7,394,635	223.08	132,677[c]	633.61	210,571	6.35	1,108[c]	5.29
2	China	1,710,000	79,824[d]	.55[d]	806[e]	4.71	2,870[d]	.02[d]	–	–
3	Brazil[f]	755,274	3,910,901[f]	183.99	29,403	389.30	121,515	5.72	183	2.42
4	Russian Federation[g]	496,791	845,443	57.93	1,224	24.64	14,058	.96	–	–
5	India	478,600	6,223,519	44.99	17,258[h]	360.59	97,529	.77	16[h]	.54
6	Thailand[i]	379,274	3,559	.51	–	–	59	.008	–	–
7	Turkey[j]	281,094	154,500	18.27	202	7.19	4,276	.51	4	.14
8	Iran[k]	240,000	453,637	53.84	–	–	25,986	3.08	–	–
9	Indonesia[l]	232,736	282,724	10.31	–	–	10,601	.39	–	–
10	Philippines[m]	215,000	309,303	28.14	–	–	5,448	.50	–	–
11	Mexico[n]	198,384	733,717	56.76	3,200	161.30	76,603	15.93	316	15.93
12	South Africa[o]	154,437	627,041	105.38	6,413	95.35	14,149	2.38	103	1.56
13	Vietnam[p]	123,697	1,094	.11	–	–	35	.004	–	–
14	Ethiopia[q]	113,727	74,584	6.45	–	–	1,191	.10	–	–
15	Egypt[r]	106,000	95,147	9.25	331	31.23	4,971	.48	17	1.60
16	Argentina[s]	103,209	723,132	159.64	304	29.45	16,113	3.56	12	1.16
17	Colombia[t]	102,637	824,042	161.53	–	–	25,828	5.06	–	–
18	Peru[u]	96,440	585,236	176.86	12,294	1,274.78	27,453	8.30	–	–
19	Myanmar[v]	92,000	12,425	2.28	–	–	284	.05	–	–
20	Bangladesh[w]	88,084	362,043	21.93	–	–	5,219	.32	–	–
21	Morocco[x]	85,767	121,183	32.74	–	–	2,152	.58	–	–
22	UK: England & Wales[y]	79,433	446,156	65.64	540	67.98	42,072	6.19	44	5.34
23	Pakistan[z]	77,275	311,516	14.04	–	–	6,474	.29	–	–
24	Poland[aa]	69,375	89,962	23.78	–	–	2,483	.66	–	–
25	Malaysia[bb]	68,603	11,135	3.43	–	–	134	.04	–	–
26	Rwanda[cc]	65,000	4,836	3.21	–	–	29	.02	–	–
26	Algeria[dd]	65,000	51,368	11.66	–	–	1,726	.39	–	–
28	Nigeria[ee]	62,258	58,647	2.83	–	–	1,111	.05	–	–
29	Saudi Arabia[ff]	61,000	334,187	95.63	–	–	4,739	1.36	–	–
30	Taiwan[gg]	60,956	513	.22	0	0	7	.003	0	0
31	France[hh]	58,695	550,690	84.32	–	–	31,893	4.88	–	–
32	Spain[ii]	58,642	758,172	162.14	–	–	31,614	6.76	–	–
33	Germany[jj]	57,600	290,466	34.64	–	–	9,556	1.14	–	–
34	Cuba[kk]	57,337	5,531	4.88	–	–	122	.11	–	–
35	Venezuela[ll]	57,096	73,528	25.88	–	–	614	.22	–	–
36	Uganda[mm]	55,229	8,017	1.74	–	–	75	.02	–	–

(Continued)

Table 3. (Continued).

Rank	Country	Prison Population Total [a]	Total Community Case Count [b]	Community Case Rate per 10,000 persons [b]	Total Prison Case Count*	Prison Case Rate per 10,000 persons*	Total Community Death Count [b]	Community Death Rate per 10,000 persons [b]	Total Prison Death Count*	Prison Death Rate per 10,000 persons*
37	South Korea[nn]	53,920	23,699	4.62	–	–	407	.08	–	–
38	Italy[oo]	53,619	313,011	51.79	–	–	35,875	5.94	–	–
39	Kenya[pp]	53,348	38,378	7.10	–	–	707	.13	–	–
40	Ukraine[qq]	52,609	143,030	32.75	113	21.48	2,979	.68	1	.19
41	Japan[rr]	48,802	82,494	6.53	–	–	1,557	.12	–	–
42	Iraq[ss]	45,000	358,290	88.60	–	–	9,122	2.26	–	–
43	Australia[tt]	44,358	27,055	10.58	–	–	882	.34	–	–
44	Canada	M = 39,579	156,856	41.47	360[uu]	90.96	9,290	2.46	2[uu]	.51
45	Chile[vv]	39,284	461,300	240.81	1,700	432.75	12,725	6.64	15	3.82
46	Ecuador[ww]	39,251	135,749	76.66	–	–	11,312	6.39	–	–
47	El Salvador[xx]	36,693	29,981	44.63	–	–	839	1.29	–	–
48	Cambodia[yy]	36,600	277	.17	–	–	0	0.00	–	–
49	Tanzania[zz]	35,803	509	.08	–	–	21	.003	–	–
50	Belarus[aaa]	32,500	78,260	82.83	–	–	828	.88	–	–

See Appendix A for citations.

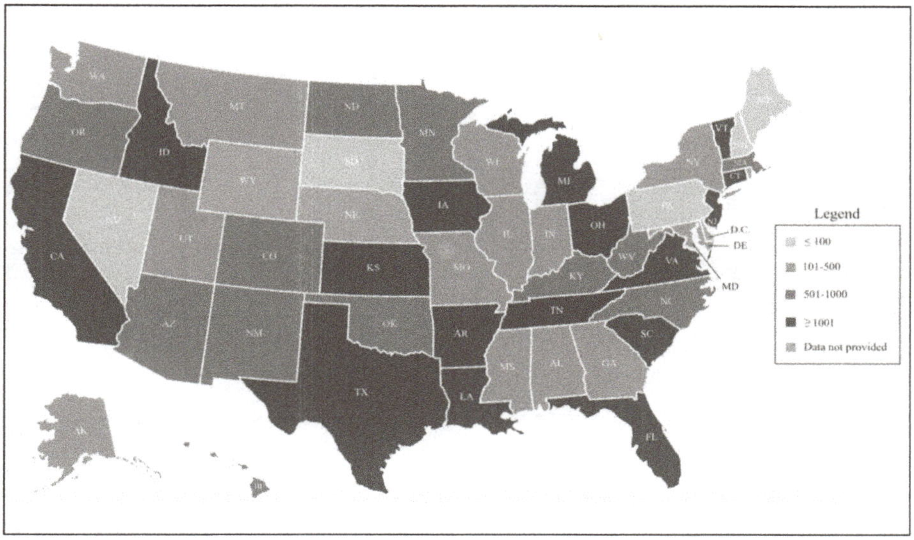

Figure 2. State-level variations in COVID-19 rates per 10,000 inmates in USA. * Rates refer to COVID-19 infection rates among inmates across the USA as of September 30, 2020.

community. Trending similarly, in Brazil, the rate of infection is reported to be twice as high in their prison system than in the general community, while in the USA, the rate of infection is 2.8 times higher, and in India, it is 8 times higher.

We recognize that country-level estimates do not capture the significant variation *within* countries in both community and prison infection rates identified in the country-level reviews (see, e.g., Ribeiro & Diniz's review of Brazil, 2020). A good example of within-country variation in prison infection rates is the United States (see Figure 2, Table 3). While infection rates rise and fall over time in both settings, what we report here (see Table 4) are the cumulative rates of infection in the general community and in each country's prison system since the start of the pandemic. Based on our assessment of cumulative COVID-19 infection and death rates, prisons are not safer than the community during the first wave of the pandemic. What we do **not** know yet is whether the rate of infections (and death) in prisons is higher or lower than the rates for individuals under community corrections control (and for workers in the community corrections system).

In sight but left out: The forgotten community corrections system

Most reviews of COVID-19 outbreaks in corrections are prison and jail-focused; they do not include any data on the nature and extent of the virus in community corrections. Given that the mitigation strategies identified by correctional administrators include both front-end alternatives and back-end early release strategies, it certainly makes sense to collect the necessary data on the rates of infection and death in community corrections, and to determine whether placement in various forms of community corrections control – either as an alternative to incarceration or pretrial detention, or as an early release mechanism – actually reduces the risk of infection and death. At present, not a single country has, to our

Table 4. State-level variations in the extent, impact, and response to the COVID-19 outbreak in USA prisons.

State	Number of Prisoner Cases^	Rate per 10,000 Prisoners^	Number of Prisoner Deaths^	Rate per 10,000 Prisoners^	Number of Staff Cases^	Number of Staff Deaths^	Reduction in population (%) March – June 2020[+]	Primary Mechanism for Population Reduction
Alabama	403[a]	195	21[a]	10	377[a]	2	7	Suspended admissions; automating releases[a]
Alaska*	54[b]	118	0[b]	0[b]	34	0	–	None
Arizona	2517[c]	612	27	7	689	1	3	None
Arkansas	5752	3655	39	25	399	1	6	Early releases[d]
California	12456[e]	1109	59	6	3388[e]	9	7	Early releases[e]
Colorado	888[f]	570	3	2	146[f]	0	12	No new admits; early releases[f]
Connecticut*	1553	1610	7	7	403	0	22	Early release[g]
Delaware*	541	–	11	26	169	1	14	None
Federal	13583[h]	902	126	8	1710[h]	2	10	None
Florida	15996[i]	1828	119[i]	13	2955[i]	3	6	None
Georgia	2259	448	59[j]	11	868[j]	2	5	None[j]
Hawaii*	300	667	0	0	92	0	4	Early release[k]
Idaho	1518[l]	1845	2	3	112	0	8	None
Illinois	1448[m]	397	14	4	704[m]	0	14	Suspended admission; Early release; medical release[m]
Indiana	1166[n]	401	24[n]	8	458[n]	2	–	None
Iowa	1003[o]	1093	4	5	132[o]	0	11	Early release[o]
Kansas	1750	2003	4	5	238	3	7	None[n]
Kentucky	897[p]	807	13	12	152[p]	1	7	Pre-trial release; Early release[p]
Louisiana	2110[q]	1306	26[q]	16	463[q]	5	3	Early release[q]
Maine	4	22	0	0	1	0	14	Early release[r]
Maryland	767[s]	405	10[s]	5	672[s]	1	–	Early release[s]
Massachusetts	420	597	8	11	207[t]	0	11	Pre-trial release; Early release[t]
Michigan	5462[u]	1543	72[u]	20	497[u]	3	6	Suspended admissions; Early release[u]
Minnesota	175[v]	680	2	3	137[v]	0	5	None
Mississippi	555[w]	350	1	–	135	0	10	Pre-trial release[w]
Missouri	1590[x]	435	1	0.4	426	0	7	Pretrial release; Early release[x]
Montana	79	202	0	0	12	0	12	None
Nebraska	184[y]	–	–	–	95[y]	0	5	None
Nevada	34	29	0	0	124[z]	0	9	None
New Hampshire	1	4	0	0	11	0	8	None
New Jersey	3009	1897	49	31	1000	3	10	Medical Release; Early release[aa]
New Mexico	525[bb]	829	4	6	82	0	.01[bb]	Early release[bb]
New York	755	201	17	5	1326[cc]	5	12	Early release[cc]

(Continued)

Table 4. (Continued).

State	Number of Prisoner Cases^	Rate per 10,000 Prisoners^	Number of Prisoner Deaths^	Rate per 10,000 Prisoners^	Number of Staff Cases^	Number of Staff Deaths^	Reduction in population (%) March – June 2020+	Primary Mechanism for Population Reduction
North Carolina	2444[dd]	701	11	3	738	1	9	Early release[dd]
North Dakota	24[ee]	97	0	0	40[ee]	0	18	Early release[ee]
Ohio	6138[ff]	1329	94[ff]	20	1123[ff]	5	5	Early release[ff]
Oklahoma	2193[gg]	728	5[gg]	0	216[gg]	3[gg]	8	Early release[gg]
Oregon	909[hh]	604	6	4	234[hh]	0	3	Early release[hh]
Pennsylvania	600[ii]	82	11	3	484[ii]	2	6	Early release[ii]
Rhode Island*	20	–	–	–	18	0	18	Early release[jj]
South Carolina	1888	1150	26[kk]	12	454	2[kk]	5	None
South Dakota	112[ll]	30	0	0	19[ll]	0	9	None
Tennessee	5190[mm]	2590	16[mm]	8	439[mm]	2[mm]	7	None
Texas	21581[nn]	7123	155[nn]	12	4651[nn]	20	9	None
Utah	60	101	0	0	29[oo]	0	11	Early release[oo]
Vermont*	240	1727	0	0	22	0	16	Early release[pp]
Virginia	3232[qq]	1111	21[qq]	6	646	0	2	Early release[qq]
Washington	451	289	2	1	167[rr]	1	7	Early release; commutations[rr]
West Virginia	319[ss]	664	2[ss]	0	117[ss]	0	18	Early release[ss]
Wisconsin	1044[tt]	423	0	0	234	0	7	Early release[tt]
Wyoming	105	–	–	–	33	0	7	None
TOTAL	**126,304**	–	**1,071**	–	**27,878**	**80**	–	–

See Appendix B for citations.

knowledge, collected or published the data necessary to answer this fundamentally important question: Is it safer to be in prison or under some form of community supervision during a pandemic? The assumption being made is that *of course* it is safer in the community, but we do not know, which means that we are developing mitigation strategies without the necessary data on comparative risk.[9] Driving blind during a storm is never a good idea; this admonition also applies to a pandemic.

As we mentioned at the outset, the pandemic has highlighted an incredible data shortfall that needs to be addressed: we do not systematically collect data on community corrections systems globally (Byrne et al., 2019; Byrne et al., 2015). In fact, it is currently not possible to provide an estimate of the *size* of the community correction system globally, let alone details on individuals under various forms of community release, the types of programs offered, and the staffing resources of these programs. In Table 5, we have attempted to bridge this gap and provide a preliminary estimate of the size of the community corrections systems in the countries with the 50 largest prison systems, using data from a wide range of official and unofficial sources, and building on the initial estimates provided by members of the Global Community Corrections Initiative.[10]

Our review reveals that there is significant variation in the size of the community corrections systems among the 30 countries with large prison systems with available data; for the remaining 20 countries, these basic data were unavailable, so we can offer no capacity estimates. For those 30 countries with both prison and community corrections data, we found that the capacity of the prison system was higher for prisons than community corrections in 16 of these 30 countries. Why does this matter in the context of the COVID-19 outbreaks in these prison systems? Our short answer: when proposing front-end or back-end mitigation strategies, capacity matters. In the 16 prison systems that we identified, front-end and back-end mitigation strategies designed to reduce prison and jail populations will require building a larger community corrections system. The mantra, "*If you build it, they will come*," appears to apply here. We will revisit this point in the next section of our review when examining the root causes of the COVID-19 outbreaks in prisons globally. Our research documenting the relative size of prisons and community corrections systems represents a tentative first step toward creating a global community corrections database similar to the database provided in the World Prison Brief, but there is much work to be done.

What we know (and do not know) about the response to COVID-19 outbreaks in community corrections

The fact that we were unable to identify a single country that can provide us with baseline data on the extent of COVID-19 outbreaks in community corrections indicates that the problem must be addressed.[11] We cannot blithely assume that the danger and harm posed by COVID-19 outbreaks is in the past or that there will not be a "second wave" to prepare for soon, because historically pandemics come in several waves with durations lasting at least 18 months.[12] In addition to the collection of baseline data on incidence rates among individuals and staff placed in community corrections programs due to front-end and back-end mitigation strategies, we need to collect baseline data on the steps being taken to protect the health of staff and program participants. One country that is already doing this is the United States (Viglione et al., 2020), but much more is required to document these in-

Table 5. Total corrections populations in top 50 countries with highest prison populations (2020).

Rank	Country	Prison Population *(Year)**	Community Corrections Population *(Year)**	Total Corrections Population
1	United States of America	2,094,000 *(2018)*	[a]4,399,000 *(2018)*	6,493,000
2	China	1,710,000 *(2018)*	[b]707,058 *(2013)*	2,417,058
3	Brazil	755,274 *(2019)*	[c]–	
4	Russian Federation	496,791 *(2020)*	[d]511,191 *(2019)*	1,007,982
5	India	478,600 *(2019)*	[e]39,199 *(2015)*	517,799
6	Thailand	379,274 *(2020)*	[f]230,107 *(2014)*	609,381
7	Turkey	281,094 *(2020)*	[d]454,599 *(2019)*	735,693
8	Iran	240,000 *(2018)*	–	
9	Indonesia	232,736 *(2020)*	[f]57,456 *(2015)*	290,192
10	Philippines	215,000 *(2018)*	[g]83,208 *(2019)*	298,208
11	Mexico	198,384 *(2019)*	–	
12	South Africa	154,437 *(2020)*	[h]71,573 *(2018)*	226,010
13	Vietnam	123,697 *(2019)*	[f]50,800 *(2015)*	174,497
14	Ethiopia	113,727 *(2020)*	–	
15	Egypt	106,000 *(2014)*	–	
16	Argentina	103,209 *(2018)*	[i]4,665 *(2018)*	107,874
17	Colombia	102,864 *(2020)*	[j]75,125*(2020)*	176,989
18	Peru	95,765 *(2019)*	[k]29,559*(2019)*	125,324
19	Myanmar (formerly Burma)	92,000 *(2018)*	[f]–	
20	Bangladesh	88,084 *(2020)*	[e]–	
21	Morocco	85,767 *(2019)*	[l]∧	
22	United Kingdom (England & Wales)	79,433 *(2020)*	[m]241,350 *(2020)*	320,783
23	Pakistan	77,275 *(2019)*	[n]44,437 *(2018)*	121,712
24	Poland	69,375 *(2020)*	[d]245,328 *(2019)*	314,703
25	Malaysia	68,603 *(2020)*	[o]∧	
26	Rwanda	65,000 *(2019)*	–	
26	Algeria	65,000 *(2019)*	–	
28	Nigeria	62,258 *(2020)*	[p]∧	
29	Saudi Arabia	61,000 *(2017)*	–	
30	Taiwan	60,956 *(2019)*	[q]11,685 *(2020)*	72,641
31	France	58,695 *(2020)*	[d]175,978 *(2019)*	234,673
32	Spain	58,642 *(2020)*	[d]60,157 *(2019)*	118,799
33	Germany	57,600 *(2020)*	[r]160,948 *(2010)*	218,548
34	Cuba	57,337 *(2012)*	–	
35	Venezuela	57,096 *(2017)*	–	
36	Uganda	55,229 *(2019)*	–	
37	Republic of (South) Korea	53,920 *(2020)*	[s]199,184 *(2013)*	253,104
38	Italy	53,619 *(2020)*	[d]81,623 *(2019)*	135,242
39	Kenya	53,348 *(2019)*	[t]450,300 *(2012)*	503,648
40	Ukraine	52,609 *(2020)*	[d]58,439 *(2019)*	111,948
41	Japan	48,802 *(2019)*	[f]40,000 *(2015)*	88,802
42	Iraq	45,000 *(2015)*	–	
43	Australia	44,358 *(2020)*	[u]80,411 *(2020)*	124,769
44	Canada	M = 39, 579 *(2018)*	[v]150,239 *(2018)*	189,818
45	Chile	46,989 *(2020)*	[w]49,723*(2020)*	96,712
46	Ecuador	39,251 *(2020)*	–	
47	El Salvador	34,949 *(2020)*	[x]1,704	36,693
48	Cambodia	36,600 *(2019)*	[f]∧	
49	Tanzania	35,803 *(2019)*	[y]175	35,978
50	Belarus	32,500 *(2018)*	[z]∧	

See Appendix C for citations.

program infection mitigation strategies, particularly in countries with large prison systems. According to Viglione and colleagues (2020), the pandemic has forced probation and parole systems administrators to reimagine probation supervision in ways that may have both short-term and long-term implications for the USA's Federal, state, and local community corrections systems.

At the core of community supervision is face-to-face contact with probationers and parolees, but the engagement and supervision strategies place both officers and supervisees at risk. According to the results of a national survey of community corrections agencies, the agencies were much more likely to provide personal protective equipment (PPE) to supervision staff than to individuals on supervision, which is concerning from a public health perspective (Viglione et al., 2020). They were also less likely to drug test supervisees and to require community service. In the short term, the COVID-19 crisis has resulted in a greater reliance on technology, in myriad forms, including the increased use of telephone calls and text-messaging, remote drug testing, and the use of electronic monitoring to provide both surveillance and control, and also to assist probationers and parolees in ways that support desistance (e.g., apps that monitor progress and provide support and resources).[13]

In USA prisons, one of the key drivers of increased prison populations over the past two decades is the community corrections system's response to individuals who violate the technical conditions of probation and parole. It is likely that in many community corrections systems, the practice of sending technical violators of probation and parole conditions (or technical violators of pretrial release conditions) to prison, has either been eliminated or significantly reduced during the first several months of the pandemic. This fundamental change in core supervision practice will need to be researched carefully; the COVID-19 crisis has provided a unique opportunity for a natural experiment on the short-term effects as well as long-term impact of this change in practice. The pandemic response in community corrections may potentially provide evidence that the imposition of a "return-to-prison" sanction for technical violations is not needed and that there are other ways to induce compliance that can be used without threatening public safety.

The root causes of the COVID-19 crisis in corrections systems

The root causes of the COVID-19 crisis in prisons can and should be viewed through both a crime control and a public health lens. Governments have a responsibility to protect the public by enforcing laws and sanctioning convicted offenders in a manner that maximizes public protection,[14] without sacrificing fairness and equity (M. H. Tonry, 2016). Governments also have a responsibility to protect the health and safety of individuals in both the institutional and community corrections systems. During the current pandemic, governments are attempting to balance these dual functions; it should come as no surprise that there is disagreement on how this can be accomplished.

One important factor to consider is the seriousness of the crime problem in each country, because sentencing and corrections policies are often justified as necessary responses to a country's crime problem. The prison sentence is certainly a card in the sentencing deck that is played more often in some countries than others to address crime. The question we raise here is a simple one: Does more prison equal less crime?[15] To examine this issue, we have reviewed 2000–2018 violent crime trends in the countries with the 50 largest prison systems and compared these trends to changes in the prison populations of these countries during the same review period.

Table 6 presents the results of our review of global crime trends over the past two decades. Violent crime rates have declined significantly over the past two decades in these

Table 6. Recent violent crime trends for top 50 countries with the highest prison population PP totals (per 100,000 persons).

				Homicide Rate			Assault Rate			Sexual Violence Rate			Robbery Rate		
Rank	*Country*	*Region*	*PP Rate (Rank)*	*2000*	*2018*	*% Change*	*2003*	*2018*	*% Change*	*2003*	*2017*	*% Change*	*2010*	*2017*	*% Change*
1	USA	North America	639 (1)	5.5	5.0	−9.1	296.4	246.8	−16.7	32.3	41.7	+29.1	119.4	98.6	−17.4
2	China	Asia	121 (129)	2.1	0.5	−76.2	NA	NA	NA	NA	NA	NA	NA	NA	NA
3	Brazil	South America	357 (21)	23.8	27.4	+15.1	346.9	65.2	−81.2	14.5[f]	28.0[m]	+93.1	552.4	806.5	+46.0
4	Russian Federation	Europe/Asia	344 (25)	28.1	8.2	−70.8	39.9[d]	15.2	−61.9	11.4[n]	11.6	+1.8	114.7	6.3	−94.5
5	India	Asia	35 (211)	4.6	3.1	−32.6	24.5[d]	26.1[m]	+6.5	5.6[d]	9.1[m]	+62.5	1.9	2.8[m]	+47.4
6	Thailand	Asia	546(4)	8.2	2.6[q]	−68.3	43.2[e]	13.3	−69.2	NA	5.0	NA	2.7	1.5[p]	−44.4
7	Turkey	Europe/Asia	335(29)	4.3[c]	2.6	−39.5	139.2	102.8[n]	−26.1	4.3	54.0[n]	+1155.8	11.9	34.0[p]	+185.7
8	Iran	Asia	294(37)	2.6[c]	2.5[o]	−3.5	NA	NA	NA	NA	NA	NA	NA	NA	NA
9	Indonesia	Asia	85 (160)	1.0	0.4[q]	−60.0	14.2[h]	4.2	−70.4	NA	2.1	NA	4.1	4.0	−2.4
10	Philippines	Asia	200 (72)	7.4	6.5	−12.2	NA	NA	NA	NA	NA	NA	38.4	15.3	−60.2
11	Mexico	Central America	158 (98)	10.9	29.1	+167.0	235.7[d]	37.1	−84.3	27.6	30.7	+11.2	647.0	196.1	−69.7
12	South Africa	Africa	259 (45)	48.4	36.4	−24.8	NA	293.6[q]	NA	NA	87.9	NA	337.3[n]	331.7	−1.7
13	Vietnam	Asia	128 (118)	1.2[b]	1.5[k]	+25.0	NA	NA	NA	NA	NA	NA	NA	NA	NA
14	Ethiopia	Africa	127 (119)	NA	7.5[q]	NA	NA	NA	NA	NA	NA	NA	NA	NA	NA
15	Egypt	Africa	166(132)	0.6[c]	2.6[l]	+333.3	0.1[f]	0.4[k]	+300.0	NA	NA	NA	0.8	NA	NA
16	Argentina	South America	230 (58)	8.4[b]	5.3	−36.9	365.4[e]	306.5	−16.1	26.6	32.5[g]	+22.2	NA	922.6	NA
17	Colombia	South America	2014 (70)	67.0	25.3	−62.2	77.3[d]	346.1	+347.7	10.3	48.7[d]	+372.8	135.9	244.4	+79.8
18	Peru	South America	290 (39)	5.0	7.9[q]	+58.0	54.4[d]	145.3	+167.1	25.4	31.1[g]	+22.4	195.7	222.9	+13.9
19	Myanmar	Asia	171 (90)	2.2	2.3[p]	+4.5	5.7[i]	8.7	+52.6	NA	NA	NA	0.03	0.3[p]	+1053.8
20	Bangladesh	Asia	52 (200)	2.6	2.4	−7.7	NA	NA	NA	NA	NA	NA	0.6[f]	NA	NA
21	Morocco	Africa	237 (51)	1.6	1.4	−12.5	163.4	309.0	+89.1	2.8	11.3	+303.6	44.1[m]	135.4	+207.0
22	UK: Engl. & Whales	Europe	133 (114)	1.5	1.1	−26.7	861.7	925.4	+7.4	92.2	257.2	+179.0	136.8	131.2	−4.1
23	Pakistan	Asia	38 (208)	6.3	3.9	−38.1	19.8[j]	12.5	−36.9	1.9	1.8[j]	−5.3	10.1	6.2	−38.6
24	Poland	Europe	183 (82)	2.2	0.7	−68.2	32.8[h]	17.4	−47.0	9.7	8.5[g]	−12.4	50.5	21.4	−57.6
25	Malaysia	Asia	212 (66)	2.4	2.1[m]	−12.5	NA	NA	NA	6.0	5.1	−15.2	81.7[f]	NA	NA
26	Rwanda	Africa	511(6)	3.5[f]	2.6[o]	−25.7	23.6[h]	30.5[m]	+29.2	NA	NA	NA	20.6	25.6[m]	+24.3
26	Algeria	Africa	153 (102)	2.0[c]	1.4[o]	−30.0	71.4	123.6[o]	+73.1	10.4[f]	8.5[o]	−18.3	51.4	65.5[o]	+27.4
28	Nigeria	Africa	30 (215)	5.4[d]	35.0[p]	+548.1	10.3[g]	9.6[m]	−6.8	1.1[g]	1.0[m]	−9.1	1.4	1.1[m]	−21.4
29	Saudi Arabia	Asia	197 (74)	0.8	1.3[q]	+62.5	NA	5.7[q]	NA	NA	0.1[o]	NA	NA	9.3	NA
30	Taiwan	Asia	258 (46)	5.1	0.8[o]	−84.3	NA	NA	NA	NA	NA	NA	NA	NA	NA
31	France	Europe	87 (157)	1.8	1.2	−33.3	224.1	375.6[p]	+67.6	42.8	64.1	+49.8	192.5	154.3	−19.8
32	Spain	Europe	124 (125)	1.4	0.6	−57.1	392.6[e]	39.2	−90.0	22.8[g]	20.3	−11.0	179.9	132.4	−26.4
33	Germany	Europe	69 (176)	1.2	0.9	−25.0	546.1	164.5	−69.9	66.9	42.1	−37.1	59.6	47.0	−21.1
34	Cuba	Caribbean	510 (7)	5.3	5.0[p]	−5.7	NA	NA	NA	NA	NA	NA	NA	NA	NA
35	Venezuela	South America	178 (88)	33.2	36.7	+10.5	NA	6.5	NA	NA	NA	NA	NA	NA	NA
36	Uganda	Africa	124 (125)	8.2[c]	10.5	+28.0	75.0	13.9[q]	−81.5	50.9[e]	49.3[p]	−3.1	18.6	16.6	−10.8
37	South Korea	Asia	105 (142)	0.8	0.6	−25.0	576.8[f]	103.3	−82.1	27.9[f]	47.2	+69.2	8.9	1.9	−78.7

(*Continued*)

Table 6. (Continued).

				Homicide Rate			Assault Rate			Sexual Violence Rate			Robbery Rate		
Rank	*Country*	*Region*	*PP Rate (Rank)*	*2000*	*2018*	*% Change*	*2003*	*2018*	*% Change*	*2003*	*2017*	*% Change*	*2010*	*2017*	*% Change*
38	Italy	Europe	89 (156)	1.4	0.6	−57.1	89.4[d]	109.4	+22.4	4.8	8.4	+75.0	80.9	51.4	−36.5
39	Kenya	Africa	105 (142)	3.4[d]	4.9	+44.1	34.7[e]	34.1	−1.7	8.1[d]	10.9	+34.6	6.8	5.4	−20.6
40	Ukraine	Europe	148 (105)	9.0	6.2[q]	−31.1	12.0	3.6[q]	−70.0	4.6	1.9	−58.7	50.9	47.5	−6.7
41	Japan	Asia	39 (2017)	0.5	0.3	−40.0	45.7	19.1[p]	−58.2	9.8	5.6[p]	−42.9	3.2	1.8[p]	−43.8
42	Iraq	Asia	126 (122)	6.5[a]	10.1[m]	+55.4	53.6[h]	83.2[m]	+55.2	1.7[h]	1.5[n]	−11.8	NA	NA	NA
43	Australia	Oceania	174 (89)	1.9	0.9	−52.6	318.9[h]	292.0	−8.4	85.1[j]	101.5	+19.3	66.1	39.0	−41.0
44	Canada	North America	107 (141)	1.8	1.8	0.0	152.9	150.8[q]	−1.4	83.0	95.3	+14.8	89.3	61.9	−30.7
45	Chile	South America	212 (66)	3.2[c]	4.4	+37.5	128.4[f]	65.2	−49.2	62.0[f]	69.5	+12.1	478.6	633.5	+32.4
46	Ecuador	South America	224 (60)	14.5	4.8	−66.9	53.0	37.6	−29.1	25.0[i]	80.5	+222.0	360.5	457.2	+26.8
47	El Salvador	Central America	566 (2)	60.3	52	−13.8	76.5[e]	58.6[q]	−23.4	31.1[i]	68.5	+120.3	87.6	59.4	−32.2
48	Cambodia	Asia	220 (63)	4.7	2.4[q]	−48.9	NA	NA	NA	NA	NA	NA	NA	NA	NA
49	Tanzania	Africa	59 (193)	7.6[c]	6.5[p]	−14.5	NA	4.6[o]	NA	NA	0.1[o]	NA	26.9	18.2[o]	−32.3
50	Belarus	Europe	344 (25)	10.3	2.4	−76.7	41.7	7.7	−81.5	8.1[d]	9.2	+13.6	50.3	16.3	−67.6

*NA denotes that data were "not available" during (or near) the displayed, designated time period. Note: All data were extracted from the United Nations Office on Drugs and Crime website: https://dataunodc.un.org/#state: 47 Sexual violence data for Malaysia were extracted from: https://wao.org.my/rape-statistics/. It is also important to note that operational definitions of different forms of violent crime (e.g., assault and sexual violence) differ cross-nationally. Data provided by each country for homicide, assault, sexual violence, and robbery rates did not always conform to the baseline (e.g., 2000, 2003, or 2010) year or "most current" year (e.g., 2017 or 2018); thus, the closest year for which these countries provided data were provided in this table and are specified with the following superscripts: [a](1994), [b](2001), [c](2003), [d](2004), [e](2005), [f](2006), [g](2007), [h](2008), [i](2009), [j](2010), [k](2011), [l](2012), [m](2013), [n](2014), [o](2015), [p](2016), and [q](2017).

top 50 prison population countries, but it should be noted that data availability varied by the type of crime under review.[16] Homicide rates declined in 38 of 49 countries providing data, with the largest declines in country-level homicide rates reported in Taiwan (−84.3%), Belarus (−76.7%), and China (−76.2%). Assault rates declined in 25 of 37 countries providing data, with the largest declines reported in Spain (−90.0%), Mexico (−84.3%), and South Korea (−82.1%). Robbery rates declined in 24 of 36 countries providing data, with the highest reported declines in Russia (−94.5%), South Korea (−78.7%), and Mexico (−69.7%). The one violent crime category that did not follow this downward overall trend was sexual violence, with only 11 of 31 countries reporting declines. One explanation for this pattern is that the countries we reviewed here have differing operational definitions of what constitutes sexual violence, which will have an impact on these reporting trends. Moreover, increased rates of sexual violence may be a reflection of increased reporting and not necessarily increased prevalence (i.e., similar rates may exist over time, while the number of individuals that report being victimized increases or decreases).

We present the results of our review of prison population changes (2000–2019) in Table 7. Given the general violent crime declines documented in Table 6, similar declines in prison populations might be expected, but this is not the case. Only 10 of 50 countries downsized their prison systems between 2000 and 2019, including only one of the 10 largest prison systems (Russia) and 2 of the top 20 largest prison systems (Russia and South Africa). The largest reported decreases in prison populations were documented in the Ukraine (−74.8%), followed by Russia (−43.2%), and Rwanda (−42.0%). Violent crime rates declined significantly in both Russia and the Ukraine during this period, which certainly supports the view that major reductions in prison population can be achieved without increasing the violent crime rate. Each of the 10 countries that reduced their prison population during this period had lower reported homicide rates. For assault, 6 of 7 countries (that reported) had declines in their prison populations, and for robbery, 8 of 9 countries (that reported) experienced decreases. It is worth noting that these 10 countries with reductions in prison populations do not include a single country from North America, South America, or Central America. It appears that governments in these regions have sentencing and incarceration policies that are driven by factors other than violent crime trends. Governments in other global regions have downsized their prison systems without increasing the risk to the public,[17] so there is certainly much to be gained by looking globally when considering potential shifts in the use of incarceration as a crime control strategy generally, in particular when developing front-end and back-end mitigation strategies to reduce harm during a public health crisis.

One consequence of increasing prison populations is that it inevitably leads to prison crowding. Table 8 highlights the level of overcrowding found in the 50 largest prison systems globally. Data on occupancy level are available from the World Prison Brief database for 44 of the 50 countries included in our review. China is the only country housing one of the 10 largest prison systems that does not report occupancy levels. Thirty-four of these 44 prison systems can be designated as operating officially above capacity, with the highest reported crowding levels for prisons in the Philippines (463.8%), Uganda (319.2%), and Peru (240.3%).

Overcrowded prisons strain correctional resources in ways that are important to understand. First, crowding places a premium on inmate control-based funding (e.g., funding for line staff and technology), which results in less funding available for treatment programming. Second, crowded prisons are more violent prisons, with prison crowding consistently

Table 7. World prison population (PP) trends for countries with 50 largest prison systems (2000–2019).

Ranking	Country	Region	PP Rate (Rank)	2019 PP Total	2000 PP Total	PP Change	% Change
1	USA	North America	639 (1)	2,094,000*	1,937,482	+156,518	+8.1
2	China	Asia	121 (129)	1,710,000*	1,427,407	+282,593	+19.8
3	Brazil	South America	357 (21)	755,274	232,755	+522,519	+224.5
4	Russian Federation	Europe/Asia	344 (25)	602,176*	1,060,404	−458,228	−43.2
5	India	Asia	35 (211)	478,600	272,079	+206,521	+75.9
6	Thailand	Asia	546(4)	366,316*	223,406	+142,910	+64.0
7	Turkey	Europe/Asia	335(29)	200,339***	49,512	+150,827	+304.6
8	Iran	Asia	294(37)	240,000*	158,000 [2]	+82,000	+51.9
9	Indonesia	Asia	85 (160)	256,051*	53,399	+202,752	+379.5
10	Philippines	Asia	200 (72)	215,000	79,299	+135,701	+171.1
11	Mexico	Central America	158 (98)	198,384	154,765	+43,619	+28.2
12	South Africa	Africa	259 (45)	164,129*	171,462	−7,333	−4.3
13	Vietnam	Asia	128 (118)	123,697	55,000 [1]	+68,697	+124.9
14	Ethiopia	Africa	127 (119)	113,727*****	55,209	+58,518	+106.0
15	Egypt	Africa	166(132)	106,000***	56,587 [2]	+49,413	+87.3
16	Argentina	South America	230 (58)	103,209*	37,885	+65,324	+172.4
17	Colombia	South America	2014 (70)	118,513*	51,518	+66,995	+130.0
18	Peru	South America	290 (39)	87,995*	27,734	+60,261	+217.3
19	Myanmar	Asia	171 (90)	92,000*	31,648 [2]	+60,352	+190.7
20	Bangladesh	Asia	52 (200)	83,350*	62,669	+20,681	+33.0
21	Morocco	Africa	237 (51)	85,767	54,288	+31,479	+58.0
22	UK: England & Wales	Europe	133 (114)	82,773*	64,602	+18,171	+28.1
23	Pakistan	Asia	38 (208)	77,275	78,938	−1,663	−2.1
24	Poland	Europe	183 (82)	72,294*	70,544	+1,750	+2.5
25	Malaysia	Asia	212 (66)	59,278*	27,358	+31,920	+116.7
26	Rwanda	Africa	511(6)	65,000	112,000 [3]	−47,000	−42.0
26	Algeria	Africa	153 (102)	65,000	33,992	+31,008	+91.2
28	Nigeria	Africa	30 (215)	71,522*	44,450	+27,072	+60.9
29	Saudi Arabia	Asia	197 (74)	61,000**	23,720	+37,280	+157.2
30	Taiwan	Asia	258 (46)	60,956	56,676	+4,280	+7.6
31	France	Europe	87 (157)	74,255*	48,049	+26,206	+54.5
32	Spain	Europe	124 (125)	59,694*	45,309	14,385	+31.7
33	Germany	Europe	69 (176)	63,643*	70,252	−6,609	−9.4
34	Cuba	Caribbean	510 (7)	47,337******	55,000 [4]	−7,663	−13.9
35	Venezuela	South America	178 (88)	57,096**	14,196	+42,900	+302.2
36	Uganda	Africa	124 (125)	55,229	21,700	+33,529	+154.5
37	Republic of (South) Korea	Asia	105 (142)	54,744*	62,959	−8,215	−13.0
38	Italy	Europe	89 (156)	59,655*	53,165	+6,490	+12.2
39	Kenya	Africa	105 (142)	53,348	40,010	+13,338	+33.3
40	Ukraine	Europe	148 (105)	55,078	218,800	−163,722	−74.8
41	Japan	Asia	39 (2017)	50,578*	61,242	−10,664	−17.4
42	Iraq	Asia	126 (122)	45,000****	7,000 [5]	+38,000	+542.9
43	Australia	Oceania	174 (89)	42,974*	21,714	+21,260	+97.9
44	Canada	North America	107 (141)	39,579	35,533	+4,046	+11.4
45	Chile	South America	212 (66)	41,689*	33,050	+8,639	+26.1
46	Ecuador	South America	224 (60)	37,996*	8,029	+29,967	+373.2
47	El Salvador	Central America	566 (2)	39,642	7,754	+31,888	+411.2
48	Cambodia	Asia	220 (63)	36,600	5,502	+31,098	+565.2
49	Tanzania	Africa	59 (193)	35,803	45,611	−9,808	−21.5
50	Belarus	Europe	344 (25)	32,500*	56,590	−24,090	−42.6

All data were extracted from the World Prison Brief database: https://www.prisonstudies.org/highest-to-lowest/prison_population_rate?field_region_taxonomy_tid=All

* One asterisk denotes that the most up-to-date prison population totals (prior to COVID-19) were released in 2018, two asterisks indicate that the most current prison population totals (prior to COVID-19) were released in 2017, three asterisks denote that the data were last released in 2016 (prior to the pandemic), four asterisks indicate 2015, five asterisks indicate 2014, and six asterisks denote 2012. In other words, 2019 data were not made available for prison population totals for some countries included in this table. In some cases, 2020 data have been updated; however, to avoid the internal threat of "history," as contamination to these prison population trends, 2020 prison population data were not included in this table. Moreover, some countries did not provide prison population data in 2000, but rather in 1998 (denoted by 1), 2001 (denoted by 2), 2002 (3), 2003 (4), and 2004 (5).

Table 8. Top 50 largest prison systems by occupancy level (%).

Rank	Country	Occupancy Level (%)	Most Recent Update (Year)
1	USA	103.9	2018
2	China	–	–
3	Brazil	170.7	2019
4	Russian Federation	72.8	2019
5	India	118.5	2019
6	Thailand	144.8	2015
7	Turkey	130.6	2019
8	Iran	153.0	2018
9	Indonesia	174.8	2020
10	Philippines	463.8	2018
11	Mexico	90.1	2019
12	South Africa	137.4	2019
13	Vietnam	–	–
14	Ethiopia	–	–
15	Egypt	–	–
16	Argentina	122.1	2018
17	Colombia	127.2	2020
18	Peru	240.3	2020
19	Myanmar (formerly Burma)	139.4	2018
20	Bangladesh	215.1	2020
21	Morocco	136.9	2018
22	United Kingdom: England & Wales	105.6	2020
23	Pakistan	133.8	2019
24	Poland	85.4	2020
25	Malaysia	131.9	2020
26	Rwanda	101.3	2017
26	Algeria	89.3	2014
28	Nigeria	146.8	2018
29	Saudi Arabia	–	–
30	Taiwan	114.8	2015
31	France	96.9	2020
32	Spain	80.0	2018
33	Germany	78.7	2020
34	Cuba	–	–
35	Venezuela	153.9	2016
36	Uganda	319.2	2019
37	Republic of (South) Korea	112.0	2020
37	Italy	106.1	2020
39	Kenya	190.5	2018
40	Ukraine	68.3	2017
41	Japan	56.6	2018
42	Iraq	139.2	2013
43	Australia	112.2	2017
44	Canada	M = 102.2	2015
45	Chile	100.4	2019
46	Ecuador	133.2	2020
47	El Salvador	215.2	2018
48	Cambodia	206.1	2015
50	Tanzania	115.7	2015
50	Belarus	83.4	2014

*All data were extracted from the World Prison Brief database: https://www.prisonstudies.org/highest-to-lowest/prison-population-total?field_region_taxonomy_tid = All

identified as the leading cause of prison violence (Byrne et al., 2008; McGuire, 2018). Third, crowded prisons are – by definition – resource poor, with major staffing quality and turnover problems, inadequate physical structure, and perhaps most germane to this review, a poorly staffed and funded health care system (Akiyama et al., 2020; Heard, 2020; Nowonty & Piquero, 2020). We view overcrowded prisons as one of the root causes that can be identified to explain why the rate of infection and death is higher in prison than in the general community.

The response of prison systems to the current COVID-19 crisis has certainly been made more challenging due to the historically understaffed and underfunded prison health care systems found in most – if not all – of the prison systems included in our review (Heard, 2019). While we do not have access to detailed data on the prison health care systems in each of these countries, it is possible to describe – in broad strokes – the likely conditions in these prison systems at the time of the initial outbreaks in several of these countries: lack of qualified health care staff, inadequate physical structure, and a lack of basic health care supplies. These problems are likely exacerbated by the privatization of health care services in many countries, although we cannot state this definitively, because a detailed comparative assessment of publicly operated versus privately contracted prison heath care has yet to be conducted (Byrne et al., 2019).

One final "root cause" of the COVID-19 crisis is that many of the individuals involved in the corrections systems of the countries included in our review often enter the corrections system with significant health deficits that increases their risk of infection while in prison. These health problems likely began before they arrived to prison, due to deficits in the health care systems within their home communities. It is well-documented that nonwhite (and foreign-born) individuals are overrepresented in corrections systems globally, and that these individuals tend to also reside in high crime, high poverty, but resource-poor communities. Heard (2019) recently reviewed the health care systems in 10 countries, including 7 of the countries that we include in our review.[18] She found that the inmates in the prison systems she reviewed entered prison with a variety of physical health problems including the following:

(1) higher infectious disease prevalence (Tuberculosis, Hepatis B, Hepatitis C, HIV/AIDS, and other infections);
(2) weaker immune systems due to poverty, homelessness, substance abuse, previous incarceration; and
(3) at higher risk for non-communicable diseases (e.g., diabetes, cancer, respiratory illness, and heart disease).

Heard (2019) has also documented the mental heath problems found among the prison populations examined in her 10-country review:

(1) higher prevalence in prison population than in general population of serious mental health conditions ("depression, personality and anxiety disorders, schizophrenia, bipolar disorder and psychosis" (Fazel et al., 2016; Heard, 2019, p. 4; World Health Organization, Regional Office for Europe, 2014)
(2) higher prevalence of intellectual disabilities in prison populations (Fazel et al., 2008), and new evidence of higher prevalence of traumatic brain injury (Williams et al., 2018);
(3) higher prevalence of drug and alcohol disorders, higher rates of comorbidity with substance abuse and mental health (Butler et al., 2011), and higher prevalence of trauma and abuse (Durcan, 2008)

Physical and mental health problems exhibited by individuals upon entering prisons and jails are often made worse during their time in prison. The prison experience may also result in *new* physical and mental health problems due to a variety of factors, including "overcrowding, violence, reduced access to medical treatment, availability of drugs, poor diet, limited opportunities for exercise, limited activity and interaction with others, reduced access to natural light and fresh air, lack of contact with family members and support networks, and high levels of boredom, tension and despair" (Heard, 2019, p. 7). Given this grim profile of what she found in each of the ten countries in her review, it is not surprising that she links these conditions to higher rates of suicide and self-harm in prison than in community,[19] and to the onset of major psychiatric disorders while in prison.

Heard (2019) goes on to note that there are differential rates of both physical and mental health problems among subgroups of the prison population, such as female inmates, inmates from the LGBTQ+ community, young inmates, older inmates, and inmates from racial and ethnic minority backgrounds, and foreign national inmates. Her major conclusion is that the prisons she examined did not have adequate resources and personnel to address the myriad of physical and mental health challenges faced by prisoners; and that we do not make communities safer by relying on prisons to rehabilitate these individuals. If individual change/rehabilitation is the desired outcome to achieve with a prison system, then a health-informed approach to prison management is required, while simultaneously reducing our reliance on prison as a sanction. Her assessment, conclusions, and reform recommendations should be given serious consideration because the situation she described has further deteriorated since the start of the pandemic, due to the mitigation strategies (e.g., lockdowns, suspension of visitation) used to respond to the COVID-19 outbreaks in our prisons. We examine these strategies in the next section of our review.

An overview of COVID-19 mitigations strategies used in prisons in each global region

There are three main types of COVID-19 mitigation strategies that have been employed by corrections managers to respond to COVID-19 outbreaks in prison – before and after the fact – that can be identified:

(1) front-end mitigation strategies designed to limit the movement of the virus into prison,
(2) in-prison mitigation strategies designed to limit the spread of the virus among inmates and staff in prison, and
(3) back-end mitigation strategies designed to reduce the risk of infection among vulnerable subgroups of both inmates and staff.

In the following section, we document the types of mitigation strategies used, and highlight variation in the utilization of these strategies within and across global regions, focusing on decisions made by corrections administrators in the five largest prison systems. We base this review on data available from 20 of the 50 countries with the largest prison populations – including the top-5 countries in terms of prison population – and from 6 other countries with smaller prison populations with available data on COVID-19 mitigation strategies.[20] Table 9 highlights the results of our review.

Table 9. Comparison of mitigation strategies in response to COVID-19 in prison systems around the world, ranked by corrections population.

Country (Rank)	Front-End	Within	Back-End
USA (1st)	Suspension of visitation and prison transfers; New intakes for federal prisons only if offender being held for federal government in a state or local facility; Preventative screening for prison staff	Federal system-wide and state-level lockdowns; Widespread testing; Disbursement of masks, dispersal of hand sanitizer and other PPE among staff and inmates; increased sanitation; Isolation of confirmed or suspected inmates; remote legal counsel; Use of "field-ready" tents to maximize social distancing; "Stay at home" policy for prison staff manifesting COVID-like symptoms, coming in contact with individuals (including inmates) that have, or are suspected of having, COVID-19	Appx. 4.29% (N = 7,000) inmates in the federal system released to home confinement; Inmates in states such as CA, AL, CO, and MA have implemented early release (for inmates with low-level offenses or who are high-risk in terms of health)
China (2nd)	Supplemental funding from federal and local governments to financially support prison responses to COVID-19; Suspension of family visitation; Sentence deferment (in some cases)	Dispersal of PPE; Testing; Increased efforts in providing medical care (including mental health services); Establishment of a formal reporting system (for prison staff); Suspension of alternating shifts among prison staff and replaced with consecutive periods of up to 14 days of work, followed by 14 days off; Grid-management approach; Isolation of inmates in contact with suspected cases; Quarantine of inmates with symptoms; Daily disinfection of surfaces; Maintained ventilation by opening windows; Mandated mask-wearing among prison staff; Suspension of certain prison activities	None
Brazil (3rd)	Suspension of family and attorney visitation; Suspension of transfers and temporary exits	Daily sanitation of cells; Increased exposure to sunlight; Isolation of symptomatic inmates; Isolation of vulnerable inmates	Appx. 4.6% (N = 32,500) released on house arrest or electronic monitoring
Russian Federation (4th)	Suspension of in-person court hearings (in some cases); Suspension of visitation (in some regions); Reduction in the use of pre-trial detention; Preventive screening of prison staff and visitors before admission to facility	Lockdowns (quarantining); Aggressive testing; Daily preventive sanitation and disinfection; Mask-wearing by prison staff and visitors; Isolation of infected inmates; Rotations of 14 consecutive days on and off work among prison staff; Newly admitted inmates in isolation for 20 days prior to assimilation with the general prison population	None

(Continued)

Table 9. (Continued).

Country (Rank)	Front-End	Within	Back-End
India (5th)	Formation of high-level committees to create processes and guidelines for early release/release on bail; Prison staff preventive screening; suspension of family visitation	Inmate and staff testing; Prison staff remaining on prison property to reduce the likelihood of contraction (i.e., not entering the community at large); Quarantining; Proper handling of food; Mandating daily medical checkups for inmates above 60 years old (in some cases)[7]; Newly admitted inmate testing and isolation	Appx. 14.3% (N = 68,264) inmates temporarily released either on parole for 4– 6 weeks or on interim bail for those being held on pre-trial with offenses worth a sanction of 7 years or less[8]
Philippines (10th)	Use of videoconferencing for hearings	Improved sanitary conditions in facilities; Expanded access to medical care; Strengthened testing and contact tracing; Established isolation centers for infected inmates	Eased the rules on parole granting and executive clemency; Expanded compassionate release for most vulnerable inmates
Mexico (11th)	Suspension of transfers; Reducing or eliminating visits; Suspended work-related activities that occurred outside of custody	Implemented policies for early detection, isolation, identification of severity, and evacuation of the seriously ill; Testing of inmates and staff; Restricted movement of people and staff inside the 525 state-level prisons, as well as suspended work and/or educational activities; Use of videoconferencing to reduce inmate trips to court	Amnesty for first-time, low level inmates, and/or inmates whose crimes were driven by poverty
South Africa (12th)	Reconsidering the sentencing of certain offenses and those awaiting pre-trial to incarceration; Non-arrest for certain offenses, particularly those that are lockdown-related	Designation of facilities to quarantine sick incarcerated individuals; Enhanced testing protocols for inmates and staff; Provision of PPE for inmates	Early release; Alterations to current sentencing policies; Engagement with community-based support
Argentina (16th)	Suspension of educational and work activities occurring outside of prisons; restriction for on-site prison visitation; restriction on transfers	Restriction on staff per unit; controls for at-risk groups; testing for inmates and staff; health kits and PPE for inmates and staff; designated areas for isolation	Appx. 13% early release to probation, parole, house arrest, or other exceptional mechanisms
Colombia (17th)	Suspension of educational and work activities occurring outside of prisons; restriction for on-site prison visitation; restriction on transfers	Restriction on staff per unit; educational campaigns regarding COVID-19; testing for inmates and staff; health kits and PPE for inmates and staff; designated areas for isolation	Appx. 20% released to house arrest or other exceptional mechanisms
United Kingdom (22nd)	Temporary suspension of visits; Suspended educational programs and non-essential work; Halted inter-prison transfers; Movement from courts to prison effectively stopped – court hearings were held remotely by video and by phone; lockdown of facilities with only essential staff permitted access to facilities	Establishment of hand washing stations and adequate supplies of soap and cleaning supplies; Distribution of personal protective equipment (PPE) to staff; Routine testing of prison officers; Isolated confinement of inmates for social distancing purposes; Movement from prisons to courts effectively stopped – court hearings were held remotely by video and by phone	Early release of some prisoners (if deemed necessary); Addition of temporary accommodations across prisons; Implementation of a "cohorting" strategy

(*Continued*)

Table 9. (Continued).

Country (Rank)	Front-End	Within	Back-End
Pakistan (23rd)	Release of pre-trial detainees on bail/surety; Police discretion to not use arrest for less serious offenses; Pre-entrance screening for all visitors	Mass testing[a]; Contact tracing[b]; On-site containment[b]; Quarantine suspected cases[b]; Restricted mobility within jails[b]; Distribution of PPE to staff (e.g., Hazmat Suits, surgical gowns, surgical gloves, respirators, eye protection goggles, caps, hand sanitizers, gloves, blankets and drip sets)[b]; Close monitoring and distribution of high-nutrition meals to infected patients[xb]	None
Spain (32nd)	Suspension of visitation, but free telephone and videoconferencing with families and attorneys; Use of pre-trial and sentencing alternatives; Electronic monitoring; Decline in the number of offenders remanded to prison by courts during the pandemic – drop of over 50% in first part of 2020 when compared to same period in 2019	All external communications and all leave exits suspended, except for reasons of force or extreme necessity; Prohibition of access to prisons of any person (volunteers, collaborating entities, etc.) who are not part of the prison staff, unless their work inside was considered essential; Suspension of teaching activity and production workshops; Suspension of inmate transfers, except for health or judicial reasons; Authorization for the inmates to stay voluntarily in their cells; Staggering of mealtimes in dining areas; Communication of mitigation efforts to inmates; Provision of PPE to inmates and staff	Extensive release to community – an increase of over 400% of the number of offenders on home confinement
Germany (33rd)	Courts limited their work and mainly dealt only with cases of alleged offenders being sent to pre-trial detention, reducing new prison admissions; Elimination of incarcerations for nonpayment of fines; Restricted visits by suspending all visits with personal contact; Implementation of video telephone calls	Provision of masks, hygiene products and other PPE to inmates; Establishment of quarantine areas in facilities; Restriction of inmates to cells for more hours per day; Suspension of activities such as work, reentry programs, and recreation	Early release or non-execution of short-term prison sentence since March (i.e., Germany's prison occupancy level has decreased from 83.3% to 78.7% since March 2020)
Republic of (South) Korea (37th)	Reduction of new incarceration-based sanctions; Restrictions placed on visitation	Provision of the prison population protective eyewear, clothing, and hand sanitizer; Isolation and medical examinations of those newly entering facilities	Modest reductions in prison populations via early release, particularly in facilities that had outbreaks
Italy (38th)	Restricted access into and out of prison facilities; Substitution of phone calls or other available technology in lieu of in-person visits with relatives or third parties (other than defense lawyers)	Temporary suspension of treatment programs that involved participation from persons in the local community; Curtailment of work related activities serving the facilities that involve people coming in from outside; Extended release time for those already out on leave	Eligible persons with 18 months or less of their sentence to serve remainder of sentence at home or at other private healthcare facilities; Expanded use of electronic monitoring for those released to the community; Measures resulted in a decrease of nearly 10% of the incarcerated population

(Continued)

Table 9. (Continued).

Country (Rank)	Front-End	Within	Back-End
Kenya (39th)	Temporary scale down of services and activities in the justice sector to curtail the number of offenders entering the system – the National Council on the Administration of Justice discouraged the arrest and detention of minor offenders; Suspension of visitation	Mandatory screening for all prison officers; Sanitization at all entry points; Regular disinfection of prison facilities; Mandatory quarantine of symptomatic inmates; Testing of all new inmates entering the prison system; Use of PPE; Maintenance of a well-organized shift system for officers	Aggressive program of deinstitutionalization implemented – an estimated 12,000 persons had been released from prison within a span of five months since March 2020
Australia (43rd)	Suspension of visitation	Screening of inmates, visitors, and staff implemented early in pandemic; Specialized medical facilities established in some prisons; Mandatory testing of inmates and staff; 14 day quarantine of all new intakes; Physical hygiene and social distancing encouraged; Staff required to use PPE where a person was suspected of having COVID-19; Programming conducted with smaller inmate groups; Increased access to telephone and video calls	Accelerated rate of inmate discharges at beginning of the pandemic
Canada (44th)	Provisional suspension of arrests and court proceedings for minor offenses; Preparation of protocols for the transfer and hospitalization of inmates with severe cases of COVID-19	Isolation of persons who are, or are suspected of being, COVID-positive; Enhanced hygiene measures and of PPE; Increased training for staff to perform their roles while COVID-19 is a threat	Release from prison of persons with the lowest risk of recidivism, of older inmates, and of persons with health problems; Identification of infected and recovered staff who may have acquired greater immunity and could therefore be assigned to duties related to the hygiene and care of COVID-positive inmates; Release of inmates with mental health problems
Chile (45th)	Expanded non-custodial sentences, to stem the flow of offenders entering Chilean prisons (e.g., probation, parole, house arrest, suspended sentences, electronic monitoring, and work release); Restriction of in-person visitation (replaced with video calling capability); suspension of educational/work activities taking place outside of prison grounds	Suspension of educational and work-related activities (in prison); Controls for at-risk groups; Prison authorities conducted preventative informational campaigns about the contagion of COVID-19; Designated spaces inside the prison for medical isolation; Implementation of in-facility testing; Restriction on staff per unit	Appx. 15% (N = 5940) early release
El Salvador (47th)	Family visitation and transfer rates to other facilities have decreased	Extensive use of lockdowns; Restriction of programming and activities; Early in the pandemic, the Salvadorian government renewed the focus on "sanitary protocols to prevent Coronavirus in the prison population"	None

(Continued)

Table 9. (Continued).

Country (Rank)	Front-End	Within	Back-End
Guatemala (57th)	Visits from court authorities to prison were suspended at the first report of an outbreak; suspension of family visitation	Inmate use of masks; Created a separate isolation unit with a capacity for housing nearly 500 inmates; thorough cleaning/disinfection of certain facilities; Isolation and recovery site (i.e. a hotel) established for infected prison staff	Early release after risk assessment based on criminal profile, age, medical conditions, and conduct reports while in custody; 140 were approved for early release and the applications for the remaining 380 persons under consideration were still being processed
Honduras (66th)	Family visitation and transfer rates to other facilities have decreased	"Rapid testing" and quarantine of new inmates coming into facilities; Isolation of staff to prevent spread both into facilities and into their communities; PPE provided to staff; staff remain in facilities leaving only once per month	Early release of high medical risk and elderly prisoners. In mid-June 2020, 1,624 prisoners were released as part of the measures being implemented to prevent the spread of the virus
Romania (70th)	Restriction of new intakes during the first weeks of the pandemic; Court hearings through videoconferencing or rescheduling upcoming hearings	Certain penitentiary units were specially designated to serve as quarantine units; Monitoring and isolating of those inmates who, after an epidemiological screening, had symptoms of coronavirus infection and/or were new to a facility; Reducing staff that come into contact with inmates by 30%. Those staff remained home while accomplishing professional tasks; psychological services provided only in critical situations; Informational campaigns for inmates; disinfection of accommodation-based areas	None
Portugal (88th)	Temporary suspension of visitation; Restriction on outside goods coming into facilities	Creation of specific facilities for COVID-positive inmates; Quarantine of new inmates coming into facilities; Suspension of transfers between facilities, other than in cases of security; Work activities with external entities and leisure activities suspended; Reassignment and differentiation of inmates' daily routines to try to separate, as much as possible, inmates considered most vulnerable (e.g., aged more than 60, with immunosuppression or chronic disease such as respiratory ailments, hypertension, or diabetics); Increased testing and monitoring of staff and inmates	Partial pardoning of sentences for those whose sentences were less than two years, 65+ years old, having mental or physical diseases, or with degrees of autonomy that are incompatible with life in prison (N = 1,289)

(*Continued*)

Table 9. (Continued).

Country (Rank)	Front-End	Within	Back-End
New Zealand (101st)	In person visitation suspended; Court hearings conducted by videoconference to limit inmate and staff movement	Staff regularly undergoing health screenings, temperature checks, and using PPE; New prisoners, and those who had been transported outside the facility, isolated for 14 days upon entry into the institution; Social distancing aided by lockdown protocols; Government quickly responded with mitigation strategies, such as hygiene, social distancing, and interaction procedures before any reported cases occurred in the NZ correctional system	None
Sweden (117th)	Cancellation of furloughs and visitation	Isolation and quarantine of new intakes; Minimizing the size of the custodial and treatment staff; Use of PPE by staff; Elimination of face-to-face contacts in probation and parole when possible; No-charge phone calls to compensate inmates for the loss of visitation and furlough as well as a way to maintain the treatment plans of many inmates who need prosocial contacts as a part of their rehabilitation; Communication with inmates to keep them informed of safety protocols	None

**For further details on mitigation efforts, see articles in this special volume.
[a]Extracted from Arab News
[b]Extracted from Butt et al. (2020).

Front-end mitigation strategies

Examination of the front-end mitigation strategies employed in the 26 countries included in Table 8 reveals variation across countries and regions that is likely a byproduct of how governments in these countries have decided to balance their crime control and public health responsibilities during the COVID-19 crisis. For example, several countries have suspended all court hearings in order to reduce the number of convicted offenders sent to prison, deferred sentencing for a period of time, and/or reduced their new jail admissions populations by expanding pretrial alternatives (e.g., electronic monitoring, bail). However, these strategies were not identified in most of the countries in our review. The most common strategy employed as a front-end mitigation strategy was suspension of prison visitation, a strategy that is designed to reduce the spread of the infection, both into and out of prison. However, one unintended consequence of this strategy – highlighted in many of the reviews in the volume – is increased isolation, which may have serious negative (short-term and long-term) impacts on individuals with (and without) mental health problems.[21]

The five largest countries in our fifty country review – the USA, China, Brazil, the Russian Federation, and India – took very different approaches to front-end mitigation. These countries based their front-end mitigation strategies on not only their assessments of the nature and extent of the problem in their prison systems, but also on their view of the efficacy of the range of front-end strategies available, given their dual mission of protection of the public and protection of the inmates and staff in custodial and community settings. In each of these countries, the timing and full implementation of front-end mitigation strategies varied from one part of the country to the other, because the COVID-19 outbreaks were officially recognized at different points in time, and the intensity and location of specific prison COVID-19 hotspots moved over time.

The most common method employed in the top 5 countries was suspension of visitation: all five countries suspended visitation from family and/or attorneys. Other front-end mitigation designed to reduce the flow of inmates into prisons and jails included the suspension of in-person court hearings (USA and Russia), deferred sentencing (China), increased use of bail and/or pretrial release as an alternative to jail (India and Russia), and the suspension of transfers from other institutions (Brazil).

In-prison mitigation strategies

There was more consensus across the countries we reviewed on the major categories of in-prison mitigation strategies used to reduce the introduction and spread of COVID-19 in their prison systems: (1) testing of inmates and staff, (2) suspension of programming (e.g., work or education), (3) quarantining infected inmates, and (4) the use of lockdowns of most or all of the prison population. Unfortunately, corrections administrators in the countries we reviewed did not publicly share details on testing criteria, levels, and/or frequency, so it is impossible to compare the reporting data provided. Lockdowns and suspension of programming designed to reduce the spread of the virus may have serious unintended consequences for prisoners, particularly those with serious mental health problems.

Prison administrators within the five largest prison systems globally provided the most detail on the various types of in-prison mitigation strategies that were used, but there is still much we do not know about the *intensity* of these mitigation efforts. For example, each prison system indicated that they tested all new admissions before entering facilities. Despite indicating that prison populations and staff were being tested, they provided few details on the extent of testing, and the number of tests conducted, thus rendering comparisons of positive COVID-19 testing rates across countries of dubious value. In three of the countries (China, Russia, India), shift realignments resulting in long required stays in prison by staff were used to reduce the risk of bringing the virus into work during shift changes. Two countries (USA, China) explicitly mentioned that all programming was canceled, and two countries developed strategies to increase the access of inmates to either air (China) or sunlight (Brazil). A variety of other strategies were noted by individual countries, including remote access to legal counsel (USA), video visitation with family (China), increased access to mental health services (China), and the use of field-ready tents to maximize social distancing (USA). With each of these in-prison mitigation strategies, we have a good sense of what they say they did, but we not know the intensity or duration of these efforts.

Back-end mitigation strategies

Early release mechanisms designed to reduce the size of the prison and jail population took a variety of forms, and varied from country to country based on a number of factors, including the level of crowding in the prison and jail system of a country, and the size and scope of available community corrections programs. As noted earlier, the use of early release mechanisms will likely reflect how a government has decided to balance public safety with prisoner health concerns. Between-country release criteria varied, with some countries targeting the release of vulnerable populations (e.g., elderly inmates, inmates with preexisting conditions), while others focused on risk level and/or conviction offense type as inclusion/exclusion criteria (e.g., low risk, low-level crimes). There was also significant within-country variation noted in several countries (see Table 9).

Among the five largest prison systems, both China and Russia indicated that early release mechanisms were not employed, most likely due to their view that the results of testing did not justify this strategy (see Li & Liu, 2020 and Ovchinnikov, this volume). The other three countries did report utilizing early release mechanisms, such as release to home confinement for medical reasons (USA), early release of low-risk inmates (USA, Brazil, India), and the temporary release of inmates in jail via parole (India). Since 69% of India's prison population is held pre-trial, this last strategy may be unique to their system.

The intended and unintended consequences of mitigation strategies

We have documented the nature and extent of the COVID-19 outbreaks in prisons, and we have also documented – based on the detailed country-level reviews included elsewhere in this volume – how governments in these countries responded to the pandemic, focusing on prison and jail mitigation strategies. The question we now ask is deceptively simple: did these strategies work? To answer this question, we examined the available data on (1) impact on inmate and staff health, (2) impact on prison/jail population total, and (3) impact on public safety.

The effectiveness/impact of mitigation strategies on inmate and staff health

Unfortunately, we cannot currently provide even a tentative assessment of the effectiveness (or impact) of these mitigation strategies, because the data necessary to do so are not (yet) available for review. However, we can identify countries that have declared that their prison systems are currently reporting that they are essentially either COVID-19 free (Romania), or who had very low reported positive test rates among their inmate and staff populations as of September, 2020 (New Zealand, China, Russia, Sweden). We urge you to examine these country-level profiles, which describe the initial impact of the pandemic in these countries' corrections systems. Of course, in a pandemic, the situation changes quickly, and once the virus enters the corrections system, it is difficult to contain.

The data on changes (increases or decreases) in positive testing rates among prisoners and staff during the first several months of the pandemic are difficult to obtain, and even when available, the accuracy of these data can (and should) be questioned. A similar caveat can be offered regarding death rates due to COVID-19 as a consequence of how the criteria for identifying a death in prison as COVID-19-related are likely to vary from country to country. To assess front-end and back-end strategies, for example, we need data on the positive testing rates and death rates of individuals released to the community; without these data, how can we know whether community release is a wise decision from an individual heath perspective? In terms of in-prison mitigation strategies, we recognize that there are likely *unintended* consequences to these strategies that are also important to examine, using measures of change in physical and mental health status linked to the in-prison mitigation strategies employed. Once again, these data were not available across the 50 countries targeted in our review.[22]

The impact of mitigation strategies on the size of the prison and jail population

We have been able to document changes in the overall prison and jail population between pre-pandemic times and amidst the pandemic for 20 of the 50 countries included in our review. We summarize the results of our review in Table 10. In 17 of the 20 countries where changes in prison and jail populations could be calculated, significant reductions in prison populations were reported. In the remaining three countries, the prison population continued to rise, despite the pandemic: Malaysia (+23.8%), Peru (+9.6%), and Thailand (+4.1%). The largest prison population reductions were reported in Nigeria (−15.4% reduction between July 2018 and August 24, 2020) and Russia (−14.8% reduction between September 2018 and August 1, 2020).[23]

The U.S. and Russia were the only two countries among the five with the largest prison systems that provided the necessary data to identify these changes in prison populations. Although Russia experienced a 14.8% reduction, the assessment period for Russia is between September 2018 and August 2020. There are likely other confounding factors influencing the decrease in Russia's prison population over the course of this 2-year time period. For instance, the World Prison Brief (2020) has documented a steady decline in Russia's prison population over the last decade, with an average decrease of 32,000 inmates per year. Front-end mitigation strategies, including alternatives to detention and suspension of in-person court hearings for certain types of offenses, may also be contributing

Table 10. COVID-19 prison population (PP) trends of 20 countries in top 50 largest prison systems with pre-pandemic and mid-pandemic data.

Ranking	Country	Region	Pre-COVID PP	Extraction Date	During-COVID PP	Extraction Date	% Change
1	USA	North America	*1,336,431	Mar. 2020	*1,179,211	Aug. 2020	−11.8
4	Russian Federation	Europe/Asia	582,889	Sept. 1, 2018	496,791	Aug. 1, 2020	−14.8
6	Thailand	Asia	364,288	Sept. 1, 2018	379,274	Aug. 1, 2020	+4.1
7	Turkey	Europe/Asia	291,959	Jan.1, 2020	281,094	Jul. 2020	−3.7
9	Indonesia	Asia	248,765	Aug. 24, 2018	232,736	Aug. 31, 2020	−6.4
12	South Africa	Africa	158,111	Jul. 4, 2017	154,437	Apr. 1, 2020	−2.3
17	Colombia	South America	118,708	Jul. 31, 2018	102,637	Aug. 31, 2020	−13.5
18	Peru	South America	87,995	Jun. 30, 2018	96,440	Apr. 30, 2020	+9.6
22	UK: England & Wales	Europe	83,014	Sept. 28, 2018	79,433	Aug. 28, 2020	−4.3
24	Poland	Europe	73,524	Aug. 31, 2018	69,375	Jul. 31, 2020	−5.6
25	Malaysia	Asia	55,413	Sept. 2017	68,603	Aug. 2020	+23.8
28	Nigeria	Africa	73,631	Jul. 16, 2018	62,258	Aug. 24, 2020	−15.4
31	France	Europe	65,084	Sept. 1, 2018	58,695	Jul. 1, 2020	−9.8
33	Germany	Europe	62,194	Mar. 31, 2018	57,600	Jun. 30, 2020	−7.4
37	South Korea	Asia	55,198	Dec. 31, 2017	53,920	Jun. 30, 2020	−2.3
38	Italy	Europe	59,135	Aug. 31, 2018	53,619	Jul. 31, 2020	−9.3
40	Ukraine	Europe	56,246	Sept. 1, 2018	52,609	Apr. 1, 2020	−6.5
43	Australia	Oceania	44,358	Mar. 2020	**41,784	Jun. 2020	−5.8
45	Chile	South America	42,683	Aug. 31, 2018	39,284	Jul. 31, 2020	−8.0
47	El Salvador	Central America	38,714	Aug. 13, 2018	36,693	Aug. 17, 2020	−5.2

Pre-pandemic baseline numbers were extracted from the World Prison Brief Population List 12th Edition (spanning between the dates of July 2017 and January 2020), if not otherwise specified. Mid-pandemic data were extracted from the World Prison Brief database (2020), if not otherwise specified.
*Data from the Marshall Project. **Data from the Australian Bureau of Statistics.

factors to Russia's reduced prison population size. Ovchinnikov (this volume) provides further context by clarifying that continued reductions in Russia's prison population is very likely attributable to the expanded use of forced labor as an alternative to incarceration.[24] The U.S.'s prison population – a combination of both federal and state prisons – has decreased by 11.8% strictly during the months between March and August of 2020. Although confounders must be considered, it is likely that mitigation strategies adopted by U.S. prisons are, by and large, responsible for this reduction. Such mitigation strategies include the reduction of newly admitted persons into prisons (unless being held in state facility in lieu of a federal prison) and the release of over 4% of inmates at the federal level and thousands more across states like California, Alabama, and Colorado (see Table 9).

The impact of mitigation strategies on public safety

What do we know about the impact of various pandemic-induced prison population reduction strategies on public safety? Is there any evidence that the use of front-end or back-end mitigation strategies has increased crime? And what do we know about the behavior of individuals (i.e. crime, recidivism) released from prison and jail during the pandemic? The current crisis has provided us with a unique opportunity to answer these questions via a series of country-specific natural experiments. To date, there is little available evidence to review, because the necessary research has yet to be completed in most countries. One country-level study that does provide a preliminary examination of changes in crime during the current COVID-19 crisis is Santiago Redondo Ilesces and colleagues' (this volume) examination of crime during the first 3 months of the pandemic in Spain. They report overall reductions in street crimes (80% reduction in Spain), with even steeper reductions in the communities hardest hit by the virus. In Durnescu's review of European crime trends during the initial stages of the pandemic (this volume), he reports that Italy's overall crime declined 70% between February/ March 2020 and June 2020. The United States has also released preliminary data on reported crime rates between February/March and June 2020. Examination of these short-term trends revealed that residential burglary decreased by 20% and drug offenses by 57% (Rosenfeld & Lopez, 2020).[25]

While these findings of crime reductions during a lockdown tell us nothing about the impact of release policies on public safety, we include them here because we predict that emerging crime trends will be used by governments to justify a return to the status quo of past pre-trial and sentencing policies if they show an increase over time. It is for this reason that we need to take this opportunity to systematically evaluate the impact of front-end and back-end release strategies on the behavior of releases; to date, this research has not been conducted.

Concluding comments and a COVID-19 inspired research agenda

The current COVID-19 outbreaks across corrections systems globally have led government leaders – often reluctantly – to recognize that they need to consider downsizing their prison and jail populations. As we have documented in this review, the trend over the past two decades is for the largest prison systems to keep expanding, often without the resources needed to protect the health and safety of inmates and staff. We find that it is not crime that is driving this increase in the largest prison systems, which suggests that sentencing and correctional policies globally are driven by other factors, including systemic racism (Byrne et al., 2015; Heard, 2020; Tonry, 2016). These policies result in the overrepresentation of poor, marginalized, nonwhite populations in prisons globally; in our view, the data on minority overrepresentation in prisons globally cannot be glibly justified, either by catch phrases such as "you do the crime, you do the time," or by unsupported arguments that more prison equals less crime.

We present evidence in this review that, in most large prison systems, the reported rates of COVID-19 infections and deaths during the first phase of the pandemic are higher in prisons and jails than in the general community. We identify three reasons for this finding: (1) prison expansion has resulted in prison overcrowding, making social distancing impossible, (2) large prison systems are characterized by inadequate prison infrastructure and health care services, and (3) the current global prison population includes a significant number of individuals with poor physical and mental health, making them more "at risk" for infection, both in prison and in their home communities.

We have provided a detailed review of the types of front-end, in-prison, and back-end mitigation strategies used to address the COVID-19 problem in the 50 largest prison systems globally. Unfortunately, we could not provide similar detail on how community corrections managers responded to the crisis among their supervision population and community corrections staff. We argue that this is a significant information deficit, especially when you consider that the reforms we describe in this review are based on the untested assumption that the community is always a safer place to be than the prison. This may not be the case for individuals residing in – and returning to – poverty pocket, resource-poor communities during the pandemic.

We concluded our review by examining the available data on the impact of reforms on the following outcomes of interest: (1) inmate and staff health, (2) the size of the prison and jail population, and (3) public safety. In terms of inmate and staff health, the data needed to document the short-term impact of mitigation strategies are not available for review. However, we found that the governments of several countries have declared their prison systems to be essentially COVID-19 free as of September, 2020 (Romania, New Zealand, China, Russia, Sweden). Without reviewing actual data on testing levels and outcomes, we are justifiably skeptical of these claims. We also point out that the reforms developed during the COVID-19 crisis designed to reduce the risk of the onset and spread of infection while in prison may achieve this intended goal, but at a price: the deterioration of the physical and mental health of inmates and staff due to the types of in-prison mitigation strategies employed (e.g., lockdowns, suspension of visitation, curtailment of programs). To address this potential issue, we need to collect data on both the intended and unintended consequences of in-prison mitigation strategies.

We were able to collect and review data documenting the short-term impact of COVID-19 inspired reforms on prison crowding for only 20 of the 50 countries included in our review. For 17 of these 20 countries, significant reductions in prison populations were identified. It will be critical to track the progress of individuals released during the pandemic to determine their subsequent health (physical, mental) and behavior (recidivism) in the community. Our review of the available research on the impact of the COVID-19 reforms described here on public safety revealed that we do not know whether these reforms have made communities less safe, or safer. We recommend that an aggressive, globally based research program be initiated to answer this question definitively. We need to determine whether the short-term reforms developed in response to the pandemic should be the foundation for longer term changes in corrections policy. We offer a possible research agenda here.

An agenda for global comparative research on the impact of pandemic- driven reforms in institutional and community corrections

The pandemic has provided a unique opportunity to conduct a natural experiment on the effects of various prison and jail reforms. In many countries, governments have reduced prison and jail populations in the short-term using a variety of front-end and back-end mitigation strategies. Researchers from countries in each global region have a unique opportunity to document the impact of this shift in policy on individual health and public safety outcomes. The pandemic has also highlighted the lack of basic information currently available globally on the community corrections systems that have been tasked with managing individuals–placed in probation, parole, or other community corrections programs due to these crisis-driven reforms–in the community. The fact that several months into the pandemic not a single country can provide an estimate of the extent of the COVID-19 problem in community corrections is illustrative of a larger problem: we currently lack basic data on community corrections systems in each global region.[26] Efforts to build a global community corrections data base are underway, but as we have documented here, there is much work to be done.

For the past few decades, prison reform advocates have made the case that prisons should be viewed as a last resort, and that a prison or jail term should be applied parsimoniously, targeting convicted offenders who commit violent crime and/or pose an immediate threat to public safety. An examination of prison population trends over the past two decades suggest that reformers have failed to convince governments to change their view on the need for incarceration; this is especially true in the countries with the largest prison populations (Byrne et al., 2015). The pandemic has led governments in many of these countries to implement some of these recommended reforms on an emergency, short-term basis. Will these reforms take root and serve as harbingers of long-term reforms in sentencing and corrections policies? We suspect that without an aggressive, global research program, we will miss an incredible opportunity to evaluate the impact of a wide range of major corrections reforms, which will increase the likelihood of governments – absent evidence to the contrary – returning to their old ways. We offer the following three-pronged COVID-19-based research agenda for consideration: (1) research on jail reform during the pandemic, (2) research on prison reform during the pandemic, and (3) research on community corrections reform during the pandemic.

Jail reform during the pandemic: A research agenda

One starting point in such a crisis-infused reassessment is jail reform. The fact that approximately one-third of the global prison population *has not been convicted of a crime* needs to be one factor considered when developing strategies to reduce the harm caused by incarceration during the pandemic (Byrne et al., 2015; Walmsley, 2016; World Prison Brief, 2020). Among the five countries with the largest prison systems, the percentage of their prison population that is being held pre-trial is as follows: USA (23.4%), China (12.1%), Brazil (30.4%), Russia (21.2%), and India ((69.1%); World Prison Brief, 2020). Furthermore, these 5 countries account for 52% (N = 1,355,487) of the world's pre-trial prison population (N = 2,620,54; World Prison Brief, 2020). Not surprisingly, we find that it is the pre-trial population that was the initial target of early release strategies devised in most countries. Policymakers in some countries fear that reducing pre-trial populations will come with a cost: more crime in the community due to their resumption of (alleged) criminal activity. However, there is little support for continuing the use of pre-trial detention on the scale being used globally based on a review of the research on the criminal behavior of individuals during pre-trial release. Safe release is not only possible, but it is probable at the pre-trial stage, based on the available data on crime commission during pretrial release (Byrne et al., 2015). Research needs to be conducted on current, crisis-driven jail population reduction strategies to determine their impact, and add to this body of research.

Prison reform during the pandemic: A research agenda

A second category of crisis-driven, short-term reforms includes the mitigation strategies designed to reduce the number of people being sent to prison and those reforms designed to let them leave prison early. It is argued that the prison sanction will serve as both a specific and a general deterrent. Examination of available research on the specific deterrence effects of incarceration provides, at best, mixed support for this view (Byrne, 2013; Nagin, 2013; Tonry, 2008), with a consensus among sentencing experts that certainty matters much more than severity/length of sentencing.[27] When viewed in the context of this body of research, early release strategies that target older inmates serving long sentences can certainly be justified, both from a public health *and* a public safety perspective.[28] We find no evidence from our review that releasing inmates early from prison during the COVID-19 crisis has (1) increased the risk of recidivism among this release cohort, and (2) made communities less safe. Of course, it is equally true that we have no evidence to refute claims that releasing individuals from jail and prison will have deleterious effects. The necessary research needs to be done now; we need evidence of the effects of current mitigation strategies on the heath and behavior of individuals released from prison and jail to help governments prepare for the likely next phase of the pandemic. Our review documents *what* is being done in response to COVID-19 outbreaks in prison systems globally; but we have also found that the data needed to assess the effectiveness of these strategies is not being systematically collected.

Another prison reform area that needs to be examined involves the impact of in-prison mitigation strategies, particularly those strategies that reduced prison access to programs designed to address documented deficits in mental health, education/employment, substance abuse, and cognitive development. What impact did a lack of programming during the pandemic have on in-prison and post-release behavior? These impacts need to be documented. In a similar vein, it will be critical to examine the impact of restrictions on visitation and the use of lockdowns on in-prison mental and physical health, in-prison behavior, and on post-release health and behavioral outcomes. Without this research, we will not be able to assess the unintended consequences of these short-term crisis management strategies.

Community corrections reform during the pandemic: A research agenda

A third component of our proposed global research agenda focuses on community corrections. We need to collect baseline data on community corrections systems globally, while also investigating and evaluating the impact of strategies used to mitigate the spread of COVID-19 among community corrections personnel and clients. One assumption that many prison reform advocates often appear to make is that "anything" is preferable to a prison or jail sentence, but even a cursory examination of return to prison rates for technical violations of probation or parole conditions underscores an important reality: in many countries, technical violators make up a significant proportion of new prison admissions each year. In the USA, for example, it is estimated that 25% of the individuals entering the country's prison system have not committed a new crime; instead, they violated the technical conditions of probation or parole supervision (Justice Center, 2020). Viglione and colleagues (2020) report that technical violators are not being admitted to prison during the first several months of the pandemic; they reported that new prison admissions for technical violations are down 75% since the start of the pandemic (Viglione et al., 2020). It will be critical to evaluate the impact of this natural reform experiment on public safety, because – if the results are positive – placing a moratorium on the use of incarceration for technical violators would have a major effect on the USA's prison population (Byrne et al., 2015).

Notes

1. Official sources include country-specific government reports and interviews with government officials. Unofficial sources include reports and reviews by advocacy and watchdog groups, newspaper reports, and other sources.
2. Authors of the country-level reviews were asked to provide data on the response to the COVID-19 outbreaks in both institutional and community corrections.
3. A grassroot effort to create a global community corrections data base was initiated last year by researchers at the University of Massachusetts Lowell and George Mason University. For more details on the Global Community Corrections initiative, go to: www.globcci.org.

4. We provide detailed profiles of the nature and extent of the COVID-19 crisis within each global region in several separate reviews. See the articles by Rapisarda et al. (this volume).
5. This saying has been linked to several politicians (e.g., Winston Churchill) and political activists (e.g., Saul Alinsky); in the USA, it has been used recently by former president Obama's Chief of Staff, Rahm Emanuael. See https://freakonomics.com/2009/08/13/quotes-uncovered-who-said-no-crisis-should-go-to-waste/
6. http://www.twainquotes.com/Statistics.html
7. See, in particular, the commentary on the low official rates of COVID-19 outbreaks in China's prisons (Li & Liu, this volume).
8. See Marmolejo et al.'s (2020) discussion of the COVID-19 outbreaks in Latin America.
9. This assumption may be drawn due to preliminary evidence suggesting that COVID-19 contraction risk/death is greater in prisons than in the community at large (as we stated above). However, the community corrections population and the community at large are **not** "the same" in terms of living conditions, resource availability, and mental and physical health profiles.
10. More details on the work of the global community corrections initiative and the country-level experts involved can be found on their website: http://www.globcci.org/
11. Viglione and colleagues (2020) state that 38% of survey respondents reported "at least one confirmed case of COVID-19 among individuals on supervision, while 15% reported at least one confirmed case among officers." They go on to note that when this occurred, remote supervision was used until the individual tested negative.
12. In our view, a "return-to-normalcy" strategy will be evidence of déjà-vu (or more precisely, we need to coin a new term, dumja-vu: making the same, and often ineffective, policy choices time and time again).
13. For an overview, see Byrne and Pattavina (2013) and Pattavina and Corbett (2019).
14. This public protection goal has been presented by some governments to explain the over-representation of nonwhite and foreign-born populations in prisons globally. For a review, see Heard (2020).
15. Here we refer to the use of prison as a sanction and the length of the prison sentence.
16. For more detail, see notes for Table 5. These data are available on the United Nations Office of Drugs and Crime website.
17. Data on the recidivism of releasees from the countries in our review should also be examined to assess impact on public safety. Unfortunately, these data are not available globally. See Byrne et al. (2015) for a review and discussion.
18. These countries are USA, Brazil, South Africa, India, Australia, Kenya, and the UK (England and Wales).
19. Heard (2019) observes that the country-level research on the link between overcrowding and various forms of self-harm, including suicide, is mixed. See, for example, the 24-country comparative review by Fazel et al. (2016).
20. The countries included in Table 8 are the countries profiled by authors included in this special issue. By including 6 smaller countries in this review we are able to offer an assessment of whether the strategies employed in the large prison systems are similar to the strategies employed in these smaller countries.
21. It has been argued that suspension of visitation has a greater impact on women in prison than men in prison, due to the provider role of women in prison. See Agoff (this volume).
22. In addition to the 6 smaller countries we included in our review of mitigation strategies (see Table 8).
23. It is important to note that particularly in the cases where data were not provided in January through March of 2020 (or closer to the start of the pandemic), makes it more challenging to attribute reductions in prison population totals solely, or predominantly, to COVID-19 back-end mitigation strategies. Policy changes and other forces leading up to 2020 may have also contributed to these prison systems' population reductions.
24. The effect of COVID-19 on the forced labor population is largely unknown (Ovchinnikov, this volume).

25. Refers to crime rates in 27 different cities in the US, and thus is not encompassing of all cities in all 50 states.
26. The one exception is Europe, which does collect annual data on the region's community corrections system. See, for example, the START surveys.
27. For an overview of sentencing research, see Byrne (2013), Nagin (2013), M. Tonry (2008), and Tonry (2016).
28. We recognize that critics often conflate risk of recidivism with the stakes involved, if even a single violent crime is committed by a released inmate. Violent criminals (e.g., murderers and individuals who were charged with sexual crime(s)) have the lowest recidivism risk of any release cohort, but it is their conviction offense, not their risk, that leads policymakers to make these groups ineligible for release, even during a pandemic when their age and underlying health problems identify them as "high risk" for infection and death while incarcerated. For many, it is not the *probability* of a new crime by these high stakes inmates that matters, but rather the *possibility*. For further discussion on this topic, see Byrne et al. (2008).

Disclosure statement

No potential conflict of interest was reported by the author(s).

References

Aebi, M. F., & Tiago, M. M. (2020). *Prisons and prisoners in Europe in pandemic times: An evaluation of the short-term impact of the COVID-19 on prison populations*. Council of Europe. http://wp.unil.ch/space/files/2020/06/Prisons-and-the-COVID-19_200617_FINAL.pdf

Akiyama, M. J., Spaulding, A. C., & Rich, J. D. (2020). Flattening the curve for incarcerated populations - Covid-19 in jails and prisons. *The New England Journal of Medicine*, *382*(22), 2075–2077. https://doi.org/10.1056/NEJMp2005687

Altaf, M., Khan, M. I. U., Ahmad, U., & Yousaf, Z. (2018). Reclamation and probation department: A saving account to the government. *International Journal of Scientific and Research Publications*, *8* (2), 318–323. http://www.ijsrp.org/research-paper-0218/ijsrp-p7440.pdf

Butler, T., Indig, D., Allnutt, S., & Mamoon, H. (2011). Co-occurring mental illness and substance use disorder among Australian prisoners. *Drug and Alcohol Review*, *30*(2), 188–194. https://doi.org/10.1111/j.1465-3362.2010.00216.x

Butt, U. I., Umar, M., Khan, W. H., & Farooka, M. W. (2020). Setting up a COVID-19 care facility at a prison: An experience from Pakistan. *Annals of Medicine and Surgery*, *57*, 343–345. https://doi.org/10.1016/j.amsu.2020.06.043

Byrne, J., Hummer, D., & Stowell, J. (2008). Prison violence, prison culture, and offender change: New directions in theory, research, and policy. *The Culture of Prison Violence*. Allyn & Bacon.

Byrne, J., Kras, K. R., & Marmolejo, L. M. (2019). International perspectives on the privatization of corrections. *Criminology & Public Policy*, *18*(2), 477–503. https://doi.org/10.1111/1745-9133.12440

Byrne, J. M. (2013). After the fall: Assessing the impact of the great prison experiment on future crime control policy. *Federal Probation*, *77*, 3. https://www.uscourts.gov/sites/default/files/77_3_1_0.pdf

Byrne, J. M., & Pattavina, A. (2013). Technological innovation and offender reentry. *Technocrime, Policing and Surveillance*. https://doi.org/10.4324/9781315743981

Byrne, J. M., Pattavina, A., & Taxman, F. S. (2015). International trends in prison upsizing and downsizing: In search of evidence of a global rehabilitation revolution. *Victims & Offenders*, *10*(4), 420–451. https://doi.org/10.1080/15564886.2015.1078186

Dunkel, F. (2020). The impact of Covid-19 on prisons and penal policy in Germany. *Victims & Offenders (This Volume)*. https://doi.org/10.1080/15564886.2020.1813230

Durcan, G. (2008). *From the inside: Experiences of prison mental health care*. Sainsbury Centre for Mental Health.

Elflein, J. (2020). *Number of cumulative cases of coronavirus (COVID-19) worldwide from January 8 to September 30, 2020, by day.* Statista. https://www.statista.com/statistics/1103040/cumulative-coronavirus-covid19-cases-number-worldwide-by-day/

Fazel, S., Hayes, A. J., Bartellas, K., Clerici, M., & Trestman, R. (2016). Mental health of prisoners: Prevalence, adverse outcomes, and interventions. *The Lancet Psychiatry, 3*(9), 871–881. https://doi.org/10.1016/S2215-0366(16)30142-0

Fazel, S., Xenitidis, K., & Powell, J. (2008). The prevalence of intellectual disabilities among 12 000 prisoners—A systematic review. *International Journal of Law and Psychiatry, 31*(4), 369–373. https://doi.org/10.1016/j.ijlp.2008.06.001

Heard, C. (2019). *Towards a health-informed approach to penal reform? Evidence from ten countries.* Birkbeck Institutional Research Online. https://eprints.bbk.ac.uk/id/eprint/27743

Heard, C. (2020). Commentary: Assessing the global impact of the Covid-19 outbreak on prison populations. *Victims & Offenders.* https://doi.org/10.1080/15564886.2020.1825583

Justice Center. (2020). *Confined and costly: How supervision violations are filling prisons and burdening budget.* The Council of State Governments. https://csgjusticecenter.org/wp-content/uploads/2020/01/confined-and-costly.pdf

Li, S. D., & Liu, T. (2020). Correctional system's response to the coronavirus pandemic and its implications for prison reform in China. *Victims & Offenders.* https://doi.org/10.1080/15564886.2020.1824159

Marmolejo, L., Barberi, D., Espinoza, O., Bergman, M., & Fondevila, G. (2020). Responding to COVID-19 in Latin American prisons: The cases of Argentina, Chile, Colombia, and Mexico. *Victims & Offenders.* https://doi.org/10.1080/15564886.2020.1827110

McGuire, J. (2018). *Understanding prison violence: A rapid evidence assessment.* London: Her Majesty's Prison and Probation Service.

Nagin, D. S. (2013). Deterrence in the twenty-first century. *Crime and Justice, 42*(1), 199–263. https://doi.org/10.1086/670398

Nowonty, K. M., & Piquero, A. R. (2020). The global impact of the pandemic on institutional and community corrections: Assessing short-term crisis management and long-term change strategies. *Victims & Offenders.* https://doi.org/10.1080/15564886.2020.1813229

Pattavina, A., & Corbett, R. P. (2019). How smartphone technology can link the theoretical, policy, and practical contexts of community supervision reform: Voices from the field. *Victims & Offenders, 14*(7), 777–792. https://doi.org/10.1080/15564886.2019.1659894

Ribeiro, L., & Diniz, A. (2020). The Brazilian penitentiary system under the threat of COVID-19. *Victims & Offenders.* https://doi.org/10.1080/15564886.2020.1827109

Rosenfeld, R., & Lopez, E. (2020). *Pandemic, social unrest, and crime in U.S. Cities.* Council on Criminal Justice. https://cdn.ymaws.com/counciloncj.org/resource/collection/D26974EF-0F75-4BDE-ADE7-86DA0741DC49/Impact_Report_-_Crime.pdf

Tonry, M. (2008). Learning from the limitations of deterrence research. *Crime and Justice, 37*(1), 279–311. https://doi.org/10.1086/524825

Tonry, M. H. (2016). *Sentencing fragments: Penal reform in America, 1975-2025.* Oxford University Press.

Viglione, J., Alward, L. M., Lockwood, A., & Bryso, S. (2020). Adaptations to COVID-19 in community corrections agencies across the United States. *Victims & Offenders (This Volume).* https://doi.org/10.1080/15564886.2020.1818153

Walmsley, R. (2016). *World prison population list.* Institute for Criminal Policy Research. https://www.prisonstudies.org/sites/default/files/resources/downloads/world_prison_population_list_11th_edition_0.pdf

Wetzel, J. E., & Janeen, M. D. (2020). The response to the COVID19 crisis by the Pennsylvania department of corrections. *Victims & Offenders.* https://doi.org/10.1080/15564886.2020.1830324

Williams, W. H., Chitsabesan, P., Fazel, S., McMillan, T., Hughes, N., Parsonage, M., & Tonks, J. (2018). Traumatic brain injury: A potential cause of violent crime? *The Lancet Psychiatry, 5*(10), 836–844. https://doi.org/10.1016/S2215-0366(18)30062-2

World Health Organization. (2020). *WHO speaks at the European parliament on the COVID-19 response.* https://www.who.int/news-room/detail/30-06-2020-who-speaks-at-the-european-parliament-on-the-covid-19-response

World Health Organization, Regional Office for Europe. (2014). *Prisons and health. WHO.* https://www.euro.who.int/en/health-topics/health-determinants/prisons-and-health/publications/2014/prisons-and-health

World Prison Brief. (2020). *World prison brief database.* Institute for Crime & Justice Policy Research. https://www.prisonstudies.org/world-prison-brief-data

Worldometer. (2020). *COVID-19 coronavirus pandemic.* https://www.worldometers.info/coronavirus/

Yang, X. (2017). Community corrections programs in China: New forms of informal punishments? *Asian-Pacific Law & Policy Journal 19*(1), 50–109.

Appendices

Appendix A

Notes to Table 3, Comparison of COVID-19 case and death counts and rates in communities and prison systems.

* COVID-19 count and rate data in prisons reflect inmates only (staff members not included). It is important to note that the prevalence of COVID-19 within prions is likely much greater, upon factoring in prison staff counts and underreporting.

[a]Most current prison population data (as of September 29, 2020) extracted from World Prison Brief database.

[b]Countrywide cumulative community-based COVID-19 count and rate data from Worldometer retrieved on September 29, 2020. It should be noted that the rates initially provided by Worldometer were denoted per 1 million persons. For the purposes of comparing community and prison-based COVID-19 rates, the community rates were converted to reflect the rate of positive cases and deaths per 10,000 persons, rather than per 1,000,000 persons.

[c]Based on data provided by the Marshall Project on September 22, 2020.

[d]In order to fairly compare rates, most recent prison data publicly released in China was aligned with community-level data from February 29, 2020 (numbers provided in this table; extracted from Worldometer). However, since then, the most recent cumulative count of COVID-19 cases in the community is 85,384 while the death count is 4,634 (Worldometer, 2020).

[e]Statistics from Yang, 2020.

[f]Prison-level data from Justiça Presente (2020). It should be noted that these data were provided on August 31st, thus, in order to align the prison-based count and rates for cases and deaths among inmates with community-based data, community-level data (case and death counts) were extracted from Worldometer from August 31st. As of September 29, Brazil has reported 4,753,410 COVID-19 cases (223.24 cases per 10,000 persons) and 142,280 deaths (6.68 deaths per 10,000 persons) within the communuty (Worldometer).

[g]Most recent count and death data within the Russian prison system was provided by Ovchinnikov (this volume) as of early August (2020), thus community counts and rates for cases and deaths in this table also reflect data from August 1, 2020. Russia has experienced a tremendous increase in COVID-19 cases and deaths within the community. As of September 29, Russia reported 1,167,805 COVID-19 cases, or a rate of 80.01 cases per 10,000 residents, and 20,545 deaths, or 1.41 deaths per 10,000 residents.

[h]Prison-level count and death data from the Commonwealth Human Rights Initiative. Please note that prison-level data provide combined totals of inmates and prison staff for COVID-19 counts and deaths.

[i]Thailand has not released official statistics indicating the total number of cases and deaths within its corrections population; however, local news articles have provided local cases (for example, see the Nation of Thailand and Forbes).

[j]Since May 22, the Turkish Ministry of Justice confirmed at least 120 inmates tested positive for COVID-19 and at least 3 died. An additional 82 positive cases and 1 death were announced in Silivri Prison by the İstanbul Bakırköy Chief Public Prosecutor's Office. In order to best compare

community and prison rates, the community-level data from Worldometer aligns with May 22, 2020. However, to date (as of September 29th), there have been 317,272 COVID-19 cases reported country-wide, for a rate of 37.52 cases per 10,000 residents, and 8,130 cumulative deaths, translating to a rate of.96 deaths per 10,000 residents.

[k]Iran has not released official data pertaining to the number of inmates and prison staff afflicted by COVID-19, in terms of case or death prevalence. Various news articles provide small glimpses of insight into suspected local outbreaks (e.g., see Iran Human Rights Monitor, Just Security, and the Los Angeles Times).

[l]Official statistics on COVID-19 case and death prevalence in Indonesian prisons have not been released. This report by the Institute for Criminal Justice Reform (ICJR) states that at least 120 inmate cases and 17 staff cases can be tallied, as well as 7 inmate deaths due to COVID-19; however, official numbers have not been made available.

[m]Official data on COVID-19 cases and deaths among Filipino prions have not been released. Various news articles cover local outbreaks (e.g., UCA News, U.S. News, and the ASEAN Post).

[n]Official data on COVID-19 cases and deaths among Mexican prions have not been released. This article released by Brookings in May provides some insight into the prevalence of COVID-19 in Mexican prisons.

[o]Prison-level data from New Frame (2020). The totals for infections and deaths in this table reflect a combination of inmate and staff cases. Because the most recent prison data were provided at the end of August, community counts and rates of COVID-19 were aligned with August 31, 2020. Since then, community-based case and death counts have risen. On September 29, 2020, South Africa reported a cumulative total of 672,572 infections, or 113.06 infections per 10,000 residents and 16,667 deaths, or 2.80 deaths per 10,000 residents (Worldometer).

[p]Official statistics on infection and death counts in Vietnamese prisons have not been released. However, Vietnam has been praised for its broad response to COVID-19 and has a relatively low cumulative community case prevalence (N = 1,094 on September 29, 2020).

[q]Ethiopia has not released official data pertaining to the number of inmates and prison staff afflicted by COVID-19, in terms of case or death prevalence. A few news articles provide information regarding suspected local correctional outbreaks (e.g., see the National Herald and VOA).

[r]To align the date at which most recent confirmed and suspected case and death totals were updated in Egyptian prisons (August 7, 2020), community infections and death totals were extracted on August 7 (reflected in this table). However, more recent community-level data have been released. On September 29, 2020, Egypt reported a nationwide cumulative infection count of 103,079 cases or 10.03 cases per 10,000 residents and a cumulative death count of 5914, translating to.58 deaths per 10,000 persons (Worldometer, 2020).

[s]Federal prison-level data from the Procuraduría de Violencia Instituciona (September 30, 2020).

[t]Colombia has not released official statistics indicating the total number of cases and deaths within its corrections population to date; however, local news articles have provided local cases (for example, see U.S. News).

[u]Prison-level infection data from En-24 News (death count not provided). The most recent prison data were provided on August 22, 2020, thus the community infection count and rate of COVID-19 were aligned with this date for comparison purposes. More recent data (as of September 29, 2020) indicates that Peru has been afflicted by a cumulative total of 808,714 infections, or 244.45 infections per 10,000 residents, in addition to 32,324 deaths, or 9.77 deaths per 10,000 residents (Worldometer).

[v]Myanmar has not released official statistics indicating cumulative case and/or death count of inmates or staff in its prison system. Reliefweb provides information about mitigation strategies used by Myanmar facilities, bolstered by the UN.

[w]Bangladesh has not released official statistics indicating cumulative case and/or death count of inmates or staff in its prison system. The International Committee of the Red Cross provides information about within-prison mitigation strategies, namely sufficient PPE dissemination, while the Business Standard describes back-end strategies, such as early release.

[x]Morocco has not released official statistics indicating the total number of cases and deaths within its corrections population to date; however, local news articles have provided local cases (for example, see Anadolu Agency).

[y]Prison-level data for the UK (England and Wales) from the Ministry of Justice (document released on August 14). Consequently, community-level data were extracted from Worldometer to align with August 14th. However, it should be noted that as of September 29, 2020, reported infections in UK's community are at 79,433 (a rate of 65.64 cases per 10,000 residents), while community deaths related to COVID-19 stand at 42,072, or 6.19 deaths per 10,000 residents.

[z]Pakistan has not released official statistics indicating the total number of cases and deaths within its corrections system to date; however, local news articles have provided local cases (for example, see Justice Project for Pakistan – JPP – and organizations like Amnesty International adamantly suggesting that Pakistan's prison system approach the pandemic with more transparency and testing.

[aa]Poland has not released official data pertaining to the number of inmates and prison staff afflicted by COVID-19, in terms of case or death prevalence. Information regarding Poland's back-end response to COVID-19 can be found here (Reuters).

[bb]Malaysia has not released official data pertaining to the number of inmates and prison staff afflicted by COVID-19, in terms of case or death prevalence. Into May, the Malaysian Correctional Department claimed to have 0 reported cases or deaths related to COVID-19. However, since then, various news articles provide small glimpses of insight into suspected local outbreaks (e.g., see Malaysiakini(a), the Star, and Malaysiakini(b)).

[cc]Rwanda has not released official country-wide data pertaining to the number of inmate sand prison staff that have tested positive or died due to COVID-19. However, sources like Duma FM estimated case totals in prisons, but not as of late (July 1st).

[dd]Algeria has not reported cumulative counts for infections or death in prisons to date. However, articles such as the Arab Weekly and France24 have been published providing contextual information regarding Algeria's correctional response to COVID-19 crisis.

[ee]Nigeria has not released official country-wide data pertaining to the number of inmates and prison staff that have tested positive or died due to COVID-19. However, sources like the International Center for Investigative Reporting have provided surface-level information insinuating that outbreaks have occurred. Other contextual information, such as lifting previously instituted preventative strategies can be found here.

[ff]Saudi Arabia has not released official statistics indicating cumulative case and/or death count of inmates or staff in its prison system. However, Reuters provides information about back-end mitigation strategies, namely releases, while the Saudi Gazette describes the punitive approach adopted in order to handle violations of not abiding to strictly outlaid COVID-19 protection measures.

[gg]Taiwan has claimed to have zero cases and/or deaths in its prison system. It has also included inmates in widespread mask production.

[hh]France has not released official statistics indicating cumulative case and/or death counts of inmates or staff in its prison system. However, France24 provides information about back-end mitigation strategies, namely releases, while RFI News verifies that cases do, in fact, exist within French prisons.

[ii]Prison-level, cumulative data for Spain in terms of cases and deaths has not been reported. For more related to Spain's response to COVID-19 in its prison system visit these sources by: Aebi & Tiago (2020), European Public Service Union (EPSU), the Center for Crime and Justice Studies, and Fair Trials.

[jj]Germany has not released official statistics indicating cumulative case and/or death counts of inmates or staff in its prison system. However, Reuters provides information about back-end mitigation strategies, namely early release.

[kk]Cuba has not released official data pertaining to the number of inmates and prison staff afflicted by COVID-19, in terms of case or death prevalence. By late July, Cuba's National Institute of Epidemiology Director announced that Cuban prisons have 0 COVID-19 cases. One mitigation strategy used by Cuba includes early release, according to the Miami Herald.

[ll]Venezuela has not released official country-wide data pertaining to the number of inmates and prison staff that have tested positive or died due to COVID-19. Sources like Fair Trials and the Guardian offer more context about Venezuelan prisons in the context of the pandemic.

[mm]Despite that Uganda has not reported official country-wide prison data, cases and outbreaks have been reported by sources such as the World Health Organization and Reuters.

[nn]Despite that South Korea has not reported official country-wide prison data, sources like Korea Biomedical Review and LA Times offer more context about South Korean prisons in the COVID-19 climate.

[oo]Italy, like many other European countries has not released unified, cumulative data on COVID-19 cases and deaths in its prison system; however, Aebi & Tiago (2020) provided preliminary, binary data on whether or not European states reported positive cases early on in the pandemic. The Global Initiative Against Transnational Organized Crime also reported on the fragile state of Italian prisons due to both the pandemic and the mafia.

[pp]Kenya has not released cumulative, official data pertaining to the number of inmates and prison staff afflicted by COVID-19, in terms of case or death prevalence. However, various news articles provide small glimpses of insight into local outbreaks (e.g., see CGTN Africa, Capital News, and Anadolu Agency).

[qq]Prison-level data for Ukraine from the Corrections Department on September 8, 2020. Consequently, community-level data were extracted from Worldometer to align with August 8th. It is important to note that community-level data counts and rates have since increased. As of September 29, 2020, the Ukraine reported 204,932 community infections, translating to a rate of 46.93 infections per 10,000 residents. Moreover, COVID-19-related deaths in the community on the same date totaled 4,065, or.93 deaths per 10,000 residents. Other sources like Open Democracy have criticized the Ukraine for underreporting true infection and death rates.

[rr]Japan has not released cumulative, official data pertaining to the number of inmates and prison staff afflicted by COVID-19, in terms of case or death prevalence. However, news articles such as the Japan Times and Kyodo News provide insight into anticipating, and instances of, local outbreaks.

[ss]Iraq has not released cumulative, official data pertaining to the number of inmates and prison staff afflicted by COVID-19, in terms of case or death prevalence. However, news articles such as Anadolu Agency provide insight into local outbreaks, VOA News questions the transparency and accuracy of reported cases relative to actual case prevalence by Iraq's health ministry, and the New Arab discusses back-end mitigation strategies.

[tt]While Australia has not yet made cumulative, official country-wide prison data available, it has released detailed procedures and guidelines regarding outbreaks in Australian correctional facilities. Moreover, as is the case with many other countries, various local news outlets have published articles describing COVID-19 outbreaks (e.g., 7 News Australia).

[uu]Canadian prison-level data (updated on September 29, 2020) extracted from Correctional Service Canada.

[vv]Chile has not released official data pertaining to the number of inmates and prison staff afflicted by COVID-19, in terms of case or death prevalence. Various news articles, however, provide small glimpses into the climate and responses within Chilean prisons as well as the extent of a few local outbreaks (e.g., see Arkansas Democrat Gazette and AlJazeera).

[ww]Ecuador has not released official data pertaining to the number of inmates and prison staff afflicted by COVID-19, in terms of case or death prevalence. Various news articles provide small glimpses of insight into suspected local outbreaks (e.g., see Fair Trials).

[xx]El Salvador has not released official data pertaining to the number of inmates and prison staff afflicted by COVID-19, in terms of case or death prevalence. Various news articles provide context and the extent of suspected local outbreaks (e.g., see National Post).

[yy]Despite that Cambodia has not reported official country-wide prison data, cases and outbreaks are likely present considering its prison system's "deplorable" conditions. Both Human Rights Watch and Amnesty International have demanded prompt and drastic responses to address COVID-19 risks in Cambodia's prisons and jails.

[zz]Tanzania has not released official data pertaining to the number of inmates and prison staff afflicted by COVID-19, in terms of case or death prevalence. Various news articles, however, provide small glimpses into the climate – e.g., confusion/mixed-messaging on behalf of the President Magufuli – and responses – e.g., the installation of hand-washing stations in 4 separate facilities – of COVID-19 within Tanzanian prisons (e.g., see Reliefweb and Devex).

[aaa]Belarus, like many other countries world-wide, has not made COVID-19 data within its prisons available. Based on a report by the International Republican Institute, COVID-19 has exposed "governance gaps" specifically within authoritarian states like Belarus. In terms of Belarus's correctional response to COVID-19, minimal information has been released. However, for broad context, CNN reported Belarus's authoritarian president as adopting a denialistic approach, dismissing COVID-19 as "psychosis," despite that he tested positive himself in July.

Appendix B

Notes to Table 4, State-Level variations in the extent, impact, and response to the COVID-19 outbreaks in USA prisons.

The table presents prison data only, no jail information is included. Suspended admissions refers to allowing no new admissions from jails to prison facilities; Medical release refers to legislation or executive orders releasing individuals with designated medical conditions; Early release refers to legislation or executive orders releasing individuals based on good-time formulas, certain low-level nonviolent convictions with a lesser amount of time remaining (such as six months), and early parole granted; Pre-trial release refers to releasing individuals held in prisons for pre-trial; None refers to no action taken to release prisoners or injunctions by the court.

^Data compiled from The Marshall Project's "A State-by-State Look at Coronavirus in Prisons" (https://www.themarshallproject.org/2020/05/01/a-state-by-state-look-at-coronavirus-in-prisons) as of 9/11/2020; *An asterisk denotes state counts that include both pre-trial detainees and sentenced prisoners under a unified system of jails and prisons.; [+]The Marshall Project, "COVID-19 Impacts Prison Populations Nationwide". Alaska, Indiana, and Maryland did not provide data for this analysis. (https://www.themarshallproject.org/2020/07/16/prison-populations-drop-by-100-000-during-pandemic); https://www.prisonpolicy.org/virus/virusresponse.html#state

[a]http://www.doc.state.al.us/COVID19NewsFeed; http://www.alabamapublichealth.gov/legal/assets/soe-covid19-corrections-063020.pdf; https://www.alreporter.com/2020/05/22/alabama-prisons-to-release-some-inmates-early-amid-covid-19-outbreak/

[b]https://doc.alaska.gov/covid-19

[c]https://corrections.az.gov/adcrr-covid-19-dashboard

[d]https://www.ualrpublicradio.org/post/covid-19-inside-arkansas-prisons-past-and-future

[e]https://www.cdcr.ca.gov/covid19/covid-19-response-efforts/#R

[f]https://www.colorado.gov/pacific/cdoc/covid-19-faq-and-updates; https://wp-cpr.s3.amazonaws.com/uploads/2020/09/D-2020-016-Suspending-Certain-Regulatory-Statutes-Concerning-Criminal-Justice.pdf

[g]https://ctmirror.org/2020/05/01/how-covid-19-is-shrinking-connecticuts-prison-population/#:~:text=More%20than%20520%20people%20were,discretionary%20releases%20in%20March%202019; https://www.ctpost.com/news/coronavirus/article/State-prisons-releasing-inmates-due-to-15182364.php

[h]https://www.bop.gov/coronavirus/

[i]http://www.dc.state.fl.us/comm/covid-19.html

[j]http://www.gdc.ga.gov/content/CVD_Dashboard; https://www.ajc.com/news/local/breaking-georgia-release-some-inmates-due-covid-fears/np6zhBrlP1oe2jOkUmWVoL/

[k]https://www.civilbeat.org/2020/08/inmates-are-released-as-covid-19-spreads-inside-hawaiis-largest-jail/

[l]https://www.idoc.idaho.gov/content/careers/covid-19

[m]https://www2.illinois.gov/Documents/ExecOrders/2020/ExecutiveOrder-2020-13.pdf; https://www2.illinois.gov/Pages/Executive-Orders/ExecutiveOrder2020-21.aspx; https://ballotpedia.org/Prison_inmate_release_responses_in_response_to_the_coronavirus_(COVID-19)_pandemic,_2020#Responses_by_state

[n]https://www.in.gov/idoc/about-idoc/idoc-facility-covid-19-statistics;https://www.kansas.com/news/politics-government/article242317396.html

[o]https://www.kcci.com/article/iowa-to-release-prisoners-to-minimize-spread-of-covid-19/32216621#; https://doc.iowa.gov/COVID19

[p]https://www.courier-journal.com/story/news/politics/2020/07/29/700-more-kentucky-inmates-may-get-early-release-after-covid-19-spike/5536075002/; https://corrections.ky.gov/Facilities/Pages/covid19.aspx

[q]https://doc.louisiana.gov/doc-covid-19-testing/; https://ballotpedia.org/Prison_inmate_release_responses_in_response_to_the_coronavirus_(COVID-19)_pandemic,_2020#Responses_by_state

[r]https://www.mainepublic.org/post/maine-released-dozens-prisoners-prevent-covid-19-spread-advocates-say-more-should-be-done; https://www.maine.gov/corrections/sites/maine.gov.corrections/files/inline-files/MDOC%20COVID19WebDashboard9-17-2020.pdf;

[s]https://www.baltimoresun.com/coronavirus/bs-md-maryland-prisons-release-inmates-coronavirus-20200421-yc52bbol5jevnbkgeqnbn47hjy-story.html; https://news.maryland.gov/dpscs/covid-19/

[t]https://ballotpedia.org/Prison_inmate_release_responses_in_response_to_the_coronavirus_(COVID-19)_pandemic,_2020#Responses_by_state; https://data.aclum.org/sjc-12926-tracker/

[u]https://www.michigan.gov/whitmer/0,9309,7-387-90499_90705-523422--,00.html; https://wwmt.com/news/i-team/michigan-prison-population-sees-record-drop-during-covid-19-pandemic; https://medium.com/@MichiganDOC/mdoc-takes-steps-to-prevent-spread-of-coronavirus-covid-19-250f43144337

[v]https://mn.gov/doc/about/covid-19-updates/;

[w]https://courts.ms.gov/appellatecourts/docket/sendPDF.php?f=700_495286.pdf&c=91465&a=N&s=2; https://www.mdoc.ms.gov/Documents/covid-19/Inmates%20cases%20chart.pdf;

[x]https://doc.mo.gov/media-center/newsroom/covid-19/data; https://ballotpedia.org/Prison_inmate_release_responses_in_response_to_the_coronavirus_(COVID-19)_pandemic,_2020#Responses_by_state

[y]https://corrections.nebraska.gov/ndcs-staff-members-positive-covid-19-13; https://corrections.nebraska.gov/ndcs-coronavirus-health-update

[z]http://doc.nv.gov/About/Press_Release/covid19_updates/; https://app.powerbigov.us/view?r=eyJrIjoiNDMwMDI0YmQtNmUyYS00ZmFjLWI0MGItZDM0OTY1Y2Y0YzNhIiwidCI6ImU0YTM0MGU2LWI4OWUtNGU2OC04ZWFhLTE1NDRkMjcwMzk4MCJ9

[aa]https://ballotpedia.org/Prison_inmate_release_responses_in_response_to_the_coronavirus_(COVID-19)_pandemic,_2020#Responses_by_state; https://njdoc.gov/pages/COVID19Updates.shtml

[bb]https://cd.nm.gov/covid-19-updates/; https://www.krqe.com/health/coronavirus-new-mexico/new-mexico-prisoners-being-released-early-to-curb-spread-of-covid-19/; https://cd.nm.gov/wp-content/uploads/2020/04/Governor-announces-executive-order-for-early-release.pdf

[cc]https://doccs.ny.gov/doccs-covid-19-report; https://ballotpedia.org/Prison_inmate_release_responses_in_response_to_the_coronavirus_(COVID-19)_pandemic,_2020#Responses_by_state;

[dd]https://www.ncdps.gov/our-organization/adult-correction/prisons/prisons-info-covid-19#data;

[ee]https://www.kfyrtv.com/content/news/More-than-100-DOCR-inmates-granted-early-parole-due-to-COVID-19-570318211.html; https://www.docr.nd.gov/covid-19-information

[ff]https://ballotpedia.org/Prison_inmate_release_responses_in_response_to_the_coronavirus_(COVID-19)_pandemic,_2020#Responses_by_state; https://coronavirus.ohio.gov/static/reports/DRCCOVID-19Information.pdf

[gg]https://oklahoman.com/article/5658504/coronavirus-in-oklahoma-over-200-nonviolent-offenders-released-from-oklahoma-county-jail-to-limit-covid-19-spread; http://doc.publishpath.com/Default.aspx?shortcut=covid-19-stats-report

[hh]https://www.oregon.gov/doc/covid19/Pages/covid19-tracking.aspx; https://www.statesmanjournal.com/story/news/crime/2020/08/26/covid-cases-prisons-oregon-gov-brown-inmate-release/3444432001/

[ii]https://www.abc27.com/investigators/investigations/a-look-at-the-numbers-pa-state-prison-inmates-released-due-to-covid-19/; https://www.cor.pa.gov/Pages/COVID-19.aspx

[jj]https://www.southcoasttoday.com/news/20200325/ri-prisons-looking-to-reduce-inmate-numbers-due-to-virus

[kk]http://doc.sc.gov/covid.html

[ll]https://doc.sd.gov/documents/COVID19PositiveCaseInformationbyFacility9172020.pdf;

[mm]https://www.tn.gov/content/dam/tn/correction/documents/TDOCInmatesCOVID19.pdf

[nn]https://txdps.maps.arcgis.com/apps/opsdashboard/index.html#/dce4d7da662945178ad5fbf3981fa35c

[oo]https://corrections.utah.gov/index.php/home/alerts-2/1237-udc-coronavirus-updates

[pp]https://www.vnews.com/Vermont-NH-prisons-working-to-reduce-population-to-prevent-virus-spread-33512589

[qq]https://vadoc.virginia.gov/media/1506/vadoc-covid19-early-release-plan.pdf;

[rr]https://www.doc.wa.gov/corrections/covid-19/data.htm#confirmed; https://www.q13fox.com/news/more-than-300-inmates-released-from-washington-prisons-due-to-covid-19-concerns

[ss]https://dhhr.wv.gov/COVID-19/Documents/COVID19_DCR_2020_09-17.pdf; https://ballotpedia.org/Prison_inmate_release_responses_in_response_to_the_coronavirus_(COVID-19)_pandemic,_2020#Responses_by_state

[tt]https://madison.com/wsj/news/local/crime-and-courts/wisconsin-doc-has-released-nearly-1-600-inmates-so-far-to-combat-covid-19-spread/article_03537daa-e1ec-5fe8-ac68-f5cf38ce8be5.html#:~:text = Waupun%20Correctional%20Institution.&text = The%20Wisconsin%20Department%20of%20Corrections,a%20DOC%20spokeswoman%20said%20Thursday.

Appendix C

Notes to Table 5, Total Corrections populations in top 50 countries with highest prison populations (2020).

*"Year" refers to the most recent year in which either prison population or community corrections data were published.

^ = Probation currently not in place.

– = Data not available, but community corrections system is in place.

All prison population data were extracted from the World Prison Brief database (2020).

[a]Data from the U.S. Bureau of Justice Statistics (BJS).

[b]Data are 2013 estimates, based on a review by Yang (2017), Figures 5 & 6 (p. 91).

[c]In 2011, an amending decree was put into motion preventing persons who have committed crimes punishable with less than four years' imprisonment from being arrested, making incarceration a last resort. With the new Law, the person can only be arrested preventively after having been sentenced. Instead of incarceration, the legislation introduces new alternatives, such as the placement of a bond that can be determined by the police authority and/or a judge; electronic monitoring; nighttime house arrest; travel bans; prohibiting travel to certain places and having contact with certain people; and suspension of the exercise of public or economic activity. Consequently, because 37% (N = 183,520) of Brazil's prison population (N = 496,000) in 2011 had not yet been tried, these inmates were to be immediately released. It is important to note that this 37% applied to Brazil's prison population count in 2011 (and not present). However, this amended decree has proved to be futile. In 2019, at least 40% of Brazil's prison population, equating to over 302,000 inmates, was comprised of pre-trial detainees who, under this decree, should have been provided an alternative sanction; however, the vast majority of persons awaiting trial in Brazil are still incarcerated with convicted inmates, despite legislation saying otherwise.

[d]Data from Table 4 of Council of Europe's Annual Penal Statistics "Persons under the supervision of probation agencies" SPACE II Report (pgs. 22–23).

[e]Data denoting the number of individuals on parole in India were extracted from a publication by the Bangladesh Judicial Service entitled, "Alternative sanctions to convicted offenders in Criminal Justice System in Bangladesh focusing on probation and parole: A lesson from India" (Rahim & Parvin, 2018). While data were not provided for Bangladesh (as of 2018), the authors stated that, "Bangladesh … [is] heading toward correctional approach in criminology and penology schemes and [has] already passed some laws which allow the concerned authorities to impose alternative sanctions to the convicted offenders including probation and parole." At the time of this publication the

authors, however, noted that "Parole and probation are rarely used in criminal administration of Bangladesh," thus insinuating that the role of alternative sanctions is in its infancy.

[f]Data from The Seminar on Promoting Community-Based Treatment in the Asean Region Report from 2015 – includes both adult and juvenile probationers and parolees. Data for Vietnam reflect cumulative totals (to date) of individuals who have experienced suspended or non-custodial sentences. No specific data were provided for Myanmar; however, the report provides further context regarding Myanmar's community-based treatment and probation as of 2015. In Japan, it is estimated that as of 2015, probation offices deal with approximately 40,000 juvenile and adult probationers and parolees at any given time. Cambodia, "At present, [has] no mechanisms to look after offenders or ex-offenders in the society, except for offenders in the prison who received services like vocational training skills . . . " (as of 2015).

[g]Data from the Philippines Department of Justice Parole and Probation Administration.

[h]This number reflects the average number of community corrections caseloads (probation, parole, and awaiting trial) in South Africa in 2018.

[i]Data from the Ministerio de Justicia y Derechos Humanos's Report: Informe Ejecutivo 2018, Sistema Nacional de Estadísticas sobre la Ejecución de la Pena (SNEEP) include totals for alternative sentences to incarceration, such as electronic monitoring (3,909) and/or house arrest (756) as of 2018.

[j]Data from the Instituto Nacional Penitenciario y Carcelario's (INPEC) Report: Informe Estadístico, Agosto 2020. Include totals for alternative sentences to incarceration, such as house arrest (70,138) and electronic monitoring (4,987).

[k]Data from the Instituto Nacional Penitenciario, Informe Estadístico, Noviembre 2019. Include totals for parole (5,978), alternatives to incarceration (949), community service orders and limitation of free days (22,632).

[l]Based on an interview conducted between Justice Trends Magazine and Moroccan Delegate General of the Correctional Department, Mohamed Salah Tamek, Morocco plans to combat prison overcrowding not through alternative sanctioning (translating to a reduced prison population), but rather through increasing the quantity of facilities and infrastructure necessary to house an ever-increasing number of inmates. Additionally, he plans to increase the number of prison staff nationwide.

[m]Data from the Ministry of Justice "National Statistics Offender management statistics quarterly: January to March 2020" (published 30 July 2020).

[n]Community corrections data for Pakistan from Altaf et al., 2018.

[o]For more about Malaysia's justice process: http://malaysia.justiceaudit.org/?page_id=28

[p]Various sources (Non-custodial sentence as a means of prison decongestion in Nigeria, Probation as a non-custodial measure in Nigeria: Making a case for adult probation service, & Appraisal of the restorative criminal justice measures in Nigeria) convey that while Nigeria has the legislation to divert individuals to community corrections-based sanctioning (in theory), noncustodial alternatives are hardly ever implemented (in practice). The follow quote best encapsulates this tension: "It is only unfortunate that probation or suspended sentence and other noncustodial measures are not yet in use in Nigeria in spite of provisions for them in some relevant statutes. It has thus been observed that: 'Nigeria has the statutory provisions for probationary sentences, but the administrators of justice hardly ever employ such provisions. Yet evidence shows that on the basis of the statutorily stipulated criteria for probationary sentences, about 40% offenders presently sent to prison should have qualified for such sentences . . . '"

[q]Data indicating the combined number of individuals on probation and parole from Taiwan's Ministry of Justice Judicial Protection Statistics page.

[r]In the Vera Institute's report entitled: "Sentencing and prison practices in Germany and the Netherlands: Implications for the United States" data from 2010 were provided on the percentage of Germany's corrections population (15%) that comprised of having received suspended sentencing as a sanction, which the authors describe as the following: "In Germany, if an offender is sentenced to a prison sentence of up to two years, the court will typically suspend the execution of that sentence and place the offender on probation." To calculate the total count of individuals with suspended sentences, the total correctional population was first calculated by multiplying Germany's total incarcerated population (N = 64,379) by 100 (the denominator of 6%) and then dividing by 6

(which represents the percentage of incarcerated individuals), thus yielding a total correctional population of approximately 1,072,983 individuals. Finally the total correctional population (N = 1,072,983) was multiplied by 15% to yield the number of individuals with suspended sentences in Germany, which equates to roughly 160,948 individuals.

[s]Data from the United Nations Asia and Far East Institute (UNAFEI)'s "Overview of the commu nity corrections system of the Republic of Korea" (2013). The types of noncustodial sanctioning in South Korea include: probation (N = 96,574), community service orders (N = 41,511), educational orders (N = 28,054), investigations (e.g., Pre-sentence investigation – requested by judge, Pre-ruling investigation – requested by judge, Pre-decision investigation -requested by prosecutor; N = 30,487), electronic monitoring (N = 2,555), and pharmacological treatment (N = 3).

[t]Data from the UNAFEI's "Overview of the community corrections system in Kenya" (2012). Types of noncustodial sanctioning in Kenya include probation (N = 72,637) and community service (N = 377,663) orders.

[u]Data from the Australian Bureau of Statistics "Key Statistics" page (last updated June 2020).

[v]Data on Canadian community corrections were extracted from Statistics Canada (2019). The number provided (above) is a summation of the adult provincial/territorial community corrections (N = 150,114) AND federal community corrections populations admitted between 2017 and 2018. It is also important to note that on any given day between 2017 and 2018, there were 94,904 adult offenders under community supervision among Australia's provinces/territories (which is 80% of Australia's total correctional population), while the daily count among adult offenders under federal community supervision was 9,043.

[w]Data from Gendarmería de Chile, Estadísticas Penitenciarias a 31 de Agosto (2020). Includes open system (48,372) and presidential pardons due to COVID-19 (1,351).

[x]Data from Estadística Penitenciaria (August 17, 2020).

[y]PRI verified that Tanzania (among other African countries) does have some level of community corrections in place, more specifically, community service order. However, specific data were only located for probation and parole in Dodoma, the national capital of Tanzania, between the years of 2010 and 2012.

[z]Belarus is not currently operating a community corrections system. According to the Prison Insider, it is considered the "last dictatorship in Europe" and is the last country in Europe to uphold the death penalty. Moreover, Belarus is the only country in Europe to not yet sign the European Convention on Human Rights.

Africa Regional Overview and Reports from Kenya and South Africa

An Examination of COVID-19 Outbreaks in African Prisons and Jails

Sabrina S. Rapisarda and James M. Byrne

ABSTRACT
This article examines country-level variations in the extent of COVID-19 outbreaks in prisons and jails across the African region. Differences in the use of front-end, in-prison, and back-end mitigation strategies are identified. We conclude our regional overview by providing a preliminary assessment of the short-term impact of these varied mitigation strategies on inmate and staff health outcomes, including both physical health and mental health. Both the intended and unintended consequences of governmental responses to COVID-19 outbreaks are considered.

Introduction and overview

The extent of reported COVID-19 outbreaks in prisons and jails varies significantly from one sub-region of Africa to the next, with the largest outbreaks in countries in the Northern and Eastern regions of Africa, and the lowest reported outbreaks in countries in the Western region (see Figure 1). Reviews of prison systems in countries in this region have revealed conditions conducive to large potential outbreaks (Heard, 2019). It appears that most African countries were already encumbered by weak healthcare systems, inadequate surveillance and laboratory capacity, and limited resources, far before the start of the pandemic (Nkengasong & Mankoula, 2020). Moreover, Africa had previously been characterized by rapid population growth, increased cross-border and cross-continental movement of people, and endemic diseases like HIV, tuberculosis, malaria, Ebola, Lassa fever, and others, all of which facilitate the rapid and widespread transmission of COVID-19 (Nkengasong & Mankoula, 2020). Surprisingly, despite being the second largest continental landmass and second most populous continent globally and facing multiple public health challenges, Africa currently[1] has between 2.8– 5.8 times fewer reported COVID-19 cases than any other continental region[2] with a regional tally of 1,212,508 positive cases (Coronavirus Resource Center 2020; Nkengasong & Mankoula, 2020).[3]

The entire region of Africa reported around 10,000 cases in early April, while the U.S. confirmed over 600,000 (Worldometer, 2020). Based on these data, an argument can be made that Africa's experience with the virus may be slower to develop than other regions of the world. Others such as Dr. Tedros, a WHO director-general, believe that Africa has been able to better contain the virus due to the "great deal of experience" in combatting infectious diseases (e.g., polio, measles, Ebola and more) in the past (Bruce-Lockhart, 2020).

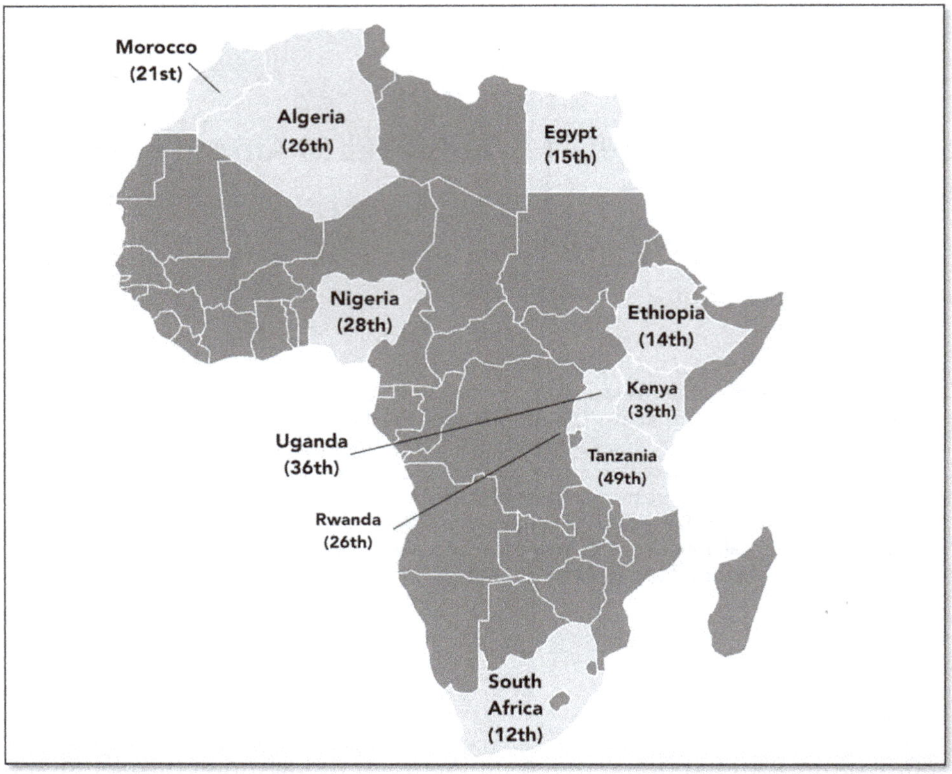

Figure 1. Africa's largest prison systems. The labeled countries in Figure 1 are among the top 50 largest prison systems globally and represent the 10 largest prison systems in Africa. See the fifth footnote (on page 9) for a closer look at the African countries' rankings (World Prison Brief, 2020).*Notes: The rankings for African countries within the top 50 largest prison systems are based on relatively current data (updated between 2019 and August of 2020); however, a few countries such as Ethiopia and Egypt have not updated their prison population data in 4 to 7 years (see Table 1).

Governments across the African region have also been credited with their rapid response to slow the spread of the virus, despite the economic cost (Bruce-Lockhart, 2020).

Notwithstanding its relatively low prevalence of positive COVID-19 cases continent-wide, certain parts of Africa have been affected more than others. For example, South Africa, Egypt, Morocco, Nigeria, and Ethiopia have borne the brunt of the virus (Worldometer, 2020). According to Coronavirus Resource Center (2020), an estimated total of 613,017 cases and 13,308 deaths have afflicted South Africa to date,[4] with Egypt at 97,619 positive cases and 5,298 deaths, and Morocco and Nigeria at over 50,000 cases (N = 55,864; N = 52,800, respectively) and around 1000 deaths each (N = 984; N = 1007, respectively; Coronavirus Resource Center, 2020). Meanwhile, other African countries like Rwanda and Somalia have reported less than 4,000 cases (N = 3,275; N = 3,537, respectively) as well as COVID-related deaths in the double-digits (N = 15; N = 95, respectively), since the inception of the pandemic (Coronavirus Resource Center, 2020).

Table 1. Africa's largest prison systems in the world's top 50.

Rank	Global Region	Country	Prison Population	Date of Most Recent Report
12	Southern Africa	South Africa	154,437	April 2020
14	Eastern Africa	Ethiopia	113,727	2013–2014
15	Northern Africa	Egypt	106,000	August 2016
21	Northern Africa	Morocco	85,767	September 2019
26	Eastern Africa	Rwanda	65,000	October 2019
26	Northern Africa	Algeria	65,000	2019
28	Western Africa	Nigeria	62,258	August 2020
36	Eastern Africa	Uganda	55,229	2019
39	Eastern Africa	Kenya	53,348	2019
49	Eastern Africa	Tanzania	35,803	December 2019

*Data were extracted from the World Prison Brief database.

COVID-19 outbreaks in countries with the largest prison populations in the African region

Some of the countries that are currently experiencing the greatest prevalence of COVID-19 infections and deaths are also home to the largest prison systems in the African region (see Table 1). According to World Prison Brief (2020), Africa accounts for 20% (N = 10) of the world's top 50 largest prison systems. Countries such as South Africa, Ethiopia, Egypt, Morocco, Rwanda, and Algeria are included in this top rank.[5] Seven of the 10 African countries found in the world's top 50 largest prison systems – South Africa, Ethiopia, Egypt, Morocco, Algeria, Nigeria, and Kenya – are also within the top 8 countries reporting the highest COVID-19 case counts across the continent (Worldometer, 2020; World Prison Brief, 2020). We have identified within-region variations in the extent of reported outbreaks of COVID-19 and the types of mitigation strategies employed in these large prison systems (see Table 2).[6]

Reported outbreaks of COVID-19 in South Africa's prisons and jails

South Africa has the largest prison population in Africa and is ranked 12th worldwide, incarcerating well over 150,000 individuals (World Prison Brief, 2020). In May, the president of South Africa announced that approximately 19,000 inmates (just over 12% of the total prison population) who are considered low-risk to public safety and have passed serving their minimum sentence periods, would be eligible for parole by mid-July to alleviate the potential threat of spreading the virus within its prisons (Mabuza, 2020). However, by July 17, 2020, just under 6,800 inmates had been released on parole, which mainly encompassed elderly individuals, those with underlying health issues, and female offenders with infants (Mabuza, 2020).

South Africa has the highest total count of COVID-19 community cases in Africa to date (Coronavirus Resource Center, 2020). Additionally, as of August 15, 2020, the Correctional Services Department of the Republic of South Africa reported 6,202 positive cases and 94 deaths among inmates and prison staff. By August 23, 2020, the department confirmed 6,448 positive cases, of which 4,116 were prison staff and 2,332 were inmates (News24, 2020). Eighty-nine percent of inmates and staff in South African prisons have recovered (News24, 2020).[7] While the virus infiltrates jails and prisons through those entering from the community (e.g., prison staff, visitors, legal representatives, etc.), it can also exit prisons in the same fashion (Ollove, 2020).

Table 2. A comparison of mitigation strategies used in Africa's prisons and jails.

Country (Rank)	Front-End	Within	Back-End
South Africa (12th)[a]	Reconsidering the sentencing of certain offenses and those awaiting pre-trial incarceration; Non-arrest for certain offenses, particularly those that are lockdown-related; Suspension of prison visitation	Designation of facilities to quarantine sick incarcerated individuals; Enhanced testing protocols for inmates and staff; Provision of PPE for inmates	Early release; Alterations to current sentencing policies; Engagement with community-based support
Ethiopia (14th)	Suspension of family and legal in-person visitation	Increased medical supplies and PPE; Increased testing	Release of 4,000 inmates who were elderly, female with children or expecting, incarcerated for minor offenses, or approaching their release date
Egypt (15th)	Suspension of family and legal in-person visitation	–[b]	Appx. 13,000 inmates released into the community between February and July
Morocco (21st)	Newly admitted inmates undergo required testing; Staff are screened prior to entering; Suspension of transportation in and out of prisons	Court hearings conducted remotely to limit inmate movement in and out of prisons	Release of 5,645 inmates in April
Rwanda (26th)	Suspension of prison visitation; Newly admitted inmates are isolated for 14 days and tested prior to integrating with general populations[c]	Limitation to staff movement outside of prisons; Frequent handwashing; Emphasis on maintaining good hygiene[c]	Appx. 3,600 inmates released into the community
Algeria (26th)	Newly admitted inmates are isolated for 14 days[d]	Some prisons have undergone isolation protocol; Movements in and out of prisons (e.g., to attend court hearings) have been suspended[e]	Appx. 15,000 inmates pardoned between February and March[d]
Nigeria (28th)	Lockdown[f]	Wearing protective equipment (masks and gloves)[f] Treatment and isolation sites within prison facilities for inmates that test positive[g]	Over 3,700 inmates released into the community[h]
Uganda (36th)	Lockdowns; Inmates are closely monitored for 2 weeks prior to transfers[i]	Received essential, donated goods from UNODC, including medical supplies and hygiene products to increase the medical response and sanitation within Ugandan prisons, as well as technology to support videoconferencing in facilitation of virtual (in lieu of in-person) court hearings[j]	Evacuating prisoners and staff who test positive to off-site treatment centers[i]

(Continued)

Table 2. (Continued).

Country (Rank)	Front-End	Within	Back-End
Kenya[k] (39th)	Temporary scale down of services and activities in the justice sector to curtail the number of offenders entering the system – the National Council on the Administration of Justice discouraged the arrest and detention of minor offenders; Suspension of visitation	Mandatory screening for all prison officers; Sanitization at all entry points; Regular disinfection of prison facilities; Mandatory quarantine of symptomatic inmates; Testing of all new inmates entering the prison system; Use of PPE; Maintenance of a well-organized shift system for officers	Aggressive program of deinstitutionalization implemented – an estimated 12,000 persons had been released from prison within a span of five months since March 2020
Tanzania (49th)	Temporary suspension of all visitation[l]	Handwashing stations installed[m]	Release of nearly 4,000 inmates into the community in April[n]

*Note: Sources regarding unmarked countries in this table can be found in the text of this article.
[a]See Kras and Fitz (this volume) for more details regarding South Africa's response to COVID-19 in its prison system.
[b]Little is known about procedures in response to COVID-19 within Egypt's prison, largely due to information blackouts.
[c]See All Africa https://allafrica.com/stories/202004010634.html.
[d]See Anadolu Agency. It is important to note that it is unknown if the release of Algerian inmates was specifically to address the pandemic https://www.aa.com.tr/en/africa/algerian-president-pardons-over-5-000-prisoners/1788147.
[e]See the Global Detention Project https://www.globaldetentionproject.org/countries/africa/algeria.
[f]See UNODC https://www.unodc.org/nigeria/en/nigerian-correctional-service-partners-with-unodc–unaids-and-eu-to-prevent-the-spread-of-covid-19-in-custodial-centres.html.
[g]See the Guardian https://guardian.ng/news/covid-19-51-medical-officers-17-inmates-test-positive-in-bauchi-state/.
[h]See the Nigerian Correctional Service https://m.facebook.com/story.php?story_fbid=295620761827295&id=101563864566320.
[i]See the World Health Organization https://www.who.int/news-room/feature-stories/detail/uganda-ministry-of-health-and-who-respond-covid-19-cases-spike-in-prison.
[j]See UNODC https://www.unodc.org/easternafrica/en/Stories/boost-to-covid19-response-in-uganda-prisons.html.
[k]See Deche and Bosire (this volume) for more information on Kenya's mitigation strategies to COVID-19 in its prison system.
[l]See Human Rights Watch https://www.hrw.org/news/2020/05/21/tanzania-prisoners-rights-ignored-covid-19-response.
[m]See Reliefweb https://reliefweb.int/report/united-republic-tanzania/covid-19-prisons-handwashing-stations-tanzania-inmates.
[n]See the Citizen https://www.thecitizen.co.tz/news/-Magufuli-pardons-3-973-prisoners-on-union-day/1840340-5534890-93usycz/index.html.

There have been conflicting reports on COVID-19 response tactics of prison administrators, depending on the source (i.e., members of the correctional department versus inmates). In Pretoria, which contains South Africa's largest correctional facility, Kgosi Mampuru II, after an outbreak of 118 inmates in mid-August, inmates accused guards of not only general neglect and brutality, but for spreading the virus while conducting unnecessary raids under fabricated allegations of contraband (Koko, 2020; Mahlangu, 2020). Inmates also alleged that social distancing is impossible (Mahlangu, 2020). A department spokesperson refuted these claims by stating that inmates within the prison were intentionally instigating prison staff as a tactic for release and ensured that necessary preventative measures had been implemented, such as isolating infected inmates and quarantining and monitoring the remaining prison population (Koko, 2020; Mahlangu, 2020). The spokesperson also detailed the current multi-pronged approach of prevention, containment, and treatment implemented across South African prisons, which includes the use of personal protective equipment (goggles, gloves, masks, gowns and more) as well as screening and testing (Mahlangu, 2020). Moreover, it was reported that over 700 additional nurses were employed to better bolster the prisons' response to COVID-19 across South Africa (Mahlangu, 2020). After months of banned visitations, on August 25, 2020, the Correctional Services Department announced the possibility of reinstituting visitations to inmates, as South Africa lifted some restrictions while moving to level 2 of lockdown measures (Mlamla, 2020).

Reported outbreaks of COVID-19 in Ethiopia's prisons and jails

Ethiopia houses the second largest prison system in Africa and ranks 14th worldwide with almost 114,000 inmates (World Prison Brief, 2020). As a country, Ethiopia has tallied 45,221 positive COVID-19 cases and 725 COVID-19 related deaths to date (Coronavirus Resource Center, 2020).[8] However, estimations of case prevalence within correctional settings have been imprecise. According to Marks and Negeri (2020), as of August 21, 2020, the Ethiopian Health Ministry would not respond with a verified number of infected inmates. Based on multiple sources, it appears that COVID-19 has been spreading throughout prisons in the city of Ziway, where 23 cases were confirmed in just two weeks (early-to-mid August); it has been reported that authorities have responded by ramping up testing (Marks & Negeri, 2020). It has also been speculated that recent spikes in positive cases within jails can be attributed to "widespread unrest" that led to almost 200 deaths and thousands of individuals incarcerated.[9] Jails reported an influx of inmates, which contributed to overcrowded conditions that were conducive to increased risk of transmission.

Despite recent rises in cases within correctional settings in Ethiopian cities such as Ziway, many initial precautions were reported to combat the virus's spread in the early stages of the pandemic. According to the United Nations Office on Drugs and Crime (UNODC, 2020), approximately 4,000 inmates who were elderly, female with children or expecting, incarcerated for minor offenses, or approaching their release date, were released in March. Prior to release, inmates were quarantined to ensure that the virus would not spread into the community (UNODC, 2020). Furthermore, the Government of Sweden, amongst other agencies such as UNODC, provided Ethiopia with essential medical supplies and PPE to aid in the effective response of frontline workers to COVID-19 in prisons and the community at large.

Reported outbreaks of COVID-19 in Egypt's prisons and jails

The third largest prison system in Africa is located in Egypt, which ranks 15th worldwide with 106,000 incarcerated individuals (World Prison Brief, 2020). To date, Egypt has confirmed almost 98,000 positive COVID-19 cases and 5,317 deaths (Coronavirus Resource Center, 2020). On February 14th, Egypt was also the first country to report a positive case in Africa (Aljazeera, 2020). As a preventative measure, approximately 13,000 inmates had been released between February and July to reduce the risk of spreading the virus (Human Rights Watch, 2020); though, critics claim that this number is far too small to effectively decongest prisons and jails, making social distancing practices near-to-impossible. Moreover, Egyptian prisons and jails were not equipped to provide sufficient medical care and had poor access to testing and symptom screening, which can be corroborated by Egypt's low testing rate (N = 1,316 per 1 million individuals, to date[10]), ranking 40th out of 57 African territories (Human Rights Watch, 2020; Worldometer, 2020). According to the Committee for Justice (2020), by August 7, 2020, Egyptian prisons had 220 suspected cases, 111 confirmed cases and 17 deaths. However, prison case counts to date have been questioned, due to perceived lack of transparency (Madhok & UNICEF, 2020).

Despite suspected outbreaks among prisons, Egypt had officially implemented a strict information blackout regarding the state of correctional sites countrywide, in addition to banning all prison visits, including meetings with lawyers, since early March (Human Rights Watch, 2020). The Egyptian government threatened to take legal action against media outlets or journalists that reported on COVID-19 in ways that departed from official statements. These intentional, isolating actions align with accusations of (and potentially reveal) corruption and mismanagement of resources allocated to respond to COVID-19, and the avoidance of transparency and accountability in these matters (Amnesty International, 2020).

Reported outbreaks of COVID-19 in Morocco's prisons and jails

Of Morocco's nearly 86,000 inmates, 5,645 were released in April as a precautionary measure (Eljechtimi, 2020). In response to hotspots of COVID-19 in some of its prisons in early July, Morocco intensified its response. For example, all incoming inmates were required to be tested before entering prison, and staff were screened before resuming their work (Mebtoul, 2020). The Moroccan judiciary continued to hold its trials remotely, rather than to transport inmates in-and-out of prisons. Three of the most affected prisons in Morocco (as of early July) were placed on quarantine to prevent further outbreaks (Mebtoul, 2020). In a similar fashion, hotspots within the community were also met with increased restrictions and augmented responses to the virus. As of August 26, 2020, Morocco had a cumulative community count of 55,864 positive COVID-19 cases and 984 deaths (Coronavirus Resource Center, 2020).

Reported outbreaks of COVID-19 in Kenya's prisons and jails

Kenya is ranked 39th in the world's top 50 largest prison systems (N = 53,348) and 8th in cumulative COVID-19 case totals among other African countries (N = 34,016).[11] Similar to other African countries, Kenya has not been immune to prison-based COVID-19 outbreaks

(Coronavirus Resource Center, 2020; World Prison Brief, 2020). In response to over 100 confirmed COVID-19 cases and 3 deaths among inmates and staff in Kenyan prisons by early April, nearly 4,000 inmates were released and monitored outside of custodial settings (Wasike, 2020). The Kenyan Commissioner General of Prisons noted that this preventative tactic was intended to achieve at least one meter in distance between inmates within prison settings to reduce the spread of the virus (Wasike, 2020).

On August 21, 2020, it was reported that a prison in Kericho, Kenya confirmed 48 positive cases among inmates and staff, which prompted a total lockdown, indefinitely suspending any members of the community from entering Kenyan prisons (Mbewa, 2020a; Rotich, 2020). This incident also prompted the Chief Justice of Kenya to address the public and propose an effective response. He announced that the judiciary would be aiding in the decongestion of prisons; however, he noted that a "fair allocation of funds" must be made available to increase the number of judicial officers and expand infrastructure for the process to be efficient and successful (Muiruri, 2020).

Reported outbreaks of COVID-19 in Uganda's prisons and jails

Uganda has reported a very small number of COVID-19 cases (N = 2,524) and deaths (N = 26) relative to other African countries and worldwide (Coronavirus Resource Center, 2020). However, this may represent the calm before the storm. On August 23, 2020, just over 150 inmates and 1 staff member tested positive in one Ugandan prison in less than 24 hours, thus spurring this Northern Ugandan prison to close for nearly a month (Agade, 2020; Mbewa, 2020b). The Ugandan Commissioner General of Prisons attributed the spike in cases within this Ugandan prison to a combination of influences, including abated lockdown restrictions, higher transmission rates in the community, and continued sentencing and incarceration (e.g., newly admitted inmates potentially infiltrating jail or prison settings with the virus, particularly in asymptomatic cases; Agade, 2020).

COVID-19 outbreaks in other countries throughout the African region

Rwanda released approximately 3,600 inmates (almost 6%) of its estimated 65,000 inmate population nationwide (Prensa Latina, 2020; World Prison Brief, 2020), while Algeria pardoned over 15,000 of its inmates between February and March,[12] which accounts for nearly a quarter of its prison population (Jibril, 2020). Interestingly, Nigeria has both a relatively small prison population size (N = 62,258) as well as total community COVID-19 case count (N = 53,021), despite that it is the most populous country on the continent (Agence France Presse, 2020).

Concluding comments

COVID-19 outbreaks in both the general community and in the largest prison systems in the African region appear to be lower than other global regions, at least during the initial several months of the pandemic. One plausible explanation for this trend is that, unlike any other global region in the world, all 10 African countries containing Africa's largest prison systems have engaged in back-end mitigation strategies with the prominent goal of reducing prison overcrowding. Nine out of 10 of the African prison systems have, to some degree, engaged in releasing thousands of inmates into the community. However, this situation may change in the coming months, as evidenced by the recent increase in reported cases in both prisons and the general community. The well-documented problems related to the pre-existence of many diseases, prison crowding, prison heath care, and prison infrastructure underscore the need to reduce the prison and jail populations in these regions, because in-prison mitigation strategies will likely be difficult to implement, due to lack of resources.

Notes

1. As of late-August (2020).
2. Not including either the Oceanic region or Antarctica.
3. Africa's total COVID-19 case count is based on data extracted from Coronavirus Resource Center on August 26, 2020.
4. As of late August (2020).
5. The African countries within the world's 50 largest prison systems include South Africa (ranked 12th), Ethiopia (ranked 14th), Egypt (ranked 15th), Morocco (ranked 21st), Rwanda (ranked 26th), Algeria (also ranked 26th), Nigeria (ranked 28th), Uganda (ranked 36th), Kenya (ranked 39th), and Tanzania (ranked 49th; World Prison Brief, 2020).
6. For more detail, see the country-specific reviews of South Africa and Kenya included in this volume.
7. As of August 23, 2020.
8. As of August 26, 2020.
9. For more detail, see Marks and Negeri (2020).
10. As of the end of August (2020).
11. As of August 26, 2020.
12. However, the Algerian president was not explicit as to whether his choice to release inmates was related to the pandemic.

Disclosure statement

No potential conflict of interest was reported by the author(s).

References

Africa: Regional cooperation needed to fight COVID-19 as cases go over one million mark. (2020, August 7). Amnesty International. https://www.amnesty.org/en/latest/news/2020/08/africa-regional-cooperation-needed-to-fight-covid19-as-cases-go-over-one-million-mark/

Agade, H. (2020, August 24). *Uganda's rising prison COVID-19 infections.* China Global Television Network. https://africa.cgtn.com/2020/08/24/ugandas-rising-prison-covid-19-infections/

Agence France Presse. (2020, April 9). *Nigeria to release 2,600 prisoners amid virus fears.* Barron's. https://www.barrons.com/news/nigeria-to-release-2-600-prisoners-amid-virus-fears-01586439903

Bruce-Lockhart, A. (2020, May 25). *Africa 'least affected' by COVID-19; hydroxycholoroquine trial suspended - WHO briefing.* World Economic Forum. https://www.weforum.org/agenda/2020/05/covid19-africa-hydroxycholoroquine-world-health-organization/

Coronavirus meter inside the Egyptian detention places. (2020, August 7). Committee for Justice. https://www.cfjustice.org/corona-alert/

Coronavirus Resource Center. (2020, August 24). *COVID-19 dashboard by the Center for Systems Science and Engineering (CSSE) at Johns Hopkins University (JHU).* John Hopkins University & Medicine. https://coronavirus.jhu.edu/map.html

COVID-19. (2020, August 15). Correctional services: Republic of South Africa. http://www.dcs.gov.za/?page_id=5070

COVID-19 cases top 10,000 in Africa. (2020, April 7). World Health Organization. https://www.afro.who.int/news/covid-19-cases-top-10-000-africa

COVID-19 Coronavirus pandemic. (2020, August 26). Worldometer. https://www.worldometers.info/coronavirus/#countries

Covid-19 in prisons: 89% of those infected have recovered, says correctional services dept. (2020, August 23). News24. https://www.news24.com/news24/southafrica/news/covid-19-in-prisons-89-of-those-infected-have-recovered-says-correctional-services-dept–20200823

Egypt: Apparent Covid-19 outbreaks in prisons. (2020, July 20). Human Rights Watch. https://www.hrw.org/news/2020/07/20/egypt-apparent-covid-19-outbreaks-prisons

Eljechtimi, A. (2020, April 21). *Moroccan prison becomes coronavirus hotspot*. Reuters. https://www.reuters.com/article/us-health-coronavirus-morocco/moroccan-prison-becomes-coronavirus-hotspot-idUSKCN223254

Heard, C. (2019). *Towards a health-informed approach to penal reform? Evidence from ten countries*. Birkbeck Institutional Research Online. https://eprints.bbk.ac.uk/id/eprint/27743

International partners support authorities in Ethiopia to prevent transmission of COVID-19 in places of detention. (2020, May 8). UNODC. http://www.unodc.org/easternafrica/Stories/supporting-ethiopia-to-prevent-covid19-transmission-in-places-of-detention.html

Jibril, H. (2020, April 1). *Algerian president pardons over 5,000 prisoners*. Anadolu Agency. https://www.aa.com.tr/en/africa/algerian-president-pardons-over-5-000-prisoners/1788147

Koko, K. (2020). *Deaths of prisoners spark fears of Covid-19 outbreak at Kgosi Mampuru*. Independent Online. https://www.iol.co.za/the-star/news/deaths-of-prisoners-spark-fears-of-covid-19-outbreak-at-kgosi-mampuru–adec7e46-6759-462d-a31d-5d93f837ab12

Mabuza, E. (2020, July 17). *6,791 inmates granted parole under lockdown dispensation*. Sunday Times. https://www.timeslive.co.za/news/south-africa/2020-07-17-6791-inmates-granted-parole-under-lockdown-dispensation/

Madhok, R., & UNICEF. (2020, August 24). *Imprisoned rights defenders in Egypt at 'grave risk' of COVID-19, warn UN experts*. UN News. https://news.un.org/en/story/2020/08/1070882

Mahlangu, I. (2020). *Fear as 118 inmates test positive for Covid-19 at Kgosi Mampuru II prison in Pretoria*. Sowetan Live. https://www.sowetanlive.co.za/news/south-africa/2020-08-13-fear-as-118-inmates-test-positive-for-covid-19-at-kgosi-mampuru-ii-prison-in-pretoria/

Marks, S., & Negeri, T. (2020). *COVID-19 spreads inside Ethiopian detention centers*. Voice of America. https://www.voanews.com/covid-19-pandemic/covid-19-spreads-inside-ethiopian-detention-centers

Mbewa, D. O. (2020a). *Kenyan prison put under lockdown after 48 inmates test positive for COVID-19*. China Global Television Network. https://africa.cgtn.com/2020/08/21/kenyan-prison-put-under-lockdown-after-48-inmates-test-positive-for-covid-19/

Mbewa, D. O. (2020b). *Ugandan prison closed after more than 150 inmates test positive for COVID-19*. China Global Television Network. https://africa.cgtn.com/2020/08/23/ugandan-prison-closed-after-more-than-150-inmates-test-positive-for-covid-19/

Mebtoul, T. (2020). *3 Moroccan prisons detect new cases, intensify covid-19 measures*. Moroccan World News. https://www.moroccoworldnews.com/2020/07/308254/3-moroccan-prisons-detect-new-cases-intensify-covid-19-measures/

Mlamla, S. (2020). *Fears monthly prison visits could increase likelihood of inmates getting Covid-19*. Independent Online. https://www.iol.co.za/capeargus/news/fears-monthly-prison-visits-could-increase-likelihood-of-inmates-getting-covid-19-56aca352-53b1-4596-a7ff-4ffe8f93bbc9

Muiruri, M. (2020). *CJ Maraga says Judiciary will help decongest prisons*. Daily Nation. https://www.nation.co.ke/kenya/news/cj-maraga-says-judiciary-will-help-decongest-prisons-1923508

Nkengasong, J. N., & Mankoula, W. (2020). Looming threat of COVID-19 infection in Africa: Act collectively, and fast. *The Lancet*, *395*(10227), 841–842. https://doi.org/10.1016/S0140-6736(20)30464-5

Ollove, M. (2020). *How COVID-19 in jails and prisons threatens nearby communities*. Pew Research Institute. https://www.pewtrusts.org/en/research-and-analysis/blogs/stateline/2020/07/01/how-covid-19-in-jails-and-prisons-threatens-nearby-communities

Rotich, B. (2020, August 21). *Panic grips Kericho GK Prison after 48 inmates, staff test positive for COVID-19*. Citizen Digital. https://citizentv.co.ke/news/panic-grips-kericho-gk-prison-after-48-inmates-staff-test-positive-for-covid-19-342713/

Rwanda releases some 3,600 prisoners through Covid-19. (2020). Prensa Latina. https://www.plenglish.com/index.php?o=rn&id=55842&SEO=rwanda-releases-some-3600-prisoners-through-covid–19

Timeline: How the new coronavirus spread. (2020). AlJazeera. https://www.aljazeera.com/news/2020/01/timeline-china-coronavirus-spread-200126061554884.html

Wasike, A. (2020, April 2). *COVID-19: Kenya frees nearly 4,000 prisoners*. Anadolu Agency. https://www.aa.com.tr/en/africa/covid-19-kenya-frees-nearly-4-000-prisoners/1789969

World Prison Brief. (2020, August). *World prison brief data*. Institute for Crime & Justice Policy Research (ICPR). https://www.prisonstudies.org/world-prison-brief-data

The Silver Lining in the Covid-19 Cloud: An Appraisal of Accelerated Prison Decongestion in Kenya

Mercy Deche and Conrad Bosire

ABSTRACT
Kenya, like most developing countries, has for a long time grappled with overcrowding in its penal institutions. Prison decongestion has hence been a key focus area of the penal reforms which were rolled out in 2002. The reforms have however been relegated to the back burner amidst competing priorities. When the country announced its first COVID-19 case on March 13, 2020, penal institutions were immediately identified as weak links in the containment of the pandemic. The Institutions were put on a total lockdown and de-congestion measures upscaled as a means of curbing the spread in prisons. So far, the exercise has resulted in the release of over 12,000 inmates. This paper discusses the implementation of the decongestion measures during COVID-19 amidst certain systemic challenges incidental to its implementation and how the gains from the COVID-19 period can be infused into long terms policies of prison decongestion.

Introduction

Kenya, like most developing countries, has for a long time grappled with overcrowding in its penal institutions (Langat et al., 2020). Consequently, prison de-congestion has, among other key reform areas, been a specific focus for penal reforms in the country. Whereas the prison reform agenda was rolled out in 2002, it is the current Constitution, which was promulgated in 2010, that consolidated these reforms by providing a strong constitutional foundation. Important changes included the recognition of bail as a constitutional right for all offenses. In addition, there are in place numerous laws and policies that provide for various non-custodial punishment options especially for minor offenses.

Despite the existence of laws and policies to facilitate decongestion, implementation of the same has not always been as effective as expected. The prison population has remained high and beyond what penal institutions in Kenya can handle. A 2003 report, for instance, indicated that prisons in the country, at the time, held up to 40,000 prisoners against a capacity of 14,000 prisoners (UNODC, 2011).

The prevailing COVID-19 situation has, however, led to an accelerated and rapid prison de-congestion initiative, mainly as a public health measure to control and curb the spread of the virus. Since Kenya officially confirmed its first COVID-19 case on March 13, 2020, penal institutions have been on an extremely high alert, mainly because of its high and vulnerable prison population. Indeed, given the nature and identified patterns of spread of COVID-19, Kenyan prisons remain "high-risk" facilities (Langat et al., 2020). With confirmed COVID-19 cases approaching 40,000 and deaths steadily approaching 700, the country's Prisons Service remains cautious and vigilant. So far, not a single case of COVID-19 has been reported among the general prison population of over 40,000 inmates. The few cases reported in the media are from the quarantine facilities that have been established to temporarily hold new inmates for fourteen days pending their release to the general prison population (Kenya Prison Service, 2020a).

The relative success of the Kenya Prisons Service in preventing the spread of the virus in the main prisons is partly linked to the current robust prison de-congestion programme. Country statistics show that as at the end of 2019, Kenyan prisons were holding a total 53, 348 (NCAJ, 2019). However, statistics from prison authorities show that by August 2020, this number had fallen sharply to 41,155. An estimated 12,000 persons had been released from prison within a span of five months since March 2020. The majority of prison population has always been those who are in pre-trial custody. With the rapid prison decongestion programme, the majority of the current prison population (25,123) comprises those serving custodial sentences as opposed to pre-trial detention (Kenya Prison Service, 2020b).

The urgency that has been created by the COVID-19 situation has yielded a coordinated response by Kenya's justice sector, with the aim of achieving the much-needed coherence in the administration of justice. This effectiveness and early positive result lay a basis for sustained future measures. This paper, therefore, discusses the implementation of the decongestion measures during COVID-19 amidst certain systemic challenges incidental to its implementation and how the gains from the COVID-19 period can be infused into long terms policies of prison decongestion.

The paper is divided into six parts. The first part is the introduction which is followed by an overview of the normative and constitutional framework of prison decongestion programs. This then gives way to part three which provides a background to the core subject by discussing the decongestion initiatives before the COVID-19 pandemic. Part four unpacks the modalities that have been put in place for the rapid decongestion of prisons during COVID-19 crisis. This is followed by the identification of the silver lining in the "COVID-19 cloud" and thereafter the conclusion. The information in this paper is mainly from desk research of primary and secondary data sourced from the library and from the database of various justice sector entities. Unpublished, but publicly available data and information, on file with the authors, which has come into possession of the authors in the course of their official engagement with the justice sector, has also been utilized.

The normative and constitutional framework for Kenya's prison de-congestion programs

The phrase "prison de-congestion" has gained currency and prominence in prison reform debates albeit with vagueness and lack of clarity. Indeed, use of the term has received criticism for not only overshadowing the broader penal reforms initiatives, but for over simplification of a complex issue to mere reduction of numbers in prisons (Nairametrics, 2011). However, the comparative use of the term, which typically goes beyond reduction of numbers, implies the totality of state obligations with regard to penal reform. It thus provides a clear lens and standard against which the effectiveness of penal reform can be measured. Applying that broader approach, prison decongestion can be used and appropriated within the context of access to justice. This is premised on the fact that persons who are held within prison facilities, whether on pre-trial detention or serving sentences, have certain rights, including access to justice. For instance, while the former Constitution precluded bail from persons accused of capital offenses, such as murder or robbery with violence, the 2010 Constitution now guarantees the right to bail for all accused persons, regardless of the offense committed. The exercise of such a right and adherence to this constitutional provision has a direct bearing on prison population, especially since majority of the prison population has always been pre-trial detainees (UNODC, 2013).

Apart from access to justice, other rights in the bill of rights section of the constitution reinforce the case for decongestion. As earlier observed, congestion creates an environment where the inherent rights of prisoners are likely to be abrogated. Griffiths and Murdoch (2009) observe that prison congestion:

> 'has a negative impact on the quality of nutrition, sanitation, programmes, health services, activities for prisoners, and the care for vulnerable prisoners or prisoners with special needs. It affects the physical and mental wellbeing of all prisoners, generates prisoner tension and violence, exacerbates existing mental and physical health problems and poses immense management challenges.'

From the above, it is clear that whereas congestion fraternizes with scarcity of resources as they are spread thin across the bloated numbers, decongestion invariably enhances the ability of the state to adequately meet its human rights obligations to persons held in lawful restriction.

Kenya's legal system is replete with constitutional and legislative provisions that are available to courts and other criminal justice sector institutions as appropriate tools to manage the numbers of those held in the penal institutions and thereby achieve their decongestion. As stated above, all offenses in Kenya are now bailable unlike under the previous constitutional dispensation where persons charged with capital offenses (such as murder and robbery with violence) were not entitled to bail. Pre-trial bail is therefore a constitutional right and it may only be denied where there are compelling reasons to do so. This right is reiterated in section 123 of the Criminal Procedure Code (2010) and unpacked in the Bail and Bond Policy Guidelines (2015). In addition, the Constitution explicitly provides that a person charged with an offense that is punishable by a fine or imprisonment of less than six months should not to be remanded in custody. Traditionally, inmates awaiting trial or appeals in custody have always outnumbered those serving custodial sentences. Bail is therefore a factor that indirectly contributes to the high number of persons remanded in custody, resulting in more prison congestion.

Beyond bail and bond, there are other entry points in the legal and policy framework meant to achieve the broad objective and purpose of prison decongestion. Where one is convicted of an offense at the end of a trial or on their own plea of guilt, the Penal Code provides for a raft of options beyond custodial sentences. These include fines, Community Service Orders, Probation Orders, and discharge.

The punishment of Community Service Orders (CSOs) is provided for and regulated by the Community Service Orders Act, which was enacted in 1998 and came into force in 1999. CSOs generally entail unpaid public work within a community for those who are found guilty of specified categories of offenses. Under section 3 of the CSOs Act, such community service is usually imposed where the offender is convicted of an offense punishable by imprisonment for a term not exceeding three years, with or without the option of a fine. They are therefore appropriate for minor offenses such as: being drunk and disorderly, petty theft, assault, creating disturbance, and being in possession of illicit brew. The assigned work has typically included activities such as afforestation, environmental protection, construction, and maintenance of public roads. Useful tangible public projects such as afforestation/tree planting, construction of public utilities such as toilets, and farming (for example, fish and poultry keeping) have been realized through the CSO sentences. (UNODC, 2013). In *Gilbert Mwangi Kiai v Republic* ([2017] eKLR), the court underscored the importance and essence of CSOs as follows:

> The Community Service Order is therefore not meant to be an easy way out of a serious sentence. It is the sentence that ensures that an offender serves his sentence within his or her community, while going on with his or her normal life. It is a path to complete reintegration of an offender, who may even have committed a serious offence and who is on the way to recovery. It is the one sentence that is expected to grow the trust of the *Mwananchi* (ordinary citizen) that the Criminal Justice System works. That is why the offender is to do public work, in the eyes of the community he offended, as a form of payback, for the benefit of the community, while benefitting from its non-custodial nature. It is a serious sentence and must be accorded its place, because in addition it saves tax payers the money spent incarcerating offenders, reducing contamination by serious offenders and congestion in the prison (*Gilbert Mwangi Kiai v Republic*, 2017).

CSOs is therefore an important tool. It not only contributes in decongestion. It also assists in ensuring that offenders are afforded a chance to carry out work with a great potential of ensuring re-integration to the society.

Probation of Offenders Act (2012) affords the courts power to issue probation orders, either as a sentence or in lieu of sentence, under certain circumstances. Unlike the Community Service Order, the Probation Order does not require the offender to render community service. It requires a person to submit themselves to the supervision of a probation officer for a period between six months and three years. In addition, it contains conditions such as residence and movement restrictions and the requirement that the offender refrains from offending.

For those already serving custodial sentences, section 46 of the Prisons Act (2009) provides for remission of one-third of their sentences. This is available through industry and good conduct to those sentenced for a period exceeding one month. It however excludes those sentenced to life imprisonment, those serving sentences for the offense of robbery, and those detained at the President's pleasure. The issue as to whether remission is a function of the Prisons Service or the court has often arisen. The court has recently clarified in *Francis Opondo v Republic* [2017] eKLR), that the power of remission lies with the Prison's authorities and not the court.

Another opportunity for convicted inmates to leave prison is found in Article 133 of the Constitution. The provision empowers the President, on advice of the Power of Mercy Advisory Committee (POMAC) to intervene in the case of a person convicted of an offense. The intervention may be through granting them a free or conditional pardon, substituting their punishment for a lesser form, or remitting the whole or part of their punishment. The enabling statute is the Power of Mercy Act enacted in 2011, which establishes the Power of Mercy Advisory Committee.

Kenya's obligation to implement prison decongestion extends to certain regional and international obligations that Kenya is party to. Article 2(5) of the Constitution provides that any treaty or convention ratified by Kenya shall form part of the law of Kenya under the Constitution. There are various international instruments that provide for prison decongestion measures, and which provide an additional layer of accountability and obligation for the Kenyan state to ensure prison decongestion is effectively implemented. Specific instruments include: the UN Standard Minimum Rules for Non-custodial Measures (the Tokyo Rules), The Kampala Declaration on Prison Conditions in Africa (1996), the Kadoma Declaration on Community Service Orders in Africa (1997), and the Ouagadougou Declaration on Accelerating Prison and Penal Reform (2002). In addition, the Standard Minimum Rules for the Treatment of Prisoners sets standards that are consistent with decongestion. These include provision of accommodation that meets health requirements and in particular the cubic content of air, floor space, and ventilation.

There is no doubt that the Kenyan state has a normative and public duty to implement prison decongestion as part of the broader penal reform initiative. This is not to minimize the necessity and place of physical custody as a form of punishment and restraint. It should be interpreted and constructed as part of a wider framework of an appropriate state response in the balancing of rights and obligations and ensuring access to justice. COVID-19 has, no doubted, presented an opportunity to test the existing legal and policy frameworks and laws put in place to ensure prison decongestion. Before analyzing the rapid implementation of decongestion measures in response to the pandemic, it is important to review the factors and effectiveness of prison decongestion before COVID-19.

Implementation of prison decongestion programmes prior to March 2020

As discussed in the section above, Kenya has always had in place a constitutional, legal, and policy framework to facilitate prison decongestion. The implementation and uptake of the framework has however not had any discernible impact on the prison population over the years. This is evident from the numbers held in Kenyan prisons since the commencement of the prison decongestion programme. An Analysis conducted between 2000 and 2016 reveals little change in prison population during these years as indicated in the Table 1 below. Indeed, even the prison population rate (prisoners per 100,000) remains comparatively high. This may be indicative, among other factors, of unsatisfactory uptake of the opportunities for decongestion provided by the existing framework.

Table 1. Prison population trends 2000–2019.

Year	Prison population	Prison population rate
2000	40,100	129
2002	35,157	108
2004	52,000	150
2006	47,036	129
2008	46,150	119
2010	49,757	122
2012	52,000	121
2014	54,579	122
2016	50,900	108
2019	53, 348	105

Source: https://www.prisonstudies.org/country/kenya (with 2019 statistics added by authors).

The narrative remains unchanged even viewed from a different perspective. The Community Service Orders programme reveals a declining number of referrals for community service (Judiciary, 2018/2019). This may be indicative of the courts' preference for custodial sentences even where non-custodial options are available. Other reasons behind the declining referrals may be lack of operationalization of the governance structures established under the CSOs Act, coupled with other administrative inefficiencies and inadequate funds to support programmes, leading to the general ineffectiveness.

While the option of Probation Orders also has the potential for prison decongestion, it faces similar challenges to those of the Community Service Orders. Probation and Aftercare Services (PACS) are generally underfunded. Their services are often hampered by a shortage of human and financial resources required to support the probation function. In many cases, court decisions are made without probation reports due to the lack of capacity in the probation department to prepare reports in time. There are also reported cases of attacks on probation officers in the course of carrying out social inquiries in the community which hampers their work (Judiciary, 2018/2019). The potential of probation services to contribute to prison decongestion has hence not been optimized.

While the Power of Mercy that is exercised by the President is one of the measures to ensure prison decongestion, the slow progress in implementation of the Advisory Committee recommendations has proved a major challenge. For instance, whereas the committee had recommended the release of a total of 18,956 prisoners in the period between 2011 and 2014 only 7000 convicts were released (*Aloise Onyango Odhiambo & 2 others v Attorney General & another* [2019] eKLR). The exercise of the power of mercy is, nonetheless, a viable route to achieve prison decongestion, where appropriate.

From the foregoing, the pre-Covid 19 uptake of prison decongestion initiatives was of negligible impact on the prison population. It has taken intentional concerted effort of all the stakeholders in the criminal justice system to achieve the results which are now evident. These have been achieved through the modalities discussed in the following section.

Rapid implementation of prison decongestion during the Covid 19 pandemic

The first COVID-19 case in the Kenya was first announced on 14th March 2020. The following day, Kenya's justice sector institutions met under the auspices of the National Council on the Administration of Justice (NCAJ, 2020a). Before delving into the modalities of the rapid implementation of prison decongestion measures, it is important to provide a picture of the operations of the NCAJ, under whose supervision and control, the decongestion measures were carried out. The NCAJ is a high-level policy-making organ that brings together critical state and non-state actors in the justice sector in order to ensure coordination, coherence, and harmony in the administration of justice. It is established under national legislation (Judicial Service Act, 2011). It has representation from the Judiciary (with the Chief Justice and the Chief Registrar of the Judiciary as the chair and secretary, respectively), Director of Public Prosecutions, Police Service, Prisons Service, Probation and Aftercare Services, Department of Children Services, the Kenyan Bar, the Executive, and Non-Governmental Organizations. Section 35 of the Judicial Service Act outlines the core responsibilities of the NCAJ to include the formulation and development of policies and strategy for the administration of justice, and the mobilization of resources to assist in the administration of justice.

The NCAJ is devolved to the smallest unit at court station level as Court User Committees (CUCs). The CUCs are typically composed of justice sector agencies at the court level who assist in decentralized decision-making in the administration of justice. CUCs have been established at each of the 128 court stations in the country, and are headed by the head of court station. At the county level, the CUCs are headed by the Presiding Judge in the county. A CUCs manager, appointed by the Judicial Service Commission and based at the Secretariat of the NCAJ, assists in coordinating the major activities of the CUCs and compiles quarterly reports of activities undertaken by CUCs. The quarterly reports assist the NCAJ to distil and understand specific issues in the administration of justice for purposes of crafting appropriate policy responses to ensure effectiveness and efficiency.

Prior to the establishment of the NCAJ in 2011, the justice sector had no formal coordination mechanism that congregated the wide players in the justice sector under a common and concrete structure for policy-making. The closest that the justice players came to coordinated engagement was through the Governance, Justice, Law and Order Sector (GJLOS). This was a donor basket fund, of an *ad hoc* nature, which directly implemented justice sector activities in partnership with justice sector agencies (McCormick et al., 2007). The programs and activities of GJLOS were mainly donor-driven, which proved unsustainable in the long-run. In addition, they took the approach of direct implementation of activities and, thus, denied justice sector agencies development of internal capacities to undertake activities that the GJLOS was performing. The NCAJ, on the other hand, does not take over or directly implement activities of the respective council member agencies. Instead, the main emphasis and approach is policy formulation on cross-cutting justice sector issues, such as prison decongestion. This approach has assisted in ensuring effective coordination of justice sector issues, including the prison decongestion measures.

It was therefore under the auspices of the NCAJ that the collective decision to temporarily scale down services and activities in the justice sector, after the confirmation of the first COVID-19 case was arrived at. The decision was announced by the Chief Justice in his capacity as the chairperson of the NCAJ. The down-scaling was for an initial period of thirty days and was meant to allow the institutions time to monitor developments and put in place measures that would guarantee the safety of those working in the justice sector as well as members of the public (NCAJ, 2020a). In addition, the Chief Justice announced the formation of a sub-committee, chaired by the President of the Court of Appeal, to review the developing situation and make proposals to the NCAJ regarding administration of justice (NCAJ, 2020b).

The immediate concern for the Kenya Prisons Service (KPS), was the congestion in all the 129 prisons across the country and the need to take immediate measures to reduce the congestion. The same concern was expressed by the National Police Service with respect to the holding cells in the police stations across the country. In response to this, the NCAJ made a collective decision directing heads of police stations to administer police bonds for minor offenses and to ensure a minimal number of persons are held in police custody during the COVID-19 period (NCAJ, 2020a). For the prison authorities, the immediate reaction was to suspend all new admission to prison facilities (Kenya Prisons Service, 2020a). This decision was, however, untenable. This is because while the NCAJ Guidelines discouraged the arrest and detention of minor offenders, they made no provision for serious offenses (NCAJ, 2020a). The COVID-19 period has seen a sharp rise in serious offenses especially gender-based violence offenses like intimate partner violence, rape, and defilement (Kombuthi-Kuria, 2020). Such offenses are not subject to police bond or bail. As a result, the decision to close all prison facilities to newcomers had the potential of transferring the congestion to police stations, which are not typically equipped to handle large numbers of persons in custody.

In order to forestall a crisis in police stations, the sub-committee that was formed to monitor justice sector operations made a recommendation to courts, through the CUCs, to allow plea-taking in serious offenses and the admission of such offenders to prison remand facilities where necessary (NCAJ, 2020c). These special arrangements ensured that there was plea-taking in cases involving serious offenses such as murder, defilement, and rape. To ensure that new admissions do not affect the vulnerable prison population, the Kenya Prisons Service designated regional facilities as quarantine facilities, or holding centers for new admissions, before they are allowed to join the general prison population. Initially, the KPS set aside a handful of these quarantine facilities to handle the new admissions. With time, this proved inadequate necessitating expansion to a total of 59 holding facilities across the country (Kenya Prison Service, 2020a). Currently, the courts are required to issue committal orders that are specific to the facilities identified for quarantine where those freshly charged with serious crimes and have compelling reasons to be denied bail are held for 14 days before they are allowed to join the general prison population.

The Prison facilities have managed to ensure zero infections among the serving inmates. The 318 COVID-19 cases detected in the Kenyan Prisons have been in the 59 holding facilities and not among the general prison facilities (Kenya Prison Service, 2020b). The success in preventing spread in prisons has mainly been as a result of the implementation of strict protocols in the management of the main prison facilities.

Other conditions put in place by the Prison authorities include mandatory screening for all prison officers (regardless of rank) and sanitization at all entry points, suspension of all visits to prisoners, regular disinfection of prison facilities, mandatory quarantine, and testing of all new inmates, use of Personal Protection Equipment (PPEs), and maintaining of a well-organized shift system for serving officers, among other measures. These conditions have ensured that there are no cases among the main prison population in the 129 prison facilities in the country (Kenya Prison Service, 2020b).

One of the earliest decisions made by the NCAJ sub-committee was to advise the High Court to review 19,000 files. The files were to be submitted by prison authorities and the review was for purposes of considering the release of deserving persons as a decongestion measure (NCAJ, 2020b). According to the National Coordinator of Community Service Orders, the Kenya Prisons submitted a list of 7,459 prisoners for sentence review during the 2019/2020 Financial Year. This covers the period when the COVID-19 cases began. Out of these 4,313 were released while 983 had their sentences reduced by 39 High Courts across the country. A further 15,433 cases were presented for consideration of CSOs out of which 15,379 offenders were placed on CSOs. The magistrates too reviewed files for accused persons remanded in custody for purposes of reviewing their bail terms. The courts then communicated the reviewed bail terms to the prison facilities where the accused persons were remanded. The prison facilities assisted in contacting their lawyers or next of kin. Those who were able to comply with the reviewed bail and bond terms were released from custody.

The upshot of the above is that while the population in Kenya's penal institutions was over 55,000 in March 2020, the number had dropped to 41,119 as at August 2020. This comprises 25,123 serving prisoners, 15,404 remandees, and 657 child offenders (Kenya Prison Service, 2020b). The categories of persons released from prisons since the onset of the Covid 19 pandemic include those who benefitted from the review of their bail terms, those serving short sentences of less than six months, and those whose longer sentences were coming to an end (remaining with 6 months or less of prison time).

There is the valid concern of the capacity of both the CSO and Probation Order systems to manage the offenders placed with them during the pandemic. The concerns stem from the fact that the systems operate within a community whose day to day processes and routines were disrupted by the pandemic. To begin with, the CSO work sites are mainly within public institutions like schools, courts, and hospitals. The CSO supervisors are drawn from the senior staff of these institutions. The schools were closed on the onset of Covid 19 while access to hospitals and courts was highly restricted. This has translated into shrinkage of available worksites for the offenders released to CSOs. For reasons yet to be ascertained, there is substantial social stigma associated with Covid 19 in Kenya. According to the immediate former National Coordinator for CSOs, M Atiang' (personal communication, September 12, 2020), most supervisors are uncomfortable with close interaction with offenders recently released from penal institutions during Covid 19. They are often wrongfully perceived as being capable of spreading the virus and shunned. The problem of scarcity of worksites for CSOs is therefore exacerbated by a shortage of supervisors.

With regard to the Probation Service Order regime, effective supervision requires access to the areas or communities that the offenders are released into. PACS however, PACS has only 84 serviceable vehicles that are shared between the headquarters in Nairobi and the 132 probation stations across the country. Their workload is heavy as during the 2019/20 Financial Year, they received 6,760 court referrals for probation supervision (SOJAR 2019/20). The already dire pre-Covid 19 situation has therefore been aggravated by the surge in numbers as a result of the decongestion program. The service is also understaffed, a situation which is likely to persist as the recruitment and promotion of 300 probation officers that was planned for the Financial Year 2019/20 did not take place due to Covid 19 related disruptions (KPAS, 2020).

Supervision of Probation Orders during the pandemic has therefore largely proceeded amidst the above resource constraints. The most viable cost-effective option has been remote monitoring by phone. Offenders with no access to phone services are required to physically present themselves to the nearest probation office periodically. Use of electronic monitoring of offenders is yet to be implemented in Kenya. Plans to introduce the same at a pilot stage in partnership with UNODC are however at an advanced stage (Probation and Aftercare Service, n.d.).

The silver lining

The pandemic has provided the much-needed thrust to decongest prisons that has eluded the justice sector players for over a decade. The fact that the system has managed to procure the release of over 13,000 inmates within a period of four months is remarkable. The first and most obvious sight of the silver lining in the overall "COVID-19 cloud" is in the numbers. Those that needed to leave prison have been facilitated to do so while those who did not need to end up there have been kept away. Only those who must be in prison for one reason or another remain. It is therefore appropriate to conclude that but for the pandemic, such accelerated decongestion would not have been realized.

Prison decongestion programs rely on multiple institutions and it is only through cooperation that results can be achieved. The rapid results mentioned above have been as a result of coordinated effective cooperation between all justice sector agencies. The respective roles played range from the review of prison records, retrieval of files from court registries, placing of files before the Court and often times tracing of relatives and next of kin to process reviewed bail. As stated earlier in this paper, the platform for the institutional coordination is provided by the NCAJ. The crisis created in the justice sector by the pandemic has given the otherwise moribund NCAJ a new lease of life. Its activities have been revamped and visibility enhanced as its meetings have attracted representation from the highest office in each organization.

The enhanced visibility of the NCAJ, through its interventions during the COVID-19 crisis is important for the institution and the justice sector generally as it holds great promise for effective national coordination on issues of administration of justice. The visibility is also timely as it coincides with proposals for reform of the Council. Proposed reforms include expansion of its membership to include representation from the legislature and Council of Governors. Other proposals include having a stand-alone statute to govern the council away from the Judicial Service Act (National Committee on Criminal Justice Reforms. The NCAJ is deemed as a platform with the potential of bringing together the heads of the three arms of government that is the President, Speakers of the two Houses, and the Chief Justice, to engage directly on issues around administration of justice (JSC, 2019). Such an engagement would be critical for outcomes which require political will like prison decongestion.

The COVID-19 crisis has illuminated the focus of stakeholders in the justice sector to hitherto unacknowledged gaps that have led to an extremely slow uptake of decongestion measures. Some of the gaps are symptomatic of lack of capacity to apply alternative sentencing. Others relate to human and financial capacity which may be addressed through targeted capacity development. Whatever their nature, the crisis presents an opportunity to identify and address these capacity gaps through institution-specific interventions.

Finally, it is clear from the rapid response that there are some institutions that need to be retrieved from the back burner to the front row due to the critical role they play in prison decongestion. This includes the Probation and Aftercare Service (PACS) and the Executive Office of the Community Service Orders. Despite the central role they play, they are grossly underfunded. In the Financial Year 2019/20, for instance, PACS was allocated a total of Ksh1,756,092,977 which is equivalent to 16,210,300 USD. Over 90% of this allocation was spent on recurrent expenditure like including salaries. The remaining 10% went into the completion of four office and two hostel construction projects (KPAS, 2020). The upshot of this is that PACS often make recommendations they have no capacity to implement as they are heavily reliant on erratic donor funding (Judiciary, 2018/2019). The National Community Service Orders Committee, which is supposed to provide policy guidance on CSOs, has not been operational since 2016 when the term of the last one expired (Judiciary, 2018/2019). Administrative inefficiencies and plain bureaucracy leads to unnecessary delay in activating the team that is meant to give guidance to the CSOs process. Other challenges, which can be traced to the lack of clear policy leadership and guidance, include: delay in gazettement of Community Service Orders District Committees, which offer supervision of implementation of CSOs. Training and capacity development initiatives have also not taken off.

Conclusion

This paper has contextualized prison decongestion within the wider initiative of prison reforms. It has interrogated it against the existing normative and constitutional framework before tracing its implementation before the COVID-19 Pandemic. The paper has established that the decongestion initiative before COVID-19 yielded scant results that had minimum impact. The paper has then discussed the initiatives that were put in place by the justice sector actors under the NCAJ and the results yielded. While the legal and institutional architecture to facilitate decongestion of penal institutions is intact, the gap is in the lack of focused implementation. The NCAJ provides a most useful platform of addressing the challenges in prison decongestion and active utilization of the platform can actually facilitate effectiveness.

It is apparent from the discussion in this paper that it has taken the COVID-19 pandemic for prison decongestion measures, which have been in place for the last decade, to be implemented to their near optimum. It is the results of the successful implementation that this paper hails as the silver lining in the "COVID-19 cloud." The gains incidental to the successful implementation are best retained, consolidated, and carried forward for posterity beyond the COVID-19 period. The starting point would be to address the gaps discussed earlier in this paper and thereafter sustain the momentum launched by the COVID-19 rapid response decongestion initiative. While it has taken a crisis to activate de-congestion measures in the prisons, the constitutional, legal, and policy gains should be identified and consolidated for longer-term action. After all, prison de-congestion is and should indeed be a long-term issue that is based on constitutional, legal, and policy foundations that go beyond a public health potential. There being no private-owned prison facilities and the state run ones being over stretched, decongestion should also not be seen as voiding punishment or undermining the core principles of criminal justice. It is an effective option of balancing justice and safety, and ultimately a sustainable way of ensuring access to justice.

Disclosure statement

No potential conflict of interest was reported by the author(s).

References

Criminal Procedure Code. (2010). s 123. Ken.

Griffiths, C. T., & Murdoch, D. J. (2009). *Strategies and best practices against overcrowding in correctional institutions.* International Centre for Criminal Law Reform and Criminal Justice Policy.

JSC. (2019). *Memorandum of the judicial service commission to the building bridges initiative.* Judicial Service Commission.

Judiciary. (2015). *Bail and bond policy guidelines.* National Council on the Administration of Justice. http://kenyalaw.org/kl/fileadmin/pdfdownloads/Bail_and_Bond_Policy_Guidelines.pdf

Judiciary. (2018/2019). *State of the judiciary and administration of justice.* The Judiciary of Kenya. https://ncaj.go.ke/wp-content/uploads/2020/01/SOJAR-REPORT-2018-_-2019.pdf

Kenya Prison Service. (2020a). *Corona virus (COVID 19) contingency measures in Kenya Prison Service (on file with author).*

Kenya Prison Service. (2020b). *Brief to the NCAJ on prison statistics, as at August 2020 (on file with author).*

Kombuthi-Kuria, J. (2020). *Domestic violence: The shadow pandemic.* The Star. https://www.amnestykenya.org/domestic-violence-the-shadow-pandemic/

KPAS. (2020). *Submission of the annual achievements and challenges of the Kenya Probation and Aftercare Service to the NCAJ (on file with the authors).*

Langat, K., Melly, J., & Nyawira, M. (2020). Impact of COVID-19 on incarcerated offenders and community reintegration challenges in Kenya prisons. *American Research Journal of Humanities Social Science, 3*(6), 55–62. https://www.researchgate.net/publication/342330224

McCormick D., Mitullah W., & Manga E. (2007). Donor proliferation and coordination in Kenya: Extent and forms, 2000–2005, paper read at Workshop on Donor Proliferation and Coordination, 26 July, Utalii Hotel, Nairobi. http://www.2.ids.ac.uk/futurestate/research/Phase2/prog3/projects/donorproliferation.html

NCAJ. (2019). *Report of the first national criminal justice reforms conference November 2019.* National Council on Administration of Justice.

NCAJ. (2020a). *Statement on the administrative and contingency management plan to mitigate COVID-19 in Kenya's justice sector of 15th March 2020.* National Council on Administration of Justice.

NCAJ. (2020b). *Statement on measures implemented by the justice sector to prevent the spread of COVID-19 of 18th March 2020.* National Council on Administration of Justice.

NCAJ. (2020c). *Statement on justice sector operations in the wake of the COVID-19 pandemic of 1st April 2020.* National Council on Administration of Justice.

Niametrics. (2011). Strategies For the Attainment of Total Prison Decongestion Within. https://nairametrics.com/wpcontent/uploads/2011/12

Probation and Aftercare Service. (n.d.). *UNODC and probation and aftercare service in joint project partnership.* http://www.probation.go.ke/news/94-unodc-and-probation-and-aftercare-service-in-joint-project-partnership.html

UNODC. (2011). *Access to legal aid in criminal justice systems in Africa survey report.* United Nations.

UNODC. (2013). *A second chance: A report on alternatives to imprisonment and the social reintegration of offenders in Kenya.* United Nations.

The Social and Environmental Implications of the Novel Coronavirus on Institutional and Community Corrections in South Africa

Kimberly R. Kras and Lincoln Fitz

ABSTRACT
South Africa is experiencing the worst outbreak of COVID-19 on the African continent. Amidst many other social and economic pressures facing the country, the surge of coronavirus cases has also disrupted operations in correctional environments. Incarcerated individuals are among the most vulnerable as they are susceptible to infectious disease due to higher rates of chronic and acute illness, close confinement, and overcrowding. Despite the advances in upholding prisoner's rights by the South African government and the pandemic responses by the Department of Correctional Services, the novelty of this virus exposes the weaknesses in systems ill-equipped to deal with a rapidly growing pandemic. This article chronicles the spread of COVID-19 in South Africa's correctional system, its response, and continued areas for improvement, highlighting the unique context of South Africa's history related to corrections and contagion.

Introduction

The year 2020 stands unforgettable as the world struggles to fight the COVID-19 pandemic. Irrespective of one's living conditions, the outbreak has negatively affected all our lives and will disrupt normal life for the foreseeable future. As the disease progresses around the globe, South Africa emerges as a coronavirus hot spot on the African continent.

South Africa is the sixth most populous country on the African continent, and 24th most populous in the world, with over 58 million citizens (Statistics South Africa, 2020; United Nations, 2019). South Africa experienced a modest economic growth by the standards of other emerging economies and is comprised of a very diverse population encompassing of a wide variety of cultures, languages, and religions (Arndt et al., 2019; Kinner & Young, 2018). The country is currently experiencing a number of challenges ranging from negative structural change, high unemployment and inequality, and persistent poverty. The high unemployment rate and poverty in rural areas have led to increased migration and population growth from the 226 local municipalities to the eight metropolitan areas. The inability of the metropolitan areas to accommodate these huge influxes has placed severe pressure on infrastructure development and the creation of uncontrollable informal settlements (Arndt et al., 2019).

In this context, the worldwide outbreak of the Coronavirus has also adversely affected South Africa. South Africa is experiencing the world's ninth highest total of COVID-19 cases and the largest outbreak in Africa, with 663,282 confirmed cases and 13,952 deaths[1] (Center for Infectious Disease Research and Policy [CIDRAP], 2020; Johns Hopkins University, 2020). Infection rates have been especially high in metropolitan areas where density limits social distance opportunities. On March 15, 2020, President Cyril Ramaphosa declared the coronavirus outbreak to be a National Disaster (Evans, 2020), and entered a nationwide lockdown for 21 days beginning midnight on Thursday, March 26, 2020 – a decisive measure to save millions of South Africans from infection (Egbe & Ngobese, 2020). The lockdown was extended through the summer, but as of September 21, 2020, the country entered Lockdown 1 Level, which eased restrictions on gathering capacities but maintained restrictions on things like sporting events (Department of Health, 2020). As added support for the country's response, the World Health Organization (WHO) deployed a 43-member, multidisciplinary surge team to South Africa on August 5, 2020, to provide necessary oversight and services to the hardest-hit provinces: Eastern Cape, Free State, Gauteng, Kwazulu Natal, and Mpumalanga (CIDRAP, 2020; World Health Organization [WHO], 2020).

The outbreak of the coronavirus has not only affected the social and economic aspects of the South African population, but all spheres of government, especially public institutions which accommodate individuals such as hospitals and correctional centers (prisons). The impact of the virus in correctional centers, which currently house over 160,000 individuals, poses serious implications for inmates and correctional officials. Since the start of the outbreak, South African correctional centers have recorded a total of 7,062 positive COVID-19 cases, 2,683 among inmates and 4,379 among staff[2] (Department of Correctional Services [DCS], 2020a). The uncertainty of the virus' characteristics and the prediction that the infection rate is most likely to peak only in September (Abdool Karim, 2020) makes South African correctional centers high-risk areas because inmates are sleeping in communal cells that accommodate ± 50 per cell. The increased infection rates in communities also make correctional centers more vulnerable as correctional officials can quickly transfer the virus to inmates.

Examining the experience of and response to the coronavirus in South Africa is also contextualized by the history of human rights in institutional settings. The United Nations (UN) Standard Minimum Rules for the Treatment of Prisoners, also known as the Nelson Mandela Rules after South Africa's most famous ex-prisoner, obliged government institutions to prevent foreseeable threats to public health and ensure that all who need vital medical care receive it (United Nations [UN], 2015). In this current time, the intersection of COVID-19 and protecting prisoner's health is all the more apparent and essential for slowing the transmission, ensuring proper health care, and ultimately protecting the public. The UN Human Rights Office has issued additional guidance on upholding the human rights of those in detention and reminding governing bodies of their mandates under the Nelson Mandela Rules (UN, 2020b).

Using data from publicly available databases, government and non-government reports and websites, global corrections resources, and news reporting, this article examines the state of the COVID-19 pandemic in South Africa's correctional system, highlighting its successes and challenges. First, we discuss the Department of Correctional Services, which operates prisons and community corrections in South Africa. Then, we consider the response to and impacts of COVID-19, as well as the current conditions of prison environment. Third, we examine the impacts of movements to release individuals from incarceration on community corrections. Finally, we consider unique issues presented by COVID-19 in the South African context.

Institutional corrections in South Africa

South Africa operates a centralized institutional and community corrections system. The fundamentals of the correctional system of South Africa derived from the Constitution (Act 108 of 1996), the Correctional Services Act (Act No. 111 of 1998) and the integrated justice system (Constitution of the Republic of South Africa [No. 108 of 1996], n.d.). In 1996, the Department of Correctional Service (DCS) transformed from a punitive military system to one aligned rehabilitation-focused practices. While safety and security remain the core of DCS, it is informed by the strategic imperatives of correcting offending behavior, rehabilitation, and correction as a societal responsibility (Government Printer SA, 2003). Under the auspices of the DCS are correctional centers and community corrections supervision.

Correctional centers (prisons)

The DCS operates 235 active corrections centers which are divided into six regions across South Africa. The country has two ultra-maximum security correctional centers, Pretoria Central and Kokstad, and two privately run centers, Mangaung in Bloemfontein (operated by British company G4S) and Kutama Sinthumule in Limpopo (operated by American company Geo Group; Byrne et al., 2019; DCS, 2020a; Makou et al., 2017). Each region is divided into different management areas that controls correctional centers in their respective jurisdictions. The correctional centers are divided into four categories: 1) remand, 2) minimum, 3) medium, and 4) maximum centers. The remand centers accommodate unsentenced individuals who are awaiting trial. The medium and minimum correctional centers accommodate mostly inmates that are in the low-risk categories whereas the maximum centers accommodate the high-risk (based on offense and behavior record) inmates. Notorious and high-profile inmates are accommodated in ultra-maximum correctional centers.

The political head of the department is the Minister of Justice and Correctional Services, who is supported by a Deputy Minister of Correctional Services. As of August 2020, the Minister is Ronald Lamola and the Deputy Minister is Patekile Holomisa. The department has about 34,000 staff who are responsible for the administration of the 235 correctional centers and community corrections offices across the country (DCA Annual Report, 2017).

There are189,748 incarcerated individuals in South Africa, the majority of whom are men (97%), and reflecting an incarceration rate of 286 per 100,000 residents (DCS, 2020b; Prison Insider, 2020a). Nearly 80% of the incarcerated population is black (DCS, 2020b). The annual cost of housing individuals in correctional centers is R133,805 (South African Rand; Prison Insider, 2020a).[3] South Africa is experiencing severe overcrowding, an overage of 29.30%, as the reported allocated bed space across facilities is 118,572 (DCS, 2020b). The main driver of overcrowding is remand detainees (pre-trial detention) which constitute 29.17% (47,526) of the total inmate population (DCS Annual Report, 2019; Makou et al.,

2017). The DCS reported that as of June 25th, 2020, more than half of individuals incarcerated were being held pre-trial (Deklerk, 2020).

The issue of overcrowding exacerbates another challenge faced by DCS: the rate of infectious disease, particularly HIV, and Tuberculosis (Beyrer et al., 2016; Makou et al., 2017). There are currently 641 Tuberculosis and 27,751 HIV reported cases in correctional centers nationally (DCS Annual Report, 2019). This dilemma is even more pronounced with the problems presented by the coronavirus pandemic. In addition to increasing positive cases, as a result of COVD-19 spread, there have been a reported 69 deaths among staff and 53 deaths among inmates[4] (DCS, 2020a). Minister of Justice Lamola stated, "We are confronted with a glaring impossibility of maintaining social distancing in our centres due to overcrowding" (Heiburg, 2020).

On March 20, 2020, DCS Justice Minister Lamola announced protocols for deeply cleaning all correctional facilities (Richardson, 2020). President Ramaphosa also suspended visitation at correctional facilities for at least 30 days to control the spread of infection into facilities (Richardson, 2020). On May 8, 2020, in a response to the United Nations' call to reduce prison populations (UN, 2020a), President Ramaphosa authorized the early release of nearly 19,000 individuals from South Africa's prisons, which is roughly 12% of the prison population (Isilow, 2020). These early releases emphasize individuals deemed low-risk and within 5 years of release, excluding individuals serving life sentences or those convicted of violent crimes, such as gender-based violence and child abuse, sexual offenses, and murder (Isilow, 2020).

Deplorable incarceration conditions

Over the course of the pandemic, reports of deplorable prison conditions have emerged. In March 2020, detainees at the St. Albans facility described inadequate protocol to disinfect the facility and allow individuals to practice proper hygiene (Kimberley, 2020a). In April 2020, journalists' reports contradicted those of the Minister of Justice, suggesting that prison officials at the "Sun City" facility in Johannesburg staged the observance of strict health protocols (Mvumu, 2020). In June 2020, reports of inmates burning themselves and others to secure placement in isolation emerged (Naik, 2020). These inmates also reported delayed testing results, staff keeping positive testing information from them, and advised that the number of staff be reduced and certain procedures be limited to lessen the exposure within the facility (Naik, 2020). In the middle of July, reports of a water shortage at the Brandvlei prison in Western Cape depicted inmates sharing a single pan of water (The South African, 2020).

Inadequate healthcare services have also plagued the DCS. The DCS is responsible for the healthcare of all persons incarcerated. In a 2017 Annual Report, DCS employed 890 nurses, 9 doctors, 42 pharmacists, and 83 psychologists and vocational counselors. But, according to recent accounts, individuals who have tested positive for COVID-19 are not receiving adequate medical care, including not being seen by doctors, not receiving medical treatment, and improper cell conditions like frigid temperatures that make the symptoms worse (Ngoepe, 2020).

Reports of unrest and riots have also emerged in South Africa. Incarcerated persons have gone on hunger strikes (Hans, 2020; Koko, 2020; Mdakane, 2020), setting fires to mattresses and clothes (Ellis, 2020; Kimberley, 2020b), engaging in damaging of prison property

(Siqathule, 2020), self-isolation and self-protection with improvised weapons (Mitchley, 2020), and most recently violence against prison officials (Singh, 2020). Inmates' complaints include overcrowding with inmates sleeping on the floor, restrictions to recreation and tobacco, a decrease in food quality, and delays in court proceedings (Postman, 2020). While some of these complaints are not new as previously uncovered by the Judicial Inspectorate for Correctional Services (see Van der Westhuizen, 2017), the coronavirus pandemic exacerbates these conditions. Most recently, on July 5, individuals incarcerated at the Sun City prison in Johannesburg and the Kgosi Mampuru Prison in Pretoria began a hunger strike to protest the alleged concealment of the actual number of sick prisoners and inadequate measures to protects individuals and staff (Koko, 2020; Makgatho, 2020). In a news story published by News24 (Gililli, 2020) about the Sun City prison, one incarcerated individual reported,

> It's a mess here to tell you the truth. We don't even have a doctor or nurses on site. We don't have PPE, we don't practice social distancing at all. The situation is very bad. People are dying, each and every day. Last week two diabetic prisoners died because they didn't get their injections. It's really bad. I even had to buy my own mask, because we are not provided with any.

Prison staff have also engaged in protests due to conditions during the pandemic. In the Voorberg prison in the Western Cape province, supervisors went on strike in response to management's unwillingness to disinfect the institution and provide support for temperature checks (Vuso, 2020). A subsequent protest by frontline officers at Qalakabusha prison in KwaZulu-Natal, demanded testing after an incarcerated person tested positive and improved temperature checks upon entry into the facility (Zincume, 2020). One area of concern for frontline staff has been the risk of exposure to family members. For example, at the East London and Port Elizabeth's St. Albans Correctional Centers, there are approximately 800 apartments on the premises where staff members and their families reside (Prison Insider, 2020b; Zuzile, 2020). Family members have expressed their concern after increased positive cases and deaths of correctional staff at the facilities. Recently, three prison staff working at the Modderbee facility died within a two-week period, generating additional fear and alarm about the inconsistent prevention measures in place (Marupeng, 2020).

Efforts to contain the virus

Prisons are epicenters for infectious diseases because of the higher prevalence of infection, the higher levels of risk factors for infection, the unavoidable close contact in often overcrowded, poorly ventilated, and unsanitary facilities, and the poor access to healthcare services relative to that in community settings. Infections can be transmitted between prisoners, staff and visitors, between prisons through transfers and staff cross-deployment, and to and from the community. As such, prisons and other custodial settings are a focus of the public health response to COVID-19.

Numerous efforts have been underway to combat transmission of the virus and adequately treat the virus, including early release, alterations to current sentencing policies, system-wide facility checks, designation of facilities to quarantine sick incarcerated individuals, and engagement with community-based support. By July 18, approximately 7,000 individuals had been released (Dube, 2020). The judicial system is also reconsidering the sentencing of certain offenses and those awaiting pre-trial to incarceration in an effort to decongest the prison population (SA News, 2020). This is due in part to the large number of financial and property crimes comprising prison sentences, and the recent estimate that 55.1% of the current population are those awaiting trial (SA News, 2020). Another judicial effort is expunging records of those who plead guilty to certain crimes committed during the lockdown. The Justice Department is considering erasing criminal records of those who are convicted of lockdown-related offenses, such as staying out after curfew as a mechanism to reduce the possibility of incarceration, having a criminal record, and the stigma of conviction (Meyer, 2020).

In April 2020, DCS Chief Operations Commissioner, Mandla Mkabela, conducted operational visits across the country to engage with staff in identifying and implementing best practices for health and safety as well as to assess levels of compliance with DCS protocols. This type of operational scan allowed administrators to "get a true picture" of the on-the-ground battle against COVID-19 (DCS, 2020c).

Special facilities dedicated to quarantining COVID-19 cases have also been established. For instance, the Barberton Medium A Correctional Center in Limpopo, Mpumalanga and North West (LMN) region is being used exclusively for the isolation and treatment of incarcerated individuals who have contracted coronavirus. While Barberton is a release center designated for low-risk individuals, during the pandemic it will house up to 100 people, increase its nursing staff, and coordinate with the local hospital to treat very severe cases of the virus (DCS, 2020i).

In addition to internal efforts to control the virus, DCS has benefitted from the support of community-based agencies. For example, the Gauteng Department of Health has provided additional COVID-19 testing support, while the local Church of Scientology supplied cleaning and disinfecting services to the correctional center offices (DCS, 2020d). Members of the organization Metropolitan, which provides staff with financial wellness support, have donated masks to staff (DCS, 2020e).

Incarcerated individuals have also been part of the effort to control the spread of the virus. In the Windhoek Correctional Center, inmates have been involved in making masks that will disseminated to other incarcerated people and members of the community (Mutanga, 2020). Parolees have also organized to contribute masks to individuals housed in the Rooigrond Medium B Correctional Center (DCS, 2020f).

Advocacy organizations have also been instrumental at improving conditions for those incarcerated and helping to reduce the prison population. While the President's release authorization of 19,000 individuals substantially reduces the prison population, the South African Prisoners Organization for Human Rights (SAPOHR) suggests releasing another 24,000 people to reduce the prison population even further (Maswaneng, 2020). SAPOHR has also demanded that incarcerated individuals with dependent children also be released (Mlamla, 2020). Similarly, the South African Sentenced and Awaiting Trial Prisoners Organization (SASAPO) has advocated for the release of incarcerated mothers to house arrest in order to slow the spread and return mothers to their children (Mlamla, 2020). In a letter penned by Edwin Cameron, Inspecting Judge of Correctional Services, and supported by a coalition of NGOs, they advocated for the early release of ill and elderly individuals (Cameron, 2020). The Law Society of South Africa has also illuminated the lack of adequate disinfecting practices and are providing legal advice to incarcerated clients, such a requesting cell changes (Evans, 2020).

Community corrections in South Africa

In the South African context, community corrections are a sub-directorate of the social reintegration component in the DCS. The purpose of community corrections is to provide services and interventions that will contribute to the reintegration of individuals as law-abiding citizens by ensuring that probationers are rehabilitated, monitored, and accepted by communities (Government Printer SA, 2003). Placement under community corrections also involves non-custodial sentence options whereby the DCS and courts can place sentenced individuals in communities as an alternative to imprisonment. There are, however, certain minimum requirements that one has to meet before being considered for this sentence options. In terms of the law, there are two alternatives to imprisonment in South Africa, namely correctional supervision and parole (Act-111-of-2008, n.d.). Parole is a discretionary placement option that is executed by the DCS to place offenders under community corrections after serving a certain portion of their sentence. Correctional supervision, or probation, is a community-based sentence which can be imposed by courts whereby individuals will serve their sentence in the community under the control and supervision of correctional officials, subject to conditions which have been set by the court or the Commissioner of Correctional Services, in order to protect the community and to prevent recidivism.

The DCS operates 218 fully fledged Community Corrections offices nationally and 201 additional service points to serve the respective communities and supervised individuals within the community corrections system. The average caseload per annum in the community corrections system is estimated at 71,573 probationers and parolees, with a daily monitoring ratio of 54,935 parolees and 15,251 probationers (DCS Annual Report, 2019). The parolee totals include 1,387 individuals awaiting trial who were placed out conditionally onto community supervision as they cannot afford bail. There are currently 1,854 personnel entrusted with the monitoring of parolees and probationers in DCS community corrections which result in 1:38 monitoring rate per supervision official–two less than the required rate as stipulated in the minimum requirement (Parliamentary Management Group [PMG], 2020).

In the wake of the pandemic and lockdown protocol, DCS has suspended physical monitoring of low- and medium-risk parolees and probationers and substituted it with telephonic monitoring. The high infection rate in certain regions across the country has negatively affected community corrections offices as some staff tested positive resulting in closure of some offices.

Community corrections are responsible for the 19,000 or so individuals expected to be released to their supervision. As of July 1, 2020, only 4,138 inmates had been released on special parole, easing overcrowding by approximately 5% (SA News, 2020). The Minister of Correctional Services cited two unmet criteria: victim-offender dialogue (VOD) and DNA samples, which are requirements before an inmate is released, as the causes for the delay (PMG, 2020). Due to the outbreak of the Coronavirus, the normal route of engagement with victims of crime cannot materialize, victims must be consulted telephonically, and some victims prefer a physical engagement with offenders. The collection of DNA prior release is also problematic due to infections rates within the South African Police Services, who are tasked with entering this information into the national database, and lockdown restrictions which limits movement of individuals within and outside of correctional centers.

The release of tens of thousands of individuals from incarceration will also place additional burdens on community corrections offices. At present, the current restrictions on community supervision practices due to the lockdown and transmission prevention guidelines will make the rapid growth of community corrections clients an incredible feat. An overburdened community corrections system will diminish the rehabilitative structures currently in place to support reentry and restorative justice practices, put community corrections officers at additional risk of exposure to the virus, and ultimately pose risks to public safety. Without innovative solutions and additional resources, community corrections may struggle to serve clients and uphold public safety.

For example, the increased caseload may prevent community corrections officers from conducting effective monitoring of probationers and parolees in communities. Prior to the lockdown, the community was already uneasy about the early release of parolees, when an 8 year-old boy was murdered by a parolee under community corrections (Kiewit, 2020). Communities also remain concerned about the increases in violent crime pre-pandemic, which mirrored trends in other countries. A recent annual crime statistics report by the South African Police Service (see Table 1) with information from April 2019 to March 2020 revealed an increase in contact crimes such as murder (1.4%), robbery (6.1%), sexual offenses (1.7%), and common assault (2.1%) (Business Tech, 2020). While these statistics reflect pre-pandemic crime rates, the trend generated public suspicion about the release of individuals from prison when President Ramaphosa made his announcement in May. Recently, data reported by the South African Police Service from April to June 2020, 3 months into the pandemic, showed substantial reductions in crime, including murder (−35.8%), robbery (−49.8%), and sexual offenses (−39.7%), compared to the same period in 2019 (South African Police Service, 2020).

While the release of individuals from correctional centers will surely reduce the transmission of COVID-19 inside facilities, recently released individuals face many challenges upon reentry to communities also ravaged by the virus. The incarcerated population consists of individuals who come from disadvantaged areas with poor infrastructures.

Table 1. Police recorded contact crime statistics (pre and post pandemic).

	Pre Pandemic*			Pandemic		
Crime category	April 2018–March 2019	April 2019–March 2020	Percent change	April–June 2019	April–June 2020	Percent change
Murder	21,022	21,325	1.4%	5,398	3,466	−35.8%
Sexual Offences	52,420	53,293	1.7%	12,094	7,296	39.7%
Attempted Murder	18,980	18,635	−1.8%	4,575	3,487	23.8%
Assault with intent to inflict grievous bodily harm	170,979	166,720	−2.5%	37,425	22,064	41.0%
Common Assault	162,012	165,494	2.1%	36,185	25,995	28.2%
Common Robbery	51,765	51,825	0.1%	12,885	6,469	49.8%
Robbery with Aggravating Circumstances	140,032	143,990	2.8%	35,705	21,599	39.5%
Total Contact Crimes	617,210	621,282	0.7%	144,267	90,376	37.4%

Data come from South African Police Service (2020).

*While the global lockdown related to the pandemic began March 15, 2020, police data are captured monthly and are not disaggregated by week.

South Africa is currently already experience problems with social distancing in underdeveloped areas (i.e. informal settlements in metropolitan areas) to minimize the spread of the pandemic. It is possible that some proportion of the 19,000 released individuals might put additional strain on law enforcement agencies to enforce lockdown regulations.

In addition to public health concerns, the economic vitality of many communities has been diminished. While South Africa has the most robust economy on the continent, it is currently facing the highest unemployment rate at 30.1% (AlJazeera, 2020). Alongside the common barriers faced by recently released individuals, the efforts to curb COVID-19 transmission in the community remains a double threat.

COVID-19 stigma in South Africa

One unique issue around coronavirus in South Africa has been stigma. South Africa, among other African nations, has a storied history of stigma associated with infectious disease (Delius & Glaser, 2005). Infectious diseases, such as HIV/AIDS and tuberculosis, have been documented by scholars as being accompanied by social exclusion, discrimination, open hostility, and rejection by community members. The stigma associated with disease comes with both physiological and psychological effects. Stigmatized individuals may experience greater rates of mental illness or maladaptive coping (Skinner & Mfecane, 2004), as well as be less likely to seek out treatment or services which would reveal their diagnosis, to themselves and others (Murray et al., 2013; Skinner & Mfecane, 2004). While the greatest degree of stigma is associated with sexually transmitted diseases (Delius & Glaser, 2005), the recent experiences with stigma related to the coronavirus appear to reflect commonly held fears and uncertainties about a disease with unclear origins, symptoms, and impacts. In fact, scholar Baldwin-Ragaven (2020, p. 33), identified addressing the public fear about COVID-19 uncertainties as the "neglected element of the treatment plan."

The advance of the novel coronavirus in South Africa cannot be disentangled from these long-held beliefs about disease. In particular, stigma experienced by frontline workers, like corrections officer and other prison staff, due to their heightened risk of contracting COVID-19, have been discussed. In one report, corrections staff have been turned away in retail and other service establishments, and even "members of the community are pointing fingers at the brown uniform" according to an official DCS statement (Independent Online [IOL], 2020). In response to these incidences of stigma, President Ramaphosa (DCS, 2020g) issued a public address, stating,

> As a society, we have a collective responsibility to stamp out the stigmatisation of people infected with the coronavirus. There have been disturbing reports of individuals being ostracised from their communities and of communities protesting against coronavirus patients being admitted to local hospitals and clinics. This must stop.

For those 19,000 individuals being granted early release, double stigma will likely challenge the reentry process (Batley, 2020; Detention Justice Forum, 2020). The reentry process for formerly incarcerated individuals is rife with barriers to success. In addition to the responsibilities of finding housing, employment, and restoring relationships with family, the stigma associated with a criminal conviction, both anticipated and real, generates an unwelcoming environment in which to reintegrate. In South Africa, this stigmatized status may then be compounded by the status associated with having been in a correctional center during the pandemic. The concern about this added stigma is important because those who feel negatively perceived by the community because of formerly incarcerated status may be deterred from seeking treatment for COVID-19 or other health conditions (DCS, 2020h). The anticipated stigma related to both infectious disease and criminal status may exacerbate already frayed relationships between communities and the formerly incarcerated. It is imperative for community corrections to better assist those reentering the community in navigating the challenges of both reentry and coronavirus.

Conclusion

As South Africa faces a growing number of positive COVID-19 cases, the response to the virus in the correctional system remains particularly challenging. The widespread transmission of the virus in communities poses a serious threat to correctional centers due to the confined conditions of incarceration. People who are gathered in close proximity may act as a source of infection, amplification, and spread of infectious diseases within and beyond correctional centers (WHO, 2020). The UN's Nelson Mandela Rules uphold the human rights of those incarcerated by engaging government institutions to prevent foreseeable threats to public health and ensure that all who need vital medical care receive it. In response the outbreak in South African correctional centers, the Minister of Justice Lamola announced several protocols to prevent or to minimize the spread of the virus, including the deep cleaning of correctional facilities, suspension of visits to correctional centers, and the early conditional release of 19,000 individuals under community corrections.

In addition to the primary health impacts of the novel coronavirus, the most notable challenge experienced worldwide in correctional centers is the ability to properly social distance. Correctional centers are considered epicenters for infectious diseases because of the higher background prevalence of infection, the higher levels of risk factors for infection, the unavoidable close contact in often overcrowded, poorly ventilated, and unsanitary facilities, and the poor access to healthcare services relative to that in community settings (Dolan et al., 2016). The overcrowding levels and population density in South African correctional centers have made social isolation almost impossible. Overcrowded cells of almost ± 50 persons per cell and the sharing of bathing facilities have placed correctional centers at risk for transmitting of the COVID virus. Information presented in this article indicates the rapid transmission of the virus after it entered correctional facilities. Contact between officials and inmates is unavoidable as it requires constant interaction on a daily basis, and infections can be transmitted between inmates, staff, and to and from the community. The prevention protocols (e.g., entry screening, personal protection measures, social distancing, cleaning and disinfection, restriction of movement, and suspension of visitation) have, to a large extent, assisted DCS to minimize the infection rate in correctional centers across the country, but more needs to be done.

The issue of overcrowding and population density exacerbates another challenge faced by DCS: the already burgeoning rate of infectious disease (Beyrer et al., 2016; Makou et al., 2017). Emerging research on the COVID-19 virus indicates that individuals with underlying conditions (comorbidities) are the most vulnerable to the COVID-19 virus. Multimorbidity is normative among inmates, often with earlier onset and greater severity than in the general population, and among aging inmate populations (Kinner & Young, 2018). The constellation of preexisting individual and structural conditions (individual comorbidity, overcrowding, flow of staff from community to correctional center) in correctional settings has magnified the negative implications of COVID-19 spread. The inability of DCS to isolate individuals with such comorbidities and those who are infected due to overcrowding have contributed to the high numbers of fatalities and infections that have been reported in correctional centers (Heiburg, 2020). These conditions, among others related to hygiene and basic care, also present the circumstances for unrest and accumulation of human rights violations. In response, numerous advocacy organizations, like SAPOHR, SASAPO, and the Law Society of South Africa, as well as the Judicial Inspector of Correctional Services, have rallied to support increased attention and resources to this vulnerable population.

The response of the Minister Lamola and the call of the United Nations to reduce prison populations (UN, 2020a), have assisted DCS in dealing with overcrowded centers and establishing protocols to slow the number of infections in correctional centers. The early release of nearly 19,000 low-risk inmates from South Africa's correctional centers, which is roughly 12% of the prison population, was necessary given the circumstances in which inmates were incarcerated. The execution of this decision has been problematic because since the initial decision in May 2020, DCS has only managed to release only about 7,000 individuals (Dube, 2020). The slow release of individuals results from the lack of resources and capacity in the community to handle to proper supervision and support of these individuals, especially related to DNA collection, engagement in restorative justice practices, and other forms of reentry support. In particular, the burden placed on community corrections offices to rapidly acclimate to supervising so many additional individuals is an unmet reality. Without additional support, this shift may compromise the success of released individuals and public safety.

As disease transmission progresses, the South African government, and particularly DCS, continues its efforts to control the impacts of the virus and support the healthy integration of individuals from prison to the community while also establishing the security, safety, and treatment of those who remain incarcerated. Fortunately, there has been substantial slowing in positive cases, and especially fatalities, affording both institutional and community corrections the opportunity to steady the response to the virus.

Notes

1. As of September 23, 2020.
2. As of September 22, 2020.
3. This amount is equivalent to $7,775 US dollars or $6,542 Euro.
4. As of September 22, 2020.

Disclosure statement

No potential conflict of interest was reported by the author(s).

References

Abdool Karim, S. S. (2020). The South African response to the pandemic. *New England Journal of Medicine, 382*(24), 95. https://doi.org/10.1056/NEJMc2014960

AlJazeera. (2020, June 23). *South Africa's unemployment rate hits record high*. Reuters. https://www.aljazeera.com/ajimpact/south-africa-unemployment-rate-hits-record-high-200623154110111.html

Arndt, C., Davies, R., & Thurlow, J. (2019). *Urbanization, structural transformation and rural-urban linkages in South Africa. 35*. International Food Policy Research Institute, National Treasury. https://csp.treasury.gov.za/Resource%20_Centre/Conferences/Documents/Urbanization%20Review%20Papers/Paper%203%20-%20RSA%20Urbanization.pdf

Baldwin-Ragaven, L. (2020). Social dimensions of COVID-19 in South Africa: A neglected element of the treatment plan. *Wits Journal of Clinical Medicine, 2*(SI), 33. https://doi.org/10.18772/26180197.2020.v2nSIa6

Batley, M. (2020, May 8). *Why the release of 19,000 prisoners is a good thing*. The Daily Maverick. https://www.dailymaverick.co.za/article/2020-05-18-why-the-release-of-19000-prisoners-is-a-good-thing/

Beyrer, C., Kamarulzaman, A., & McKee, M. (2016). Prisoners, prisons, and HIV: Time for reform. *The Lancet, 388*(10049), 1033–1035. https://doi.org/10.1016/S0140-6736(16)30829-7

Businesstech. (2020, July 31). *South Africa crime stats 2020: Everything you need to know*. https://businesstech.co.za/news/government/421424/south-africa-crime-stats-2020-everything-you-need-to-know/

Byrne, J., Kras, K. R., & Marmolejo, L. M. (2019). International perspectives on the privatization of corrections. *Criminology & Public Policy, 18*(2), 477–503. https://doi.org/10.1111/1745-9133.12440

Cameron, E. (2020, April 20). *Open letter to minister of correctional services Lamola*. Detention Justice Forum. https://www.groundup.org.za/media/uploads/documents/JICS_DJF%20COVID-19%20release%20of%20prisoners_23%20April%202020%20djf-1.pdf

"DCS-Act-111-of-2008.pdf". (n.d.). http://www.dcs.gov.za/wp-content/uploads/2016/08/DCS-Act-111-of-2008.pdf

"Constitution of the Republic of South Africa [No. 108 of 1996]". (n.d.). (38):107.

Center for Infectious Disease Research and Policy. (2020). *Novel coronavirus (COVID-19) resource center*. University of Michigan. https://www.cidrap.umn.edu/covid-19

Deklerk, A. (2020, June 25). *Awaiting-trial prisoners hogging jail space: Lamola*. TimeLive. https://www.timeslive.co.za/politics/2020-06-25-awaiting-trial-prisoners-hogging-jail-space-lamola/

Delius, P., & Glaser, C. (2005). Sex, disease and stigma in South Africa: Historical perspectives. *African Journal of AIDS Research, 4*(1), 29–36. https://doi.org/10.2989/16085900509490339

Department of Correctional Services. (2017). *DCS annual report 2016-2017*. https://nationalgovernment.co.za/department_annual/176/2017-department:-correctional-services-annual-report.pdf

Department of Correctional Services. (2019). *DCS annual report 2018-2019*. http://www.dcs.gov.za/wp-content/uploads/2019/12/DCS-Annual-Report-_web-version.pdf

Department of Correctional Services. (2020a). http://www.dcs.gov.za/

Department of Correctional Services. (2020b). *DCS in numbers*. http://www.dcs.gov.za/?page_id=4601

Department of Correctional Services. (2020c). *Let's hold hands together and find better ways to fight the coronavirus, says chief operations commissioner*. http://www.dcs.gov.za/?page_id=5592

Department of Correctional Services. (2020d). *Kgoši Mampuru II management area forges ahead with efforts to combat spread of COVID-19*. http://www.dcs.gov.za/?page_id=5507

Department of Correctional Services. (2020e). *Metropolitan donates cloth face masks to DCS as part of youth month*. http://www.dcs.gov.za/?page_id=5612

Department of Correctional Services. (2020f). *Parolees join fight against Covid-19*. http://www.dcs.gov.za/?page_id=5600

Department of Correctional Services. (2020g). *President Ramaphosa calls for an end to stigmatization amid rising coronavirus cases*. http://www.dcs.gov.za/?page_id=5734

Department of Correctional Services. (2020h). *Western Cape amplifies fight against Covid-19 stigmatisation*. http://www.dcs.gov.za/?page_id=5608

Department of Correctional Services. 2020i. *Construction of quarantine centre for Mpumalanga inmates underway*. http://www.dcs.gov.za/?page_id=5688

Department of Health. (2020). *Disaster management act regulations: Alert level 1 during coronavirus COVID-19 lockdown*. https://sacoronavirus.co.za/2020/09/18/disaster-management-act-regulations-alert-level-1-during-coronavirus-covid-19-lockdown/

Department of Statistics South Africa. (2020). *Mid-year population estimates*. Stats South Africa. http://www.statssa.gov.za/publications/P0302/P03022020.pdf

Detention Justice Forum. (2020, May 12). *Open letter to the minister of correctional services*. Restorative Justice Center. https://www.facebook.com/RestoreSA/posts/10157321685417253?__xts__[0]=68.ARBNEH0o6_vveJ7L4Wtn06wiuq7AmcALzjaMNPC-BlPFepAQAOdTx2OMJe_qqsVH7UE9g75FxrDg2YjkIG-cd3x6xXqjaDA4hSzUFszck6zx4–zzRytR7xDHGqHdpXODwc-8gN1Uy6orCpz31ywjpMFmxA7XdobWBRy2Ciz4be0XE_wQcBfn7RjVFZxiBGzYr0lEEwdBf0PNSmz3kkSw7pkf20OYffsh5-go49jxFeJQrjLXTCv0pFZ_RKCDPrhPzDMBMvpZ5YUmIjW_Bghgzn9UoarW8-qw5BUoHmYLhBB5OdTp_8kQKetOKCJpURdsiQWfRxPCByqdw

Dolan, K., Wirtz, A. L., Moazen, B., Ndeffo-mbah, M., Galvani, A., Kinner, S. A., Courtney, R., McKee, M., Amon, J. J., Maher, L., Hellard, M., Beyrer, C., & Altice, F. L. (2016). Global burden of HIV, viral hepatitis, and tuberculosis in prisoners and detainees. *The Lancet*, *388*(10049), 1089–1102. https://doi.org/10.1016/S0140-6736(16)30466-4

Dube, P. (2020, July 18). Covid-19: South Africa releases 7,000 inmates to decongest prison. *Daily Nation*. https://www.nation.co.ke/kenya/news/africa/covid-19-south-africa-releases-7-000-inmates-to-decongest-prisons-1900922

Egbe, C. O., & Ngobese, S. (2020, May 18). COVID-19 lockdown and the tobacco product ban in South Africa. *Tobacco Induced Diseases*, *18*(May), 39–40. https://doi.org/10.18332/tid/120938

Ellis, E. (2020, April 23). *Prison riots about cellphones and cigarettes not coronavirus, authorities claim*. The Daily Maverick. https://www.dailymaverick.co.za/article/2020-04-23-prison-riots-about-cellphones-and-cigarettes-not-coronavirus-authorities-claim/

Evans, J. (2020, March 21). Coronavirus: Law society sounds alarm over the slow pace of sanitising courts, prisons. *News24*. https://www.news24.com/news24/southafrica/news/coronavirus-law-society-sounds-alarm-over-the-slow-pace-of-sanatising-courts-prisons-20200321

Gililli, C. (2020, July 31). Prisoners fear for their lives at Sun City as Covid-19 wave spreads. *News24*. https://www.news24.com/news24/southafrica/news/prisoners-fear-for-their-lives-at-sun-city-as-covid-19-wave-spreads-20200730

Government Printer SA. (2003). *Draft White paper on corrections in South Africa. V. 2006*. Department of Correctional Services. https://www.gov.za/sites/default/files/gcis_document/201409/correct1.pdf

Hans, B. (2020, June 20). *'Nudity, hunger strike' expected in prisons over visitation ban induced by the coronavirus*. Independent Online. https://www.iol.co.za/saturday-star/news/nudity-hunger-strike-expected-in-prisons-over-visitation-ban-induced-by-the-coronavirus-49653234

Heiburg, T. (2020, May 8). *South Africa to parole 19,000 prisoners to curb coronavirus*. Reuters. https://www.reuters.com/article/us-health-coronavirus-safrica/south-africa-to-parole-19000-prisoners-to-curb-coronavirus-idUSKBN22K1I8

Independent Online. (2020, May 5). *Prison staff being turned away from shops because of Covid-19 stigma*. https://www.iol.co.za/news/south-africa/prison-staff-being-turned-away-from-shops-because-of-covid-19-stigma-47586967

Isilow, H. (2020, May 8). *COVID-19: South Africa grants parole to 19,000 inmates*. Andalou Agency. https://www.aa.com.tr/en/africa/covid-19-south-africa-grants-parole-to-19-000-inmates/1833867

Johns Hopkins University. (2020). *Coronavirus resource center*. https://coronavirus.jhu.edu/map.html

Kiewit, L. (2020, March 4). South Africa's parole system has failed child victims. *Mail & Guardian*. https://mg.co.za/article/2020-03-04-south-africas-parole-system-has-failed-child-victims/

Kimberley, K. (2020a, March 28). St Albans prison a ticking time bomb. *Daily Dispatch*. https://www.dispatchlive.co.za/news/2020-03-28-st-albans-prison-a-ticking-time-bomb/

Kimberley, K. (2020b, May 6). Frustrated inmates at St Albans set fire to parts of the building. *Herald Live*. https://www.heraldlive.co.za/news/2020-05-06-watch-frustrated-inmates-at-st-albans-set-fire-to-parts-of-the-building/

Kinner, S. A., & Young, J. T. (2018). Understanding and improving the health of people who experience incarceration: An overview and synthesis. *Epidemiologic Reviews, 40*(1), 4–11. https://doi.org/10.1093/epirev/mxx018

Koko, K. (2020, July 8). *Riots erupt in prisons as inmates say they fear getting Covid-19*. Independent Online. https://www.iol.co.za/the-star/news/riots-erupt-in-prisons-as-inmates-say-they-fear-getting-covid-19-50597004

Makgatho, L. (2020, July 11). *Riots erupt in prisons as Covid-19 infections rise*. Independent Online. https://www.iol.co.za/sundayindependent/news/riots-erupt-in-prisons-as-covid-19-infections-rise-50868586

Makou, G., Skosana, I., & Hopkins, R. (2017, July 18). *FACTSHEET: The state of South Africa's prisons*. Africa Check. https://africacheck.factsheets/factsheet-the-state-of-south-africas-prisons/

Marupeng, P. (2020, July 6). Deaths of three prison warders spark health fears. *Sowetan Live*. https://www.sowetanlive.co.za/news/south-africa/2020-07-06-deaths-of-three-prison-warders-spark-health-fears/

Maswaneng, K. (2020, May 20). Prisoner rights organisation calls for release of 24,000 more inmates. *Sunday Times*. https://www.timeslive.co.za/news/south-africa/2020-05-20-prisoner-rights-organisation-calls-for-release-of-24000-more-inmates/

Mdakane, B. (2020, April 19). *Prisoners threaten hunger strike if Covid-19 fears are not addressed*. City Press. https://www.news24.com/citypress/News/prisoners-threaten-hunger-strike-if-covid-19-fears-are-not-addressed-20200419

Meyer, D. (2020, May 18). Justice department could scrap criminal records after lockdown. *The South African*. https://www.thesouthafrican.com/news/criminal-record-could-be-scrapped-after-lockdown-admission-of-guilt-2020/

Mitchley, A. (2020, June 17). Detainees face action after blocking cell, arming themselves with makeshift weapons. *News24*. https://www.news24.com/news24/southafrica/news/detainees-face-action-after-blocking-cell-arming-themselves-with-makeshift-weapons-20200617

Mlamla, S. (2020, June 8). *Covid-19 outbreak: 'Put moms in prison under house arrest'*. Independent Online. https://www.iol.co.za/capeargus/news/covid-19-outbreak-put-moms-in-prison-under-house-arrest-49114529

Murray, E. J., Bond, V. A., Marais, B. J., Godfrey-Faussett, P., Ayles, H. M., & Beyers, N. (2013). High levels of vulnerability and anticipated stigma reduce the impetus for tuberculosis diagnosis in Cape Town, South Africa. *Health Policy and Planning, 28*(4), 410–418. https://doi.org/10.1093/heapol/czs072

Mutanga, M. (2020, May 4). *Prisoners produce face masks for country*. Informante. https://informante.web.na/prisoners-produce-face-masks-for-country/

Mvumu, Z. (2020, April 12). 'Sun City' accused of staging Covid-19 preparedness 'act' for Lamola. *Sunday Times*. https://www.timeslive.co.za/sunday-times/news/2020-04-12-sun-city-accused-of-staging-covid-19-preparedness-act-for-lamola/

Naik, S. (2020, June 13). *Inmates resort to desperate measures to force social distancing in crowded prisons*. Independent Online. https://www.iol.co.za/saturday-star/news/inmates-resort-to-desperate-measures-to-force-social-distancing-in-crowded-prisons-49331172

Ngoepe, K. (2020, June 27). *Prisoners tested positive for Covid-19 say they are not getting proper medication*. Independent Online. https://www.iol.co.za/news/south-africa/gauteng/prisoners-tested-positive-for-covid-19-say-they-are-not-getting-proper-medication-50049865

Parliamentary Management Group. 2020. *Lockdown case backlogs; overcrowding & release of inmates: Minister's briefing | PMG*. Parliamentary Management Group.org. https://pmg.org.za/committee-meeting/30529/

Postman, Z. (2020, May 25). Covid-19: Lockdown makes access to justice for prisoners even more difficult. *The Daily Maverick*. https://www.dailymaverick.co.za/article/2020-05-25-covid-19-lockdown-makes-access-to-justice-for-prisoners-even-more-difficult/

Prison Insider. (2020a). *Country profile: South Africa.* https://www.prison-insider.com/countryprofile/prisonsinsouthafrica

Prison Insider. (2020b). *Coronavirus: Africa.* https://www.prison-insider.com/en/articles/afrique-coronavirus-la-fievre-des-prisons#afrique-du-sud-5e81fd6b2aacd

Richardson, J. (2020, March 20). Prisons to undergo deep cleaning to limit the spread of coronavirus. *The South African.* https://www.thesouthafrican.com/news/prisons-undergo-deep-cleaning-limit-coronavirus/

SA News. (2020, June 25). *South Africa is rethinking jail time as a punishment for low-risk crimes.* Business Tech. https://businesstech.co.za/news/government/410789/south-africa-is-rethinking-jail-time-as-a-punishment-for-low-risk-crimes/

Schnirring, L. (2020, August 5). *Global COVID-19 deaths top 700,000; WHO team heads to South Africa.* Center for Infectious Disease Research and Policy, University of Minnesota. https://www.cidrap.umn.edu/news-perspective/2020/08/global-covid-19-deaths-top-700000-who-team-heads-south-africa

Singh, O. (2020, August 13). Westville Prison wardens stabbed by prisoners after morning meal. *Times Live.* https://www.timeslive.co.za/news/south-africa/2020-08-13-westville-prison-wardens-stabbed-by-prisoners-after-morning-meal/

Siqathule, S. (2020, May 12). *Prison riot in Lusikisiki.* Ground Up. https://www.groundup.org.za/article/prison-riot-lusikisiki/

Skinner, D., & Mfecane, S. (2004). Stigma, discrimination and the implications for people living with HIV/AIDS in South Africa. *Sahara-j: Journal of Social Aspects of HIV/AIDS, 1*(3), 157–164. https://doi.org/10.1080/17290376.2004.9724838

South African Police Service. (2020). *Crime statistics.* https://www.saps.gov.za/services/crimestats.php

The South African. (2020, July 20). *Western Cape prison without water for over a week.* https://www.thesouthafrican.com/news/western-cape-prisons-correctional-services-tuesday-22-july-2020/

United Nations. (2015). *Resolution 70/175.* https://undocs.A/RES/70/175

United Nations. (2019). *World population prospects.* https://population.un.wpp/

United Nations. (2020a, March 25). *Advice of the subcommittee on prevention of torture to states parties and national preventive mechanisms relating to the coronavirus pandemic.* https://www.ohchr.Documents/HRBodies/OPCAT/AdviceStatePartiesCoronavirusPandemic2020.pdf

United Nations. (2020b). *Covid-19 human rights dispatch – Number 2: Covid-19 and protection of right to life in places of detention.*

Van der Westhuizen, J. (2017). *Annual report for the period 01 April 2015 to 31 March 2016 "people are living there".* Judicial Inspectorate for Correctional Services.

Vuso, S. (2020, May 12). *Western Cape warders strike, demand mass testing at prison.* Independent Online. https://www.iol.co.za/capetimes/news/western-cape-warders-strike-demand-mass-testing-at-prison-47876492

World Health Organization. (2020, August 5). *World Health Organization surge team to arrive in South Africa.* https://www.afro.who.int/news/world-health-organization-surge-team-arrive-south-africa

Zincume, M. (2020, June 5). *First Covid-19 case at Qalakabusha Prison in Empangeni.* Zululand Observer. https://zululandobserver.co.za/226441/first-covid-19-case-at-qalakabusha-prison-in-empangeni/

Zuzile, M. (2020, April 16). Prison officials fear for their families' lives amid Covid-19 outbreak. *Sowetan Live.* https://www.sowetanlive.co.za/news/south-africa/2020-04-16-prison-officials-fear-for-their-families-lives-amid-covid-19-outbreak/

Asia Regional Overview and Reports from China, South Korea, Pakistan, India, and the Philippines

An Examination of COVID-19 Outbreaks in Prisons and Jails Throughout Asia

Sabrina S. Rapisarda and James M. Byrne

ABSTRACT
This article highlights regional variation in the extent of COVID-19 outbreaks in prisons throughout Asia. Stark differences in the utilization of front-end, in-prison, and back-end mitigation strategies designed to prevent and control COVID-19 outbreaks in these prison systems are identified. We conclude by offering our assessment of the nature and (true) extent of COVID-19 outbreaks within countries and across the region; and in the process, we offer a tentative explanation for the large variation we have found in the response to reported COVID-19 outbreaks in prisons and communities across Asia.

Introduction and overview

Asia contains more prison systems within the world's top 50 largest prison systems than any other continental region (see Table 1). Seventeen of the 50 largest prison systems in the world are located in Asia, including countries such as China, India, Thailand, Iran, Indonesia, the Philippines, Vietnam and more (World Prison Brief, 2020).[1] We document the extent of COVID-19 outbreaks in these prison systems, and then describe the types of mitigation strategies implemented by governments throughout this region, focusing on the following countries: China, India, Pakistan, South Korea, and the Philippines (see Table 2).[2] Our review of the available data on the extent of the COVID-19 outbreaks suggests that some governments in this region (e.g., China) have been reluctant to provide estimates of the extent of the problem, both in prison and in the community. Without these data, it is difficult – and impossible – to assess the impact of the mitigation strategies that they officially report.

COVID-19 outbreaks and mitigation strategies used in China's prison system

China has the largest prison population in Asia and has the second largest prison system worldwide, incarcerating more than 1.7 million individuals (World Prison Brief, 2020). According to the World Health Organization (WHO) and John Hopkin's Coronavirus Resource Center, as of August 24, 2020, China had confirmed approximately 90,000 positive COVID-19 cases and around 4,700 deaths nationwide since the virus's initial outbreak in late December of 2019 (Coronavirus Resource Center, 2020). In late March, China reported a cumulative total of almost 82,000 positive cases (Secon et al., 2020), thus translating to a mere 9% increase in cases over a five month period (between late March and late August).

Table 1. Asia's largest prison systems in the world's top 50.

Rank	Global Region	Country	Prison Population	Date of Most Recent Report
2	Eastern Asia	China	1,710,000	2018
5	Southern Asia	India	478,600	December 2019
6	South-Eastern Asia	Thailand	379,274	August 2020
8	Southern Asia	Iran	240,000	2018
9	South-Eastern Asia	Indonesia	232,736	August 2020
10	South-Eastern Asia	Philippines	215,000	November 2018
13	South-Eastern Asia	Vietnam	123,697	2019
19	South-Eastern Asia	Myanmar	92,000	2018
20	Southern Asia	Bangladesh	88,084	February 2020
23	Southern Asia	Pakistan	77,275	September 2019
25	South-Eastern Asia	Malaysia	68,603	August 2020
29	Western Asia	Saudi Arabia	61,000	June 2017
30	Eastern Asia	Taiwan	60,956	December 2019
37	Eastern Asia	South Korea	53,920	June 2020
41	Eastern Asia	Japan	48,802	October 2019
42	Western Asia	Iraq	45,000	2015
48	South-Eastern Asia	Cambodia	36,600	November 2019

*Data were extracted from the World Prison Brief (2020).

According to Patranobis (2020), in late July, the northwest province of Xinjiang had been declared a hotspot for the virus, where at least 105 new cases were reported.

Official reports of the prevalence of COVID-19 cases within Chinese prisons have not been released since late February. Additionally, it is speculated that the Chinese Ministry of Justice was intentionally lacking transparency even prior to February when the first instances of COVID-19 were confirmed in China's prisons (Yang, 2020). Presumably, one of the first occurrences of COVID-19 amongst inmates outbroke on January 21, 2020 (Yang, 2020), despite being publicized over a month later. It is plausible that Chinese officials willingly chose to conceal information pertaining to these outbreaks in order to support public statements about the declining trend of new COVID-19 cases (Yang & Thompson, 2020). Given the size of China's prison population (1.7 million), it is certainly possible that the number of reported cases among inmates in China is substantially higher than actual counts, but we have no evidence available to further investigate this issue.[3]

In the following section, we examine the available, yet limited data on the extent of COVID-19 in Chinese prison systems and the mitigation strategies instituted to address it. As of February 21, 2020, over 500 positive cases were reported across three Chinese provinces, with more than half of these cases originating in the Hubei province and the remaining in the Shandong and Zhejiang provinces (Mahbubani, 2020; Yang, 2020). The number of infected inmates continued to rise, thus contributing to a cumulative total of 806 infections among inmates in Wuhan alone (the capital of China's province, Hubei) as of February 29, 2020 (Yang, 2020). China attributed these outbreaks, in part, to prison staff and officials' lack of willingness to be forthcoming about their own potential exposure(s) to COVID-19 (e.g., while traveling) in combination with lax management, which allowed for staff to enter facilities regardless of potential infection (Mahbubani, 2020; Xinhua News Agency, 2020a). These outbreaks led to a spike in the national count of COVID-19 cases, which triggered public fear and prompted several local officials to be fired (Mahbubani, 2020). However, Yang and Thompson (2020) recommend putting more of an emphasis on improving the prison healthcare system than on management accountability (e.g., firing). They advocate for intensified education for inmates and prison staff, increased funding

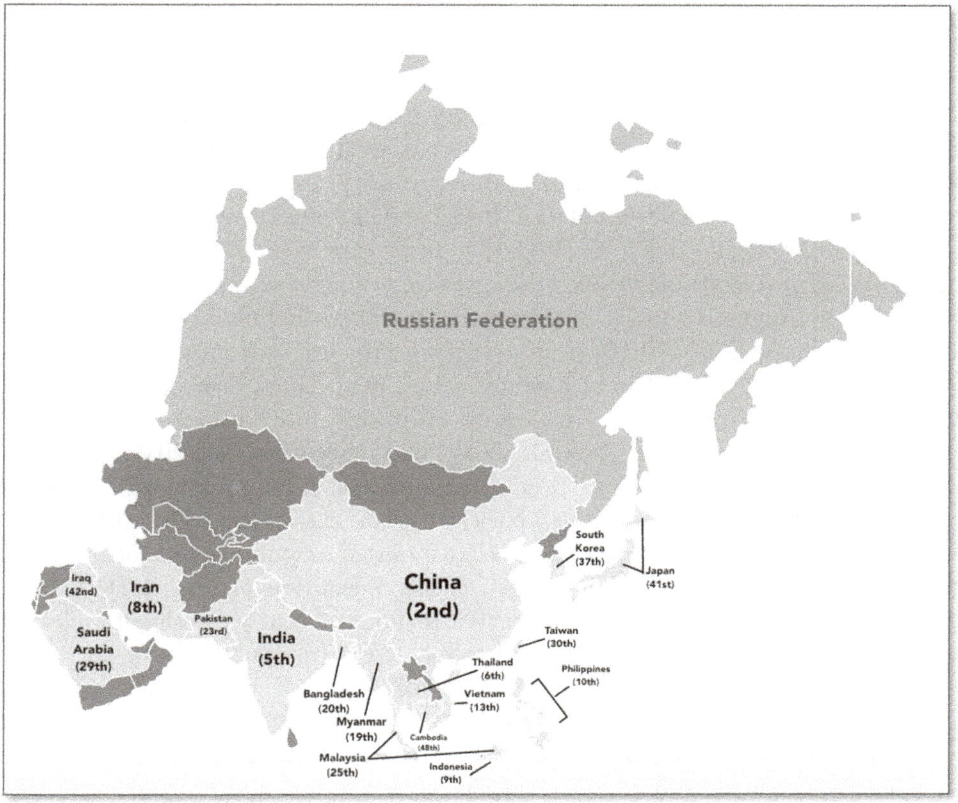

Figure 1. Asia's largest prison systems. The labeled countries in Figure 1 are among the top 50 largest prison systems globally and represent the 17 largest prison systems in Asia.*Notes: The rankings for Asian countries within the top 50 largest prison systems are based almost entirely on current data (within the past 2–3 years); however, a few countries (e.g., Iraq) have not (yet) updated their prison populations in 5+ years (see Table 1). For the purposes of categorization, the Russian Federation is included as part of Europe; however, it should be noted that the Russian Federation is a transcontinental country belonging to both Asia and Europe.

invested in preventative and treatment-based approaches, and decongesting prisons in order to reduce the potential for outbreaks.[4]

COVID-19 outbreaks and mitigation strategies used in India's prison system

India houses the second largest prison system in Asia with 478,600 inmates nationwide (World Prison Brief, 2020). Thus, it is unsurprising that India, as a country, is ranked third globally for the highest prevalence of COVID-19 cases, with 3,106,348 positive cases and 57,542 deaths so far (as of late August; World Health Organization [WHO], 2020). A number of prisons across India have emerged as COVID-19 hotspots (Trivedi, 2020). Again, this is predictable considering that India's prisons are overcrowded by up to 150%, thus making social distancing near-to-impossible and transmission more likely (Trivedi, 2020). For example, among the 8,819 inmates in Assam's prisons, around 1300 inmates had tested positive for COVID-19 by August 5, 2020 (News Live, 2020). The situation is especially poor in Guwahati Central Jail, where as many as 435 inmates were infected (Trivedi, 2020). Another Indian state, Andhra Pradesh, reported an outbreak on August 7, 2020 in its largest prison, Rajamahendravaram Central, with 247 new cases amongst inmates and staff (Express News Service, 2020a). A total of 928 prison inmates and 167 staff within Andhra Pradesh jails tested positive for COVID-19 by August 21, 2020 (Jain, 2020). On August 9, 2020, while the state of Jharkhand had already reported 16,534 infected individuals and 189 deaths due to COVID-19 in the community, 248 of 350 inmates tested positive in a jail in Godda, while 60 more cases were verified in Ranchi and 40 in Pakur (Rani, 2020). By August 12, 2020, 17 prison staff members had tested positive in Odisha, while Bihar reported 200 COVID-19 cases among inmates, staff members, and security personnel (TNN, 2020a). In one of Kashmir state's main cities, Srinagar, by August 14, 2020, one in five (102 out of 480) inmates tested positive for the virus (Bukhari, 2020). Furthermore, the community of Kashmir Valley, had reported at least 20,000 cases at this point in time (Bukhari, 2020). Within a similar timeframe, as many as 449 jail officials and 77 prison officials had tested COVID-19 positive to date in Punjab (TNN, 2020b).

In another Indian state, Maharashtra, jails had reported a combined total of at least 1,478 positive cases (1,166 inmates and 312 jail staff) and 6 deaths as of August 21, 2020 (PTI, 2020). Cases still remain regardless of the 10,536 inmates that were already released as a preventative measure in slowing the spread of the virus, pulling back the total jail population of Maharashtra to 26,408 (PTI, 2020). In a jail in the state of Kerala – Thiruvananthapuram – by August 21, 2020, at least 476 inmates tested positive after rapid testing was conducted (Jain, 2020). Conversely, by August 21, 2020, no COVID-19 positive inmates resided in three of Delhi's jails: Tihar, Rohini and Mandoli, which Tihar officials claim was a consequence of the extensive mitigation measures taken (Express News Service, 2020b; Lama, 2020). Only 63 cases were confirmed among inmates in Delhi's jails (Express News Service, 2020b). Delhi's success can be juxtaposed to the state of Uttar Pradesh where, on August 22, 2020, the Mathura District Jail reported a total count of 1831 positive COVID-cases and 43 deaths, with 24 of the positive cases having emerged within 48 hours (Jaiswal, 2020). The Mathura district jail is operated at three times its intended capacity (Jaiswal, 2020). Also, in Uttar Pradesh, Basti jail reported at least 419 inmates having tested positive, 191 of which tested positive over the course of one week in mid-August (Lama, 2020).

Responses to COVID-19 in prison systems throughout India vary in both the quantity and quality of measures implemented. Due to the outbreak of cases, jail/prison authorities in Godda and Tihar have banned visitors (Lama, 2020; Rani, 2020). Godda's jails have also provided herbal juice, vitamin C, warm water with lemon juice and other herbs to inmates to improve their immune systems (Rani, 2020). Tihar's prison started in-house production of masks and sanitizers, and therefore preventing a shortage of essential items (Lama, 2020).

With a significant number of prison guards testing positive in Jharkhand and Uttar Pradesh – and thus leaving prisons at a deficit in terms of staffing – remaining prison staff have since been asked to remain on the premises with exceptions and are required to undergo screening before reentering (Rani, 2020; TNN, 2020a). Staff that feel unwell have been asked to stay home (TNN, 2020a). Furthermore, all court hearings and meetings with lawyers in Tihar have been virtual to reduce the risk of exposure among inmates (Lama, 2020).

In consideration of, and accommodation for, the number of inmates increasing (again) in custodial settings, likely due to "loosening up" of the lockdown, on August 10, 2020, a three-member panel suggested that Punjab's jail populations be reduced to 50% of their authorized capacity, which would require that the current population of 23,800 be reduced by 4000–5000 (Gopal, 2020). By August 12, 2020, the panel confirmed its decision to release 3,500 inmates (TNN, 2020b). Punjab's jail departments had previously responded by releasing 11,000 inmates between March and May (Gopal, 2020). The state of Odisha decongested its prisons as fast as possible by releasing 16,789 inmates from 85 prisons (TNN, 2020a), while Tihar released 4,000 inmates on interim bail and parole (Lama, 2020). Contrary to the rationale of early release and an emphasis on public health, some Indian states are taking a punitive approach of (ironically) threatening to impose prison sentences for not abiding by social distancing measures (Trivedi, 2020).

In addition to other response tactics, Punjab had implemented a three-tier testing system, which included (1) testing upon entrance to the jail, followed by a 2-week quarantine at a separate, off-site jail; (2) testing upon completion of the 2-week quarantine and if negative returning to the original jail to be held in a separate part of the jail for another 2 weeks, and if positive, inmates are to remain for another 2 weeks at the original quarantine site and repeat the process, and (3) if testing negative after quarantining on site at the jail, the inmates can return to the general jail population.[5] In a much less complex fashion, the Mathura district jail's outbreak prompted a quarantine of at least 500 inmates (Jaiswal, 2020) while prisons including Kashmir's Srinagar and Delhi's Tihar are testing and then quarantining their newly admitted inmates for two weeks (Bukhari, 2020; Lama, 2020). The outbreak in Bihar prompted 18 jails to be allocated for the sole purpose of quarantining COVID-19 positive inmates (TNN, 2020a). However, Bihar did not act on the Supreme Court of India's directive to relieve overcrowded prisons (Trivedi, 2020).

COVID-19 outbreaks and mitigation strategies used in Iran and Saudi Arabia's prison systems

A few countries in the Middle East, which include two in the world's top 50 largest prison systems – Iran and Saudi Arabia – have also released inmates to curb the spread of COVID-19 in their prisons (Das, 2020). According to the World Prison Brief (2020), Iran holds the 8th largest prison system in the world, incarcerating around 240,000 inmates. In mid-March, Iran's judiciary minister announced the release of 85,000 prisoners as a preventative measure to reduce the risk of transmission in prisons (Das, 2020).

John Hopkin's Coronavirus Resource Center reported Iran as the most COVID-19-affected country in the Middle East with 361,159 confirmed cases and 20,776 deaths as of August 24, 2020. The large prevalence of cases in Iran, as a country, despite proactive measures such as releasing 85,000 inmates, may be attributable to the continued movement (coming and going) of inmates to courthouses and thus an increased risk of exposure, as well as to the Ministry of Health's lack of response to Iran's prison administrators' pleas for personal protective equipment, disinfectants and detergents, and other key medical equipment through the months of late February into early July (Amnesty International, 2020; Iran Human Rights Monitor, 2020a). Additionally, overcrowding still appears to be an issue in some Iranian prisons, as one previously incarcerated activist in the Evin prison (Tehran) noted that 17 inmates were jammed into a 12-foot square room, and that there were only 5 toilets for 150 inmates in the prison (Iran Human Rights Monitor, 2020b).

Saudi Arabia – ranked 30th out of the world's top 50 prison systems – contains about 61,000 inmates (World Prison Brief, 2020) and a confirmed 308,654 positive COVID-19 cases nationwide as of August 24, 2020, in addition to 3,691 COVID-19-related deaths (WHO, 2020). Due to mounting pressure from human rights groups, in late-March, Saudi Arabia released hundreds of prisoners from Al-Shumaisi Prison, in addition to around 250 immigration offenders, to lower the risk of spreading the virus (Das, 2020). Also in early March, the Middle Eastern country of Bahrain released 1,486 prisoners, including 300 political inmates on "humanitarian grounds" (Das, 2020).

COVID-19 outbreaks and mitigation strategies used in South, East, and Southeast Asia's prison systems

A handful of countries in Southern, Eastern, and Southeastern Asia reside in the world's top 50 largest prison systems, including Thailand (N = 379,274), Indonesia (N = 232,736), the Philippines (N =215,000), Myanmar (N = 92,000), Bangladesh (N = 88,084), Pakistan (N = 77,275), Malaysia (N = 68,603), South Korea (N = 53,920), and Cambodia (N = 36,600; World Prison Brief, 2020). By August 24, 2020, Indonesia had reported 157,859 positive COVID-19 cases and 6,858 COVID-related deaths, the Philippines had confirmed 197,164 positive cases and 3,038 deaths countrywide, Bangladesh had confirmed experiencing 297,083 positive cases and 3983 deaths, and Pakistan reported 293,361 infections and 6,244 deaths (WHO, 2020). At the same point in time, South Korea reported significantly less infections with 17,665 reported cases and 309 deaths, and Thailand reported only 3,402 positive COVID-19 cases and 58 deaths, despite having the world's 6th largest prison system (WHO, 2020; World Prison Brief, 2020). Malaysia reported 9,274 cases and 175 deaths, Vietnam at 1,029 confirmed cases and 27 deaths, while Myanmar and Cambodia reported 474 and 273 positive cases and 6 and 0 deaths, respectively (WHO, 2020). Laos had only 22 confirmed COVID-19 cases and 0 deaths by late August (WHO, 2020).

One speculation as to why Asian countries like Thailand, Myanmar, Vietnam, Cambodia, and Laos have relatively low counts of COVID-19 cases and deaths, takes on a cultural angle (Beech & Dean, 2020). For example, the Thai culture already practices social distancing and greetings unfold in a prayer-like motion and at a distance, rather than via full-contact embraces. Others theorize that there may be genetic components influencing the immune systems of individuals in this region of the world (Beech & Dean, 2020). It has been reported that administrations in Thailand, Indonesia, the Philippines, Myanmar, and Cambodia have also all stopped prison visitations, while ramping up screening and hygiene protocol (Turton & Bopha, 2020). These mitigation strategies may be related to lower reported outbreaks within the prison systems of these countries.

While some Asian countries have reported low prevalence of COVID-19 cases countrywide during the first several months of the pandemic, their prison systems are still in much need of reform to prevent future outbreaks. Prisons throughout this region have been identified in recent reviews[6] as seriously overcrowded and lacking resources (particularly in the realm of health care); for this reason, they are potential breeding grounds for the future spread of COVID-19 in prisons. Due to these preexisting weaknesses, screening staff and new inmates cannot alone prevent an outbreak (Kinner et al., 2020). Kinner et al. (2020)

recommend that countries reduce prison population sizes as soon as possible, in anticipation of the next wave of outbreaks in this region.

In several countries in this region, governments have instituted prison population reduction strategies in order to reduce crowding.[7] Without significant decongestion of prison populations across many Asian countries in the region, social distancing is an unrealistic in-prison mitigation strategy, at least until the number of individuals in prison is dramatically reduced. South Korea is an example of a country that currently has a prison occupancy level of approximately 112% (World Prison Brief, 2020), yet has enacted downsizing of its prison population in a modest fashion (see Lee, this volume). Despite over capacity and modest downsizing efforts, South Korea has managed to report a very small number of infections, which may be attributed to South Korea's multi-faceted approach to combatting COVID-19 in its prisons (see Lee, this volume). In a more aggressive manner, Indonesia paroled 36,500 inmates, targeting inmates who had completed nearly 70% of the length of their sentences. It is important to note that no explicit protocols had been established for those freed, potentially creating further risk for spreading the virus in the community as they return home (Turton & Bopha, 2020). In Myanmar, the prison system has an official total capacity of 66,000 people amongst all prisons and detention centers, but these facilities are currently holding an estimated 92,000 inmates (Turton & Bopha, 2020). However, due to persistent pressure, that number is reportedly set to drop dramatically, utilizing early release mechanisms (i.e., by nearly 24,000 inmates; Lynn, 2020; Turton & Bopha, 2020).

According to Penal Reform International, in a 10 work-day window, 33,287 bail applications were heard, and 20,938 inmates were released from detention on bail in Bangladesh (Ali, 2020). As of mid-August, the Bangladesh government released an additional 329 inmates who served sentences of 20 years or more for murder convictions (United News of Bangladesh, 2020). Like other densely-packed South-East Asian countries' prison systems, Filipino jails and prisons were housing five times as many inmates as their operating capacity, making it the most overcrowded prison system in the world, according to the World Prison Brief (2020). To mitigate the effects of overcrowding (and more), 21,858 inmates were released as part of the Philippines's efforts to decongest the country's crowded jails, and thus, ultimately aiding in the reduction of COVID-19 transmission among inmates and staff (Ankara, 2020; Xinhua News Agency, 2020b).

Other governments in this region have been slower to respond to the COVID-19 outbreaks in prisons through prison population reduction. For example, Thai prisons are overcrowded, with a population of almost 380,000, in a prison system designed to house 255,000. Malaysia's prisons are also overcrowded, with a surplus of 16,000 inmates above the intended capacity (Bernama, 2020; Turton & Bopha, 2020). There are no plans for early release reported in either country.

Concluding comments

There are conflicting reports on the extent of the COVID-19 outbreaks across this region, but several countries officially report low rates of infection, both in the general community and in the prison system. Cultural differences related to the acceptance of social distancing norms have been identified by some researchers as a possible explanation for the low official rates; while others have argued that the authoritarian governments in these regions are

Table 2. *A comparison of mitigation strategies used in Asia's largest prison systems.*

Country (Rank)	Front-End	Within	Back-End
China (2nd)[a]	Supplemental funding from federal and local governments to financially support prison responses to COVID-19; Suspension of family visitation; Sentence deferment (in some cases)	Dispersal of PPE; Testing; Increased efforts in providing medical care (including mental health services); Establishment of a formal reporting system (for prison staff); Suspension of alternating shifts among prison staff and replaced with consecutive periods of up to 14 days of work, followed by 14 days off; Grid-management approach; Isolation of inmates in contact with suspected cases; Quarantine of inmates with symptoms; Daily disinfection of surfaces; Maintained ventilation by opening windows; Mandated mask-wearing among prison staff; Suspension of certain prison activities	None
India (5th)[b]	Formation of high-level committees to create processes and guidelines for early release/release on bail; Prison staff preventive screening	Inmate and staff testing; Prison staff remaining on prison property to reduce the likelihood of contraction (i.e., not entering the community at large); Quarantining; Proper handling of food; Mandating daily medical checkups for inmates above 60 years old (in some cases) newly admitted inmate testing and isolation	Appx. 14.3% (N = 68,264) inmates temporarily released either on parole for 4– 6 weeks or on interim bail for those being held on pre-trial with offenses worth a sanction of 7 years or less
Philippines (10th)[c]	Use of video conferencing for hearings	Improved sanitary conditions in facilities; Expanded access to medical care; Strengthened testing and contact tracing; Established isolation centers for infected inmates	Eased the rules on parole granting and executive clemency; Expanded compassionate release for most vulnerable inmates
Pakistan (23rd)[b]	Release of pre-trial detainees on bail/surety; Police discretion to not use arrest for less serious offenses' Pre-entrance screening for all visitors	Mass testing; Contact tracing; On-site containment; Quarantine suspected cases; Restricted mobility within jails; Distribution of PPE to staff (e.g., Hazmat Suits, surgical gowns, surgical gloves, respirators, eye protection goggles, caps, hand sanitizers, gloves, blankets and drip sets); Close monitoring and distribution of high-nutrition meals to infected patients	None
Republic of (South) Korea (37th)[d]	Reduction of new incarceration-based sanctions; Restrictions placed on visitation	Provision of the prison population protective eyewear, clothing, and hand sanitizer; Isolation and medical examinations of those newly entering facilities	Modest reductions in prison populations via early release, particularly in facilities that had outbreaks

*The Asian prison systems included in this table are underscored here not only because they comprise some of Asia's largest prison systems, but also because they are the focus of a few of the country-level articles reported on in this volume; [a]See Li and Liu (this volume) for more detail regarding China's mitigation strategies to combat COVID-19 within federal and state prisons; [b]See Dmello and Ranjan (this volume) for more information on India and Pakistan's response to COVID-19 within their prison systems; [c]See Cahapay (this volume) for more details regarding the Philippines' response to COVID-19 in its prison system; [d]See Lee (this volume) for more detail regarding South Korea's mitigation strategies in response to COVID-19.

better equipped to enforce mitigation strategies in community and in prison settings (Li and Liu, this volume). Another possible explanation for low reported infection rates is that governments in this region lack transparency. We find that the most common mitigation strategies being used by governments in this region involve both front-end alternatives to incarceration and pretrial detention (e.g., India), and back-end early release strategies (e.g., Iran). However, it should be noted that the largest country in this region, China, reports that early release strategies are not necessary because the in-prison mitigation strategies employed have been effective enough to combat the virus.

Notes

1. The Asian countries within the world's 50 largest prison systems include China (ranked 2nd), India (ranked 5th), Thailand (ranked 6th), Iran (ranked 8th), Indonesia (ranked 9th), Philippines (ranked 10th), Vietnam (ranked 13th), Myanmar (ranked 19th), Bangladesh (ranked 20th), Pakistan (ranked 23rd), Malaysia (ranked 25th), Saudi Arabia (ranked 29th), Taiwan (ranked 30st), South Korea (ranked 37th), Japan (ranked 41st), Iraq (ranked 42nd), and Cambodia (ranked 48th; World Prison Brief, 2020).
2. Detailed country-specific reviews are included in this volume.
3. Some have attributed the lower rates of infection reported in China's prisons to the ability of the central government's authoritarian regime to respond decisively to early outbreaks. See Li and Liu (this volume) for a more detailed discussion.
4. See Table 2 for more details on China's mitigation strategies toward COVID-19 in its prison system.
5. See Table 2 for more details on India's mitigation strategies in addressing COVID-19 in its prisons.
6. See Kinner et al. (2020).
7. Examples of countries that have not adopted this back-end mitigation strategy within this region include China and Pakistan.

Disclosure statement

No potential conflict of interest was reported by the author(s).

References

329 prisoners to be released. (2020, August 13). United News of Bangladesh. http://www.unb.com.bd/category/Bangladesh/329-prisoners-to-be-released/55955

Ali, I. (2020, June 11). *Releasing 20,000+ people from prison in Bangladesh in 10 days – The view from a judge.* Penal Reform International. https://www.penalreform.org/blog/releasing-20000-people-from-prison-in-bangladesh-in/

Ankara. (2020, July 22). *COVID-19: Philippines releases nearly 22,000 inmates.* Anadolu Agency. https://www.aa.com.tr/en

Assam: 31 jails hit by COVID-19, 1300 prisoners infected. (2020, August 5). News Live. https://newslivetv.com/assam-31-jails-hit-by-covid-19-1300-prisoners-infected/

Beech, H., & Dean, A. (2020, August 20). *No one knows what Thailand is doing right, but so far, it's working.* The New York Times. https://www.nytimes.com/2020/07/16/world/asia/coronavirus-thailand-photos.html

Bernama. (2020, August 8). *Prisons swell with 16,000 extra inmates.* FMT News. https://www.freemalaysiatoday.com/category/nation/2020/08/08/prisons-swell-with-16000-extra-inmates/

Bukhari, F. (2020, August 4). *One in five at Kashmir jail tests positive as India COVID cases soar*. Reuters. https://fr.reuters.com/article/healthcareSector/idUKL4N2FG1SM

Coronavirus Resource Center. (2020, August 24). *COVID-19 dashboard by the Center for Systems Science and Engineering (CSSE) at Johns Hopkins University (JHU)*. John Hopkins University & Medicine. https://coronavirus.jhu.edu/map.html

Crisis in Taybad prison: Infection of guards wreaks havoc among inmates. (2020a, August 13). Iran Human Rights Monitor. https://iran-hrm.com/index.php/2020/08/13/crisis-in-taybad-prison-infection-of-guards-wreaks-havoc-among-inmates/

Das, H. J. (2020, April 3). *COVID-19: Developments in West Asia*. Vivekanada International Foundation. https://www.vifindia.org/article/2019/april/03/covid-19-developments-in-west-asia?slide=$slideshow$

Detained activist sheds light on Evin prison conditions during the pandemic. (2020b, August 17). Iran Human Rights Monitor. https://iran-hrm.com/index.php/2020/08/17/activist-sheds-light-on-evin-prison-conditions/

Express News Service. (2020a, August 7). *Andhra Pradesh's biggest prison reports 247 Coronavirus cases*. The New Indian Express. https://www.newindianexpress.com/states/andhra-pradesh/2020/aug/07/andhra-pradeshs-biggest-prison-reports-247-coronavirus-cases-2180201.html

Express News Service. (2020b, August 22). *After two deaths, no more COVID-19 positive cases in Delhi prisons*. The New Indian Express. https://www.newindianexpress.com/cities/delhi/2020/aug/22/after-two-deaths-no-more-covid-19-positive-cases-in-delhi-prisons-2186727.html

Gopal, N. (2020, August 10). *Panel wants jails further decongested, suggests releasing another '4000-5000'*. The Indian Express. https://indianexpress.com/article/cities/chandigarh/panel-wants-jails-further-decongested-suggests-releasing-another-4000-5000-6547748/

Iran: Leaked letters revealing COVID-19 crisis in prisons. (2020, July 31). Amnesty International. https://www.amnesty.org/download/Documents/MDE1328112020ENGLISH.PDF

Jain, A. (2020, August 21). *As COVID-19 hits India's prisons, expert explains why decongestion is not enough*. Huffpost. https://www.huffingtonpost.in/entry/covid-19-prisons-decongestion_in_5f3e4dd6c5b66346158130cf

Jaiswal, A. (2020, August 22). *Uttar Pradesh: Two dozen prisoners in Mathura district jail test positive for COVID-19*. The Times of India. https://timesofindia.indiatimes.com/city/agra/two-dozen-prisoners-in-mathura-district-jail-test-positive-for-covid-19/articleshow/77695956.cms

Kinner, S. A., Young, J. T., Snow, K., Southalan, L., Lopez-Acuna, D., Ferreira-Borges, C., & O'Moore, E. (2020, March 17). Prisons and custodial settings are part of a comprehensive response to COVID-19. *The Lancet*, *5*(4), e188–e189. https://doi.org/10.1016/S2468-2667(20)30058-X

Lama, P. (2020, August 22). *In the time of COVID-19, Tihar allows virtual meetings between prisoners, families*. Hindustan Times. https://www.hindustantimes.com/india-news/in-the-time-of-covid-19-tihar-allows-virtual-meetings-between-prisoners-families/story-IRlB7nQzJQcJII0GI4vJnN.html

Lynn, K. Y. (2020, April 17). *Myanmar pardons more than 24,000 prisoners in amnesty*. Anadolu Agency. https://www.aa.com.tr/en/asia-pacific/myanmar-pardons-more-than-24-000-prisoners-in-amnesty/1808054

Mahbubani, R. (2020, February 21). *Chinese jails have become hotbeds of coronavirus as more than 500 cases have erupted, prompting the ouster of several officials*. Business Insider. https://www.businessinsider.com/500-coronavirus-cases-reported-in-jails-in-china-2020-2

Patranobis, S. (2020, July 30). *China logs another 105 COVID-19 cases in new surge, silent about virus link in Xinjiang*. Hindustan Times. https://www.hindustantimes.com/world-news/china-logs-another-105-covid-19-cases-in-new-surge-silent-about-virus-link-in-xinjiang/story-urh9MMWvnq1rO9cR8thmiP.html

PTI. (2020, August 21). *COVID-19: 27 Maharashtra jails record 1,478 cases; six deaths*. Financial Express. https://www.financialexpress.com/lifestyle/health/covid-19-27-maharashtra-jails-record-1478-cases-six-deaths/2061660/

Rani, L. (2020, August 9). *COVID-19: Alarm as 248 out of 350 prisoners in Jharkhand jail test positive*. Gulf News: World ASIA. https://gulfnews.com/world/asia/india/covid-19-alarm-as-248-out-of-350-prisoners-in-jharkhand-jail-test-positive-1.73085236

Secon, H., Woodward, A., & Mosher, D. (2020, June 30). *A comprehensive timeline of the coronavirus pandemic at 6 months, from China's first case to the present*. Business Insider. https://www.businessinsider.com/coronavirus-pandemic-timeline-history-major-events-2020

TNN. (2020a, August 12). *As more cops & prison staff test positive, states come up with Plan B*. The Times of India. https://timesofindia.indiatimes.com/india/as-more-cops-prison-staff-test-positive-states-come-up-with-plan-b/articleshow/77495670.cms

TNN. (2020b, August 12). *Punjab to release over 3,500 prisoners*. The Times of India. https://timesofindia.indiatimes.com/city/chandigarh/punjab-to-release-over-3-5k-prisoners/articleshow/77493673.cms

Trivedi, D. (2020, August 28). *Prisons become breeding grounds for coronavirus*. Frontline: India's National Magazine. https://frontline.thehindu.com/the-nation/tinderbox-prisons/article32296969.ece

Turton, S., & Bopha, P. (2020, April 21). *Asian prisons are ticking time bombs for coronavirus outbreaks*. Nikkei Asian Review. https://asia.nikkei.com/Spotlight/Coronavirus/Asian-prisons-are-ticking-time-bombs-for-coronavirus-outbreaks

WHO Coronavirus disease (COVID-19) dashboard. (2020, August 24). World Health Organization. https://covid19.who.int/

World Prison Brief. (2020, August). *World prison brief data*. Institute for Crime & Justice Policy Research (ICPR). https://www.prisonstudies.org/world-prison-brief-data

Xinhua News Agency. (2020a, March 4). *China concludes investigation on prison COVID-19 outbreak*. China.org.cn http://www.china.org.cn/china/2020-03/04/content_75774142.htm

Xinhua News Agency. (2020b, July 22). *Philippines frees nearly 22,000 inmates to prevent COVID-19 infections in crowded jails*. China.org.cn. http://www.china.org.cn/world/Off_the_Wire/2020-07/22/content_76299735.htm

Yang, H., & Thompson, J. R. (2020, April 2). *Fighting COVID-19 outbreaks in prisons*. The BMJ. https://www.bmj.com/content/369/bmj.m1362

Yang, Z. (2020, March 9). *Cracks in the system: COVID-19 in Chinese prisons. The spread of the disease in prisons reveals flaws in China's epidemic countermeasures*. The Diplomat. https://thediplomat.com/2020/03/cracks-in-the-system-covid-19-in-chinese-prisons/

Correctional System's Response to the Coronavirus Pandemic and Its Implications for Prison Reform in China

Spencer D. Li and Tzu-Hsuan Liu

ABSTRACT

Large outbreaks of coronavirus infections occurred in several prisons in China in February 2020. Since then, the authorities on the national and local levels have introduced a series of measures to prevent more COVID-19 infections in correctional institutions. This article reviews those strategies and explores their ties to past prison reforms and their potential influences on future directions. First, it provides an overview of the changes in prison management and operation that foreshadowed some of China's approaches to COVID-19 in the prison system. Second, it examines the strategies undertaken by the prison system to stop the spread of COVID-19. Finally, the article discusses the implications of the COVID-19 response for prison reforms and the challenges the Chinese prison system faces in its continuous efforts to contain COVID-19.

Prisons and jails are intensively vulnerable to infectious diseases because they are highly crowded places where social distancing is difficult. Also, incarcerated populations are at higher risk of exposure because correctional officers and supportive personnel frequently leave and return to the facility (Liebrenz et al., 2020). China has one of the largest incarcerated populations in the world. According to World Prison Brief, the rate of incarceration in China was 119 per 100,000 by mid-2014. There are 1,657,812 sentenced prisoners in the Ministry of Justice prisons, excluding individuals held in detention centers, which are reported to be in excess of 650,000. The inclusion of the detainees would raise the incarceration rate to 166 per 100,000 (Walmsley, 2020).

Large outbreaks of coronavirus infections have occurred in many prisons around the world since February 2020. China was no exception. By February 25, there were 555 confirmed infected cases in five prisons, including 271 cases in Hubei province, the epicenter of COVID-19 in China, and 284 cases outside Hubei (Z. Li et al., 2020). The confirmed cases in China's prisons continue to rise in the days following. On February 29, the total number of infected inmates in Wuhan city's prisons alone rose to 806 (Z. Yang, 2020). Since then, the authorities on the national and local levels have introduced a series of measures to speed up the efforts to stop the spread of coronavirus and to improve case management and healthcare services in the prison system that had already been underway before the coronavirus pandemic. This article reviews these efforts and assesses its potential implications for prison reforms in China. First, it provides an overview of two major prison reforms undertaken in recent years that underpinned some of China's approaches to COVID-19 in the correctional settings. Second, it examines the measures taken by the prison system to minimize the risks and consequences of the coronavirus pandemic. Lastly, the article discusses the implications of the COVID-19 strategies and experiences for prison reforms and the challenges the Chinese prison system faces in the continuous efforts to improve its COVID-19 response.

Chinese prison management and reforms

The Chinese prison system is a top-down system (S. D. Li & Liu, 2019). The Ministry of Justice sets policies and guidelines for the structure and operation of all prisons. It also supervises the performance of prisons of all levels and has ultimate control over personnel management in those facilities. As safety is the top concern in all correctional institutions, the first priority of the system is to keep inmates under strict control to prevent any disorderly conduct and accident (e.g., suicide) from happening (Huo, 2020; Sun, 2020). Under the safety-first principle, the system launched a series of reform efforts to improve case management and provide better services to inmates in the correctional facilities in recent years. Two of the most notable ones have been grid management with integrated risk assessment[1] and restructuring prison healthcare services. Both efforts were innovations initially developed on the local levels and endorsed by the central government for national promotion.

Worldwide, prison management has become progressively more professionally oriented and more reliant on actuarial approach to justice during the era of soaring prison population (McSherry, 2020; Rothschild-Elyassi et al., 2018). Prisons around the world, including China, have placed increasingly more emphasis on risk assessment, classification, and control (Byrne & Dezember, 2016). Since 2015, the central government of China has promoted grid management in the correctional system (General Office of the CPC Central Committee of the People's Republic of China, 2015). With this approach, the authority divided the facility into a number of segments, which were further divided into grid cells. Prison staff collected inmates' information, such as crime history, conviction records, sentences served, risk of escape, potential harms to the community, in-facility performance, and personality profiles through interview, questionnaire, and observation. Based on the assessment, they classified inmates into different risk levels and assigned them the grid cells appropriate for their levels of risk (Beijing Bureau of Prisons, 2016; Pang, 2016; Wang & Xu, 2019).

Inmates in similar subgroups were routinely shuttled between different activities, such as work assignments, meals, educational programs, and physical exercises throughout the prison. Each grid cell was equipped with prison guards who were responsible for monitoring inmates, supervising and educating them, and attending to their needs (Beijing Bureau of Prisons, 2016; Pang, 2016; Wang & Xu, 2019). They were also responsible for submitting regular reports to designated authorities about the conditions of their grid cells and the behaviors of the inmates assigned to the cells. Through grid management, prison authorities at the higher levels could obtain up-to-date information about every cell in real time and monitor daily activities performed at lower levels (J. Li, 2020). The management system provided the authorities the ability to identify anything unusual in the prison, keep dangerous inmates under control, and prevent potential riots. It coincided with the major principles of actuarial justice that rely on risk assessment and targeted control to effectively manage mass incarceration (Baker & Roberts, 2005).

Another prison reform that has spread to many areas of China in the recent years was the effort to improve healthcare services for prison inmates. Chinese prison law mandated healthcare services in all prisons (Ke, 2014). However, the types and quality of healthcare services varied significantly from region to region, and sometimes from prison to prison in the same region. Common problems faced by all prisons were shortages of qualified physicians and medical equipment. As a result, most prisons were unable to provide adequate healthcare for all inmates (Cheng, 2020). Mental health services were especially lacking. Most prison hospitals and clinics did not have licensed mental health professionals. In the absence of psychiatrists and clinical psychologists, prison staff with experiences dealing with inmate emotional and psychological problems, such as those running educational and counseling programs, often filled the vacuum and provided limited services. Insufficient funding was another problem that nearly all prisons had to deal with. For example, the national budget allocated for healthcare services in 2011 for all prisons was 224 RMB (about 34 USD) per inmate, compared to the actual expenditure of 425 RMB (65 USD) per inmate. This mismatch resulted in a budget deficit of nearly 400 million RMB (about 67 million USD) (Cheng, 2020). Prisons across the country have been experimenting with various ways to solve these problems in healthcare in general and mental health services in particular. To address shortages in medical equipment and physicians, correctional institutions partnered with local hospitals to outsource some of the care, especially the treatment of inmates with serious illness. To improve mental health services, some prisons worked with service providers in surrounding communities to bring psychologists and psychiatrists to the facility to treat inmates with psychiatric problems. However, these services were generally limited to developed areas where governments could afford to provide supplemental funding for health services to incarcerated offenders. For less developed areas, Internet-based healthcare has been promoted as cost-effective ways of overcoming financial constraints and lack of resources. In this type of approach, prison hospitals and clinics collected patient data and shared them with a network of physicians working in similar healthcare settings and community hospitals. Through remote diagnostics and consultation, prison staff could obtain timely diagnosis of the symptoms and arrange appropriate treatment for the sick inmates. The Internet-based services were especially suitable for mental health treatment. An inmate with a mental health problem could receive assessment and evaluation by a mental health professional through remote access. Treatment sessions could also be administered online with real-time interaction between the patient and the doctor (Chen, 2017).

Overall, prior to the coronavirus pandemic, the Chinese government had stepped up the efforts to accelerate the structural reform to improve efficiency of prison management and to provide better healthcare services to a correctional population that increasingly demanded more attention to their basic rights, including the rights to healthcare when incarcerated. Coincidently, these efforts, including the implementation of grid management and risk assessment as well the innovations in healthcare, helped prepare the system to deal with the larger crisis brought about by the pandemic.

Measures taken by Chinese prison system in response to COVID-19

Since the outbreaks of coronavirus infections in several prisons, the Chinese correctional system has taken a series of measures to minimize the risks of COVID-19 infections and their consequences. Unlike prisons in many other countries, Chinese prisons have not released inmates to the community to prevent coronavirus inflections, although there have been reports of sentences being deferred to reduce new admissions to prisons (Liu, 2020). Rather, the Chinese system has concentrated on efforts inside the prisons to prevent the virus from entering the facility and stop it from spreading once it was there. Although the protocols developed by the correctional institutions varied significantly from one another, there were some common elements.

First, taking advantage of the top-down organizational structure of the system, the authorities promoted a systematic approach to tackle the public health emergency. The governments on the national and provincial levels provided supplemental funding to prisons to support work related to the coronavirus pandemic. For instance, the Communist Party Committee of Bureau of Prisons in Hubei Province allocated around 55,000 U.S. dollars to 30 prisons in Hubei for pandemic prevention and control. The central and provincial authorities also sent protective equipment, testing supplies, and medical professionals to the facilities to help with the efforts to prevent and stop coronavirus infections (Liu, 2020). Moreover, the Chinese Communist Party (CCP) set up emergency party branches to coordinate the activities in every prison. The party branches were responsible for establishing rules and procedures and supervising work performed by prison officers and guards in response to COVID-19 (C. T. Yang, 2020b). The correctional institutions also established a formal reporting system as means to monitoring staff performance and strengthening accountability (Zhu, 2020b). Frontline officers were responsible for collecting the information and reporting it to their supervisors, who in turn were required to submit regular reports of the epidemic status in the prison to higher-ranking authorities. Those who neglected their responsibilities might face serious consequences. For example, several high-ranking administrators in Shandong Province, including the Director of Department of Justice, were fired because of their failure in implementing adequate control that led to a large number of confirmed infections in a prison. In a separate case, the government dismissed the head of a woman's prison in Hubei province for the large number of COVID-19 infections discovered in that facility (Z. Li et al., 2020). There were also many successful stories. For example, Guangdong Province in south China, the most populated province with jurisdiction over 25 prisons, has reported no coronavirus infection in their facilities. The authority attributed their successes to strict organizational control imposed by the communist party committees at the highest level and the "wartime" effort to strengthen interagency cooperation and coordination to achieve high efficiency in system-wide response to COVID-19 prevention and incident management operations (C. T. Yang, 2020c, p. 1). The authority also implemented tough accountability measures to ensure that all prison management and staff followed the rules and procedures specially developed for COVID-19 prevention and control (Xue, 2020).

Second, considering that the rapid spread of COVID-19 infections in several prisons were primarily caused by infected prison guards importing the virus into the facilities, the authorities developed a series of preventive measures to block this route of infection. Every prison had to have a plan on suspending shift work and quarantining prison guards and officers. For example, in some provinces, such as Hubei and Guangdong, individuals from outside were not allowed to enter the prisons until the pandemic was determined to be under control. Prison officers presently on duty stopped working in alternative shifts. Instead, they had to remain on duty for an indefinite period until further notice. In some prisons, guards worked 14 days consecutively and then took 14 days off. When they got back to work, they had to be quarantined for 14 days before returning to duty. Many prisons adopted this 14–14–14 model or some variant of it when scheduling work assignments (G. Li, 2020).

Third, in collaboration with other government agencies, the prison system accelerated its deployment of grid management with particular emphasis on risk assessment and control. In consistency with the management principles, the Chinese Center for Disease Control and Prevention (CHINACDC) officially issued "The Technological Plan of Novel Coronavirus Prevention and Control in Prisons" in March 2020 (CHINACDC, 2020). According to the guidelines, every correctional facility should categorize inmates into several groups, including seriously ill inmates, normally ill inmates with COVID-19, minor ill inmates with COVID-19, suspected cases, inmates with close contact to a positive COVID-19 case and normal inmates, and implement grid management based on their health conditions. Depending on the distribution of inmates in those categories, they should designate segments of the prison as patient zone, quarantine zone, isolated observation zone, and/or normal zone. Generally, inmates showing serious symptoms of COVID-19 should stay in patient zone. Inmates with minor symptoms should be quarantined. Inmates with close contacts to positive cases and those suspected to be carriers of the virus should be observed in isolated observation zone. Only healthy inmates and those tested negative at the end of the quarantine should be allowed to stay in the normal zone. Prisons with poor health conditions and those who could not meet the guidelines should transfer confirmed and suspect cases to hospitals. Chinese prisons seldom release detailed management data as those are generally considered politically sensitive. However, there are concrete examples. For instance, in mid-February, Qianchuan Prison in Anhui Province moved all 700 inmates admitted to the facility before January 25, the day of Chinese New Year, who had been quarantined for at least 14 days to cell blocks deemed appropriate for them. The management then placed all 1,320 newly admitted inmates under isolated observation. They checked the body temperature of the inmates twice a day and immediately quarantined those who showed any sign of potential infection (G. Li, 2020). In April, Zhejiang Province and the city of Wuhan, where COVID-19 first emerged late last year, tested all prison inmates to identify infected COVID-19 cases and assigned them to appropriate grid cells based on the results of the tests (Guo & Dai, 2020; Zhou, 2020).

Facing common challenges, correctional institutions also strengthened cross-regional collaboration and partnership with other social institutions to form society-wide efforts to contain the spread of the coronavirus (G. Li, 2020). In these joint efforts, the prisons served as a grid in a comprehensive approach to address the public health crisis affecting the society as a whole. For example, prisons collaborated with local government and businesses to ensure that the facilities were protected from the community spread of the virus and their needs for medical supplies and other critical recourses were attended to (C. T. Yang, 2020a). Prisons also stepped up their collaboration with community correctional agencies by promoting "seamless connection" (Luo, 2020, p. 1). In these joint operations, the prison ensured that inmates who were completing their sentences or transitioning to community supervision would be quarantined for at least 14 days before they were handed over to community correctional agencies. Once they were in the community, they would continue to be supervised by the community agencies to monitor their health conditions and their risks of catching and spreading the coronavirus to others in the community (C. T. Yang, 2020c).

Correctional institutions also developed good hygiene protocols to address various risks posed by different environmental conditions inside the prison. For example, staff cleaned and disinfected hard surfaces daily. They opened windows multiple times a day at regular intervals to maintain good room ventilation. They were required to wear face masks while on duties, especially when they were supervising sick inmates (Zhu, 2020b).

Fourth, to prevent the spread of the virus among incarcerated populations, prisons suspended all family visits during the coronavirus pandemic. To help inmates stay connected with their family members, prisons found other ways for prisoners to communicate with their families. For example, some prisons in Jiangsu province contacted the inmates' families and arranged officers to visit them and make videos to share with the inmates. Moreover, many prisons provided virtual visits through remote access via the Internet for the inmates to see and talk to their loved ones (Zhu, 2020d).

Fifth, prisons significantly stepped up their efforts in providing medical care, especially mental health services. In many prisons, physical and mental health promotion became a focus of the prison treatment curriculum during the pandemic. While in-class instructions were canceled, treatment staff made videos and online materials available to inmates to teach them how to improve individual cardiopulmonary function, strengthen immune system, combat sleep disorder, relieve anxiety and depression, and overcome fear. The institutions continued to provide treatment to seriously ill inmates in prison hospitals and clinics, and in community hospitals through referrals.

As the coronavirus pandemic swept through several prisons and across the country, it caused worries, stress, and uncertainties among prison inmates, exacerbating mental health problems that had already been prevalent in the incarcerated population (Duan & Zhu, 2020). To address this problem, many prisons provided inmates with the opportunities to talk to a clinical psychologist or psychiatrist in person or online through remote access. Some of them also set up a 24-hour hotline that inmates could use to seek psychological consulting (Zhu, 2020a, 2020c). These services were intended to prevent accidents or disruptive behavior caused by severe mental disorder during the time of the coronavirus pandemic. As mentioned previously, to reduce stress and loneliness, some prisons made videos with the family members of the inmates and shared the videos with the inmates in an effort to connect them with their loved ones.

Discussion

The Chinese prison system has made many efforts to address the problems created by the coronavirus pandemic. Some of these steps were emergency measures intended to stop the spread of infection in correctional settings. Others were built on longer-term endeavors to reform the correctional system. The coronavirus pandemic provided a strong impetus to improve the operation of the prison system through risk management and more humanitarian response to inmates' healthcare needs. It is in these two areas where the campaign to stop COVID-19 and decades-long drive to reform the prison system converged. Because of their experience in grid management, Chinese prison management has been keen to classify inmates into different risk groups and apply appropriate screening and supervision procedures to reduce the inmates' exposures to coronavirus and prevent infections. Recognizing the risk presented by prison staff who might bring the virus to the facility from the outside, prison management developed rules and procedures to minimize staff movement and their risk of being infected and infecting others. Another critical link between prison reform and the war against COVID-19 was the quest to improve healthcare in the correctional settings. Many prisons struggled with providing better care for prison inmates. To make meaningful changes, they had to lobby higher authorities for more funding while building partnerships with local government and hospitals. In the meantime, they made significant progresses in adopting new technology to provide remote consultation, diagnostics, and treatment. Coincidently, all of these experiences served as good preparation for the tasks involved in COVID-19 prevention and control. The coronavirus crisis, after all, is a public health emergency. To manage it well, the prison system needs to work with governments of all levels and forge strong partnerships with the communities. The successes of the Chinese prison system in combatting COVID-19 are attributable to their continuous effort to manage risks and enhance healthcare services in the correctional setting. It is safe to assume that these reforms will continue not only because the war against COVID-19 is ongoing but also for the fact that all of these changes serve the "safety first" principle of the Chinese prison system. Grid management based on actuarial assessment of risks and targeted intervention has shown to increase the efficiency of correctional supervision and reduce in-prison conflicts and accidents. In the context of public health crisis, such as COVID-19, prison healthcare has also become a safety issue as infections occurred inside the prison can endanger the health and wellbeing of all involved and cause significant disruption to the operation of the facility. In addition to the safety concern, these changes also serve other objectives of prison reform, including improving treatment outcomes and constructing smart prisons through the application of artificial intelligence and Internet-based technology. For all of these reasons, grid management and healthcare services are likely to remain as major focuses of prison management in the foreseeable future.

The Chinese prison system has made significant progresses in response to COVID-19. Since February, there has been no report of new coronavirus outbreak in Chinese prisons either from Chinese sources or by Western media. The lack of new cases could be due to official coverup. But more likely, it reflected China's overall successes in keeping the pandemic under control. Since the beginning of March, the daily count of new coronavirus cases throughout China, including Hong Kong, has been ranging from 0 to less than 150, until a recent outbreak in Hong Kong in late July that pushed the total number of new cases to over 200 on some days (Baidu, 2020). Despite the progresses, major challenges remain. First, the common practice of holding the top management of the prison system responsible for a virus outbreak in any of their facilities regardless of the actual circumstance may lead to lack of transparency in case reporting. For fear of punishment or job loss, prison administration may resort to hiding information of confirmed cases in order to avoid negative exposure. Lack of transparency with regard to the number of individuals infected in the facilities and steps taken to stop the spread of the virus may lead to more problems because public health experts are unable to access the information and use it to help the administration develop effective countermeasures to control the outbreak.

Another challenge is to address the complex medical needs of vulnerable individuals incarcerated in the prisons during the pandemic, including the elderly, inmate with a mental health condition, and those with a chronic condition, such as asthma, diabetes, or high blood pressure. Providing continuous medical care and mental health services to these individuals is essential for the purposes of protecting human rights, promoting offender rehabilitation, and reducing coronavirus-related fatalities. Moreover, medical referral is a complex issue for the correctional system. Early coordination between prison authorities, prosecutors, public security, hospitals, and others is vital. The prison system should work with other agencies to develop clear guidelines on referrals (Liebrenz et al., 2020).

Third, from the resource management perspective, it is difficult to sustain the massive control effort in all facilities for a long period of time. Social distancing is hard to implement in correctional institutions due to the crowded nature of the facilities (Liebrenz et al., 2020). In addition, prisons and jails have fast and unexpected population turnover. Newly convicted offenders and those completing their sentences continue to move in and out of the facilities as long as the legal processes remain operating. To reduce overcrowding in correctional institutions during the pandemic, the United Nations and human rights advocates have called for the releases of selected prisoners to stem the spread of COVID-19 (Human Rights Watch, 2020). Many countries have adopted this strategy. To date, there has been no report of early or temporary release of prison inmates to prevent coronavirus infection in Chinese prisons. It is an option that the Chinese prison system should consider if COVID-19 continues to pose a serious threat to the incarcerated population.

Fourth, maintaining mental health through social support became more challenging than ever during the lockdown. Family support is important for inmates' rehabilitation because it helps them stay connected with the outside world and feel being valued by their loved ones. During the lockdown, correctional institutions suspended family visits. The loss of connection with their family members may lead to mental distress, maladaptive behavior, suicide, and self-harm. The virtual meetings provided by some prisons have their limits. For example, some families did not know how to use the Internet technology. Also, correctional facilities in poor rural areas do not have recourse to utilize the communication technology (G. Li, 2020). Governments should do more to strengthen family support for the incarcerated offenders during the public health crisis.

Another challenge is to protect the health and wellbeing of the correctional staff. Prison officers are responsible for enforcing all of the measures for the prevention and control of COVID-19 in the facilities. Long working hours and extended duty time during the pandemic have a negative impact on their physical health, mental health, work performance, and their relationships with their families. Because of the difficulties in practicing social distancing in correctional settings, prison officers are at a heightened risk of being infected (Liebrenz et al., 2020). Staff turnover and absenteeism are low in Chinese prisons, which contributed to the stability in the operation of the facilities. However, prison management should make stronger efforts to ensure a healthy and motivated workforce that is ready to take on some of the most difficult and unpredictable problems that the correctional institutions may encounter during the pandemic.

In conclusion, Chinese prisons have been under emergency management since the outbreaks of the coronavirus infections in February. The Chinese government adopted the risk management model to contain the spread of the virus and prevent new infections. Correctional facilities categorized inmates based on their health conditions and risk of infection and used public health protocols including cleaning, social distancing, personal protection equipment, testing, and medical isolation to minimize the risk of mass infections among the incarcerated population. The system also paid special attention to the healthcare needs of the staff and inmates, including the needs for mental health services during the pandemic. Through the collaboration of the governments, correctional institutions, hospitals and public health professionals, the system developed and implemented a series of strategies to address the public health emergency while improving mental health services to staff and inmates. Given that no further cluster infection has been reported from the correctional system, it seems that the Chinese control and preventive measures are effective, at least in terms of their own objectives. The crisis brought about by the pandemic has been both a challenge and an opportunity. On the one hand, it created enormous problems for prison management. On the other hand, it provided an impetus for more innovative approaches in prison management, stronger humanitarian responses to the needs of the inmates and closer cooperation among corrections systems, healthcare institutions, local enterprises, and government agencies aiming at achieving broad-based public safety and health.

Note

1. Grid management has been under development as a system of social control in China since 2013. In the prison setting, this system applies risk assessment to categorize prison inmates and places them in a network of supervision and control to promote management efficiency. Beijing Bureau of Prisons (2016) provides a good review of this strategy.

Disclosure statement

No potential conflict of interest was reported by the author(s).

References

Baidu. (2020). *Realtime big data report of coronavirus pandemic*. https://voice.baidu.com/act/newpneumonia/newpneumonia/?from=osari_pc_3

Baker, E., & Roberts, J. (2005). Globalization and the new punitiveness. In J. Pratt, D. Brown, M. Brown, S. Hallsworth, & W. Morrison (Eds.), *The new punitiveness: Trends, theories, perspectives* (pp. 121–138). Willan.

Beijing Bureau of Prisons. (2016). *Changing concept and operating mechanism in grid management in prisons*. http://jyj.beijing.gov.cn/lldt/201912/t20191211_1068260.html

Byrne, J., & Dezember, A. (2016). The research director perspective on the design, implementation and impact of risk assessment and offender classification systems in USA prisons: A national survey. In F. Taxman (Ed.), *Handbook on risk and need assessment: Theory and practice* (pp. 49–64). Routledge.

Chen, S. (2017). The construction of prison medical model under the Internet plus initiative. *China Prison Journal*, *2017*(1), 58–62.

Cheng, K. (2020). Construction of medical security system for prison inmates. *South Forum*, *2020*(4), 62–67.

CHINACDC. (2020). *The technological plans of novel coronavirus prevention and control in prisons*. http://www.chinacdc.cn/jkzt/crb/zl/szkb_11803/jszl_2275/202003/t20200310_214270.html

Duan, L., & Zhu, G. (2020). Psychological interventions for people affected by the COVID-19 epidemic. *The Lancet Psychiatry*, *7*(4), 300–302. https://doi.org/10.1016/S2215-0366(20)30073-0

General Office of the CPC Central Committee of the People's Republic of China. (2015). *The opinions on strengthening social public security prevention and control system*. http://www.gov.cn/xinwen/2015-04/13/content_2846013.htm

Guo, Y., & Dai, Q. (2020). *To consolidate the outcomes of pandemic prevention and control, Zhejiang expanded orderly nucleic acid and antibody testing in orderly*. People.cn. http://zj.people.com.cn/BIG5/n2/2020/0427/c228592-33980454.html

Human Rights Watch. (2020). *Asia: Reduce prison populations facing COVID-19 overcrowding, unsanitary conditions threaten catastrophe*. https://www.hrw.org/news/2020/04/06/asia-reduce-prison-populations-facing-covid–19

Huo, Z. (2020). On construction of offender risk assessment and control system. *Justice of China, 2020*(5), 78–83.

Ke, S. Z. (2014). Prison medical dilemma and construction of medical socialization model. *Journal of Fujian Police College, 2014*(4), 40–46.

Li, G. (2020, February 15). Keeping Covid-19 out of the prison gate. *Legal Daily*. http://www.legaldaily.com.cn/zt/content/2020-02/15/content_8118023.htm

Li, J. (2020). Research on the prison reform. *Legality Vision, 2020*(7), 15–18.

Li, S. D., & Liu, T. (2019). Problem-solving courts in China: Background, development and current status. *Victims & Offenders: An International Journal of Evidence-based Research, Policy, and Practice, 14*(3), 360–374. https://doi.org/10.1080/15564886.2019.1595246

Li, Z., Qing, M., Ni, H., Wei, H., & Liu, Y. (2020, February 22). Holes exposed in the prevention and control of coronavirus in prison. *Global Times*. http://m.fx361.com/news/2020/0222/6384129.html

Liebrenz, M., Bhugra, D., Buadze, A., & Schleifer, R. (2020). Caring for persons in detention suffering with mental illness during the Covid-19 outbreak. *Forensic Science International: Mind and Law, 1* (2020), 1–2. https://doi.org/10.1016/j.fsiml.2020.100013

Liu, Z. (2020, June 8). Strengthening criminal justice response in normalcy of coronavirus prevention and control. *Legal Daily*. http://www.legaldaily.com.cn/Personnel_matters/content/2020-06/08/content_8215387.htm

Luo, X. (2020). *Keeping Covid-19 out of the prison gate: COVID-19 prevention and treatment practices in Hunan prions*. Legal Weekly. https://xw.qq.com/amphtml/20200411A0B4KO00

McSherry, B. (2020). Risk assessment, predictive algorithms and preventive justice. In J. Pratt & J. Anderson (Eds.), *Criminal justice, risk and the revolt against uncertainty* (pp. 17–42). Palgrave Macmillan.

Pang, Y. (2016). *Promotion of innovative supervision models and grid management in prisons in Sichuan Province*. Sichuan Daily. http://scnews.newssc.org/system/20160109/000638053.html

Rothschild-Elyassi, R., Koehler, J., & Simon, J. (2018). Actuarial justice. In M. Deflem (Ed.), *The handbook of social control* (pp. 194–206). John Wiley & Sons.

Sun, H. (2020). *Implement "Five Major Reforms" and construct school-like new type of prisons*. Ministry of Justice of People's Republic of China. http://www.moj.gov.cn/Department/content/2020-01/06/606_3239235.html

Walmsley, R. (2020). *World prison population list, eleventh edition*. World Prison Brief. https://www.prisonstudies.org/sites/default/files/resources/downloads/world_prison_population_list_11th_edition_0.pdf

Wang, J., & Xu, M. (2019, July 3). Using smart applications to improve job performance in Beijing women's prison. *Legal Daily*. http://www.legaldaily.com.cn/zt/content/2019-07/03/content_7924528.htm

Xue, J. H. (2020). Behind "zero infection" in Guangdong prisons: Their 58-day closed duty inside the high walls. *Yangcheng Evening News*. http://gdjyj.gd.gov.cn/ztbd/yqfk/content/post_2964705.html

Yang, C. T. (2020a). *Liaoning prison administration is determined to defeat the coronavirus epidemic with the highest standards, strongest measures, and biggest resolution*. Ministry of Justice of People's Republic of China. http://www.moj.gov.cn/subject/content/2020-03/12/1457_3243845.html

Yang, C. T. (2020b). *The no. 2 prison in Yunnan Province adheres to seven "battle plans" and constructs seven "defense lines"*. Ministry of Justice of People's Republic of China. http://www.moj.gov.cn/Department/content/2020-03/30/606_3245159.html

Yang, C. T. (2020c). *Guangdong prisons achieved notable results in big recognization prompted by COVID-19 prevention and control*. Ministry of Justice of People's Republic of China. http://www.moj.gov.cn/subject/content/2020-04/24/1457_3246846.html

Yang, Z. (2020). Cracks in the system: COVID-19 in Chinese prisons. *The Diplomat*. https://thediplomat.com/2020/03/cracks-in-the-system-covid-19-in-chinese-prisons/

Zhou, F. (2020). *Wuhan is expanding nucleic acid testing, covering all individuals in several categories*. YICAI. https://www.yicai.com/news/100588214.html

Zhu, J. (2020a). *The Chang Tai prison in Tianjin implemented "four battles" plans to improve inmate psychological treatment programs*. Ministry of Justice of People's Republic of China. http://www.moj.gov.cn/Department/content/2020-03/13/606_3243912.html

Zhu, J. (2020b). *Ding Shan prison in Jiangsu Province takes strong hold of the management of inmate emotional problems*. Ministry of Justice of People's Republic of China. http://www.moj.gov.cn/Department/content/2020-05/14/606_3248573.html

Zhu, J. (2020c). *Prevent and control coronavirus with full strength and strong strategies in Jiangsu prison system*. Ministry of Justice of People's Republic of China. http://www.moj.gov.cn/Department/content/2020-02/12/606_3241234.html

Zhu, J. (2020d). *The remote video interviewing project in Anhui prisons shows strong effectiveness*. Ministry of Justice of People's Republic of China. http://www.moj.gov.cn/Department/content/2020-05/14/606_3248572.html

Lock Unlock: The Impact of COVID-19 on Health Security in Pakistani and Indian Prisons

Jared R. Dmello and Sheetal Ranjan

ABSTRACT

This paper assesses the state of COVID-19 in the Pakistani and Indian prison systems. Using publicly available data, governmental documents, media, and non-profit organization reports, and scholarly literature, we provide an overview of COVID-19 in each country and the current state of each nation's prison system. We then analyze the impact of the novel coronavirus on the corrections systems and each government's response to the virus in its prison infrastructure. The pandemic provides both Pakistan and India with the opportunity to change course and move toward a more sustainable prison system that protects human rights while bolstering health security.

Introduction

On December 31, 2019, the World Health Organization (WHO) was notified of a cluster of pneumonia cases with an unknown cause originating in Wuhan, China. One week later, China identified a new coronavirus (2019-nCoV) as the cause of the quickly spreading outbreak. Nepal reported its first case of 2019-nCoV on January 24, 2020, marking the first confirmed case in South Asia. Sri Lanka and India followed with confirmed cases three and six days later respectively. Within weeks, COVID-19 had evolved into a global health crisis, being declared a global pandemic by WHO on March 11, 2020. As the pandemic progressed, much attention was paid to COVID-19 from the lens of health security, specifically of nations. In some nations, debates over virus-mitigation plans quickly coalesced around economic priorities, while others took a stronger non-traditional security approach, which emphasizes the promotion of human-focused security (Caballero-Anthony, 2016).

Within the criminal justice system, detention facilities create unique populations that are often more susceptible to the spread of disease. These centers approximate small-world networks, where residents can often be connected to one another using relatively short distance lengths; however, the constant flow of staff entering from the outside world creates opportunities for COVID-19 to be introduced into the system. Based on the theory of hyperdyadic contagion, once introduced into the system, a contagion would be expected to quickly diffuse through a network, creating ripple effects toward new individuals, increasing infection (*see*: Christakis & Fowler, 2009). This principle has been applied in multiple contexts, including the spread of violence, resources, and most relevant, viruses (*see*:

Bichler et al., 2019; Firestone et al., 2011; Green et al., 2017; Van Mieghem et al., 2008). Thus, theoretically and practically, prison populations are at heightened risk for exposure to the novel coronavirus. This paper assesses the state of COVID-19 in the Pakistani and Indian prison systems. Although eight countries are commonly included operationalization of the South-Asian region,[1] the current manuscript focuses primarily on India and Pakistan. In the subsequent sections, we discuss COVID-19, the prison systems, and the impact of the pandemic on the prisons in both countries. Although both nations have worked to forge unique identities, the ongoing prison conditions and the current health crisis underscores similar challenges, perhaps representative of the South Asian region.

COVID-19 in Pakistan

COVID-19 precipitated a severe health crisis in Pakistan. The International Crisis Group (2020) places Pakistan among the twelve countries hardest hit by coronavirus, largely attributed to the federal government reopening the country too early. As was the case in multiple countries, the pandemic hurt Pakistan's economy, which prompted Prime Minister Imran Khan to prematurely lift the nation-wide lockdowns on May 9, despite a continued surge in positive tests for the virus throughout the country (Gannon, 2020; TRT World, 2020b). Even Pakistan's Supreme Court weighed economic concerns in its ruling that all stores and shopping malls could immediately open, stating that the government cannot keep stores closed (Shah, 2020). However, lifting restrictions catalyzed existing trends, severely expanding the health security threat for the country. In fact, observers note that this policy decision has done little to improve the country's economic situation. On the contrary, Pakistan's already "ill-equipped and under-funded health systems" (International Crisis Group, 2020, p. 1) were quickly overwhelmed, threatening hostility and resentment amongst the citizenry. In the month following the easing of restrictions, Pakistan reported over 100,000 new cases, with media reporting that some hospitals closed their gates as they were at maximum capacity and medical care providers were contracting the virus at increasing rates (ur-Rehman et al., 2020). This is particularly problematic, as it provides ammunition for fringe and militant elements operating within the state to garner support for their political objectives.

Predicting a depression of growth by 2.5%, the United Nations Development Programme (2020) called for a political commitment from all countries to combat severe economic consequences while ensuring that the most vulnerable populations receive the aid they needed. However, country-level responses to the pandemic around the globe became grid-locked due to conflict between political factions. Specifically, the Pakistani Prime Minister's Tehreek-e-Insaf government maintained somewhat strained relations with the country's largest opposition parties (*see*: Mukhtar, 2020), the Muslim League and the Pakistan Peoples Party, resulting in conflicting policy and mixed messaging.

For example, on March 23, Sindh Province, the only territory held by opposition parties, clashed with the central government when it became the first territory to implement a province-wide lockdown (International Crisis Group, 2020). This ran contrary to PM Khan's fear that a country-wide lockdown would result in the roughly 25% of Pakistanis already living below the poverty line being forced to remain at home without means of income (Maqsood, 2020). However, just one week later, Khan was forced to reckon with increasing case counts and moved the country into a national lockdown. In an attempt to provide direct relief to those affected by the lockdown and ongoing health crisis, the government issued payments to a large number of citizens (Maqsood, 2020), a policy implemented by multiple countries, such as Spain, Denmark, France, and the United States (Kaplan, 2020). Citing economic reasons, Khan opened the country back up on May 9, and in the month after, cases quadrupled in Pakistan, bringing the total death count up to 2,356 people (ur-Rehman et al., 2020). The Prime Minister cited economic reasons for reopening, noting that his government could not afford to continue providing cash handouts to the approximately 150 million people affected by Pakistan's shutdowns, noting also an anticipated 30% shortfall in government revenues. Khan cited rhetoric from American president Donald Trump, describing that 100,000 deaths occurred in the United States but that country also had decided it would also collapse if under a lockdown (Ray, 2020); however, in doing so, the Prime Minister failed to account for the fact that the health systems of the two countries have extremely different capacities, though in many of the U.S.'s hardest hit areas, hospitals also were unable to meet the needs of their local communities (*see*, e.g. Hutchinson & Margolin, 2020). In early July 2020, Pakistan opened its borders for trade, once again increasing the possibility of cross-border spread. The ongoing crisis has seriously impacted all Pakistani citizens. However, given the focus of this paper, in the next few sections we describe the prison system in Pakistan followed by how the pandemic has impacted it.

Prisons in Pakistan before COVID-19

Pakistan is the fifth most populous country in the world with a population of 220 million (Worldometer, 2020b). Pakistan's five provinces each have four categories of prisons: central prisons, special prisons, district prisons, and sub-jails (Zhang, 2017). Pakistan has a total prison population of 77, 275 with an occupancy rate of 133.8% in 2019 (World Prison Brief, 2020). Pakistan's prisons are over-populated by nearly 34%, holding approximately 20,000 incarcerated individuals over capacity across Pakistan's 114 jails (Human Rights Watch [HRW], 2020a; Justice Project for Pakistan [JPP], 2020a; World Prison Brief, 2020). At least 62% of prisoners are currently under trial,[2] meaning that over half of the country's incarcerated population has not even been convicted of a crime. JPP (2020a) reports that at least 1,500 incarcerated individuals are at the age of 60 or over. Females represent 1.6% of Pakistan's prison population, while juveniles represent 1.7%.

These numbers starkly indicate the over-crowding in prisons which could lead to unhygienic conditions even in normal times. The Justice Project for Pakistan (JPP) (2020a) reported that justice-involved individuals in Pakistan are subject to over-crowded prisons, where they are "cramped in tiny cells with no proper hygiene facilities, making them more vulnerable to contagious diseases." Past reports have documented severe deficiencies within Pakistani prisons, including inadequate toilet facilities and lack of access to clean drinking water (Dawn, 2013). Based on these reports, prisoners in Pakistani are subjected to conditions that do not promote proper hygiene and health behaviors.

While the prison system is already under-staffed generally, the total number of health-care vacancies is approximately one per jail. This could be problematic for organizational climate, decreases in which have been correlated with decreased commitment to the organization by staff (Kras et al., 2019). There are currently 108 vacant positions for medical officers in Pakistan's prisons (JPP, 2020a; United Nations Office on Drugs and Crime

[UNODC], 2020), indicating the lack of proper healthcare available to the prisoners. Consequently, in addition to prisons themselves posing an increased risk to those housed within them, current data suggest that the system is ill-prepared for outbreaks within the institutions. This effect is magnified because Pakistani prisons are already deficient in providing proper hygiene to incarcerated individuals. This problem is further exacerbated at the local level. For example, 10% of the prisons in Punjab do not have access to ambulances (JPP, 2020a); this means that these facilities are unable to transport individuals for emergency care.

Community corrections in Pakistan

Pakistan's community corrections system primarily includes probation and parole which are attached to the provincial Home Departments in Punjab, Sindh, Balochistan, and Khyber Pakhtunkhwa. A Director of Reclamation and Probation heads each Provincial Directorate, supported by Deputy Directors and Assistant Directors, probation and parole officers, office superintendents, and other administrative and support staff (Penal Reform International, 2012). While each province has some differences in operations, they are governed by the Probation of Offenders Ordinance 1960/Rules 1961.

The Good Conduct Prisoners' Probational Release Act, 1926, and its Rules, 1927, along with certain executive orders for implementation govern parole releases in Pakistan. These releases are primarily to allow prisoners to serve the last portion of their sentence in the community after completing a mandatory period in the prison. The main difference between probation and parole in Pakistan is that probation is given/revoked by the judiciary and parole is authorized/revoked by the Executives. The probation and parole population is not uniformly reported across all provinces. Punjab, the most populated province of Pakistan, reported 44,437 probationers and parolees under their jurisdiction in 2017-2018 compared to a prison population of 50,226 (Altaf et al., 2018). The introduction of the National Judicial Policy (NJP) 2009 led to significant progress in the use of probation as an alternative measure to detention in the country with steadily an increasing number of probationers leading to an almost even split in parole/probation and prisoner populations in the Punjab province (Mahmood, 2016).

However, probation and parole are grossly underfunded compared to prisons. Altaf et al. (2018) report that the annual spending of the Prisons Department per prisoner in 2017-2018 was 18,561 Pakistan Rupee (US $111.92), whereas the annual spending of the Reclamation and Probation Department per probationer/parolee was 3,381 Pakistan Rupee (US $20.39) clearly indicating the cost-savings of community corrections. The scarcity of official data makes it difficult to assess whether probation and parole are uniform within and across provinces and these alternative approaches have been largely neglected in the criminal justice system of Pakistan (Mahmood, 2016).

Prisons in Pakistan during COVID-19

Given the overcrowding in prisons, it would be almost impossible to enforce recognized best practices – such as social distancing, increased use of hand sanitizer, washing hands with soap and water – for minimizing risk in prisons. Overcrowding in prisons coupled with poor hygiene has longitudinally posed significant risks to health security in the country's prisons. The COVID-19 pandemic tests the limits of the Pakistani prison system's ability to mitigate threats for its population. Because of structural problems in the system, the high levels of positive cases during the pandemic were not unexpected.

Pressure has been mounting on Pakistani authorities to engage in transparent reporting of the prevalence of COVID-19 and testing protocols within the country's prison system. Amnesty International (2020a) reported that on April 21, 2020, one month after the first reported case of COVID-19 in a jail in Lahore, the government confirmed at least 97 incarcerated individuals nationwide had contracted COVID-19; however, the government revised this number to 86 just five days later without explanation. This abrupt revision undermined the legitimacy of the government's official reporting, raising concerns of biases in the official data being presented. This is in contrast to calls from prisoners where approximately 150 prisoners were expected to have contracted the virus in March 2020 (TRT World, 2020a). While Amnesty International (2020a) reports no additional official updates from the government, the Justice for Pakistan Project (2020a) reports that at least 1,890 Pakistani prisoners have tested positive and three have died of COVID-19.[3] No official reports have been released by the Pakistani government on the number of justice-involved individuals who have recovered from the virus.

A descriptive analysis of the available data suggests a disproportionate prevalence of the virus within Pakistan's prison population, as shown in Table 1. While the Pakistan prison population accounts for approximately 0.035% of the Pakistani population, incarcerated individuals represent over 18.31 times that ratio for testing positive for the novel COVID-19. This is theoretically expected through the lens of network science, as contagions are expected to diffuse through networks more quickly when the 'shortest path' when traveling from person-to-person remains quickly traveled (i.e. betweenness centrality, *see*: Freeman, 1977). Death rates amongst incarcerated individuals, based on available data, approximate similar trends to the broader Pakistani population. Thus, Amnesty International's (2020b) warning from March 2020 when the first inmate in Lahore was confirmed to be positive for COVID-19 that "Pakistani prisons and detention centers could become hotspots for the transmission of coronavirus" appears to have been merited. However, more reliable data and further analysis are needed to draw definitive conclusions of trends within the prison system.

Care should be taken to contextualize these figures. Specifically, data on prisoner positive rates and fatalities are reliant on data compiled by the Justice for Pakistan Project. This is currently the best available data to assess the impact of COVID-19 on Pakistan's prison system, but it is highly likely that reported cases do not account for the 'dark figure of COVID-19,' a concern that is heightened by the Pakistani government's failure to release transparent data on testing protocols and administration within the prison system. Thus, we

Table 1. Comparing Pakistan's general and prison populations against COVID-19 measures.

Category	Pakistan Prison Population	Population of Pakistan	Ratio (%)
Population	77,275	220,892,340	0.035
COVID-19 Positive Tests	1,890	294,638	0.641
Death from COVID-19	3	6,274	0.048

Data on Pakistan's population and COVID-19 case and death counts was pulled from the Worldometer data and represents the reporting as of 7:15PM CST on August 27, 2020 (Worldometer, 2020a, 2020b). Data on Pakistan's prison population comes from the Justice for Pakistan Project (JPP, 2020a).

should consider these figures to be conservative estimates, with ratios representing minimum thresholds though likely far higher in reality.

Because of the exorbitant risk Pakistan's prisoners face, various groups have called for the Government to take immediate steps to protect vulnerable populations. For example, the Legal Rights Forum [LRF] (2020) cites the International Covenant on Economic, Social and Cultural Rights (ICESCR) as the foundation for justifying why the Government has a duty to protect prisoners in the country. Similarly, the Justice Project for Pakistan (2020b) cites the Nelson Mandela Rules declaring prisoner healthcare as a responsibility of the state (*see also*: UN General Assembly, 2015). Both reports highlight several recommendations that the government could implement to better address safety during the health crisis. Among others, both reports argue that prison populations could be reduced, with special care taken to release those most at risk.

Specifically addressing this issue, in March 2020, the Islamabad High Court ordered the release of "under-trial prisoners alleged to have committed offences falling within the ambit of the non-prohibitory clause are admitted to bail, subject to furnishing such surety or security as may be deemed appropriate by an officer authorised in this regard by the Deputy Commissioner, Islamabad Capital Territory," also directing Islamabad police to not arrest individuals for petty offenses (Asad, 2020). While a somewhat controversial decision, the ruling would have resulted in at least 408 prisoners convicted of minor offenses being released from Adiala jail (Geo News, 2020). Additionally, the court ordered police to refrain from "unnecessary events" (Asad, 2020). Such a move is a drop in the ocean in the context of the country's 20,000 incarcerated individuals above the maximum operating capacities of Pakistani prisons. However, it set legal precedent for other states to follow suit, which could result in a larger long-term impact on Pakistan's justice system. The Sindhi High Court also ordered the release of just over 800 prisoners that had not yet been convicted (JPP, 2020b). In addition to reducing the risk of contracting COVID-19 for a large number of individuals, many of whom are not yet actually convicted of a crime, the prison reductions could help address the overcrowding in the system more broadly, creating opportunity for the implementation of a framework for increased sanitation standards. The Islamabad High Court's decision was promptly appealed to the Supreme Court of Pakistan sparking criticism from the Pakistan Bar Council (Geo News, 2020).

In April 2020, the Supreme Court recommended the release of prisoners currently under trial who are charged with "offences under non-prohibitory clauses, vagrancy law, or offences carrying less than three years sentence may be considered for bail: 1) Persons suffering from ailments or physical or mental disability, 2) All women and juvenile under-trial prisoners, 3) Under-trial prisoners who are 55 years of age or older, and 4) Other male UTPs provided there is no history of past convictions" (JPP, 2020b). Although it contributes to prison population reduction, the order excludes several categories of at-risk populations. For example, the Supreme Court explicitly addresses those currently under trial, but provides no provision for those who have been convicted. Past research has found that prisons have engaged in risk-based assessments in determining which prisoners could be released during the pandemic (Lofaro & McCue, 2020), bolstering the case for including non-violent offenders in such orders. The Supreme Court's intervention to block the release of prisoners ordered by a High Court is not unique to the Pakistani context. In June 2020, the U.S. Supreme Court blocked an order from a federal judge that would have released over 800 prisoners at risk of COVID-19 in Ohio (COVID-19 World News, 2020). In both situations, the politicization of criminal justice reform likely impacted decision-making, with the Supreme Court of the respective countries handing victories to the governing parties.

Advocacy groups have urged for Pakistan to take even further steps to protect prisoners, including releasing all individuals convicted for minor or non-violent offenses, release all individuals awaiting trial, and to release all prisoners over the age of 60 who meet specific criteria (LRF, 2020). Additionally, groups have called for increased release of prisoners who are mentally ill or disabled and for women and children who have yet to be convicted (JPP, 2020b; LRF, 2020). Ultimately, concerns remain for the safety of Pakistan's prison population, with heightened frustration over the country's lack of protections for its vulnerable populations and the reopening of the nation while unable to stop the spread of COVID-19 within its borders.

COVID-19 in India

India is the world's second most populous country with a population nearing 1.37 billion (Worldometer, 2020d). At the time of writing this paper, India's recorded coronavirus case total surpassed that of Brazil, making it the second worst-affected country in the world after the United States (Pathak, 2020). India recorded 90,802 new cases and the highest one-day increase in new cases anywhere in the world since the pandemic began. India's total cases are now more than 4.2 million (Pathak, 2020). Indian politicians widely tout the current rate of deaths per hundred thousand people (5.3) being lower than that of United States (57.75), United Kingdom (62.63), & Peru (92.80), but India's rate is much higher than its immediately neighboring countries such as Pakistan (2.99), Bangladesh (2.78), and Nepal (1.03) (John Hopkins University, n.d.).

On January 31, 2020, in its first situation report of the novel coronavirus (2019-nCoV), WHO (2020a) declared the virus a Public Health Emergency of International Concern (PHEIC). At that time, India had one case of COVID-19 in the State of Kerala as a result of travel to China. Since then, the numbers have increased exponentially with the 209th WHO situation report dated August 17th, 2020 confirming 2,589,682 cases and 49,980 deaths in India (WHO, 2020b). Testing has significantly improved with 969 labs in the government sector and 501 private labs testing about 30,041,400 samples to date with 731,697 samples tested on a single day on August 16, 2020 (WHO, 2020b). These numbers, however, may not reflect the true magnitude of cases in India. The stigma resulting from testing positive has resulted in many people trying to manage their symptoms without subjecting themselves to testing. A recent antibody study conducted in five areas of Pune (a city in Western India) revealed that 51.5% of residents tested positive, with one of the areas reporting 65% (the threshold for herd immunity). A similar study conducted a few weeks back in the nation's capital city, New Delhi, indicated positive antibody tests for 29% of people which translates to about 6 million infections. In sum, the number of cases confirmed positive tests, antibody tests, and projected increases point to a grim few months ahead (Thevar, 2020). The large youth population of India (35% of its population of 1.2 million) aged between 18 and 24 years is expected to mitigate the deaths resulting from the COVID-19 virus, the question that remains to be answered in the forthcoming weeks is whether India will lead the world in the total number of cases and total number of deaths.

The government's response in India has been characterized by dramatic moves without much forethought. India did a test-run of a national 14 hour "Janata Curfew" on March 22 and went into full national lockdown on March 24, putting restrictions on the movement of nearly one-and-half billion Indians for two months. These actions were taken without foresight and had a devastating impact on millions of unorganized migrant daily-wage workers who live from hand to mouth. Left without a source of income, or means to travel, there was a mass exodus of almost ten million people returning to their villages, many of them walking or cycling hundreds of miles. The nationwide lockdown imposed by the Government of India banned people from stepping out of their homes; closed all shops and services except for pharmacies, hospitals, groceries, and essential services; closed all commercial and private businesses allowing only work-from-home; suspended all educational institutions; closed all religious institutions and places of worship; suspended all non-essential transport and prohibited all kinds of public activities including political, social, religious, cultural, and entertainment. This early closure was lauded by experts and health officials, but the impact on the economy resulted in the government relaxing these measures much before the pandemic could be contained.

The lockdown and unlock dates shown in Table 2, observed in relation to the growth of number of cases as indicated in Figure 1, clearly indicate that, like with Pakistan, while India did well in initiating the lockdown, it opened up too soon. Given the large population of the country and high population density, opening up of the country through its UNLOCK phases has been largely unsuccessful with new cases rising at a rapid rate since the country launched its first opening up through UNLOCK-1 on June 1, 2020.

COVID-19 is predicted to plunge the global economy into its worst recession since World War II and its impact on India will prove to be catastrophic. Despite the economic recovery packages put forth by the Indian government, the International Labour Organization (2020) projects that 400 million people in India are likely to fall into poverty

Table 2. Timeline of India's lockdown and reopening phases.

Nationwide lockdown:
Phase 1: 25 March 2020 – 14 April 2020 (21 days)
Phase 2: 15 April 2020 – 3 May 2020 (19 days)
Phase 3: 4 May 2020 – 17 May 2020 (14 days)
Phase 4: 18 May 2020 – 31 May 2020 (14 days)
Unlock:
Unlock 1.0: 1 June 2020 – 30 June 2020 (30 days)
Unlock 2.0: 1 July 2020 – 31 July 2020 (31 days)
Unlock 3.0: 1 August 2020 – 31 August 2020 (29 days)

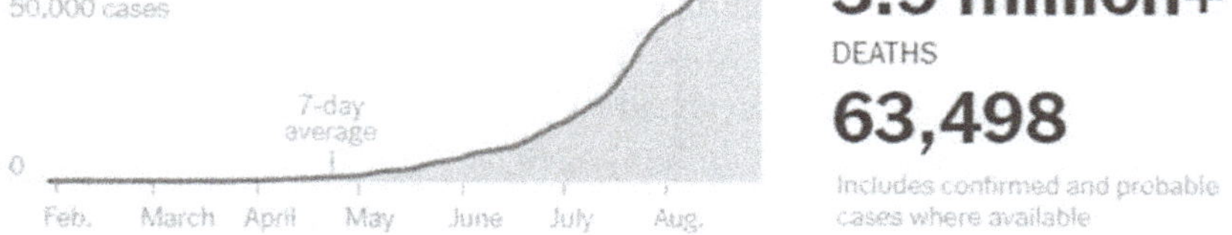

Figure 1. Growth Curve of India's COVID-19 cases.
Note: Image credit: (The New York Times, 2020).

as a result of the economic stoppage caused by the pandemic. While the global GDP is expected to contract by 5.2% (The World Bank, 2020), it is projected that India's economy will contract by 20% in the first quarter of the fiscal year (PTI, 2020). In an effort to mitigate the financial losses and bolster the country's economic security, the government's UNLOCK-4 plans will allow metro trains to resume services from September 7 and political, social, and religious congregations of up to 100 people will be permitted from September 21 (Arora, 2020).

The initial hotspots of COVID-19 in India were in large metropolitan areas, but the pandemic has now diffused to the farthest corners of the country. India's prisons are also now looking at the possibility of becoming the biggest virus clusters given the large number of people living in close proximity.

Prisons in India before COVID-19

In India, the State Governments are exclusively responsible for the management and administration of prisons. They are guided by the Prisons Act of 1894 and each state government has its own prison manual (Ministry of Home Affairs, n.d.). The individual states have the primary responsibility of prisons and have the authority to change any prison laws or policies in their respective state prison systems. For the past two decades, India has been trying to reform its prison system with advisory committees, commissions, and training institutes. The primary issues driving the reform are "overcrowding, prolonged detention of undertrials, unsatisfactory living conditions, staff shortage, poor training, corruption and extortion, inadequate social reintegration programs, poor spending on healthcare and welfare, lack of legal aid and allegations of indifferent and inhuman approach of prison staff among others" (Lok Sabha Secretariat, 2017, pp. 3–4).

In 2019, there were about 478,600 people in prisons and jails in India at an occupancy rate of 118.5% (NCRB, n.d.). The 1,350 prisons referenced in the 2019 data include 617 Sub Jails, 410 District Jails, 144 Central Jails, 31 Women Jails, and other specialized types of jails. The highest number of inmates were lodged in various Central (46%) and District Jails (43%) whose occupancy rates exceeded capacity. Overcrowding and high occupancy rates have been a consistent problem in Indian prisons as demonstrated by the data in Table 3.

Most prisoners in India are male (96%), and 70% of the total prison population comprises under-trial prisoners. India ranks 15th out of 217 countries in under-trial incarceration (Tata Trusts, 2019). Table 4 shows the annual ratio of prisoners undertrial to those convicted of a crime. This statistic is rather alarming as it represents those who have been locked up without a conviction. Illiteracy, poverty, and lack of understanding of the

Table 3. India's prison type & occupancy.

Year	No. of Prisons	Actual Capacity of Prisons	No. of Prisoners at the End of the Year	Occupancy Rate at the End of the Year
2017	1,361	391,574	450,696	115.1%
2018#	1,339	396,223	466,084	117.6%
2019#	1,350	403,739	478,600	118.5%

Image credit: Recreated from NCRB (n.d.). Numbers represent data provided by States/UTs. #Due to no data being received from West Bengal in 2018 and 2019, data provided for 2017 was used. Figures represent levels as of December 31st for each respective year.

Table 4. India's prisoner types & demography.

Year	No. of Convicts	No. of Under-trial Prisoners	No. of Detenues	No. of Other Inmates	Total No. of Prisoners
2017	139,149	308,718	2,136	693	450,696
2018#	139,488	323,537	2,384	675	466,084
2019#	144,125	330,487	3,223	765	478,600

Image credit: Recreated from NCRB (n.d.). Numbers represent data provided by States/UTs. #Due to no data being received from West Bengal in 2018 and 2019, data provided for 2017 was used. Figures represent levels as of December 31st for each respective year.

prison system coupled with police corruption and the huge backlog in court cases results in many prisoners languishing in the prison for a very long time without legal recourse.

Prisoners consistently have lower life expectancy and higher health risks due to unsanitary conditions in prisons and lack of healthcare. As noted in the recent Tata Trust (2019) study, prison populations have comparatively higher rates of diseases such as HIV, STD, Tuberculosis, and Hepatitis B & C compared to the general population (Tata Trust, 2019). In 2016, the death rate (per 100,000 prisoners) had consistently increased over the years to 382.2.

The Supreme Court of India has recognized the overcrowding of prisons and tried to address it in the past few years through directives to States. In response to an amicus curiae brief the court was informed that many prisons were functioning at 150% capacity with one prison at 609% capacity. The court emphasized that prisoners have 'human rights' and cannot be kept in jails 'like animals' (PTI, 2018). The Supreme Court had directed the States, in 2016 to submit a plan of action to address overcrowding of prisons and noted that not a single State had submitted a plan by the deadline of March 2017. This indicates a complete lack of interest by authorities to tackle the issue. More recently, in February 2020, the chief justice of the supreme court clearly stated that overcrowding in jails is connected to "performance of courts" and held courts squarely responsible for not handling cases quickly to reduce the number of under-trial prisoners (The Print, 2020).

The problem of overcrowding is further exacerbated by the poor staffing in jails which is purported to be at, on average, 30% to 40% of sanctioned strength (The Print, 2020). The Tata Trust (2019) report which, for the first time in India, analyzed data across the four pillars of the criminal justice system (police, prisons, judiciary, and legal aid) states that there are just 621 correctional staff across India's 1,421 jails. Uttar Pradesh has only one sanctioned correctional staffer for 95,366 inmates. The new Model Prison Manual (Ministry of Home Affairs, 2016) stipulates one medical officer for every 300 prisoners and requires central prisons to have a doctor available at all times. Most often, these positions are left unfilled and medical staff are unavailable for prisoners; for example, the Uttarakhand jail has a vacancy for 10 medical officers and does not have a single officer available at the facility. More than 12 states in India are operating at less than 50% capacity of medical officers. Further, the prison manual requires prison systems to have a cohort of correctional staff geared toward rehabilitation of prisoners. These correctional staff can include welfare officers, social workers, counselors, psychologists, and lawyers to ensure the well-being of prisoners providing individualized care to ensure their needs are met. However, according to the 2019 Prison Statistics of India, four states with prison populations ranging from 7,000 to 25,000 had no such staff, and few others had only one or two staff for prison populations ranging from 15,000 to 100,000 (NCRB, n.d.). Despite vacancies and funds allocated for hiring of staff, these positions remain unfilled primarily because these staff are grossly underpaid.

Even without the pandemic, India has been contending with serious issues in its prison system. Operating over capacity with acute shortage of staff often results in prisoners being forced and locked up in crowded small spaces for long periods of time even though space may be available in other areas of the prison. This results in poor sanitary conditions. Additionally, this makes separation of convicted prisoners from undertrial prisoners, non-violent, or first offenders impossible. Reform and educational activities or prison industries are impossible to operate with the shortage of staff. Many prisons have been using long-term inmates as free labor inside prisons to manage various tasks to act as warders, convict officers, or night watchmen. This enables some convicts to have power over other prisoners and allows for exploitation, violence, and collusion in many illegal activities, including corruption in the prison system. In this milieu, the COVID-19 pandemic has further exacerbated the human rights violations in the Indian prison system.

Community corrections in India

The two community corrections in India are probation and parole. In India probation is granted under *The Probation of Offenders Act (Act No. 28 of 1958)* which contains elaborate provisions relating to probation of offenders, applicable throughout the country. The intent of this ACT was to reform amateur offenders by providing rehabilitation in society and to prevent the conversion of youthful offenders into obdurate criminals under environmental influence by keeping them in jails along with hardened criminals. There are no official statistics about how often probation is implemented by the courts, however, the popular notion is that it is not uniformly implemented. Further, the lack of probation-officers due to open vacancies makes it extremely difficult to implement and therefore is not an option of choice used by judges. Parole in India is administered by the rules of the Prison Act, 1894, and Prisoner Act, 1900. Each state in India has its own parole rules with some minor alternations from each other. During the year 2019, a total of 26,390 persons were released on parole and only 205 prisoners (less than 1%) released on parole have absconded (NCRB, n.d.). Similar to Pakistan, community corrections in India face a pending crisis due to staffing, and it is likely that the effects of COVID-19 will add further stress on the system.

Prisons in India during COVID-19

Media reports have referred to India's prisons as 'ticking time bombs' with more than 70% of prisoners (and their children) residing in enforced proximity either due to overcrowding or shortage of staff (The New Indian Express, 2020). These conditions are further worsened by the inability of prisoners to maintain personal hygiene, the single largest protector from the virus. India's prisons are looking at the possibility of becoming the biggest virus clusters and in response jails have been racing against time to put in place measures to avoid this situation. The first step taken to address this issue was a directive to all States by the Supreme Court of India on March 23, 2020. The court ordered each State to form high-level committees to put in place processes and guidelines to release convicted prisoners on parole for four to six weeks; and to consider interim bail for undertrial prisoners with offences that required a sentence of less than seven years. On April 13 2020, in response to various public interest lawsuits that demanded clearer guidelines and better conditions for prisoners, the court clarified that it was not 'compulsory' for States to release prisoners and its earlier directive was intended to prevent overcrowding of prisons in view of the pandemic.

As States started forming high-powered committees at the direction of the Supreme Court, the policies and processes varied from State to State, making it impossible to implement a uniform national response. For example, the 18 member high-powered committee in Maharashtra State, charged with selecting prisoners for release excluded people charged under the Maharashtra Control of Organised Crime Act, Prevention of Money Laundering Act, Maharashtra Protection of Interest of Depositors Act, Narcotics Drugs and Psychotropic Substances Act, Unlawful Activities Prevention Act, and foreign nationals (Chaudhari, 2020).

Based on data gathered by the Commonwealth Human Rights Initiative (2020), which relies on media reports to compile state-by-state statistics, as of August 26th, 2020, including prisoners and staff the total number of COVID-19 cases in Indian prisons is 6,621 with 15 related deaths, as shown in Table 5. The total number of prisoners released since these measures were implemented is 61,100 representing about 15.4% of the total prison population in India. Even with these releases, the occupancy rate of Indian prisons remains above capacity at 103.1%.

In comparing the ratios in Tables 1 and 5, we see similar findings for both Pakistan and India. For both countries, roughly 0.035% of the population is incarcerated; however, it should be noted that while proportions are the same, India has a far greater number of individuals within its corrections system, given the sheer volume of its population. While inter-country direct comparisons cannot be made about the proportion of COVID-19 positives, in India, the ratio is far lower. Even though the Indian data suggest a ratio approximately one-third less than Pakistan, officially reported data for this field include staff and prisoner positive cases – thus, the true proportion of prisoners who test positive out of all Indian positive cases would be even smaller. In India, the proportion of COVID-19-related deaths is actually smaller than the proportion of the prison to the general population. While these numbers may look promising based on the available data, it is yet to be seen what the official statistics (when available) will reveal and if the data collected from media reports line up with it.

There have been many criticisms of the approach taken by the Indian Supreme Court, mainly because it created a climate of imperfect and unequal justice in the country. By allowing the individual States to define the criteria for release, a person with the same charges would be treated differently depending on where they were imprisoned. Some States used the pandemic as an opportunity to imprison or refuse to release activists and human

Table 5. Comparing India's general and prison populations against COVID-19 measures.

Category	India Prison Population	Population of India	Ratio (%)
Population	478,600	1,382,347,512	0.035
COVID-19 Positive Tests	6,621	3,687,939	0.180
Death from COVID-19	15	65,435	0.022

Data on India's population and COVID-19 case and death counts was pulled from the Worldometer data and represents the reporting as of 3:48 PM CST on August 31, 2020 (Worldometer, 2020c, 2020d). Note: The prison population field represents all prisoners, but data for COVID-19 positives in prisons aggregates prisoners and staff. Data on India's prison population COVID-19 data comes from the Commonwealth Human Rights Initiative (2020), while data on total number of prisoners comes from the NCRB (n.d.).

rights workers. Many students and activists who participated in peaceful protests against India's recent discriminatory citizenship laws based on religion continue to be unfairly detained (Amnesty International, 2020c). Amnesty International released a report citing India as one of the countries where many human rights defenders were kept in pre-trial detention under the Unlawful Activities (Prevention) Act (UAPA), legislation which has often been liberally and unjustly used to imprison critics of the government. For example, the case of Safoora Zargar, a pregnant activist who protested against laws that discriminate against Muslims, was detained as an undertrial prisoner and was finally released in June after much campaigning on her behalf. Similarly, other activists continue to be detained despite health concerns or other illnesses (Amnesty International, 2020d). Another major criticism of the Supreme Court's response was that the court merely directed the formation of high-powered committees to determine the categories of prisoners. The actual task of releasing them was at the initiative of the offenders or their families as application for bail had to be filed, and hearings conducted before a release could occur. All of this during the pandemic made the task onerous and difficult for prisoners and their families as the courts had restricted their work during the pandemic to urgent cases only (Jain, 2020).

Given that the occupancy rate of prisons and jails still lurks above the 100% mark, and the staffing shortfall is yet to be remedied, merely releasing prisoners to decongest the prison is going to be insufficient. Proper measures and safety precautions have to be put in place for those still in the prisons as inmates or staff. Also, the suspension of family visits, legal aid services created isolation among prisoners who could not access the legal help they needed to take advantage of the bail options. This is a violation of human rights. It was only towards the end of June 2020 that video-conferencing facilities were introduced in jails. Even this information is not publicly available on websites of the prisons. Families with little or no access to the internet have no way of knowing how their relative is doing in the prison.

In sum, India's response to COVID19 in prisons has laid bare the inefficiencies and injustices in the criminal justice system. It has highlighted the problems caused by letting States make their own decisions about who to release and who not to. Further, the high-handed attitude of the government to human rights workers using pandemic-related restrictions towards activists and critics of the government demonstrates the shrinking of civic space and suppression of voices that are uncomfortable to the government (Amnesty International, 2020e).

Conclusion

Stemming from a unified polity prior to 1947, India and Pakistan have also been intimately connected, despite both nations striving to develop distinct identities. Past work has found this nation-building mentality forged into the very core of the nation, such as the school system (Lall, 2008). The COVID-19 pandemic, in some ways, is a test of how similar they still are. In examining the response of both the countries to the pandemic, it can be seen that prison systems in the two countries face similar circumstances, including overcrowding, understaffing, and concerns over hygiene and prisoner safety. Specifically, both India and Pakistan face a critical shortage of medical staff in prisons to the extent that the safety and well-being of incarcerated individuals are at severe risk.

Additionally, both countries took the consequential step of reopening the nation before they fully controlled the spread of COVID-19 as a step to stabilize economic security.

Conversely, each country's political elite largely controlled the COVID-19 response, shaped by the political, cultural, and economic changes that have taken place in each country. For example, Pakistan's Prime Minister Khan clashed with Sindh Province's decision to institute lockdown protocols only to reverse course later. Similarly, succumbing to calls to stabilize the economy, India's Prime Minister Modi prematurely reopened the country, resulting in a dramatic increase in positive cases. Ironically, each country has accused the other of engaging in unlawful or unjust imprisonment of activists (*see, e.g.*: BBC News, 2020; HRW, 2020b), ignoring their own use of similar tactics. Although both countries have taken steps to address the historically rooted, systemic issues that plague their corrections systems, inadequate policies have been implemented, resulting in limited protections for some of the populations most vulnerable for exposure to the novel coronavirus through closed networks. The pandemic offers an opportunity to both countries to evaluate their own approaches and to recognize the similarities still connecting them, rooted through common memories of colonization, embedded in the Weberian (1978) framework for ethnicity.

The pandemic has offered both India and Pakistan an opportunity for a natural experiment to test what happens if large numbers of undertrial prisoners or convicts with shorter sentences are released? If there are no increases in crime rates despite the large number of releases, or if the number of absconded individuals remains as low as the statistics indicate (less than 1%), it goes to prove that such large numbers of undertrials really do not need to be incarcerated in the first place. The justice system can still function without incarcerating them. This will then allow the existing prisons to function at or below capacity, with staffing that meets the requirements of the model code. Further, both countries need to make the conditions of work in prisons more conducive thereby attracting more applicants and filling up vacancies sooner. If these measures are coupled with increased funding and wider implementation of community corrections, the COVID pandemic offers both countries a chance to truly reform its prison systems.

Notes

1. The eight member states of the South Asian Association for Regional Cooperation are: Afghanistan, Bangladesh, Bhutan, India, the Maldives, Nepal, Pakistan, and Sri Lanka (Dmello, 2019; NTI Nuclear Security Index [NTI], 2011).
2. The trial status of some prisoners was unavailable.
3. JPP collected data from official government figures, leaked reports, and media reports. For a full list of sources, see: (JPP, 2020a).

ORCID

Jared R. Dmello http://orcid.org/0000-0001-8805-1061
Sheetal Ranjan http://orcid.org/0000-0002-7991-3472

References

Altaf, M., Khan, M. I. U., Ahmad, U., & Yousaf, Z. (2018). Reclamation and probation department: A saving account to the government. *International Journal of Scientific and Research Publications*, *8* (2), 318–323. http://www.ijsrp.org/research-paper-0218/ijsrp-p7440.pdf

Amnesty International. (2020a, May 7). *Pakistan: Authorities must be transparent about COVID-19 cases in prisons.* https://www.amnesty.org/en/latest/news/2020/05/pakistan-authorities-must-be-transparent-about-covid-19-cases-in-prisons/

Amnesty International. (2020b, March 26). *Pakistan: Punjab prisoners at heightened risk of COVID-19.* https://www.amnesty.org/en/documents/asa33/2032/2020/en/

Amnesty International. (2020c, August 6). *Virus-hit prisons still full of human rights defenders, as attacks continue.* https://www.amnesty.org/en/latest/news/2020/08/attacks-on-hrds-during-pandemic-report/

Amnesty International. (2020d). *Daring to stand up for human rights in a pandemic.* https://www.amnesty.org/download/Documents/ACT3027652020ENGLISH.PDF

Amnesty International. (2020e). *Human rights defenders: We need them more than ever! States worldwide must protect human rights defenders in the current COVID-19 crisis.* https://www.amnesty.org/download/Documents/ACT3021022020ENGLISH.pdf

Arora, N. (2020, August 29). *India to reopen underground train networks even as coronavirus cases jump.* Reuters. https://www.reuters.com/article/us-health-coronavirus-india-cases/india-to-reopen-underground-train-networks-even-as-coronavirus-cases-jump-idUSKBN25P0AJ

Asad, M. (2020, March 21). IHC orders release of under-trial prisoners. *Dawn.* https://www.dawn.com/news/1542607

BBC News. (2020, January 27). *Manzoor Pashteen: Activist who dared to challenge Pakistan y held.* https://www.bbc.com/news/world-asia-51262639

Bichler, G., Norris, A., Dmello, J. R., & Randle, J. (2019). The impact of civil gang injunctions on networked violence between the bloods and the crips. *Crime & Delinquency, 65*(7), 875–915. https://doi.org/10.1177/0011128717739607

Caballero-Anthony, M. (2016). *An introduction to non-traditional security studies.* Sage Publications.

Chaudhuri, K. (2020, May 12). *Maharashtra panel decides to release 50% of prisoners on temporary bail to prevent spread of Covid-19.* Hindustan Times. https://www.hindustantimes.com/india-news/maharashtra-panel-decides-to-release-50-of-prisoners-on-temporary-bail-to-prevent-spread-of-covid-19/story-U2yob9EHSa5TJXai12tHEI.html

Christakis, N. A., & Fowler, J. H. (2009). *Connected: The surprising power of our social networks and how they shape our lives.* Little, Brown.

Commonwealth Human Rights Initiative. (2020). *State/UT wise prisons response to COVID 19 pandemic in India.* https://www.humanrightsinitiative.org/content/stateut-wise-prisons-response-to-covid-19-pandemic-in-india

COVID-19 World News. (2020, June 4). *Supreme Court blocks order to remove inmates at prison infected with COVID-19.* https://covid19data.com/2020/06/04/supreme-court-blocks-order-to-remove-inmates-at-prison-infected-with-covid-19/

Dawn. (2013, June 26). Lack of drinking water, sanitation found major issues in prisons across Sindh. *Dawn.* https://www.dawn.com/news/1020875

Dmello, J. R. (2019). *Friends, foes, and unknowns: Investigating the dynamics of relationships between actors in ethnic conflicts* (Publication No. 13898086) [Doctoral dissertation]. University of Massachusetts Lowell. ProQuest Dissertations and Theses Global.

Firestone, S. M., Ward, M. P., Christley, R. M., & Dhand, N. K. (2011). The importance of location in contact networks: Describing early epidemic spread using spatial social network analysis. *Preventive veterinary medicine, 102*(3), 185–195. https://doi.org/10.1016/j.prevetmed.2011.07.006

Freeman, L. C. (1977). A set of measures of centrality based on betweenness. *Sociometry*, 35–41.

Gannon, K. (2020, June 23). As virus cases soar, Pakistan says it must keep its economy open. *The Diplomat.* https://thediplomat.com/2020/06/as-virus-cases-soar-pakistan-says-it-must-keep-its-economy-open/

Geo News. (2020, March 28). Pakistan bar council 'dismayed' at petition challenging IHC's decision to release prisoners. *Geo News.* https://www.geo.tv/latest/279683-pakistan-bar-council-dismayed-at-petition-challenging-ihcs-decision-to-release-prisoners

Green, B., Horel, T., & Papachristos, A. V. (2017). Modeling contagion through social networks to explain and predict gunshot violence in Chicago, 2006 to 2014. *JAMA Internal Medicine, 177*(3), 326–333. https://doi.org/10.1001/jamainternmed.2016.8245

Human Rights Watch [HRW]. (2020a, March 19). *Pakistan: Prisoners at risk of COVID-19.* https://www.hrw.org/news/2020/03/19/pakistan-prisoners-risk-covid-19

Human Rights Watch [HRW]. (2020b, April 15). *India: Activists detained for peaceful dissent.* https://www.hrw.org/news/2020/04/15/india-activists-detained-peaceful-dissent

Hutchinson, B., & Margolin, J. (2020, April 5). With coronavirus apex still to come, some US hospitals reeling from capacity crunch. *ABC News.* https://abcnews.go.com/US/coronavirus-apex-us-hospitals-reeling-capacity-crunch/story?id=69987748

International Crisis Group. (2020, August 6). *Pakistan's COVID-19 crisis.* International Crisis Group. https://www.crisisgroup.org/asia/south-asia/pakistan/b162-pakistans-covid-19-crisis

International Labour Organization. (2020). *ILO Monitor: COVID-19 and the world of work. Second edition - Updated estimates and analysis.* https://www.ilo.org/wcmsp5/groups/public/—dgreports/—dcomm/documents/briefingnote/wcms_740877.pdf

Jain, A. (2020, August 21). As Covid-19 Hits India's prisons, expert explains why decongestion is not enough. *Huffington Post.* https://www.huffingtonpost.in/entry/covid-19-prisons-decongestion_in_5f3e4dd6c5b66346158130cf

John Hopkins University. (n.d.). *Mortality analyses.* https://coronavirus.jhu.edu/data/mortality

Justice Project for Pakistan [JPP]. (2020a). *COVID-19 and prisoners.* https://www.jpp.org.pk/covid19-prisoners/

Justice Project for Pakistan [JPP]. (2020b). *Policy recommendations: Safeguards for Pakistani prisoners during COVID-19.*

Kaplan, J. (2020, May 8). *14 countries that are paying their workers during quarantine — and how they compare to America's $1,200 stimulus checks.* Business Insider. https://www.businessinsider.com/countries-offering-direct-payments-or-basic-income-in-corona-crisis-2020-4

Kras, K. R., Dmello, J. R., Meyer, K. S., Butterfield, A. E., & Rudes, D. S. (2019). Attitudes toward punishment, organizational commitment, and cynicism: A multilevel analysis of staff responses in a juvenile justice agency. *Criminal Justice and Behavior, 46*(3), 475–491. https://doi.org/10.1177/0093854818810857

Lall, M. (2008). Educate to hate: The use of education in the creation of antagonistic national identities in India and Pakistan. *Compare, 38*(1), 103–119. https://doi.org/10.1080/03057920701467834

Legal Rights Forum [LRF]. (2020, March 25). *Policy paper: Protection of Pakistani prisoners during COVID-19 pandemic.* http://lrfpk.org/wp-content/uploads/2020/04/Policy-Paper-Protection-of-Pakistani-Prisoners-during-COVID-19-Pandemic.pdf

Lofaro, R. J., & McCue, C. (2020). Salient target populations and the subcategorization of deviants in the release of inmates during the COVID-19 pandemic. *Administrative Theory & Practice*, Online First, 1–15. https://doi.org/10.1080/10841806.2020.1794745

Lok Sabha Secretariat. (2017). *Prison reform in India.*

Mahmood, A. (2016, February 9). The neglected probation system. *The Tribune.* https://tribune.com.pk/story/1043366/the-neglected-probation-system#:~:text=The%20Probation%20and%20Reclamation%20Department,and%20five%20female%20parole%20officers

Maqsood, N. (2020, May 11). On the coronavirus, Pakistan's government is missing in action. *Foreign Policy.* https://foreignpolicy.com/2020/05/11/on-coronavirus-pakistans-government-is-missing-in-action/

Ministry of Home Affairs. (2016). *Model Prison Manual 2016. Government of India: Ministry of Home Affairs.* https://bprd.nic.in/WriteReadData/CMS/PrisonManualNew.pdf

Ministry of Home Affairs. (n.d.). *About prison reforms.* https://www.mha.gov.in/MHA1/PrisonReforms/home.html

Mukhtar, I. (2020). PRI congratulates itself after two years in office. *The Nation.* https://nation.com.pk/19-Aug-2020/pti-congratulates-itself-after-two-years-in-office

NCRB (n.d.). *Prison statistics India - 2019.* https://ncrb.gov.in/sites/default/files/Executive-Summary-2019.pdf

NTI Nuclear Security Index [NTI]. (2011, October 26). *South Asian Association for Regional Cooperation (SAARC).* NTI: Building a Safer World. https://www.nti.org/learn/treaties-and-regimes/south-asian-association-regional-cooperation-saarc/

Pathak, S. (2020, September 7). *India moves into 2nd place for COVID-19 cases.* NPR. https://www.npr.org/sections/coronavirus-live-updates/2020/09/07/910401174/india-moves-into-2nd-place-for-covid-19-cases

Penal Reform International. (2012). *Probation and parole system in Pakistan: Assessment and recommendations for reform.*

PTI. (2018, March 30). Supreme Court shocked at over 600 per cent overcrowding in jails. *Times of India.* http://timesofindia.indiatimes.com/articleshow/63546393.cms?utm_source=contentofinterest&utm_medium=text&utm_campaign=cppst

PTI. (2020, August 19). India's GDP to contract by 20 per cent in first quarter of FY21: Care ratings. *The Economics Times.* https://economictimes.indiatimes.com/news/economy/indicators/indias-gdp-to-contract-by-20-per-cent-in-first-quarter-of-fy21-care-ratings/articleshow/77637707.cms?utm_source=contentofinterest&utm_medium=text&utm_campaign=cppst

Ray, M. (2020, June 2). Imran Khan lifts lockdown amid rising COVID-19 cases, urges Pakistan to 'live with the virus'. *Hindustan Times.* https://www.hindustantimes.com/world-news/imran-khan-lifts-lockdown-amid-rising-covid-19-cases-urges-pakistan-to-live-with-the-virus/story-9lmwJzHv9zc0owqy3GQW4M.html

Shah, S. (2020, May 18). Pakistan court says stores can reopen, weighing economic concerns. *The Wall Street Journal.* https://www.wsj.com/articles/pakistan-court-says-stores-can-reopen-weighing-economic-concerns-11589831323

Tata Trusts. (2019). *India justice report: Ranking states on police, judiciary, prisons & legal aid.* https://www.tatatrusts.org/upload/pdf/overall-report-single.pdf

The New Indian Express. (2020, July 28). Our country's prisons are a ticking coronavirus time bomb. *The New Indian Express.* https://www.newindianexpress.com/opinions/editorials/2020/jul/28/our-countrys-prisons-are-a-ticking-coronavirus-time-bomb-2175641.html

The New York Times. (2020). India coronavirus map and case count. *The New York Times.* https://www.nytimes.com/interactive/2020/world/asia/india-coronavirus-cases.html

The Print. (2020, February 5). *Supreme Court says overcrowding in jails related to courts' performance, to pass orders.* https://theprint.in/judiciary/supreme-court-says-overcrowding-in-jails-related-to-courts-performance-to-pass-orders/360393/

The World Bank. (2020). *ILO Monitor: Global economic preferences.* https://www.worldbank.org/en/publication/global-economic-prospects

Thevar, S. (2020). Pune Covid-19 sero survey suggests 51.5% have antibodies. *Hindustan Times.* https://www.hindustantimes.com/india-news/pune-survey-suggests-51-5-have-antibodies/story-9MlFUJfmiWnNOrzujCwKIP.html

TRT World. (2020a, April 7). *Dozens of prisoners contract coronavirus, doctors demand PPE in Pakistan.* https://www.trtworld.com/asia/dozens-of-prisoners-contract-coronavirus-doctors-demand-ppe-in-pakistan-35194

TRT World. (2020b, June 22). *Economy forces Pakistan to reopen even as COVID-19 cases spike.* https://www.trtworld.com/asia/economy-forces-pakistan-to-reopen-even-as-covid-19-cases-spike-37480

UN General Assembly. (2015). *United Nations standard minimum rules for the treatment of prisoners (the Nelson Mandela rules): resolution/adopted by the General Assembly.* https://www.refworld.org/docid/5698a3a44.html

United Nations Development Programme [UNDP]. (2020). *High level of political commitment needed to fight COVID-19.* UNDP. https://www.undp.org/content/undp/en/home/stories/highest-level-of-political-commitment-needed-to-fight-covid-19.html

United Nations Office on Drugs and Crime [UNODC]. (2020). *Prisons and pandemic: Inaction is not an option.* Advocacy Brief 1.

ur-Rehman, Z., Masood, S., & Abi-Habib, M. (2020). Pakistan's lockdown ended a month ago. Now hospital signs read 'full'. *The New York Times.* https://www.nytimes.com/2020/06/15/world/asia/pakistan-coronavirus-hospitals.html

Van Mieghem, P., Omic, J., & Kooij, R. (2008). Virus spread in networks. *IEEE/ACM Transactions On Networking, 17*(1), 1–14. https://doi.org/10.1109/TNET.2008.925623

Weber, M. (1978). *Economy and society.* University of California Press.

World Health Organization. (2020a). *Novel coronavirus* (2019-nCoV)*: Situation Report - 1.* https://www.who.int/docs/default-source/coronaviruse/situation-reports/20200121-sitrep-1-2019-ncov.pdf?sfvrsn=20a99c10_4

World Health Organization. (2020b). *Novel coronavirus disease (COVID-19): Situation update report - 29.*

World Prison Brief. (2020, August 27). *World prison brief data: Pakistan.* https://www.prisonstudies.org/country/pakistan

Worldometer. (2020a, August 27). *Pakistan coronavirus cases.* https://www.worldometers.info/coronavirus/country/pakistan/

Worldometer. (2020b, August 27). *Pakistan population.* https://www.worldometers.info/world-population/pakistan-population/

Worldometer. (2020c, August 31). *India coronavirus cases.* https://www.worldometers.info/coronavirus/country/india/

Worldometer. (2020d, August 31). *India population.* https://www.worldometers.info/world-population/india-population/

Zhang, Y. (2017).Corrections in Pakistan. In *The encyclopedia of corrections* (1st ed., pp. 1–9). Wiley-Blackwell. https://doi.org/10.1002/9781118845387.wbeoc045

National Responses for Persons Deprived of Liberty during the COVID-19 Pandemic in the Philippines

Michael B. Cahapay

ABSTRACT

The main purpose of this paper is to review the national responses for persons deprived of liberty (PDLs) during the coronavirus disease 2019 (COVID-19) pandemic in the Philippines. The researcher discusses the major responses that have been carried out such as easing the rules on parole grant and executive clemency, providing human consideration to the vulnerable segments, and improving the corrections facilities health management. These responses are expected to decrease the growth of virus infection inside the corrections facilities, protect the condition especially of the vulnerable segments, and ensure the overall safety of the community. This paper specifically recommends for the need to expand the virtualization of judiciary functions to the provincial zones, place the release of the vulnerable segments in priority order, and technically improve the health management of corrections. However, as current responses may just represent temporary measures due to the crisis, this paper further urges for responses that will eventually lead to long-term decongestion of corrections facilities or reduction of the perennially high prison population of the country.

Introduction

The world continues to grapple with the crisis brought by the COVID-19, a respiratory syndrome caused by a new strain of coronavirus. As of July 26, the World Health Organization (2020) reported a total of 15,581,009 confirmed positive cases across the globe. There is no codified treatment that has been discovered to cure the infection but authorities have long distinguished the importance of physical distancing as one of the approaches to prevent the virus transmission. However, in closed environments of corrections facilities such as jails, prisons, detention centers, and community corrections, people have no option but to share inadequate spaces and spend most of their time locked in the cells. Thus, the recommended physical distance is almost an impossible measure in these areas plagued by structural challenges. When one is exposed to the virus, the entire corrections facilities become fragile grounds of concentrated infections. A population that has become vulnerable, especially in countries with a congested penal system like the Philippines, is the group of PDLs.

As a background for the term based on the Mandela rule, prisoners shall be called PDLs who, under the guideline of the United Nations, are entitled to minimum humanitarian treatment (Echeminada, 2017). Under Article 10 of the International Covenant on Civil and Political Rights that provides for the respect for the essential dignity of the human person, the term PDLs is adopted with the purpose that such neutral term will prevent branding by the use of derogatory words like "prisoner" and others. The new term PDLs in the Philippines appeared in the Revised Implementing Rules and Regulations, according to Section 23 of Republic Act No. 10575, otherwise known as the "The Bureau of Corrections Act of 2013." It legally defines PDLs as "detainee, inmate, or prisoner, or other person under confinement or custody in any other manner."

The Philippine penal system is considered as one of the most concentrated systems in the world (McCarthy, 2020). Based on the relevant data gathered from the World Prison Brief (2020), an increasing trend in the prison population of the country can be observed. In 2012, the total prison population was 106,323 with a prison population rate of 111. In 2016, the total prison population increased to 142,168 with a prison population rate of 140. In 2019, the total prison population ultimately reached 215,000 with a prison population rate of 200. The present national prison population cannot be accurately determined at the moment but based on available data, the Bureau of Corrections reported the congestion rate in its facilities at 310% in January while the Bureau of Jail Management at 534% in March (Cabrera & Nonato, 2020). This overcrowding has since been exacerbated by the drug war program that has seen thousands sent to prison. Because of the upward trend in the national prison population, which is aggravated by the deplorable structural condition of the corrections facilities, there has been a public expression of heightened fears that the spaces occupied by the PDLs may soon emerge as the epicenter of the COVID-19 infection (Santos, 2020).

Looking at the COVID-19 epidemiological status of the country, the surge of COVID-19 cases began when quarantine measures eased up. As of reports on July 15, the total national COVID-19 infection was recorded at 70,764 confirmed positive cases, including 45, 646 active cases, 23,281 recoveries, and 1,837 deaths. When accounting for the number of COVID infection in the corrections facilities supervised by the Bureau of Jail Management in about the same period, there are 1,086 confirmed positive cases which include 180 active cases, 895 recoveries, and 11 deaths (Sajid, 2020). It should be noted that it does not include the cases in the corrections facilities under the Bureau of Corrections. There is further a concern that the real number of cases could be higher as some authorities were unable to establish the cause of the recent mortality of some PDLs who died inside the facilities (Siu, 2020). As of this September 10, the COVID-19 figures of the country recorded 241,987 confirmed positive cases with 52,893 active cases, 185,178 recoveries, and 3,916 deaths (Umali, 2020). It can be observed, however, that there have been no reports of a significant increase in corrections facilities nationwide.

Amid the COVID-19 crisis overwhelming many parts of the world, the United Nations Office on Drugs and Crime (2020) has issued a position paper for the safety of the confined population of PDLs as well as workers and officers who are involved in ensuring their custody. It underscored the rights of PDLs to equal care standards and suggested the adoption of alternative measures without prejudice to their legal status. Recalling its past stance, it urged countries to respond to overcrowded corrections facilities and ease imprisonment measures so that states can assume its responsibility of care when removing people of their right to liberty. At the national level in the Philippines, there have also been urgent calls to safeguard the PDLs. Many human rights individuals and groups such as Amnesty

International (2020), Human Rights Watch (2020), and Commission on Human Rights (2020) have demanded the authorities to take immediate measures such as decreasing the population in corrections facilities and improving the access to medical services.

A discussion of the various responses for PDLs confined in the corrections facilities amid the COVID-19 crisis has been globally provided emerging attention in research (e.g., Cingolani et al., 2020; Franco-Paredes et al., 2020; Hawks et al., 2020). A particular attention to the national responses for PDLs amid the COVID-19 crisis is significant for some reasons especially in countries with challenging structural contexts like the Philippines. For one, it will primarily assess the possible impacts of these national responses with consideration of the complex situation of overcrowded jail system in the country and the current COVID-19 crisis. If such a research goal is achieved, it will draw recommendations for the improvement of future responses. The researcher believes though that with or without the current crisis, it should be a top concern for the government to decongest the corrections facilities or reduce the prison population of the country whether by structurally expanding such facilities or developing measures to efficiently release the PDLs.

Thus, the overall purpose of this paper is to discuss the national responses for PDLs during the COVID-19 pandemic in the Philippines.

National responses for PDLs during COVID-19 pandemic

When responding to the current crisis in the corrections facilities, the equilibrium between human rights and public health is a complex issue. Three key national responses have been undertaken and are continuously being considered by the government to secure the conditions of PDLs amid the COVID-19 pandemic. The data collected from various reports show that the accumulated numbers of the released PDLs were 9,731 in May; 21,858 in July; and 58,625 in August (Cabrera & Nonato, 2020; Sajid, 2020; Macairan & Porcalla, 2020).

Easing the rules on parole grant and executive clemency

Given the current crisis and the need to decongest the corrections facilities, specified measures such as early, temporary, or conditional release of PDLs with consideration of the gravity of the charge are being most often considered in the decision spaces. The Philippine government, in connection, has been easing the rules on parole grant and executive clemency to facilitate these measures. It has approved simplified rules for probation and parole and released guidelines on the reduction of bail for indigent PDLs (Patinio, 2020) and adopting remote processes.

As a result, in May, it was initially reported that 9,731 PDLs have been released. These are PDLs for crimes punishable with the incarceration of 6 months and below (Siu, 2020). Moreover, based on the data of released PDLs in July, there were 15,102 paralegal releases through bail, bargain, parole, or probation. At the same time, 6,756 were legal releases through acquittal or served sentence (Sajid, 2020). The most recent data in August further showed that the total number of released PDLs has increased to 58,625. However, these numbers should be carefully analyzed within the context of regional differences. It should be noted that such a response just mostly occurred in the regions of Metro Manila, Calabarzon,

Central Luzon, and Central Visayas which have the highest confirmed virus cases (Macairan & Porcalla, 2020).

Moreover, to support the continuity of the judiciary functions as a further response to hasten the release process of the PDLs amid the crisis, the government has initiated efforts to conduct video conference hearings. Through the European Union and its Governance in Justice program, 70 units of laptops have been distributed to the Supreme Court. Additionally, 120 units of tablets have been provided to the Bureau of Jail Management to facilitate the participation of the PDLs in the video conference hearings (GOJUST, 2020).

Amid the calls and responses to release the PDLs, there is another side of the issue arguing that simply releasing them has other unintended possible impacts to the community. It is known that PDLs in the country suffer from contagious health problems either caused or worsened by congestion. For example, tuberculosis is widespread, although authorities have always repelled questions about how many PDLs are infected or how much of the mortality rate can be attributed to the disease. Thus, simply releasing them without proper medical attention may place far more people at risk to the community (The Manila Times, 2020). At any normal rate, employment for released PDLs is a huge challenge. Thus, with the reported surge of national unemployment rate caused by the crisis, the conditional or final release of PDLs without assistance for entry into the labor market would just add to the jobless population.

If the response to make the justice process efficient for PDLs is coupled with assistance for medical treatment and economic entry, it is expected to curb the immediate concern on virus transmission at the same time. It can be both a desirable human rights policy and public health policy. On one hand, it will efficiently resolve cases given due process under existing laws. On the other hand, it will address the perennial problem on congestion, thus feasibly make the recommended physical distance possible inside the corrections facilities.

Providing human considerations to the vulnerable segments

Furthermore, another response to decongest the corrections facilities is the temporary arranged release of vulnerable segment of PDLs based on humanitarian grounds. These vulnerable segments of PDLs include senior citizens, sick people, persons with disabilities, and pregnant women who are considered at high risk of virus infection. It also includes the children in conflict with the law, offenders of low risk, and other persons arbitrarily detained (Patinio, 2020).

From March until July, it was reported that a total number of 21,858 PDLs in the Philippines have been released to prevent the spread of the COVID-19 in the different corrections facilities. Of this total number, 409 were senior citizens, 621 were sick people, and 24 were pregnant women (Sajid, 2020). The scheduled release of some children in conflict with the law in detention centers has been coordinated earlier with the high court (Abad, 2020). The record of the recent release of 58,625 PDLs included children in conflict with the law as well as PDLs who have served the least of their prison terms (Macairan & Porcalla, 2020).

Aside from contributing to the reduction of the population inside the corrections facilities, this response will specifically improve the condition of this vulnerable segment of PDLs such as senior citizens, sick people, persons with disabilities, and pregnant women. They must have already suffered because of their physiological status and exacerbated by psychological anxieties caused by the high risk of virus infection. Thus, their conditional release will greatly diminish their burdens.

Improving the corrections facilities health management

While all PDLs cannot be released and to protect corrections workers and officers, various national agencies and private organizations have combined efforts to improve the health management in corrections facilities. For one, since the government has started an expanded testing program, it has also been working with appropriate authorities to implement "targeted testing" in corrections facilities (Santos, 2020). This response and others have primarily aimed to provide PDLs access to medical care including access to preventive, curative, and palliative services.

Specifically, the Bureau of Jail Management has intensified measures in institutional corrections. For example, in one of the most critically infected provincial jails, it has gathered swab samples of PDLs and officers, established isolation centers, and strengthened contact tracing (Gregorio, 2020). The accumulated number of tests administered in corrections facilities is not recorded, but there has been a significant increase in the daily national testing capacity which covers several corrections facilities. Furthermore, the World Health Organization, International Committee of the Red Cross, and the Department of Health have also been closely working to provide technical expertise and establish quarantine facilities for the infected PDLs (See, 2020).

As with response for PDLs in community corrections, there have been few reports and mostly focused on the response for PDLs in drug treatment and rehabilitation centers. The drug treatment and rehabilitation centers are an important component of the Philippine Correctional System which ensures community corrections especially for the PDLs involved in illegal drugs. As a measure of COVID-19 control after their reported closures in the previous months, the Dangerous Drugs Board (2020) has implemented prevention protocols in the admissions in drug treatment and rehabilitation facilities all over the country. Such new restriction necessitated for engineering controls like isolation corners and ventilation facilities. Essential environmental controls were also implemented such as sanitation and disinfection of all areas. The facilities have been urged to meet visitation guidelines, provide personal protective equipment, and observe physical distance.

Given that such a response in institutional and community corrections facilities will be continuously provided attention, the safety not only of the PDLs but also of the outside community will be secured. It should be noted that virus infection in corrections facilities is also a menace to workers, officers, and visitors, which can potentially lead to virus transmission to the outside community. Thus, the management of the corrections facilities is a concern not only of the penal system but also of the outside community.

Conclusion

It should be underscored that the state must uphold the rights of its citizens regardless of their legal status especially in times of social crisis. This paper provides a discussion as regards the national responses for PDLs during the COVID-19 pandemic in the Philippines. The most often used measure specifically involves early, temporary, or conditional release. This measure is hastened by responses such as easing the rules on parole grant and executive clemency, providing human consideration to the vulnerable segments, and improving the corrections facilities health management. Considering that there will be continued national responses undertaken by the authorities, it is expected to have positive implications in connection to addressing the current crisis. These responses are hoped to decrease the growth of virus infection inside the corrections facilities, improve the condition especially of the vulnerable segments, and ensure the overall safety of the community.

Furthermore, looking back at the available numbers gathered and discussed in this paper, if the previous prison population and the recent number of released PDLs are to be considered, a significant decrease of around 25% in the prison population can be estimated. This decrease can be remarkably attributed to the recent national responses. However, considering the earlier negative stance of the solicitor general and justice secretary on the release of prisoners amid the crisis (Cabrera & Nonato, 2020), such a decrease in prison population may only represent a short-term reduction. It should be further noted that most of the releases occurred in four regions with the highest confirmed positive virus cases (Macairan & Porcalla, 2020), indicating that the government may primarily be just responding to the immediate danger posed by the current crisis. With this matter on hand, there is still a significant need for national responses that will eventually lead to long-term decongestion or reduction of the prison population all over the country in the future. The current national responses being considered to present a timely signal for all offices and agencies of the government to address this need.

Overall, this paper recommends for the continued inclusion of the PDLs, as well as workers and officers, in the current government decision spaces not only to combat the COVID-19 crisis but also to decongest the corrections facilities or reduce the prison population in the country. Specifically, the following recommendations, anchored also on pieces of evidence of good practices in other countries, are offered:

(1) There is a need to expand the virtualization program of the judiciary functions to the provincial zones. This measure has been implemented in countries like the UK and the USA which were badly impacted as early as the acute phase of the crisis. Such a measure included allowing civil procedures in magistrate courts to be conducted through a telephone and using online live links in criminal procedures (Zou, 2020). This measure in the Philippine context, considering challenges in technological access, can be addressed through cross-sectoral engagements with organizations that have a shared vision for enhanced governance especially judiciary functions.

(2) More efficient actions are required to immediately release the vulnerable segments of PDLs such as the senior citizens, sick persons, pregnant women, and youth in conflict of the law. The initiative has been ordered by authorities in countries with a similar case of overcrowded penal system (e.g., Matengo, 2020 on the release of female and older PDLs in Uganda) and high level of virus transmission rate (e.g., Carneiro et al., 2020 on the release of medically compromised and older PDLs in Brazil). These vulnerable segments in the Philippines must be prioritized also as far as their physiological and psychological needs are concerned.

(3) Technical improvement of the health management of the corrections facilities must be continuously supported to prevent the possible new wave of virus infection. For example, Clarke et al. (2020) reported the government initiative in Ireland to establish an approach of contact tracing in prisons in which all prisons, and two support agencies, have fully operative internal teams that conduct contact tracing

and manage quarantine procedures among the PDLs. On the other hand, as more PDLs are released in the Philippines, there is also a demand to improve the community corrections that will supervise them once they are outside.

Disclosure statement

The author confirms that there are no relevant financial or non-financial competing interests to report for this paper.

References

Abad, M. (2020, May 19). *Children deal with abuse, fears of coronavirus in 'houses of hope'.* Rappler. https://rappler.com/newsbreak/

Amnesty International. (2020). *Philippines: Jail releases a matter of life and death.* https://www.amnesty.org/download/

Cabrera, R., & Nonato, V. (2020, May 1). 804 Inmates qualified for release – BJMP. *One News.* https://www.onenews.ph/

Carneiro, M., Seto, G., & Abbud, B. (2020) *CNJ fala em crescimento de 800% de casos de Covid-19 em presi dios e renova recomendação para soltura.* Folha de S. Paulo. https://www1.folha.uol.com.br/colunas/painel/

Cingolani, M., Caraceni, L., Cannovo, N., & Fedeli, P. (2020). The COVID-19 epidemic and the prison system in Italy. *Journal of Correctional Health Care*, 107834582092973. https://doi.org/10.1177/1078345820929733

Clarke, M., Devlin, J., Conroy, E., Kelly, E., & Sturup-Toft, S. (2020). Establishing prison-led contact tracing to prevent outbreaks of COVID-19 in prisons in Ireland. *Journal of Public Health, 42*(3), 519–524. https://doi.org/10.1093/pubmed/fdaa092

Commission on Human Rights. (2020). *Human rights advisory on protecting the rights of persons deprived of liberty (PDLs) during the COVID-19 crisis and early release of older persons, low risk inmates and persons with chronic medical condition or bailable offenses.* http://chr.gov.ph/wp-content/uploads/

Dangerous Drugs Board. (2020). *Admission to drug treatment and rehabilitation centers to resume with strict health and safety protocols amid the pandemic.* https://www.ddb.gov.ph/newsroom/

Echeminada, P. (2017, April 20). Convicts now called 'persons deprived of liberty'. *The Philippine Star.* https://www.philstar.com/headlines/

Franco-Paredes, C., Jankousky, K., Schultz, J., Bernfeld, J., Cullen, K., Quan, N. G., Hotez, P., Henao-Martínez, A. F., Krsak, M., & Kon, S. (2020). COVID-19 in jails and prisons: A neglected infection in a marginalized population. *PLOS Neglected Tropical Diseases, 14*(6), e0008409. https://doi.org/10.1371/journal.pntd.0008409

GOJUST. (2020). *The European Union provides equipment to the Philippine courts in aid of COVID-19 response.* https://gojust.org/news/

Gregorio, X. (2020, May 25). *517 prisoners contract COVID-19 in jails.* CNN Philippines. https://cnnphilippines.com/news/

Hawks, L., Woolhandler, S., & McCormick, D. (2020). COVID-19 in prisons and jails in the United States. *JAMA Internal Medicine, 180*(8), 1041. https://doi.org/10.1001/jamainternmed.2020.1856

Human Rights Watch. (2020). *Philippines: Reduce crowded jails to stop COVID-19.* https://www.hrw.org/news/

Macairan, E., & Porcalla, D. (2020, August 17). SC: Inmates freed due to COVID-19 reach 58,625. *The Philippine Star.* https://www.philstar.com/nation/

The Manila Times. (2020, May 2). *Prisoners need medical intervention, not release.* Author. https://www.manilatimes.net/2020/05/02/opinion/editorial/

Matengo, D. (2020, April 7). *Uganda prisons identify 2,000 inmates for release amid COVID-19 outbreak*. CGTN. https://africa.cgtn.com/

McCarthy, J. (2020, May 5). *As COVID-19 fears grow, 10,000 prisoners are freed from overcrowded Philippine jails*. NPR. https://www.npr.org/sections/

Patinio, F. (2020, April 30). *CBCP backs release of vulnerable inmates amid health crisis*. Philippine News Agency. https://www.pna.gov.ph/articles/

Sajid, I. (2020, July 22). *COVID-19: Philippines releases nearly 22,000 inmates*. Anadolu Agency. https://www.aa.com.tr/en/

Santos, A. P. (2020, May 4). 'Waiting to die': Coronavirus enters congested Philippine jails. *Al Jazeera News*. https://www.aljazeera.com/news/

See, A. B. (2020, May 4). *Before Covid-19, Philippine jails already a death trap*. Philippine Center for Investigative Journalism. https://pcij.org/article/

Siu, P. (2020, June 13). Chinese inmates in Philippines fear the worst as coronavirus deaths rise. *South China Morning Post*. https://www.scmp.com/week-asia/health-environment/article/

Umali, R. (2020, September 8). *Philippines logs 3,281 new COVID-19 cases, tally nearing 242,000*. Xinhua. http://www.xinhuanet.com/english/

United Nations Office on Drugs and Crime. (2020). *COVID-19 preparedness and responses in prisons*. https://www.unodc.org/documents/

World Health Organization. (2020). *Coronavirus disease (COVID-19) pandemic*. https://www.who.int/emergencies/

World Prison Brief. (2020). *World prison brief data*. https://www.prisonstudies.org/country/

Zou, M. (2020, March 20). *Virtual justice in the time of COVID-19*. Oxford Business Law Blog. https://www.law.ox.ac.uk/business-law-blog/blog/

South Korea's Responses regarding Mitigating the COVID-19 Crisis behind Bars

Claire Seungeun Lee

ABSTRACT

As one of the earliest countries to identify cases of COVID-19 infection, South Korea is often considered a success story in responding to the global pandemic. This article examines South Korea's responses in terms of its incarcerated population during the crisis, provides a snapshot of how the coronavirus has impacted prisons, and outlines the mitigation strategies used to create COVID-19-safe spaces in the country. With correction officers being identified as some of the earliest COVID-19 cases in the country, South Korea has striven to manage the coronavirus in correctional facilities as part of the ecosystem of the entire country. This paper discusses South Korea's unique strategy, which focuses less on the size of the prison population and more on treating correction officers and prisoners, who also need to be protected from the virus. In particular, this paper analyzes the multifaceted strategies adopted by South Korea to mitigate the spread of the coronavirus within the criminal justice system, and specifically to protect inmates and correction officers from infection. Strategies centered on public health and human rights were implemented, combined with in-prison strategies, modestly downsizing the prison population and/or maintaining the status quo during the pandemic.

Introduction

The first case of SARS-CoV-2 (widely known as COVID-19, or coronavirus) was reported in Wuhan, China, in December 2019. Subsequently, in January 2020, the virus was introduced to that country's neighbor South Korea through an infected person who flew from China to Incheon. In February 2020, one of the early COVID-19 cases identified in South Korea was a correctional officer, who turned out to be a devotee of the Shincheonji church – a secretive religious sect of Christianity, located in the city of Daegu, that became a primary source for spreading the virus.[1] This case garnered attention in the country not only because of the correctional officer's religiosity but also because of the role of prisons and detention centers as potential COVID-19 hotspots. These concerns over prisons aligned with the belief that correctional officers could be potential transmitters of the disease as a result of the time they spend and contact they have in the outside world (Pyrooz et al., 2020). Along with the country's COVID-19 mitigation strategy, South Korea has striven to manage the virus in correctional facilities as part of the ecosystem of the entire country since then.

South Korea, one of the earliest countries to identify cases of COVID-19 infection, has been considered a success story in its response to the global pandemic (United Nations Development Programme Seoul Policy Centre, 2020). Key factors of its success include the central government's concerted efforts with various ministries and other local governments on mitigating the COVID-19 public health crisis, the daily briefings, the universal, rapid COVID-19 testing, the recommended social-distancing measures, and the mask-mandating policy. These efforts were not only aimed at mainstream society and the general population, but they also exist for those who are distanced from society because of their criminality. While increasing attention has been paid to Korea's COVID-19 story in terms of the country, people behind bars are often not discussed.

It is widely believed that correctional facilities are vulnerable as potential epicenters of the COVID-19 pandemic. Mitigating the spread of the virus to these facilities' populations is a public health issue. The ability of the corrections system to contain the virus and mitigate its spread is increasingly important. A collective lifestyle is a necessity in prisons and correction facilities. While outside factors that contribute to COVID-19 infection can be controlled, the communal nature of everyday life, including the impossibility of social distancing, essentially contributes to and increases the vulnerability of prison populations and correctional officers to the virus. In the first half of 2020, an increasing number of confirmed cases of COVID-19 were reported in correctional facilities around the world, particularly in the United States, Brazil, and the Philippines (International Drug Policy Consortium, 2020; Santos, 2020). There are conventionally three approaches that can be taken to address this double crisis of the pandemic and its impacts on prisons: downsizing, status quo, and upsizing (Byrne et al., 2015; Lux et al., 2015; Turner et al., 2015). Downsizing efforts include the early release (or shift to house confinement) of certain prisoners based on bail, misdemeanor charges, and underlying health conditions. This approach has been taken in Turkey, Cyprus, Slovenia, and some parts of the United States (American Bar Association, 2020; Letzing, 2020). Efforts to either maintain the status quo or upsize the prison populations, which are less commonly used so far, result in a greater emphasis on the public health concerns of the general population.

This article examines South Korea's responses to prisons and prison populations during the COVID-19 crisis and provides a snapshot of the impact of the coronavirus on prisons and the mitigation strategies for creating a COVID-19-safe space in the country. This research uses data compiled from the official websites of the Ministry of Justice and the Korea Correctional Service, newspaper articles, and publicly available sources concerning COVID-19 cases in the Korean corrections system. As there are no available databases tracking COVID-19 in prisons and detention centers in South Korea, estimates of confirmed cases presented in this paper, which provides an overview of COVID-19 behand bars in the country, are inherently preliminary. This paper further discusses South Korea's unique approach to its criminal justice system during the global pandemic. The country's strategy focuses less on the size of the prison population and more on treating correctional officers and the incarcerated populations, who may need more protection and attention than the general population. In particular, this paper analyzes South Korea's multifaceted strategy to prevent the virus from spreading among prison populations, in terms of two specific goals: (1) protecting correctional officers from the coronavirus and (2) protecting inmates from the coronavirus by amending visiting policies and providing public health supports to them. This paper also presents South Korea's in-prison strategies and the implications of maintaining status quo and/or modestly downsizing the prison population during the pandemic.

The following section of the paper outlines the South Korean context, in particular, the country's prisons and corrections facilities. The next section discusses Korea's in-prison and out-of-prison mitigation strategy for prison populations and correctional officers, which is primarily to maintain the status quo with a modest downsizing of the prison population during the pandemic. This research summarizes South Korea's successful mitigation strategy. This paper ends with reflections for future study and implications of understanding this case as an intersection of public health, public safety, and human rights of the prison community in the COVID-19 and post-COVID-19 era.

South Korea's criminal justice system

In South Korea in 2020, the prison system comprises 53 institutions: 38 correctional institutions, 1 private correctional institution, 11 detention centers, and 3 detention branches. There are four regional headquarters: 16 in Seoul, 18 in Daegu, 10 in Daejeon, and 9 in Gwangju Headquarter. The official capacity of Korea's prison system was 54,744 in 2018. While the number of people incarcerated increased steadily from 2012 to 2017, the number of inmates started to decrease in 2018, when the occupancy level went down from 0.111% to 0.106% (Institute for Crime & Justice Policy Research, 2019; Korea Correctional Service, 2019). The number of correctional staff in South Korea amounted to 15,999 people as of December 31, 2019, representing 3.4 inmates per officer (Korea Correctional Service, 2019; see Table 1).

COVID-19 cases and estimates of incarcerated populations in South Korea's prison system

COVID-19 cases in South Korea's correctional facilities

As of July 2020, 6 of the 53 correctional facilities in South Korea had confirmed cases of COVID-19 infection, with the total number of cases amounting to 14,305 in the country (Ministry of Health and Welfare, 2020). Table 2 presents the number of and details of contracted COVID-19 cases by facility. Because closed, indoor settings such as seniors' nursing homes, prisons, and jails are reported to be more vulnerable to COVID-19

Table 1. Trends of incarcerated population and correctional officers in South Korea.

	Korea's population	Prison population	Incarcerated population (% of country's population)	Correctional officers	Inmates per officer
2010	48,746,000	47,471	0.097	15,221	3.1
2011	48,876,000	45,845	0.092	15,478	3.0
2012	49,779,000	45,488	0.091	15,757	2.9
2013	50,004,000	47,924	0.094	15,476	3.1
2014	51,141,000	50,128	0.097	15,934	3.1
2015	51,529,000	53,892	0.105	15,887	3.4
2016	51,696,000	56,496	0.109	15,892	3.6
2017	51,778,000	57,298	0.111	15,871	3.6
2018	51,826,000	54,744	0.106	15,999	3.4

Source: Korea Correctional Service (2019).

Table 2. Number of contracted COVID-19 cases by facility.

Location/ Jurisdiction	Date	Prison	Inmates tested	Number of COVID positive inmates	Staff tested	Number of COVID positive staff	Total cases
Daegu	February 2020	Daegu Prison	40	-	62	2	2
Daegu	February 2020	Daegu Detention Center	-	1		4	
Gyeongsang -bukdo	March 2020	Kimcheon juvenile prison	29	3	18	1	3
Gyeongsang -bukdo	February 2020	Gyeongbukbukbu No.2 Prison	83	-	18	1	1
Jeonllabuk-do	June/ July 2020	Jeongeup Prison	49[a]	-	-	-	-
Seoul	May 2020	Seoul Detention center	301 or 254	-	100 or 23	1	1

[a]Whether this number of people administered COVID-19 tests were staff or inmates is not clear. However, all these people were COVID-19 negative.

transmission than other settings (Heo, 2020), each facility where infected individuals were discovered carefully took multiple steps to mitigate the further spread of the virus to the inmates and officers.

Chronologically, COVID-19 cases were identified in two facilities in February, another two in March, one in May, and one in June/July. On February 21 and February 28, 2020, two correctional officers who worked at Daegu Prison tested positive for the coronavirus. Sixty-two staff and 40 inmates were then tested. On February 25, 2020, a 27-year-old correctional officer at Kyungbuk bukbu No. 2 prison, located in Cheongsong, who was a member of the Shincheonji church, tested positive; subsequently, 18 staff and 83 inmates were administered tests, and their results were negative (Kookmin Ilbo, 2020).

In early March, a 60-year-old inmate at Gimcheon male juvenile prison[2] in Gyeongsang-bukdo contracted COVID-19 (Jeong, 2020). His cellmates, one man aged 44 and one in his 50s, were tested and found to be infected as well. All three of the infected prisoners were released on bail and self-quarantined after release. A 36-year-old staff member at the facility was also infected. Prisoners and correctional officers, who used to commute from home, are staying within the institutions due to COVID-19 infection concerns. At the juvenile prison in Gimcheon, doctors had to go home for self-quarantine immediately after confirmed cases were reported, and they could not provide education on prevention of infectious disease for Justice Ministry officials, according to Jeon (2020).

In early March, several COVID-19 cases were identified in the Daegu Detention Center, including four staff members. One inmate, who had committed burglary, was infected when he visited a hospital for an ankle treatment; a nurse at that hospital was diagnosed with COVID-19. The prisoner's sentence was suspended and he was ordered to stay in his home with supervision. On March 18, 2020, three guards and four cooks at Daegu prison, which houses 3,000 prisoners, tested positive for COVID-19. As a result, all movements, activities, and visits in the facility were suspended. Two nonresidential doctors were monitoring daily the prisoners who showed symptoms of the virus (Prison Insider, 2020).

On May 15, 2020, a 28-year-old correctional officer at the Seoul Detention Center tested positive. The officer had attended a wedding with a friend, who had visited a karaoke in Seoul. Infections have been reported at the karaoke facility where an acquaintance of the officer who went to an Itaewon club, which was one of the recent sources of COVID-19 high infections in the country, had visited. Officials at the detention center immediately disinfected the facility and quarantined 29 other employees and 254 inmates; all staff and inmates were administered COVID-19 tests, but all of their results were negative (Korea Times, 2020). In order to minimize the potential risk of infection, prisoners' meetings with both visitors and lawyers have been suspended. As a result of this case, trials that were scheduled at the Seoul Central District Court and Seoul High Court were also postponed (Korea Times, 2020; Prison Insider, 2020).

On July 2, 2020, a correctional officer at Jeongeup Prison in Jeolla province who had retired on June 29, 2020, gathered with his former colleagues. The retired officer had attended a church in Gwangju on June 28, where new COVID-19 cases were reported. Because of the potential risk of infection through this connection, 49 people from the prison were tested; all the results turned out to be negative. As of August 2020, no further hot spots had emerged, despite the national surge of COVID-19-infected cases in South Korea.

Estimates of incarcerated populations during the COVID-19 pandemic

Conditions of confinement in a country's criminal justice system impact the damages of COVID-19 on their correctional facilities, staff, and inmates. In particular, people behind bars are one of the most vulnerable, and often forgotten, populations in terms of the spread of diseases such as COVID-19. They live in a communal space, where social distancing is virtually impossible. They often have preexisting conditions (e.g., drug use, mental illness) for which treatment is delayed or improper. Therefore, in a number of countries, including the United States and India, jails and prisons became coronavirus incubators.

Although it would be useful to pinpoint the number of infections in a country's prison system, achieving an accurate estimate of cases among prison and staff populations is difficult during this global pandemic. South Korea's situation contrasts with that of most other countries with large prison populations. First, the spread of COVID-19 in South Korea is rather different from the majority of countries, which are experiencing high infection and death rates not only among the general population but also among the prison population (e.g., the United States). South Korea's relatively small case number, lower infection and mortality rates, and relatively quick flattened curve of the pandemic at large has made its criminal justice system less vulnerable than other countries' equivalent population. Thus, in South Korea, where prisons and jails have not been a primary source of COVID-19 infection, reducing prison populations for the sake of lowering the infection rate has not been necessary. The South Korean system is relatively good in terms of incarceration rate per 100,000 population, access to health care, extent of crowding, and other relevant matters. Although there are no official data about the impact of COVID-19 on South Korea's criminal justice system, such data may not be needed owing to a very small number and remote chance of infection among offenders in the country.

Within the very small number of cases among the country's prison populations, South Korea's COVID-19 infection rates were higher in terms of correctional staff than of inmates: 3 of 54,744 inmates were infected, which accounts for 0.005% of the total prison population, while 9 of 15,999 correctional officers were infected, or 0.06% of the total correctional staff population, in 6 of the 53 South Korean correctional facilities (11.3%).

South Korea's approaches to COVID-19 mitigation

South Korea's multifaceted strategy of mitigating the spread of the coronavirus within its criminal justice system involves both correctional staff and prison populations. While some measures taken by the Korean government apply to both groups, other measures are specific to one or the other group.

Mitigation strategies for inmates

South Korea's in-prison strategies, aimed primarily at protecting incarcerated individuals from the virus, are as follows: (1) the size of prison populations adjustment, (2) public health and human rights-based dimension, (3) social distancing-oriented dimension, and (4) front-end mitigation strategies for sentencing options and detainees and parolees.

The first in-prison COVID-19 mitigation strategy involves a combination of modest downsizing of the prison population with maintenance of the status quo. The country has pursued downsizing in certain facilities where infections were reported, while overall it has been maintaining the status quo. For example, a 60-year-old from Gimcheon Prison and a man in his 50s from Daegu Prison were granted early release from their sentences; not only were they considerably older than the other infected inmates but they had been convicted of misdemeanor crimes and were also close to having served their time. The government's use of minor downsizing along with status quo was a strategy performed in the spirit of public health.

The second in-prison COVID-19 mitigation strategy involves a dimension of public health and human rights. First, correctional facilities have secured and provide the prison population with personal protection equipment (PPE) (e.g., N95 masks, gloves, protective eyewear, and clothing) and hand sanitizer. While South Korea never experienced a shortage of PPE, masks were in high demand and initially, at the early stage of the pandemic, it was not easy to secure enough for each facility in the country. Some facilities started to produce their own masks, for self-sufficiency and as part of their prison labor. These were distributed to inmates, some of whom may not have been able to purchase masks otherwise. In relation to the distribution of PPE to the prison population, the prisons began to broadcast programs aimed to educate prison populations about best practices concerning prevention of transmission, causes of the coronavirus, infection routes, and preventive measures that had been initiated. Such information is still broadcast to the facilities on a daily basis (see Pyrooz et al., 2020).

Second, for prevention, prisons strengthened their isolation measures and medical examination of new people entering the facilities. While for the most part admission and transport of prisoners has ceased, there are cases of newcomers arriving in another facility. Upon arrival, they are given a medical examination and asked about symptoms and about potential contact with people who have the virus. At first, a three-day segregation policy was applied to these newcomers; since it became known that COVID-19 has a presumed asymptomatic period of 14 days, the newcomers are subject to a 14-day period of isolation in a one-person room. Those who may potentially be probable cases of infection live in a different place (annex to the main building) and they are offered the use of N95 masks, thermometers, etc. After use, these are sanitized or disposed of. Third, prisoners who require urgent hospital treatment wear protection clothing and, upon returning to the prison after the hospital visit, are put in protective isolation.

The third in-prison COVID-19 mitigation strategy entails a threefold social distancing-oriented dimension. First, prison admissions have been reduced to lessen potential contact with the virus. There has been a suspension of newly incarcerated people and those transferred from one facility to another to minimize the possibility of spreading coronavirus. This strategy is also endorsed by agencies in other countries, such as the Centers for Disease Control and Prevention in the United States (see Center for Disease Control and Prevention, 2020). Second, visitation rules have changed and visiting, except under very exceptional circumstances, has been discontinued in correctional facilities by May 2020. With the progress of COVID-19 infection in South Korea, visiting rules changed as follows[3]: (1) from May 11, one visitor for each visit (offender classification) for pretrial detainees and class 1 inmates (S1) twice a week, the rest (class 2, 3, 4 inmates (S2, S3, S4)) were allowed to have visitors for 6, 5, 4 times per month, respectively; and (2) from June 15, one visitor for each visit was allowed. Some places where the number of infections is on the rise have amended their visiting policy. For those places, pretrial detainees and S1 have a chance to have visitors once a week, whereas class 2, 3, 4 inmates (S2, S3, S4) are allowed to have visitors twice a month. On August 24, 2020, due to the recent surge of COVID-19 infection cases in South Korea, all prisons and jails started to limit the number of visitors and visitations. Pretrial detainees and S1and S2 inmates may have visits once a week, while S3 and S4 inmates are allowed to have visits once every other week (Korea Correctional Service, 2020).

In the pre-COVID-19 era, more than one visitor at a time could visit an inmate, but in the post-COVID-19 era, only one visitor was initially allowed per inmate to minimize the risk of inmates' infection; in August 2020, this number was increased to two people per visit (Korea Correctional Service, 2020). Third, training programs for incarcerated populations have been discontinued. The Korean government and the correctional institutions believe that the sources of coronavirus infection are outside of the facilities. By the very nature of training programs – which include training and educational opportunities, lectures, religious services, and job-matching sessions – contact with outside populations is inevitable. These programs have therefore been suspended.

Lastly, we are seeing front-end mitigation strategies for sentencing options and detainees and parolees. While previously mentioned measures were aimed primarily at the status quo, this final set of strategies is more related to decarceration. At present, the Korean correction system is not systematically creating and implementing front-end mitigation strategies around sentencing. This is largely because the country's prisons and jails have not been greatly affected by COVID-19 infection and, more importantly, because more cases have been reported among corrections officers than among inmates so far. Releases of inmates resulting from COVID-19 were granted on a case-by-case basis, considering their status within the criminal justice system (e.g., how far along in their sentences they were); regardless, these circumstances are worth mentioning. As of August 2020, there had been two cases of COVID-19-related (temporary) releases of inmates, involving different options. On the one hand, inmates at Gimcheon male juvenile prison infected with COVID-19 were granted full release because of their ages, which carry potential risks of being infected and infecting others, and the duration remaining in their sentences. On the other hand, Daegu Detention Center's infected inmate was released, temporarily, on terms of house supervision with suspended sentencing because he had underlying medical conditions, which may not be related directly to COVID-19 but require regular visits to hospitals.

Inmates in these two cases occupied fundamentally different positions in South Korea's corrections system, and the sentencing options for COVID-19-related releases are reflected in such differences. Convicted inmates are sentenced to a length of prison time, which can potentially be shortened owing to their good behavior, appeal results, and/or (special) parole. In contrast, pretrial detainees technically have not been convicted, but they are supposed to be held in detention centers during trial for a designated duration. Considering these contexts, the first inmates in the first case had served almost all of their prison terms, whereas the inmate in the second case had not been convicted and therefore his sentence (if convicted) had yet to be determined.

Mitigation strategies for correctional officers

Infection by COVID-19 has affected more staff than offenders in South Korea's prison system, which confirms the belief that the source of such infection is outside of a closed setting. In line with strategies targeted at inmates, South Korea's strategies for protecting correctional staff from the virus are public health-oriented and geared toward social distancing.

First, in terms of a public health dimension, the government's mitigation strategy includes the installation of thermal imaging cameras. One of the key symptoms of COVID-19 is a fever or high temperature; therefore, in order to control or mitigate the coronavirus spread, 52 correctional facilities in the country installed these cameras. Correctional officers, who are in charge of who enters and exits the facilities, observe symptoms of people who enter the main gate of each facility. Not only are thermal imaging cameras used but contactless thermometers are also used to measure temperature and facilities have mandated that entrants answer questionnaires, wash their hands, and wear masks. Staff are equipped to perform temperature checks on any group of people (staff, visitors, or incarcerated/detained persons) or provide medical care to asymptomatic quarantined persons. Staff present during a procedure on a confirmed or suspected COVID-19 case, they use respiratory aerosols. Staff receive essential PPE support such as N95 respirator, face mask, eye protection, gloves, gowns/coveralls. Staff, those who have direct contact with asymptomatic incarcerated/detained persons, are put into quarantine. Also, staff are discouraged from traveling (overseas) and from being in facilities where many people are. Public health doctors who regularly enter the prisons are also advised not to travel during the pandemic.

Second, to promote social distancing, correctional staff are encouraged to minimize travel inside and outside of the country, minimize their commute to work, and avoid any group activities. Some prisons enabled their staff to stay in the facilities in an effort to mitigate transmission of the virus. Unlike inmates, correctional staff have contact with the outside community, such as their family and their social life away from work. Thus, it is important that they practice social distancing and thereby minimize opportunities for contact with COVID-19 and avoid spreading the virus to their workplace.

Assessing mitigation strategies

Overall, the consequences of the COVID-19 pandemic for public health conditions in South Korea's prisons, and the impact of the coronavirus on the size of the country's prison population, were minor. Thus, the primary, overarching goal of South Korea's strategy was not so much to modify the size of the prison population (i.e., to downsize/upsize the prison population) as to treat corrections officers and incarcerated populations as embedded in the ecosystem of the country. Back-end release options (i.e., sentence adjustments) were adopted in certain cases, but above all the Korean response to the pandemic centered around front-end alternatives as successful mitigation strategies.

South Korea's mitigation strategies that targeted both inmates and officers were in accordance with ensuring health, safety, and human dignity, ensuring access to continued health services, and respecting human rights, as suggested by the joint statement on COVID-19 in prisons and other closed environments released by the Joint United Nations Programme on HIV/AIDS (UNAIDS), the UN Human Rights Office (OHCHR), the UN Office on Drugs and Crime (UNODC), and the World Health Organization (WHO) (World Health Organization, 2020; World Health Organization, Regional Office for Europe, 2020). Strategies specifically targeted at inmates can be understood as a combination of downsizing the population and maintaining the status quo. One element of South Korea's strategies for inmates – a mitigation strategy that has been frequently suggested and employed elsewhere in the world – is to decarcerate populations in correctional facilities in order to reduce overcrowding, among other issues. To achieve this, South Korea took the following measures: (1) sentence adjustments (applicable to prisoners who were infected with COVID-19, who were at risk of infection due to age or underlying conditions, and who had light sentences); and (2) reductions in populations, admissions, and transports of prisoners. Decarceration as a mitigation strategy is also observed in some countries, like the United States, where overcrowding in prisons and jails could potentially contribute to the spread of the virus (Prison Policy Institute, 2020). Another part of mitigating the transmission of coronavirus among inmates, which is more predominantly used than the previous strategy, is maintaining the status quo while keeping up with safety, health, and human rights. This is done through such measures as distributing PPE, offering adequate public health services, keeping the facilities safe, healthy, and clean, and discontinuing visitations to the incarcerated population. These measures are also applicable to correctional staff as well; in addition, officers practice social distancing and careful behavior when outside of their workplace. Altogether, South Korean responses to such settings and populations are in accordance with the humane approaches suggested by international human rights organizations.

Conclusion

This article examines South Korea's responses to the COVID-19 pandemic crisis in relation to its correctional system and incarcerated populations. It provides a snapshot of how COVID-19 has impacted prisons and of the mitigation measures the country put in place to create a safer space. With correctional staff being identified as some of the earliest COVID-19 cases in the country, South Korea has striven to manage the potential spread of coronavirus in correctional facilities as part of the ecosystem of the entire country.

This paper discussed South Korea's unique strategy, which focused less on the size of the prison population and more on treating the vulnerable populations who live in and work in those institutions – and who also deserve the same protection from the virus as the general population. South Korea's multifaceted mitigation strategy included protecting both corrections officers and inmates from the coronavirus. For inmates, South Korea's in-prison strategy was to largely maintain the status quo while modestly downsizing the size of the prison population during the pandemic. Thus the country's mitigation strategies aimed at inmates and correctional officers offer comprehensive public health insights into South Korea's responses to COVID-19 behind bars.

South Korea's measures related to COVID-19 in the criminal justice system are very much in line with the guidelines of global agencies such as UNODC, WHO, UNAIDS, and OHCHR. While it is unknown whether South Korea based its strategy directly on the guidance of these agencies, it is worth mentioning the guidelines and the similarities they share. The joint statement by UNODC, WHO, UNAIDS, and OHCHR on COVID-19 in prisons and other closed environments include the following recommendations: reducing overcrowding, ensuring health, safety, and human dignity, ensuring access to continued health services, respecting human rights, and adhering to United Nations rules and guidance (WHO, 2020). These guidelines play a role in putting recommendations to South Korea's approach to its prison system in this COVID-19 era.

The infection and mortality rates for South Korea's general population are relatively low, and this trend is also observed in its incarcerated populations. While more cases were found among correctional officers than inmates, the number of cases is considered extremely low in terms of a global standard. Thus, perhaps because of this small number, official data on coronavirus-related infections and deaths in South Korea's corrections system do not exist. South Korea has implemented public health-oriented, humane, human rights-based approach to both inmates and correctional staff in terms of its prisons, jails, and detention centers, institutions that are known to be a potentially dangerous epicenter of COVID-19.

While the pandemic has yet to come to an end, and thus it is rather early to draw conclusions as to the impacts of COVID-19 on the Korean criminal justice system, this paper presents a preliminary analysis of an ongoing, rapidly changing public health crisis in the country and the world. South Korea's strategy for combating COVID-19 among people in the criminal justice system has several implications: First, the system needs to better prepare for a pandemic or communal disease crisis. Second, if possible, incarceration rates should be managed as reasonable, while other options such as house imprisonment and social services can be offered to misdemeanants. Third, the Korean criminal justice system is highly state-oriented with minimal privatization (Byrne et al., 2019). The centralized system has worked well in situations like COVID-19, which is highly transmittable. The prisons and detention centers in South Korea were well coordinated with the Ministry of Justice and government agencies at central and local levels. However, if prisons and/or community corrections are increasingly privatized in the future, those facilities would also need to align with usual practices of the nationwide criminal justice system to mitigate the potential risks of viruses and diseases and to provide adequate materials and care for populations behind bars.

While the current study is presumably the first on the impact of the COVID-19 pandemic on South Korea's criminal justice system, the research is not without limitations, which can inform further research. First, as discussed earlier, given that there are no existing public data about the number of coronavirus cases in Korea's corrections system, as of July 2020, it is difficult to provide an accurate estimate of the exact number of such cases among offenders. While acknowledging that the number of cases in the corrections system is relatively low compared with other countries, it is still valuable and important for the government to make such data publicly available to researchers. The United States, for example, where the infection rate among inmates is high and prison populations have been downsized to prevent further infection, maintains a database on COVID and prisons; this database is a valuable source for researchers (e.g., Federal Bureau of Prisons, 2020; Marshall Project, 2020) and might be useful as a model elsewhere, including South Korea. Second, once transmission of the coronavirus slows and becomes manageable, future research should present a more comprehensive view of the pandemic's impact on Korea's criminal justice system. Such studies could evaluate correctional performance, the existing criminal justice system, and public health risk management in prisons and detention centers in both the public and the private sector. Lastly, COVID-19's impacts on criminal justice systems and their populations can be further examined within and across Asia.

Notes

1. Confirmed cases associated with the church are 5,175 cases as of April 2020 (Park, 2020).
2. Typically, teenagers are held in juvenile detention centers, but for exceptions, some older inmates are also assigned to be in the juvenile facilities in South Korea.
3. South Korea uses an offender classification of four classes: Class 1, 2, 3, 4 inmates are referred to as S1, S2, S3, and S4. The higher number of a class indicates a severity of criminal offenses.

Disclosure statement

No potential conflict of interest was reported by the author(s).

ORCID

Claire Seungeun Lee http://orcid.org/0000-0002-0355-8793

References

American Bar Association. (2020, April 3). *COVID-19 and the compassionate release of the elderly, infirm or high risk*. Retrieved July 11, 2020, from https://www.americanbar.org/groups/crsj/events_cle/program-archive/covid-compassionate-release/

Byrne, J., Kras, K. R., & Marmolejo, L. M. (2019). International perspectives on the privatization of corrections. *Criminology & Public Policy*, *18*(2), 477–503. https://doi.org/10.1111/1745-9133.12440

Byrne, J., Pattavina, A., & Taxman, F. S. (2015). International trends in prison upsizing and downsizing: In search of evidence of a global rehabilitation revolution. *Victims & Offenders: An International Journal of Evidence-based Research, Policy, and Practice*, *10*(4), 420–451. https://doi.org/10.1080/15564886.2015.1078186

Center for Disease Control and Prevention. (2020, May 7). *Interim guidance on management of Coronavirus disease 2019 (COVID-19) in correctional and detention facilities*. Retrieved July 11,

2020, from https://www.cdc.gov/coronavirus/2019-ncov/community/correction-detention/guidance-correctional-detention.html

Federal Bureau of Prisons. (2020). *COVID-19 Coronavirus*. Retrieved July 28, 2020, from https://www.bop.gov/coronavirus/

Heo, J. Y. (2020, April 1). Clinical and epidemiological characteristics of Coronavirus disease 2019 in the early stage of outbreak. *The Korean Journal of Medicine*, *95*(2), 67–73. https://doi.org/10.3904/kjm.2020.95.2.67

Institute for Crime & Justice Policy Research. (2019). *Republic of (South) Korea*. World Prison Brief Data. Retrieved July 11, 2020, from https://www.prisonstudies.org/country/republic-south-korea

International Drug Policy Consortium. (2020). *Leave no one behind bars in the time of Covid-19*. Retrieved July 28, 2020, from https://idpc.net/blog/2020/05/leave-no-one-behind-bars-in-the-time-of-covid-19

Jeong, S.-I. (2020, March 18). [Report from Daegu] Doctors guard prisons against COVID-19. Korea Biomedical Review. Retrieved July 11, 2020, from http://www.koreabiomed.com/news/articleView.html?idxno=7750

Kookmin Ilbo. (2020). *Cheongsong first COVID-19 infected person ... Gyeongbukbukbu No. 2 prison's officer*. Retrieved July 3, 2020, from http://news.kmib.co.kr/article/view.asp?arcid=0014278887&code=61121111&cp=nv

Korea Correctional Service. (2019). *Korea correctional service statistics 2019*. Ministry of Justice.

Korea Correctional Service. (2020). *A notice on COVID-19-related changes on visits*. Retrieved August 29, 2020, from http://www.corrections.go.kr/corrections/index.do

Korea Times. (2020). *Seoul courts close after prison officer catches coronavirus*. Retrieved July 11, 2020, from https://www.koreatimes.co.kr/www/nation/2020/05/119_289568.html

Letzing, J. (2020, June 25). *Outbreak or breakout? How to protect prison populations from COVID-19*. World Economic Forum. Retrieved July 14, 2020, from https://www.weforum.org/agenda/2020/06/outbreak-or-breakout-how-to-protect-prison-populations-from-covid-19/

Lux, J. L., Schweitzer, M., & Chouhy, C. (2015). Downsizing juvenile institutions in Ohio: Five innovations. *Victims & Offenders: An International Journal of Evidence-based Research, Policy, and Practice*, *10*(4), 379–400. https://doi.org/10.1080/15564886.2015.1078181

Ministry of Health and Welfare. (2020). *Coronavirus disease-19, Republic of Korea*. Retrieved July 31, 2020, from http://ncov.mohw.go.kr/en/

Park, J. W. (2020, April 3). *Corona from numbers ... more 20s and females, 19% of 80s were dead*. Chosun Ilbo. Retrieved July 31, 2020, from https://biz.chosun.com/site/data/html_dir/2020/04/03/2020040301710.html

Prison Insider. (2020, July 10). *Asia: Coronavirus, prison fever*. Retrieved July 11, 2020, from https://www.prison-insider.com/en/articles/asie-coronavirus-la-fievre-des-prisons#coree-du-sud-5e8206fbbff89

Prison Policy Institute. (2020, July 8). *Responses to the COVID-19 pandemic*. Retrieved July 28, 2020, from https://www.prisonpolicy.org/virus/virusresponse.html

Pyrooz, D. C., Labrecque, R. M., Tostlebe, J. J., & Useem, B. (2020). *Using social science to understand and respond to Covid-19 in jails and prisons*. Retrieved June 30, 2020, from https://items.ssrc.org/covid-19-and-the-social-sciences/society-after-pandemic/using-social-science-to-understand-and-respond-to-covid-19-in-jails-and-prisons/

Santos, A. P. (2020). *'Waiting to die': Coronavirus enters congested Philippine jails*. Al Jazeera. Retrieved July 28, 2020, from https://www.aljazeera.com/news/2020/05/die-coronavirus-enters-congested-philippine-jails-200504025823176.html

The Marshall Project. (2020). Retrieved June 28, 2020, from https://www.themarshallproject.org/2020/05/01/a-state-by-state-look-at-coronavirus-in-prisons

Turner, S. F., Davis, L. M., Fain, T., Braithwaite, H., Lavery, T., Choinski, W., & Camp, G. (2015). A national picture of prison downsizing strategies. *Victims & Offenders: An International Journal of Evidence-based Research, Policy, and Practice*, *10*(4), 401–419. https://doi.org/10.1080/15564886.2015.1078185

United Nations Development Programme Seoul Policy Centre. (2020, March 23). *Korea's rapid innovations in the time of COVID-19*. Retrieved June 8, 2020, from https://www.undp.org/content/seoul_policy_center/en/home/presscenter/articles/2019/korea_s-rapid-innovations-in-the-time-of-covid-19.html

World Health Organization. (2020, May 13). *UNODC, WHO, UNAIDS and OHCHR joint statement on COVID-19 in prisons and other closed settings*.

World Health Organization, Regional Office for Europe. (2020, March 23). *Preventing COVID-19 outbreak in prisons: A challenging but essential task for authorities*. Retrieved July 11, 2020, from https://www.euro.who.int/en/health-topics/health-determinants/prisons-and-health/news/news/2020/3/preventing-covid-19-outbreak-in-prisons-a-challenging-but-essential-task-for-authorities

Latin and South America Regional Overview and Reports from Mexico, Argentina, Columbia, Chile, Brazil, El Salvador, Guatemala, and Honduras

An Examination of COVID-19 Outbreaks in South American Prisons and Jails

Sabrina S. Rapisarda, James M. Byrne, and Lina Marmolejo

ABSTRACT

This article highlights intra-regional variation in the extent of the COVID-19 outbreaks in South America generally and then provides an assessment of the nature and extent of outbreaks in South American prisons. Country-level differences in front-end, within-prison, and back-end early release mechanisms are also described. The article concludes with an assessment of two alternative future directions for prison reform across this region.

Introduction: The nature and extent of the prison crisis in South America

A significant proportion of the world's prison population is housed in South American prisons. As Figure 1 and Table 1 illustrate, 7 of the top 50 largest prison systems in the world are located in South America (World Prison Brief, 2020). Brazil has the largest prison population among all South American countries, and it currently has the third largest prison system worldwide, behind the USA and China, housing over 750,000 inmates (World Prison Brief, 2020). Of the remaining South American countries, Argentina ranks 16th (N = 103,209), Colombia 17th (N = 102,637), Peru 18th (N = 96,440), Venezuela 35th (N = 57,096), Chile 45th (N = 39,284), and Ecuador 46th (N = 39,251; World Prison Brief, 2020). When aggregated, 11.4% of the world's prison population resides in South American prisons.[1]

Proportionately, South American nations are characterized by large prison systems and high inmate populations (see Figure 1). While correctional systems and prisons in South America vary greatly from country to country on a number of metrics, most prisons in the region are notorious for their high level of overcrowding, lack of adequate infrastructure, unsanitary conditions, poor maintenance of hygiene amongst inmates, poor ventilation, and limited access to basic goods and services, such as food, running water, and health care. South American prisons are also reported to be underfunded and understaffed and lacking adequate and effective programming and services (Bergman, 2018; Burki, 2020; Carranza, 2009; Dammert & Zuniga, 2008; Darke & Karam, 2016; UNDP, 2013). As we discuss in a separate review, it is our view that a combination of prison crowding and unhealthy prison conditions, in conjunction with the preexisting health problems of inmates, created the "perfect storm" for the large COVID-19 outbreaks reported in South American prisons.

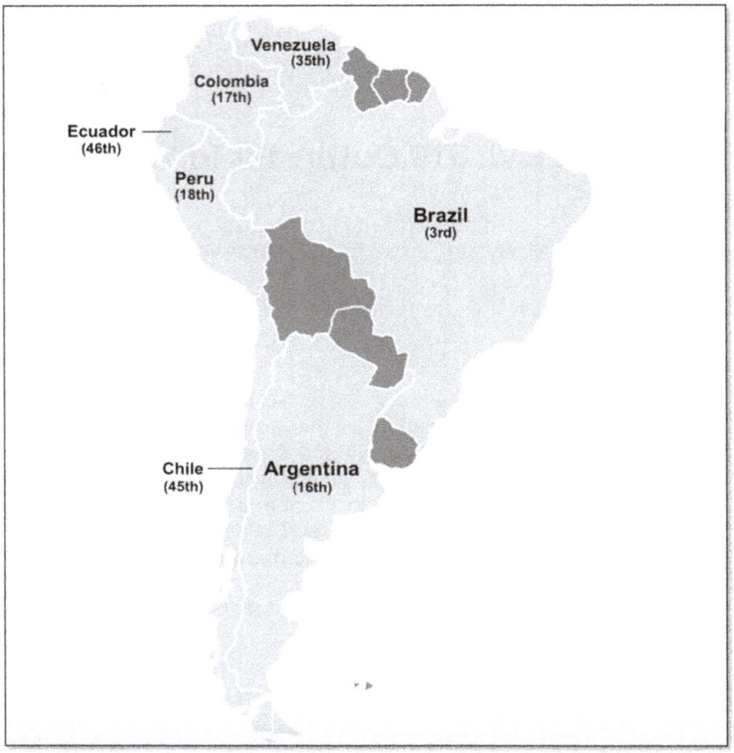

Figure 1. South America's largest prison systems. The labeled and ranked countries in Figure 1 are among the top 50 largest prison systems globally and represent the 7 largest prison systems in South America (World Prison Brief, 2020). Note: The rankings for South American countries within the top 50 largest prison systems are based on relatively current data spanning from 2017 to August of 2020.

Table 1. South America's largest prison systems in the world's top 50.

Rank	Global Region	Country	Prison Population	Date of Most Recent Report
3	South America	Brazil[1,2]	755,274	December 2019
16	South America	Argentina[1,3]	103,209	December 2018
17	South America	Colombia[1,2]	102,637	August 2020
18	South America	Peru[1,3]	96,440	April 2020
35	South America	Venezuela[1,4]	57,096	2017
45	South America	Chile[1,2]	39,284	July 2020
46	South America	Ecuador[1,2]	39,251	January 2020

**Note: Data were extracted from the World Prison Brief database,[1] National Prison Administration,[2] Ministry of Justice,[3] and Observatorio Venezolano de Prisiones[4]*

The extent of the problem: COVID-19 outbreaks in South America

As of late July, Latin America and the Caribbean (as a region) – which includes all of South America, Central America, the Caribbean, and Mexico – led the world in total cases of COVID-19, slightly ahead of North America,[2] comprising nearly 27% of worldwide cases (Reuters, 2020). Countries such as Brazil, Peru, Colombia, and Argentina have more recently experienced a surge of infections, which has likely increased their share of the worldwide infection total (Reuters, 2020).

According to Americas Society/Council of the Americas (AS/COA), Brazil has the highest reported number of COVID-19 cases and deaths amongst all South American countries with at least 3,910,901 confirmed cases and 122,515 COVID-19-related deaths, as of August 31 (Horwitz et al., 2020; World Health Organization [WHO], 2020). Of this total, less than 1% of all confirmed cases ($\approx$ 0.75%) and deaths ($\approx$ 0.15%) occurred within prisons (inmates and staff), while estimates of the extent of the outbreak in community corrections are unknown. However, it is arguably more important to compare the *rates* of COVID-19 cases and deaths between Brazil's total population and its prison population because, while Brazil houses the third largest prison system in the world, its prison population (N = 755,274) comprises less than 1% ($\approx$ 0.36%) of Brazil's total population (N = 212,559,417). Thus, while Brazil's community infection rate is approximately 184.0 positive COVID-19 cases per 10,000 residents, its prison population's rate is 389.3 positive cases per 10,000 inmates (Justiça Presente, 2020; WHO, 2020; Worldometer, 2020). This translates to greater than 2 times higher COVID-19 prevalence rate within Brazil's prisons than in the community at large. Conversely, Brazil's community COVID-19-related death rate equates to 5.8 deaths per 10,000 individuals, whereas its prison population has been afflicted by approximately 2.4 COVID-19-related deaths per 10,000 inmates (Justiça Presente, 2020; WHO, 2020; Worldometer, 2020). We can only speculate at this point, but it is possible that the lower reported death rates from COVID-19 among inmates may be explained by underreporting.[3]

The extent of the outbreaks has varied from country to country across this region, and there is preliminary evidence to support the claim that countries that moved proactively during the early stages of the pandemic (e.g., Argentina) have had fewer outbreaks than those countries that waited longer and relied on reactive containment strategies (e.g., Brazil, Mexico). For example, the Colombian government was quick to respond to the pandemic with a strict lockdown that spanned between March 17 and August 15 in some cities and August 31 in Bogota. The lockdowns were imposed earlier than in other countries, and it was also one of the strictest lockdowns in South America. In contrast, Mexico and Brazil were slow and waited longer to impose lockdowns. However, the lockdowns proved non-effective in controlling the virus. Other measures such as contact tracing, the availability of intensive care units, and testing were not developed as fast as the virus evolved and it caused cases and deaths to increase.[4]

Given the well-documented problems found in prisons throughout this region, it is unsurprising that the inmates and staff in South American prisons have experienced major and sustained COVID-19 outbreaks. Despite claims to the contrary made by leaders in some South American countries (Shadmi et al., 2020; Marmolejo et al., this volume), we can find no evidence supporting the claims that the likelihood of contracting the virus is lower in prison than in society at large. Thus, as the pandemic continues, it will be important for researchers to examine and address these claims, because they most certainly have an impact on how to best and safely proceed.[5]

After first reporting an inmate case of COVID-19 in March, Brazil had reported over 6,000 positive cases and 66 deaths among its prison population between May and July (De Oliveira Andrade, 2020). However, many advocacy groups and researchers were hesitant to believe that these counts were valid, stating that the number of cases reported is a "gross underestimation" given factors such as their own statistical projections, current prison conditions, the low priority status of prisons within the Brazilian government, and the lack of systematic diagnostic testing among inmates (De Oliveira Andrade, 2020). As of August 31, 2020, Brazil reported 29,403 confirmed cases and 183 deaths (Justiça Presente, 2020) among its prison population, a nearly 5-fold increase in reported cases since July.

Similar to other South American countries that are experiencing a rise in the incidence of COVID-19 cases, prisons throughout Colombia also continue to battle outbreaks of the virus. In mid-May, the Villavicencio prison reported over 800 positive cases, which is nearly half of the facility's population (Justice for Colombia, 2020; Robbins, 2020). At the Villahermosa prison in Cali, as of June 17, approximately 480 inmates and 48 staff had contracted the virus (Justice for Colombia, 2020). By late July, La Picota prison in Bogota had approximately 300 confirmed cases of COVID-19 among staff and inmates, despite repeated pleas for measures to prevent the spread of the virus and assured access to medical treatment (Justice for Colombia, 2020).

Brazil had the largest total count of COVID-19 cases in South America as of August 31, 2020, but Chile (N = 378,168 confirmed cases) and Peru (N = 489,680 confirmed cases) had the highest *rates* of COVID-19 cases per 100,000 individuals (Horwitz et al., 2020).[6] Colombia had a cumulative count of 410,453 COVID-19 cases, Argentina's with a total of 260,911, and Ecuador with 95,563 confirmed cases as of August 11, 2020 (Horwitz et al., 2020). It is plausible that Argentina's total count is between one-third to one-half the size of surrounding South American countries due to the proactive, swift, and "no-nonsense" response of the newly elected president (inaugurated in December 2019) and government (WHO, 2020). The Argentinian president made it clear that he prioritized public health over the economy stating that, "You can recover from a drop in the GDP, but you can't recover from death" (WHO, 2020).

Conversely, despite being in close geographic proximity to countries with very high positivity rates like Colombia and Brazil, Venezuela had reported only 27,938 confirmed COVID cases as of August 11, 2020 (Horwitz et al., 2020). We are skeptical about the accuracy of these data. According to AS/COA, Chirinos (2020), and Human Rights Watch (2020), an explanation for Venezuela's extremely low prevalence of positive cases initially reported, relative to other South American countries, is that its government may have been suppressing official tallies and has even threatened and arrested medical professionals, journalists, and academics who report higher figures.

Root causes of COVID-19 outbreaks in South American prisons

What factors can explain the large number of COVID-19 cases reported in South American prisons? The short answer is that the prison systems with the largest outbreaks in this region are the systems that have been criticized in the past for their inadequate physical conditions, insufficient staffing, poor health care, and extreme crowding (Heard, this volume). A case in point is Brazil, the country housing the region's largest prison system. In addition to the appalling physical conditions, some Brazilian prisons operate at as high as 300% over design capacity. Brazil's health care system within prisons was already weak with high rates of death among inmates with tuberculosis, an infectious disease that is highly contagious, but very curable (Sánchez et al., 2020). Furthermore, like other countries, Brazil's prison system exacerbates disparities along racial and socioeconomic lines (Fraga Arantes, 2020). Individuals who are black and/or from lower socioeconomic backgrounds are disproportionately represented in Brazil's prisons (Fraga Arantes, 2020; De Oliveira Andrade, 2020).

Brazil is struggling to contain the spread of COVID-19, and its prison population is facing the brunt of a non-proactive and unresponsive government in tandem with the absence of a coordinated response between different levels of government, states, and local prisons (De Oliveira Andrade, 2020; Fraga Arantes, 2020; Sociedad de Criminología Latinoamericana, 2020). According to Shadmi et al. (2020), Brazil's president, Bolsonaro, insisted on a "denialist" approach in March, making public announcements that were contrary to the scientific evidence, despite the Ministry of Health recommending preventative measures such as quarantining. Bolsonaro went as far as to publicly discourage the public from quarantining, purporting that there was not a public health emergency in place and that the economy must be preserved (Shadmi et al., 2020). Further, Bolsonaro believed that inmates should not be released, affirming that they were "safer" inside (Fraga Arantes, 2020).

Front-end, within-prison, and back-end mitigation strategies

There is certainly variation in the types and, more importantly, the timing of mitigation strategies used by prison systems in South America (see Table 2), but there does appear to

Table 2. A comparison of mitigation strategies used in South American prisons.

Country	Front-End	Within	Back-End
Brazil[1]	Suspension of family and attorney visitation; isolation of vulnerable inmates; suspension of transfers and temporary exits	Daily sanitation of cells; increased exposure to sunlight; isolation of symptomatic inmates	Appx. 4.6% (N = 32,500) released on house arrest or electronic monitoring
Argentina[2]	Suspension of educational and work activities; restriction for on-site prison visitation; restriction on transfers	Restriction on staff per unit; controls for at-risk groups; testing for inmates and staff; health kits and PPE for inmates and staff; designated areas for isolation	Appx. 13% early release to probation, parole, house arrest, or other exceptional mechanisms
Colombia[2]	Suspension of educational and work activities; restriction for on-site prison visitation; restriction on transfers	Restriction on staff per unit; educational campaigns regarding COVID-19; testing for inmates and staff; health kits and PPE for inmates and staff; designated areas for isolation	Appx. 20% released to house arrest or other exceptional mechanisms
Peru[3]	Suspension of all prison visitation; suspension of new intakes	Aggressive testing; inmates serving as health care monitors	Appx. 1.5% (N = 1,500) early release
Venezuela[4]	Suspension of all prison visitation	Intensive disinfection of imported goods & supplies; meticulous food preparation and handling protocol	Appx. 3.7% (N = >2,100) released, including political prisoners
Chile[2]	Suspension of educational and work activities; restriction for on-site prison visitation	Restriction on staff per unit; Vaccination campaign against influenza; educational campaigns regarding COVID-19; controls for at-risk groups; testing for inmates and staff; designated areas for isolation	Appx. 15% (N = 5940) early release
Ecuador[5]	Suspension of all prison visitation	Designated areas for isolation; testing for inmates and staff	Appx. 2.5% (N = 971) granted prerelease

[1]See Ribeiro (this volume) for more detail regarding Brazil's mitigation strategies to combat COVID-19.
[2]See Marmolejo and colleagues (this volume) for more detail regarding Argentina, Colombia, and Chile's mitigation strategies in response to COVID-19.
[3]See Iglesias Osores (2020) and VOA News (2020) for more detail on Peru's response to COVID-19 in its prison system.
[4]See D'Hoy (2020), Mozo Zambrano (2020), and PERFIL (2020) for limited details pertaining to Venezuela's mitigation strategies in prisons.
[5]See Puente (2020) for details surrounding the prerelease of inmates in Ecuadorian prisons and Sociedad de Criminología Latinoamericana (2020) for more information regarding Ecuador's front-end and within-prison mitigation strategies.

be similarities in both front-end and in-prison mitigation strategies. The biggest within-region difference we have identified is in the scale of the prison population reduction strategies employed: reductions in overall prison populations via early release strategies ranged from only 1.5% (in Peru) to 20% (in Columbia). It will be important to examine the impact of these early release strategies on both the health of releasees, and the subsequent behavior of these individuals (i.e., recidivism) during this period of early release.

At the front-end, it appears that prison managers in South America attempted to minimize the importation of the virus by limiting who can enter prisons. Thus far, measures to protect inmates in Brazilian prisons, as well as the vast majority of prisons in South America, have been limited to suspending visits, temporary releases, and following general guidelines issued by the Ministry of Health regarding health care (Fraga Arantes, 2020). Even more troubling, because of the lack of basic necessities (e.g., clean water, food, medications, etc.) provided to inmates, family members and loved ones are often relied upon to compensate for the lack of resources by bringing items into the prisons (Shadmi et al., 2020). Banning prison visitations is likely counterproductive because the deprivation experienced by inmates (e.g., hunger, thirst, weakened immune systems, etc.) may ultimately make them more susceptible to the virus.[7]

The link between COVID-19 outbreaks and violence in South American prisons

It is important to consider how and why inmates in South American prisons have expressed their concerns about the strategies used by prison officials to mitigate outbreaks within facilities. Due to overcrowded, unsanitary, and under-resourced conditions, in addition to countries' unwillingness to take action to prevent the spread of coronavirus (e.g., releases), inmates in several South American countries have engaged in collective violence and/or attempted to escape. Since the onset of the pandemic erupted, several prison rebellions have taken place in response to the governments' lack of transparency and lack of aid/security to vulnerable prison populations. It should be noted that some of the riots and protests were a consequence of the lack of action at the outset of the pandemic, and arguably pushed governments to do more, such as in the case of Colombia, while others were reactions to the measures implemented to reduce the pandemic, such as limiting visitations. One caveat is in order at this point: while violent reactions to the pandemic make the news, there have been other nonviolent protesting methods that have occurred too, including families that have organized petitions, and demonstrations (Marmolejo et al., this volume).

In early May 2020, Puraquequara Prison, in Manaus, Brazil, faced riots allegedly out of fear that guards could transmit COVID-19 throughout the facility (De Oliveira Andrade, 2020). In March 2020, inmates in Venezuelan, Colombian, Peruvian, and Argentinian prisons rioted and/or attempted to escape out of fear of contracting the virus, which in some cases, led to death (Prison Insider, 2020). Eighty-four inmates escaped a Venezuelan prison and 10 were later killed by law enforcement after authorities canceled access to visitors that normally provided the inmates with food (Prison Insider, 2020). Twenty-three inmates were killed and 83 were injured in a Colombian prison after inmates protested unsanitary conditions, lack of access to clean water, overcrowding, and inadequate measures to protect them from COVID-19 (Prison Insider, 2020). In Peru, 2 inmates were killed and 6 inmates and 11 staff were injured during protests that attempted to secure better protection for inmates against COVID-19 (Prison Insider, 2020). Lastly, five inmates in Argentina died during a protest over unsanitary conditions (Prison Insider, 2020).

Assessing the impact of current mitigation strategies on reducing COVID-19 outbreaks and on the reducing size of the prison population

One response to the outbreak in South American prisons was to expand both front-end and back-end early release mechanisms, while simultaneously taking steps to control outbreaks within prisons among inmates and staff. Preliminary evidence of the relative effectiveness of these strategies in reducing outbreaks of COVID-19 in prisons is difficult to obtain at this stage of the pandemic. While we can identify reductions in prison populations as a result of various front-end and back-end mitigation strategies, it is too early to state that by reducing the prison population, we have reduced the risk of contracting the virus for either the released population or the inmates and staff who remain in prison. It should also be pointed out that we currently know remarkably little about the outbreak of COVID-19 among South America's community corrections population (and among community corrections staff).

According to a study conducted by the Center for Latin American Studies on Insecurity and Violence in conjunction with the Latin American Society of Criminology, in mid-June, up to 15% of Chile's inmates had been released in response to the pandemic, which is one of the highest release rates relative to other Latin American countries (Robbins, 2020). While this action may have helped to mitigate the effects of overcrowding in Chilean prisons to some degree, it appears that countrywide, Chile has continued to struggle in combatting the spread of the virus with a total of 378,168 confirmed cases by August 11, 2020 (Horwitz et al., 2020). In an article published on May 21, 2020 by the Human Rights Watch, it was reported that at least 700 Chilean inmates and staff members tested positive (Vivanco & Munoz, 2020); however, more recent COVID-19 case tallies – as of early September – reflect totals nearer 1700 (inmates) and 1300 (staff) positive cases as well as 15 deaths (Gendarmería de Chile, 2020).

On August 22, 2020, the Peruvian Minister of Justice and Human Rights announced that as part of an initiative to provide systematic diagnostic testing to inmates, 27,000 tests were administered within Peru's prison systems thus far (EN24, 2020). Of those tests, 12,294 inmates tested positive for COVID-19 amongst its 96,000+ incarcerated population housed within 68 facilitates (EN24, 2020). Another means by which Peru has attempted to respond to COVID-19 within its prisons, much like other countries, is to release low-risk inmates in order to reduce overcrowding. On April 14 of 2020, the Peruvian government pledged to release 3,000 inmates, which equates to just over 3% of Peru's total incarcerated population (TRTWorld, 2020). However, as of mid-June, only 1,500 inmates had been released (TRTWorld, 2020).

On April 14 of 2020, the Colombian government approved the release of 4,000 at-risk inmates to house arrest, including pregnant women, inmates over 60-years-old, mothers with children under 3-years-old, individuals who are disabled, inmates whose sentences were under 5 years or who were being detained pre-trial, and inmates with specified health conditions such as HIV, cancer, and diabetes (Horwitz et al., 2020; Justice for Colombia, 2020). In some cases, inmates that had served more than 40% of their sentence were eligible to be transferred to house arrest in lieu of incarceration (Justice for Colombia, 2020).

Regardless of the new decree's intent, it appears that the conditions for release were too restrictive and ineffectively implemented, because as of mid-July, only 889 inmates had met conditional release requirements (Horwitz et al., 2020; Instituto Nacional Penitenciario y Carcelario [INPEC], 2020). However, to date, under ordinary practice, Colombia has released nearly 21,000 inmates to house arrest or to freedom for completing or exceeding their pretrial detention (INPEC, 2020). By early September, Colombia reported not only a rise in cases, but also a rapid increase, and consequently surpassed the prevalence of positive COVID-19 cases in other Latin American countries such as Mexico.

Concluding comments: COVID-19 and corrections reform

All of the countries in South America reviewed here demonstrate issues with access and quality of data that make it difficult to frame the COVID-19 situation inside prisons. Hopefully, one of the "lessons learned" from the pandemic will be a recognition that in order to plan effectively, prison administrators need to improve their information systems, producing better prison data, not only for internal decision-making, but also to increase the system's credibility via transparency. Apart from a clarion call for more and better data, it is certainly possible that the pandemic's impact on inmates and staff in South American prisons will be a catalyst for real change in sentencing and corrections policies and practices in several South American countries. If this occurs, it may be the result of new, yet-to-be-conducted research demonstrating that community safety was not jeopardized in countries that significantly reduced their prison populations during this period. Unfortunately, it is equally plausible that once (if and when) this latest pandemic subsides, the leaders of countries in this region will simply instruct corrections officials to return to normal practices, which will mean a return to overcrowded, understaffed, poorly managed, and unhealthy prisons. Research on the impact of this natural experiment in prison downsizing will likely play a critical role in determining which way the reform pendulum will swing.

Notes

1. South American countries include Brazil, Argentina, Colombia, Peru, Venezuela, Chile, Ecuador, Bolivia, Paraguay, Uruguay, Guyana, Suriname, and French Guiana, and, together, they account for 1,244,527 of the 10,911,380 inmates that comprise the total global prison population.
2. To calculate this proportion, we include Mexico with other Latin American countries, including South America, Central America and the Caribbean. North America's COVID-19 total used in this comparison is based on data for the USA and Canada.
3. Further research on changes in Brazil's death in prison rates – for any reason – will need to be conducted to investigate this suspected under-reporting issue.
4. For more information on Columbia's response, see Marmolejo et al., this volume; and https://www.cgdev.org/publication/covid-19-colombia-impact-and-policy-responses.
5. Our own preliminary review of the available data comparing COVID-19 infection rates in prison versus the general community in the country-level reviews included in this special issue do not support this claim (see Marmolejo, this volume; Pitts and Inkpen, this volume; Ribeiro, this volume).
6. Chile and Peru also have the highest prevalence of testing among South American countries.

7. Agoff (this volume) argues that there are critical gender-specific differences in the impact of suspended prison visitation on males versus female inmates.

Disclosure statement

No potential conflict of interest was reported by the author(s).

References

Argentina: There is no economy without health. (2020, July 29). World Health Organization. https://www.who.int/news-room/feature-stories/detail/argentina-there-is-no-economy-without-health

Bergman, M. (2018). *More money, more crime: Prosperity and rising crime in Latin America.* Oxford University Press.

Brazil Population (LIVE). (2020, August). Worldometer. https://www.worldometers.info/world-population/brazil-population/#:~:text=The%20current%20population%20of%20Brazil,of%20the%20total%20world%20population

Burki, T. (2020). Prisons are "in no way equipped" to deal with COVID-19. *Lancet (London, England), 395*(10234), 1411–1412. https://doi.org/10.1016/S0140-6736(20)30984-3

Carranza, E. (2009). *Cárcel y Justicia Penal en América Latina y el Caribe. Instituto Latinoamericano de las Naciones Unidas para la Prevención del Delito y Tratamiento del Delincuente (ILANUD).* Siglo XXI editores.

Chirinos, M. (2020, July 27). *Covering the pandemic: Arrests of journalists and healthcare workers in Venezuela.* Pulitzer Center. https://pulitzercenter.org/reporting/covering-pandemic-arrests-journalists-and-healthcare-workers-venezuela

Cómo desinfectan las cárceles para que los presos no se contagien de coronavirus. (2020, April 15). PERFIL. https://www.perfil.com/noticias/policia/coronavirus-como-desinfectan-carceles-para-que-lo-presos-no-se-contagien-covid19.phtml

Coronavirus: What is the impact in Colombia? (2020, August 19). Justice for Colombia. https://justiceforcolombia.org/news/coronavirus-what-is-the-impact-in-colombia/

D'Hoy, C. (2020, June 22). *OVP denuncia irregularidades en la liberación de más de dos mil presos.* El Universal. https://www.eluniversal.com/sucesos/73845/ovp-denuncia-irregularidades-en-la-liberacion-de-mas-de-dos-mil-presos

Dammert, L., & Zuñiga, L. (2008). *La cárcel: problemas y desafíos para las Américas.* Facultad Latinoamericana de Ciencias Sociales (FLACSO), Chile.

Darke, S., & Karam, M. L. (2016). Latin American prisons. In Y. Jewkes, B. Crewe, & J. Bennett (Eds.), *Handbook on prisons* (pp. 460–474). Routledge.

De Oliveira Andrade, R. (2020). Covid-19: Prisons exposed in Brazil's crisis. *BMJ, 370.* https://www.bmj.com/content/370/bmj.m2884

Desantis, D., & Leria, J. (2020, July 26). *Latin America leads world in coronavirus cases, Reuters count shows.* Reuters. https://www.reuters.com/article/us-health-coronavirus-latin-america/latin-america-leads-world-in-coronavirus-cases-reuters-count-shows-idUSKCN24R0JL?emci=9d70c11e-02d0-ea11-9b05-00155d03bda0&emdi=dbf92327-03d0-ea11-9b05-00155d03bda0&ceid=4606001

Fraga Arantes, M. H. (2020, July 7). *COVID-19 in Brazilian prisons: Pandemic or a necropolitical project?* openDemocracy. https://www.opendemocracy.net/en/democraciaabierta/covid-19-brazilian-prison-pandemic-or-necropolitics/

Gendarmería de Chile. (2020). *Plan de Acción de Gendarmería para enfrenta al Coronavirus.* https://www.gendarmeria.gob.cl/corona2020.html

Horwitz, L., Nagovitch, P., Sonneland, H. K., & Zissis, C. (2020, August 12). *The Coronavirus in Latin America.* Americas Society/Council of the Americas. https://www.as-coa.org/articles/coronavirus-latin-america

Iglesias Osores, S. (2020). Transmission and prevention of SARS-CoV-2 (COVID-19) in prisons. *Revista Española de Sanidad Penitenciaria, 22*(2), 87–90. https://doi.org/10.18176/resp.00015

Inmates in Peru's largest prison help authorities identify others infected by Coronavirus. (2020, August 20). VOA News. https://www.voanews.com/covid-19-pandemic/inmates-perus-largest-prison-help-authorities-identify-others-infected

Instituto Nacional Penitenciario y Carcelario (INPEC). (2020). *Informe Estadióstico No 2, Poblacioón privada de la libertad.* Ministerio de Justicia y el Derecho. https://www.inpec.gov.co/web/guest/estadisticas/-/document_library/TWBuJQCWH6KV/view_file/1135415?_com_liferay_document_library_web_portlet_DLPortlet_INSTANCE_TWBuJQCWH6KV_redirect=https%3A%2F%2Fwww.inpec.gov.co%2Fweb%2Fguest%2Festadisticas%2F-%2Fdocument_library%2FTWBuJQCWH6KV%2Fview%2F965447%3F_com_liferay_document_library_web_portlet_DLPortlet_INSTANCE_TWBuJQCWH6KV_redirect%3Dhttps%253A%252F%252Fwww.inpec.gov.co%252Fweb%252Fguest%252Festadisticas%252F-%252Fdocument_library%252FTWBuJQCWH6KV%252Fview%252F49294

Justiça Presente. (2020). *Covid-19 no Sistema Prisional.* Conselho Nacional de Justiça. https://www.cnj.jus.br/wp-content/uploads/2020/09/Monitoramento-Semanal-Covid-19-Info-02.09.20.pdf

Mozo Zambrano, R. (2020, March 23). *Ministerio Penitenciario oficializa suspensión de visitas a las cárceles para evitar el COVID-19.* Effecto Cocuyo: Periodismo que Ilumina. https://efectococuyo.com/coronavirus/ministerio-penitenciario-oficializa-suspension-de-visitas-a-las-carceles-para-evitar-el-covid-19/

Peru frees 1,500 inmates over Covid-19 fears. (2020, June 15). TRTWorld. https://www.trtworld.com/americas/peru-frees-1-500-inmates-over-covid-19-fears-37289

Peru: [DATOS Minsa] Coronavirus Peru LIVE | Official figures, news, c. (2020, August 22). EN24. https://www.en24.news/2020/08/peru-datos-minsa-coronavirus-peru-live-official-figures-news-c-2.html

Puente, D. (2020, June 20). *Un total de 971 presos dejaron la cárcel en Ecuador por dos beneficios.* El Comercial. https://www.elcomercio.com/actualidad/presos-carcel-prelibertad-beneficios-coronavirus.html

Robbins, S. (2020, July 22). *Coronavirus unrest sparks surge in riots in Latin America's prisons.* InSight Crime. https://www.insightcrime.org/news/analysis/coronavirus-unrest-prison-riots/

Sánchez, A., Simas, L., Diuana, V., & Larouze, B. (2020). COVID-19 in prisons: An impossible challenge for public health? *Cadernos de Saúde Pública, 36*(5), 1–5. https://doi.org/10.1590/0102-311X00083520

Shadmi, E., Chen, Y., Dourado, I., Faran-Perac, I., Furler, J., Hangoma, P., Hanvoravongchai, P., Obando, C., Petrosyan, V., Rao, K. D., Lorena Ruano, A., Shi, L., Eugenio de Sousa, L., Spitzer-Shohat, S., Sturgiss, E., Suphanchaimat, R., Villar Uribe, V., & Willems, S. (2020). Health equity and COVID-19: Global perspectives. *International Journal of Equity in Health, 19*(104), 1–16. https://doi.org/10.1186/s12939-020-01218-z

Sociedad de Criminología Latinoamericana. (2020). *Los efectos del coronavirus en las cárceles de Latinoamérica.* Centro de Estudios Latinoamericanos sobre Inseguridad 7 Violencia (CELIV). https://drive.google.com/file/d/1LVfsl69ZRty9JVsNnYIEp8SvJa-OrC4J/view

South America: Cut prison crowding to fight Covid-19. (2020, April 14). Prison Insider. https://www.prison-insider.com/en/articles/amerique-du-sud-cut-prison-crowding-to-fight-covid-19

United Nations Development Program (UNDP). (2013). *Citizen security with a human face: Evidence and proposals for Latin America.* Regional Human Development Report 2013–2014.

Venezuela: A police state lashes out amid Covid-19 (Arbitrary arrests, prosecutions of critics, abuses against detainees). (2020, August 28). Human Rights Watch. https://www.hrw.org/news/2020/08/28/venezuela-police-state-lashes-out-amid-covid-19

Vivanco, J. M., & Munoz, C. (2020, May 21). *How to prevent Covid-19 outbreaks in Latin America's prisons.* Human Rights Watch. https://www.hrw.org/news/2020/05/21/how-prevent-covid-19-outbreaks-latin-americas-prisons

World Health Organization (WHO). (2020, August 17). *Coronavirus disease (COVID-19) dashboard.* https://covid19.who.int/

World Prison Brief. (2020, August). *World prison brief data.* Institute for Crime & Justice Policy Research (ICPR). https://www.prisonstudies.org/world-prison-brief-data

The Brazilian Penitentiary System under the Threat of COVID-19

Ludmila Ribeiro and Alexandre M. A. Diniz

ABSTRACT

This paper seeks to identify the chief factors behind the incidence of COVID-19 cases and deaths inside the Brazilian prison system, testing the hypotheses that better equipped and better-staffed systems and the adoption of the prophylactic measures lead to lower incidence and death rates. Results show partial support for these expectations, as certain infrastructure-related measures such as the number of medical appointments held at the prison facility, the percentage of establishments not directly managed by the State, and the number of laboratory tests by inmate are statistically associated with the number of recorded COVID-19 cases. In turn, the number of provisional detainees, and the percentage of prison units without educational facilities are significant predictors of COVID-19 deaths. Nonetheless, not a single measure adopted to prevent COVID-19 inside prisons and jails stood the empirical testing. These results have important policy and research implications.

Introduction

By the beginning of September 2020, COVID-19 had caused the deaths of more than 900 thousand individuals and infected close to 29 million people worldwide (JHC, 2020). Although there is a lot of controversy regarding the reliability of these numbers (Williams et al., 2020), high ranking countries in COVID-19 infection and mortality also display high numbers of confirmed cases and deaths due to coronavirus inside their penitentiary systems (Franco-Paredes et al., 2020).

Brazil ranks second in the COVID-19 death lists, with more than 130,000 deaths recorded by September, 2020 (JHC, 2020). When the first case was confirmed, in February 2020, Brazil suffered from a lack of political coordination at the Federal level, given president Bolsonaro's administrative inability and his antagonistic approach toward the Congress and the Supreme Court (Ortega & Orsini, 2020). To make matters worse, Bolsonaro stubbornly downplayed the disease, calling it "just a little flu", championing hydroxychloroquine for treatment and prophylaxis, despite the lack of scientific backup (Ricard & Medeiros, 2020). He has also suggested the adoption of vertical isolation – quarantining exclusively high-risk groups (elderly, those with chronic diseases, i.e.), while keeping the rest of the population moving about freely for the sake of the economy (Ortega & Orsini, 2020).

The discourse adopted by Bolsonaro had implications inside the penitentiary system (Costa et al., 2020), as Brazil displays one of the highest rates of infections and deaths by coronavirus among the prison population in the world (Oliveira Andrade, 2020). By the beginning of September 2020, 108 people had lost their lives inside jails and prisons due to the disease, leading to a rate of 14.45 deaths per 100 thousand inmates (DEPEN, 2020), making the country an important case study.

Brazil holds the third-largest number of inmates in the world (World Prison, 2020), and has over 1,400 jail and prison units (DEPEN, 2019). Its penitentiary system is complex and decentralized, being marked by major discrepancies in terms of infrastructure (Siqueira et al., 2020). In general, prison units suffer from overcrowding, growing presence of criminal organizations, recurring rebellions, and several human rights violations (Dias, 2017). COVID-19 pandemic made matters even worse.

This paper seeks to understand the factors behind the spread of coronavirus inside the Brazilian penitentiary system. We argue that the number of deaths and confirmed cases of COVID-19 ought to be explained by the detention conditions and by the preventive measures adopted in each state. Using data made available by the National Penitentiary Department (DEPEN, acronym in Portuguese), an agency of the Ministry of Justice and Public Safety, we test two hypotheses. First, better-equipped prison systems have lower morbidity and mortality rates due to COVID-19. Second, the adoption of the preventive measures leads to a lower incidence of COVID-19 within the state penitentiary systems.

Methodology

Every year, DEPEN carries out a national penitentiary survey (Infopen, acronym in Portuguese) to assess the number of people held in custody, the overall infrastructure within prison units, and the services provided to inmates.[1] Information are made available at the prison unit level covering the available infrastructure, human resources, capacity, prisoner profiles, vacancies, labor, and educational services, health care, visits, among other indicators (Alcântara et al., 2018). Since COVID-19 reached Brazil, DEPEN has developed a monitoring panel,[2] where data on confirmed cases, as well as deaths inside detention facilities, are presented exclusively at the state level. This agency also discloses the measures adopted by each state penitentiary system to prevent the spread of coronavirus, including normative instructions and other precautionary actions (Oliveira Andrade, 2020).

Infopen and COVID-19 Panel are fed by prison managers based on a standardized web form, which makes data comparable across prison units and state penitentiary systems. These data sources have been criticized due to underreporting of COVID-19 cases (Siqueira et al., 2020, p. 39). However, since underestimation is a problem that affects all 27 state penitentiary systems, we can assume that this bias is equally distributed across them.

Hypotheses testing was conducted based on December 2019 DEPEN data, and September 7,th 2020 COVID-19 panel information (DEPEN, 2019, 2020). Data were aggregated at the state level, which comprises the unit of analysis of this study. Infopen and COVID-19 databases were merged in an Excel file, which was imported into IBM-SPSS. Then, we ran normality tests on the dependent variables: the number of

COVID-19-confirmed cases, and the number of deaths due to COVID-19 inside the penitentiary system. Results showed highly skewed distributions which were normalized using Templeton's (2011) Two-Step Approach. In this procedure, the variable is first converted into a percentile rank, with uniformly distributed probabilities, followed by an inverse-normal transformation which leads to a variable consisting of normally distributed z-scores.

We expected that better equipped and staffed prison systems are better prepared to face the pandemic and should have a lower number of COVID-19 cases and deaths. We also assumed that the adoption of various preventive measures by different state penitentiary systems have a dampening effect on the number of COVID-19 cases and deaths. To test these hypotheses, we used two sets of independent variables, one contemplating infrastructure and services provided by the state penitentiary systems, and another related to preventive measures adopted by each system. Since all state penitentiary systems have adopted the suspension of visits at different points in time, we opted to include the number of days without external visits as reference.

To calibrate the OLS models, the forward stepwise method was deployed. For an initial simulation, all independent variables were subjected to the forward stepwise regression method to identify the best fit model, given the small number of observations (27 states). At each stage of the process, a different variable was included in the model, and the algorithm gaged the associated error and its impact upon R2. The procedure stopped when no remaining regressor improved the model.[3]

Before we explore the OLS results it is of paramount importance to discuss how the Brazilian penitentiary system functions, emphasizing how COVID-19 has changed life in prison.

The Brazilian penitentiary system in the last thirty years

Brazil displays an atomized penitentiary system comprising 26 different state penitentiary systems, in addition to the Federal District. When we mention the Brazilian penitentiary system throughout this paper, we refer to the combination of the abovementioned 27 subsystems, including the five federal prisons.[4] The regulation of the system is relatively new, established in 1984 by the Penitentiary Executions Law (LEP, acronym in Portuguese), also known as Law # 7,210 (Lermen et al., 2015).[5] Nevertheless, despite being regulated by the same federal legislation, prison units present varying infrastructures, and often very different problems.

Overall, the country has 1,422 prison and jail units unevenly distributed among its states (DEPEN, 2019). The states of Minas Gerais, São Paulo, Rio Grande Sul, and Goiás have over 100 units each, whereas Roraima has only five. The gap among the penitentiary system becomes more pronounced when we examine the installed capacity. São Paulo concentrates about 1/3 of all prison vacancies in Brazil (147,942), followed by Minas Gerais (41,573), and Rio de Janeiro (31,485). Nonetheless, the largest rate of prison units per 100,000 inhabitants lies in northern Brazil, in the states of Rondônia and Tocantins (Table 1).

In December 2019, Brazil reached more than 748 thousand inmates, comprising the third-largest prison population on Earth (Carvalho et al., 2020). While the world imprisonment rate lies at 145 detainees per 100,000 inhabitants, this country displays an incarceration rate of 356 per 100,000 inhabitants, ranking

Table 1. Brazilian state penitentiary systems.

Brazilian States and Federal District	# of prison units	# of inmates	Resident population	Prision units per 100.000 inhabitants	Incarceration rate per 100.000 inhabitants	Total Capacity	Occupancy rate (inmates/ vacancy)
Acre	15	8,414	881,935	1.70	954.04	4,069	2.07
Alagoas	10	9,161	3,337,357	0.30	274.50	3,724	2.46
Amazonas	19	10,890	4,144,597	0.46	262.75	3,511	3.10
Amapá	7	2,750	845,731	0.83	325.16	1,546	1.78
Bahia	25	15,108	14,873,064	0.17	101.58	11,983	1.25
Ceará	33	31,569	9,132,078	0.36	345.69	11,867	2.66
Distrito Federal	7	16,586	3,015,268	0.23	550.07	7,606	2.18
Espírito Santo	34	23,427	4,018,650	0.85	582.96	13,784	1.70
Goiás	110	25,761	7,018,354	1.57	367.05	14,108	1.83
Maranhão	52	12,346	7,075,181	0.73	174.50	9,345	1.32
Minas Gerais	223	74,712	21,168,791	1.05	352.93	41,573	1.80
Mato Grosso do Sul	41	17,423	2,778,986	1.48	626.96	8,256	2.11
Mato Grosso	52	12,519	3,484,466	1.49	359.28	8,709	1.44
Pará	48	20,825	8,602,865	0.56	242.07	10,199	2.04
Paraíba	75	13,326	4,018,127	1.87	331.65	7,912	1.68
Pernambuco	75	33,641	9,557,071	0.78	352.00	12,696	2.65
Piaui	16	4,433	3,273,227	0.49	135.43	2,419	1.83
Paraná	68	29,690	11,433,957	0.59	259.67	21,824	1.36
Rio de Janeiro	50	50,822	17,264,943	0.29	294.37	31,485	1.61
Rio Grande do Norte	18	10,155	3,506,853	0.51	289.58	7,597	1.34
Rio Grande do Sul	111	41,189	11,377,239	0.98	362.03	27,733	1.49
Rondônia	50	13,419	1,777,225	2.81	755.05	7,318	1.83
Roraima	5	3,688	605,761	0.83	608.82	924	3.99
Santa Catarina	52	23,470	7,164,788	0.73	327.57	19,033	1.23
Sergipe	10	6,244	2,298,696	0.44	271.63	3,089	2.02
São Paulo	176	231,287	45,919,049	0.38	503.68	147,942	1.56
Tocantins	40	4,481	1,572,866	2.54	284.89	2,097	2.14
Brazil	**1,422**	**747,336**	**210,147,125**	**0.68**	**355.63**	**442,349**	**1.69**

Source: DEPEN, Ministry of Justice and Public Safety (2019)

among the top 20 largest in the world (World Prison, 2020). This rate varies widely among the Brazilian states. Bahia displays the lowest rate of incarceration, with an average of 102 inmates per 100 thousand inhabitants (Table 1), a number similar to Luxembourg (World Prison, 2020). Rondônia has an incarceration rate higher than the United States of America, with 755 inmates per 100 thousand inhabitants. Acre overshadows all Brazilian states with 954 people behind bars per 100 thousand inhabitants, an unmatched rate in the world (World Prison, 2020).

The large number of detainees is a relatively recent phenomenon in Brazilian history. Thirty years ago, the country's imprisonment rate was 61/100,000, implying that in three decades the rate has increased six-fold (Graph 1). During the 2000s, the average annual prison population growth was 7.5%, while the Brazilian population expanded at 1.5% per year (Carvalho, 2016).

A range of factors explains this linear growth in incarceration rates. In the early 1990s, democratically elected governments promised to end crime with mass imprisonment (Ratton, 1996). The legacy of the authoritarian regime (1964–1985) and the

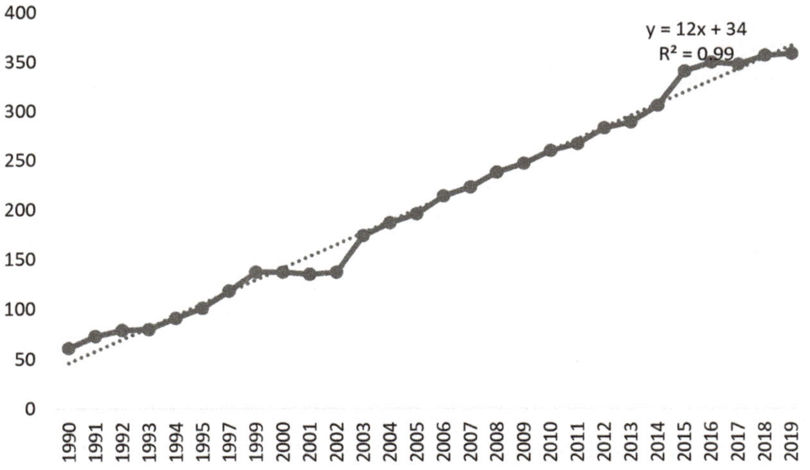

Graph 1. Incarceration rate per 100,000 inhabitants (Brazil, 1990 to 2019).
Source: DEPEN, Ministry of Justice and Public Safety (various years)

institutional framework that came into force with the Federal Constitution of 1988 allowed public safety policies to be based exclusively on the punitivist ideology carried out by police organizations (Lima et al., 2016). This situation was aggravated by increasing pressure from different social segments for effective anti-crime policies (Cruz et al., 2013), pushing the adoption of a managerially oriented and rigid penal control, targeting specific social groups, namely the black urban poor (Sinhoretto, 2018). As a result, poor and afro-Brazilians are overrepresented among arrestees, pretrial detainees and convicted inmates.

Such social pressure resulted in the approval of a series of laws allowing pretrial detention for a myriad of crimes, while warranting longer incarceration periods (de Azevedo, 2017). An example of such policy reorientation was the Heinous Crimes Law of 1990 (Law #8,072), that established not only longer incarceration periods for those committing crimes with cruelty, but also prohibited the progression of prison regime (Macaulay, 2002).[6] Soon after this Law was passed, pre-trial detainees became 1/3 of the prison population, a proportion that remained stable in subsequent decades (Cifali & de Azevedo, 2017).

During the 1990s, Brazil made international news with several headlines about the precarious conditions of its prison system (Cruz et al., 2013). One specific event shocked the world, forever changing the history of the penitentiary system: the Carandiru's massacre, which took place in 1992 (Manso & Dias, 2017). A rebellion in the Carandiru prison complex led to the arrival of the São Paulo Military Police (Dias & Salla, 2013). Police troops entered the detention center and, under the argument that inmates were armed, used lethal force resulting in 111 dead and 108 wounded inmates (Biondi & Marques, 2010). This brutal intervention has never been legally solved, and those responsible for the carnage have never been adequately punished (Macaulay, 2002). This event is an important milestone in the structuring one of the largest and most influential Brazilian criminal organization, the so-called "First Command of the Capital" (PCC – Portuguese acronym).

In the early 2000s, a small inflection in incarceration rates was noticed (Graph 1), most likely in consequence of the I National Plan for Public Safety (Brazil says no to violence). This program aimed at regaining control over crime inside and outside prison units (Adorno, 2008), exhibiting a more preventive tone and advocating the humanization of the prison system (Madeira & Rodrigues, 2015). The emphasis on preventive measures was maintained in the II National Public Security Plan (2003) and the National Citizenship Security Program (PRONASCI, Portuguese acronym) (2007) (Cifali & de Azevedo, 2017). Both initiatives highlighted the citizen security paradigm, implying that actions and decisions emanating from the Ministry of Justice should promote and warrant human rights (Madeira & Rodrigues, 2015). These national public safety plans were never translated into lower rates of incarceration, due to the approval of two contradicting legislative bills, namely Law #10,792 in 2003; and Law #11,343 in 2006.

Law #10,792 was published in 2003 creating the Differentiated Disciplinary Regime (RDD, Portuguese acronym) that subjects detainees to more stringent prison regime depending upon their affiliation with criminal organizations, such as the PCC, making their prison length inside correctional facilities longer (Cruz et al., 2013).[7] As a result, the Federal Government announced the creation of a series of federal penitentiaries to detain the more dangerous criminals, including various PCC members (Dias & Salla, 2013, 2019). By creating new penitentiaries and transferring PCC leaders, Brazilian authorities inadvertently contributed to the expansion and strengthening of the organization (Duarte & de Araújo, 2020).[8]

Law #11,343 came into force in 2006 strengthening the war on drugs boosting the rate of incarceration (Cifali & de Azevedo, 2017). The legislation exempted drug users from prison terms, granting them medical treatment and alternative penalties (Campos & Alvarez, 2017), while tightening the punishments for drug dealers, including a minimum of five years and a maximum of 15 years of imprisonment (Campos, 2014). Nonetheless, Law #11,343 failed to specify the amount of drugs necessary to classify subjects as drug dealers or drug users, leaving the differentiation up to state officials (Grillo et al., 2011). Art. 28 of this law establishes that "to determine whether the drug is intended for personal consumption, the judge will take into account the nature and the quantity of the seized substance, the place, and conditions in which the action was carried out, social and personal circumstances, as well as the conduct and background of the agent". Given the possibility of taking into account the "social and personal circumstances", the socially disadvantaged young and poor black individuals, regardless of the amount of drugs under their possession, (and sometimes even without it) were framed as drug dealers (Sinhoretto, 2018); whereas, individuals with different social profiles were classified as drug users (Campos & Alvarez, 2017).

There were two major consequences of Law #11,343. Firstly, the explosion in the number of individuals arrested for drug trafficking, adding immense pressure to the precarious prison system (Cifali & de Azevedo, 2017). Since 2007, this offense has accounted for nearly one-third of all incarcerations carried out in Brazil (Dias, 2017), involving mainly young black residents from poor urban areas (Sinhoretto, 2018). Secondly, it has enhanced the growth of PCC and its spread to most states (Manso & Dias, 2017), which often led to disputes for domination within and outside the detention facilities with other criminal organizations (Dias & Salla, 2013, 2019).[9]

In summary, the combination of the Heinous Crimes Law (1990), the RDD law (2003) and the Drug Law (2006) triggered the accelerated growth of the inmate population over the last three decades (Cifali & de Azevedo, 2017). The prison system was unable to keep up with the growing demand, and despite the creation of new prison units across the country, overcrowding remains a dominant feature (Dias, 2017). With the rapid expansion of the prison systems, new and old units coexist, with significant differences in terms of infrastructure and services provided to inmates. Hence, we hypothesize that better-equipped state prison systems are better prepared to face the pandemic and will display lower numbers of cases and deaths due to COVID-19.

Surviving in scarcity: the measures adopted to contain COVID-19

Following the increase in incarceration rates, state and federal governments invested in the creation of new prison units (Cruz et al., 2013). This policy was financed by DEPEN through agreements that aimed to reduce overcrowding and to improve the housing conditions (Madeira & Rodrigues, 2015). This movement started in São Paulo with the inauguration of numerous units in smaller cities that simultaneously sought to contain overcrowding and increase containment capacity (Godoi et al., 2019). This policy was also carried out in states such as Rio de Janeiro and Minas Gerais expanding the number of detention facilities. In Minas Gerais, the state was the pioneer in creating partnerships with the private sector and NGOs to manage some prisons units (Ribeiro & Lopes, 2018).

Despite these efforts, the deficit remained high and reasonably stable throughout the last three decades, with a national average of 1.69 prisoners per vacancy. Overcrowding, however, is highly variable among Brazilian states (Table 1), with the worst situation found in northern Brazil. In Roraima, for example, there are almost four inmates for each vacancy, a rate similar to Guatemala, which holds one of the most overpopulated prison systems in the world (World Prison, 2020). Overcrowding is only the tip of the iceberg when it comes to the subhuman conditions to which detainees are subjected to (Lermen et al., 2015; Rangel & Bicalho, 2016).

One cannot overlook the shortage of prison officers responsible for their custody, and the lack of educational, work and health facilities that should mimic life outside the walls, as Goffman's (1958) total institution concept suggests. As a result, the ability to balance precarious resources, demands for better living conditions, and access to public policies within the penitentiary units is different across states (Franco-Paredes et al., 2020; Godoi, 2015). For example, some detention facilities have physicians available for detainee's consultation, while others lack of them, increasing the likelihood of disease spread or rebellion due to the absence of these services (Oliveira Andrade, 2020).

Due to the lack of basic services and items, detainees rely mainly on what their families can bring on visitation days, including personal hygiene items, food and medicine, in heavy bags subjected to inspection and, sometimes, to confiscation of items (Silvestre, 2012). Information regarding the inmates' trials, meetings with lawyers, and the possibility of near parole are also brought by family members on these weekly visits (Godoi, 2015). They also bring news about loved ones who are unable to pay a visit, such as small children or other inmates (Biondi, 2016). Visitation bags are important sources of income for inmates (Darke, 2014), as the items and the information brought in can be interchanged for services and goods, including the illegal ones (Darke & Garces, 2017). To guarantee order inside the overcrowded and understaffed units, the administration empowers certain detainees (Darke, 2014; Dias & Salla, 2019). As noted by Darke (2013), in several prison units the inmates are in charge of supervising and carrying out numerous activities, such as cleaning, food preparation, and distribution. These inmates have a hold on the rest preventing conflicts.

If life in the prison system naturally threatens the health of individuals, in units as overcrowded as the Brazilian ones, these challenges are even greater (Costa et al., 2020; Sánchez et al., 2020). Precarious conditions associated with overpopulated, unhealthy environments, idleness, lack of health professionals, social services, and education potentialize inequities and the likelihood of contamination inside the detention facilities (Gabriel et al., 2019). In an attempt to improve the detention conditions, the National Policy for Integral Health Care of the Private Person of Liberty (PNAISP, Portuguese acronym) was instituted in 2014, with the goal of ensuring the care of people deprived of liberty, expanding and organizing the prison health teams (Carvalho et al., 2020).

Despite the PNAISP, data made available by DEPEN (2019) indicate that only 36.2% of all prison units had a designated doctor's office, while 22.7% of prisons lacked health service facilities. This enormous shortage of medical services explains why Brazil had death rates of 144 per 100,000 inmates last year (DEPEN, 2019), a number 20 times higher than the mortality rate for the Brazilian population as a whole (6.2/100,000) (IBGE, 2020). In general, "populations involved with the criminal justice system have an increased prevalence of infectious diseases such as HIV and Hepatitis C virus (HCV) infections and tuberculosis" (Akiyama, Spaulding & Rich, 2020, p. 2075). Inside the penitentiary system, diseases like scabies have an incidence rate that is thirty times higher than the ones found in the general population, leading to a substantial number of deaths behind prison walls (Sánchez et al., 2020).

With the arrival of COVID-19, the challenges regarding the provision of adequate health services became greater (Matos, 2020; Oliveira Andrade, 2020). Overcrowded penitentiary systems, with poor levels of general hygiene and sanitation practices jeopardize COVID-19 prevention (Abraham et al., 2020, p. 782). In this environment is impossible to implement even the most rudimentary cleaning and social distancing practices (Franco-Paredes et al., 2020). Making matters worse, inmates exhibit overall high rates of morbidity conditions, increasing the likelihood of deaths due to the disease (Souza, 2020). Specifically, due to RDD Law, older incarcerated individuals comprise the fastest growing population (Oliveira Carmo & Oliveira Araújo, 2011) being the ones more likely to get infected and suffer with coronavirus.

Brazil recorded the first COVID-19 case on February 26th, 2020. When the World Health Organization declared the pandemic, president Bolsonaro decided not to issue a plan to curb the virus (Ortega & Orsini, 2020). As a result, the 26 states, the Federal District, and the 5,570 municipalities received the burden of dealing with the problem (Ricard & Medeiros, 2020). On March 17th, 2020 two cases of deaths due to coronavirus were recorded. On that same day, the National Council of Justice (CNJ, Portuguese acronym) issued the Recommendation 62/2020, listing several measures that could be adopted by Brazilian states to prevent death by coronavirus inside prisons (Costa et al., 2020). These measures are listed in Table 2.

The actions suggested by the CNJ are consistent with those proposed by the World Health Organization (Williams et al., 2020), and similar to those adopted in penitentiary systems elsewhere in the world (Akiyama, Spaulding & Rich, 2020). However, recommendation 62/2020 is not a law. Judges and prison authorities have discretionary power over these measures. When this recommendation was released, the Minister of Justice and Public Safety declared that COVID-19 should not be an excuse for freeing criminals (Costa et al., 2020).

The Brazilian penitentiary system is seen as the major school of crime, as it "generates serious criminal activity, acts as an institution of discriminatory social control and discipline, and is unable to fulfil its allotted task of crime reduction or offender rehabilitation" (Macaulay, 2002, p. 11). Most public opinion surveys show that Brazilians are generally against the release of inmates from prisons and jails (Beato Filho et al., 2020), preventing the adoption of the measures recommended by CNJ. As a result, on April 2020, DEPEN consolidated some preventive measures in a manual, instructing states about actions to be implemented (Siqueira et al., 2020). The contingency plans released by state authorities had more restrictive measures than those suggested by Recommendation 62/2020, which were interpreted as offering undeserving benefits for "dangerous criminals" (Sánchez et al., 2020).

All state penitentiary systems had suspended family visits by the beginning of April, with several implications for the management of prison routine. On April 17th, 2020, the Brazilian penitentiary system registered two deaths due to COVID-19 (DEPEN, 2020);

Table 2. Measures advised by recommendation 62/2020 of the national council of justice to prevent the spread of COVID-19.

Measure	Actions
Release of detainees with comorbidities, members of risk groups: • pregnant, • nursing mothers, • those caring for children aging up to 12 years • disabled individuals, • elderly (above 60 years of age), and • indigenous	(1) Reassessment of pretrial detainees that have exceeded 90 days or that are related to crime without violence or serious threat to the person; (2) Grant early exit giving priority to people arrested in criminal institutions that are overcrowded or do not have a healthcare team assigned to the institution; (3) Maximum exceptionality of new pretrial detention orders, observing the protocol of the health authorities; (4) House arrest for people arrested for child support debt; (5) Extension of the period of return or postponement of the granting of the temporary exit benefit; (6) Alternative measures (such as house arrest, electronic monitoring) for prisoners.
Circulation reduction	(1) Suspension of the duty of periodic submission to the court of persons on pretrial release; (2) Suspension of judicial hearings and prisoner removal from one unit to another; (3) Avoid shared transportation of people deprived of liberty (4) Restriction of visits to prisoners.
Preventive measures	(1) Uninterrupted supply of water to persons deprived of liberty and public servants of the units (2) Education campaigns on the novel coronavirus (3) Increased frequency of cleaning of cells and common spaces (4) Temporary replacement of prison officers who are part of the risk group (5) Supply of personal protective equipment (PPE) to employees (6) Screening of prisoners, staff and visitors (7) Isolation of suspected or confirmed cases in prison

Source: Adapted from Carvalho, Santos & Santos (2020)

a month after the first death was recorded among the general population. Since then, prisoners' families started advocating early releases and news about inmates, as external visits are still prohibited in all states (FGV, 2020).

On April 23rd, to cope with the political pressure to block the spread of the disease, the Minister of Justice and Public Safety suggested that detainees with COVID-19 symptoms should be placed in containers (Souza, 2020). Prisoners were to be housed in these spaces without beds and proper ventilation, living like animals in cages with scarcely food (Siqueira et al., 2020). This endorsement was unwaveringly rejected by the National Council for Criminal and Penitentiary Policy in May 2020, but it gives an idea of how public authorities sought to deal with coronavirus in Brazil (Costa et al., 2020).

By July 2020, all states had published contingency plans to prevent the spread of COVID-19 inside prisons and jails. These are often palliative actions in view of the overcrowded prison system, as in the case of daily asepsis of cells (Carvalho et al., 2020). Others are seen as measures that suppress the rights of persons deprived of liberty, such as the total ban on visits or legal assistance (Oliveira Andrade, 2020). Table 3 summarizes the main actions implemented by each Brazilian state.

Contrary to the measures adopted elsewhere, in Brazil the suspension of family visits was not followed by an increase in telephone time or other means of communication (Franco-Paredes et al., 2020; Sánchez et al., 2020; Williams et al., 2020). The justification for the total suspension of external visits was to avoid the comings and goings of people from outside the prison environment (Matos, 2020). This measure has been proven to be futile, as family members are not the only contact prisoners have with the outside world (Abraham et al., 2020). Moving back and forth daily are the prison employees, members of religious organizations and lawyers, as well as outsourced service providers, present in 72% of Brazilian prisons (DEPEN, 2019).

Although only three states have not included domiciliary arrests in their contingency plans, it is possible to assert that there was a huge rejection of the prisoner release policy (Costa et al., 2020). Few progressive judges decided to substitute prison services with house arrests or electronic monitoring, removing only 32,500 inmates from detention facilities until September 2020 (CNJ, 2020). This number corresponds to only 4.6% of the total prisoner population, a figure that neither reduces overcrowding nor improves social distancing. It is worth noting that under normal circumstances, more than 222,000 individuals are released from prisons and jails annually (DEPEN, 2019), which means that COVID-19 may not have promoted any early release.

Other measures adopted by the states were seen as a strategy to reduce the prisoners' rights, being justified by the need to contain the PCC's power. Among them is the suspension of assistance from lawyers and temporary exits implemented by the majority of the states. With the rationale that important members of organized crime could be released during the pandemic, this suspension increased the tensions and, in some units, the likelihood of rebellions (Siqueira et al., 2020).

The evidence that the main concern is not the spread of coronavirus relies on the fact that not every Brazilian state isolates detainees with COVID-19 symptoms (Sánchez et al., 2020). Alagoas, Amapá, Espirito Santo, and Piauí are examples of states that have not put this measure into force (Table 3). In some states, not even longer sunbathing times or the daily cleaning of cells are part of the COVID-19 prevention protocol (DEPEN, 2020). As a result, 14 of the 27 state penitentiary systems have already experienced some form of rebellion over

Table 3. Measures adopted by the state penitentiary systems in Brazil to contain COVID-19.

State	Day of total suspension of families' visits	Domiciliar arrest	Daily cell asepsis	Increased sunbathing time	Suspension of Attorney Attendance	Suspension of transfers	Suspension of temporary exits	Isolation of prisoners over the age of 60/chronic diseases	Isolation of symptomatic prisoners
Acre	3/16	Yes	Yes	Yes	Yes	Yes	Yes	Yes	Yes
Alagoas	3/16	No	No	No	Yes	No	No	No	No
Amapá	3/17	Yes	No	No	No	Yes	No	Yes	No
Amazonas	3/14	Yes	Yes	No	Yes	Yes	Yes	Yes	Yes
Bahia	3/18	Yes	No	No	Yes	Yes	No	No	No
Ceará	3/16	Yes	Yes	Yes	Yes	Yes	Yes	Yes	Yes
Distrito Federal	3/12	Yes	Yes	Yes	Yes	Yes	Yes	Yes	Yes
Espírito Santo	4/1	Yes	No	No	No	No	Yes	No	No
Goiás	3/13	Yes	No	No	Yes	Yes	No	Yes	Yes
Maranhão	3/23	Yes	Yes	Yes	Yes	Yes	Yes	No	Yes
Mato Grosso	3/19	Yes	Yes	Yes	Yes	Yes	No	Yes	Yes
Mato Grosso do Sul	3/19	Yes	No	Yes	No	Yes	Yes	No	Yes
Minas Gerais	3/20	Yes	Yes	Yes	Yes	Yes	Yes	Yes	Yes
Pará	3/23	Yes	Yes	No	No	Yes	Yes	Yes	Yes
Paraíba	3/20	Yes	Yes	Yes	Yes	Yes	Yes	Yes	Yes
Paraná	3/13	No	No	No	No	No	No	No	Yes
Pernambuco	3/21	Yes	Yes	No	Yes	Yes	Yes	Yes	Yes
Piauí	3/17	Yes	Yes	Yes	Yes	Yes	Yes	Yes	No
Rio de Janeiro	3/13	Yes	Yes	No	Yes	No	No	Yes	Yes
Rio Grande do Norte	3/14	No	Yes	Yes	Yes	Yes	Yes	Yes	Yes
Rio Grande do Sul	3/17	Yes	Yes	Yes	Yes	Yes	No	No	Yes
Rondônia	3/21	Yes	Yes	Yes	No	Yes	No	Yes	Yes
Roraima	3/16	No	No	No	Yes	No	Yes	Yes	Yes
Santa Catarina	3/18	Yes	Yes	No	No	Yes	Yes	Yes	Yes
São Paulo	3/20	Yes	Yes	Yes	No	Yes	Yes	Yes	Yes
Sergipe	3/16	No	Yes	Yes	Yes	Yes	Yes	Yes	Yes
Tocantins	3/14	Yes	Yes	No	Yes	Yes	Yes	Yes	Yes

Source: DEPEN, Ministry of Justice and Public Safety (2020)

the past months,[10] in response to the adoption of such restrictive measures, combined with the absence of procedures for testing, isolating, and treating COVID-19 patients (symptomatic and asymptomatic). For some researchers, it is a matter of time before blood spills again amid the chaos inside prison units, (Costa et al., 2020).

Since the Brazilian penitentiary system presents poor sanitary conditions, being characterized by overcrowding and the absence of proper health assistance (Dias, 2017; Gabriel et al., 2019; Lermen et al., 2015), the contingency plans adopted by each state are not seen as appropriate to deal with COVID-19 (Oliveira Andrade, 2020; Sánchez et al., 2020). So, we expect that penitentiary systems that have adopted real preventive measures (instead of only suppressing inmates' rights) are more able to cope with COVID-19, having lower numbers of confirmed cases and mortality.

Confirmed cases and deaths by COVID-19 in the detention facilities: numbers seeking an explanation?

The measures used to prevent COVID-19 were erratic across Brazilian states, widening the gap between the state prison systems in terms of infrastructure and quality services, with significant repercussions on the incidence of cases and deaths due to the disease. The number of cases inside the Brazilian penitentiary system has been increasing every week and the number of deaths has experienced a sharp rise, indicating the ineffectiveness of the adopted preventive measures. The tendency line of the number of deaths indicates that the worst is yet to come (Graph 2).

The overall disease rate among prisoners (30.85/1,000 inmates) is higher than the national average (19.74/1,000 inhabitants) (Table 4). This difference is probably generated

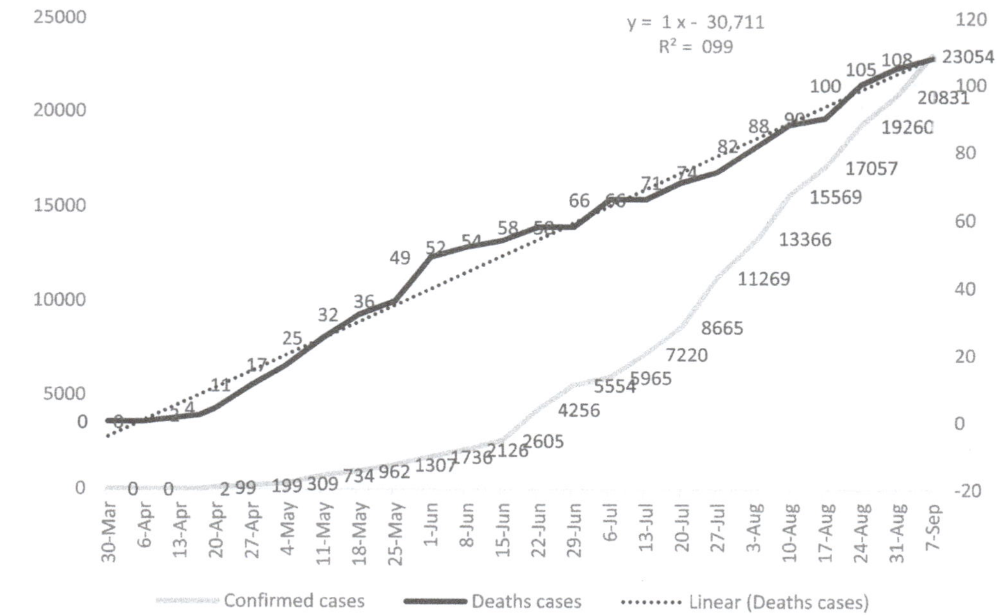

Graph 2. Cumulative number of COVID-19 Confirmed and Death Cases (03/30/20 to 09/07/20). Sources: DEPEN, Ministry of Justice and Public Safety (2020)

Table 4. COVID-19 cases and deaths across the Brazilian states until September 7th, 2020.

States	Prison Population					Total population				
	Confirmed cases	Deaths	Prison population	Confimed cases/ 1,000 inmates	Mortality rate/ 100,000 inmates	Confirmed cases	Deaths	Total population	Confimed cases/1,000 inhabitants	Mortality rate/100,000 inhabitants
Acre	228	3	8,414	27.10	35.65	58,237	1,187	881,935	66.03	134.59
Alagoas	44	0	9,161	4.80	0.00	25,469	624	3,337,357	7.63	18.70
Amazonas	163	1	10,890	14.97	9.18	123,905	3,849	4,144,597	29.90	92.87
Amapá	170	1	2,750	61.82	36.36	45,253	598	845,731	53.51	70.71
Bahia	520	0	15,108	34.42	0.00	208,259	6,257	14,873,064	14.00	42.07
Ceará	632	3	31,569	20.02	9.50	44,863	673	9,132,078	4.91	7.37
Distrito Federal	1,794	4	16,586	108.16	24.12	55,906	754	3,015,268	18.54	25.01
Espírito Santo	1,883	5	23,427	80.38	21.34	158,310	3,518	4,018,650	39.39	87.54
Goiás	882	5	25,761	34.24	19.41	82,282	1,901	7,018,354	11.72	27.09
Maranhão	233	1	12,346	18.87	8.10	222,445	8,566	7,075,181	31.44	121.07
Minas Gerais	327	10	74,712	4.38	13.38	63,810	2,294	21,168,791	3.01	10.84
Mato Grosso do Sul	1,350	1	17,423	77.48	5.74	109,706	2,550	2,778,986	39.48	91.76
Mato Grosso	1,355	2	12,519	108.24	15.98	132,420	7,721	3,484,466	38.00	221.58
Pará	649	0	20,825	31.16	0.00	80,786	1,936	8,602,865	9.39	22.50
Paraíba	259	2	13,326	19.44	15.01	73,846	1,898	4,018,127	18.38	47.24
Pernambuco	1,424	8	33,641	42.33	23.78	271,963	5,693	9,557,071	28.46	59.57
Piaui	494	0	4,433	111.44	0.00	236,012	5,851	3,273,227	72.10	178.75
Paraná	48	1	29,690	1.62	3.37	115,793	3,268	11,433,957	10.13	28.58
Rio de Janeiro	422	16	50,822	8.30	31.48	233,052	16,593	17,264,943	13.50	96.11
Rio Grande do Norte	527	0	10,155	51.90	0.00	857,330	31,377	3,506,853	244.47	894.73
Rio Grande do Sul	1,317	7	41,189	31.97	16.99	143,952	3,756	11,377,239	12.65	33.01
Rondônia	545	2	13,419	40.61	14.90	143,853	3,577	1,777,225	80.94	201.27
Roraima	212	8	3,688	57.48	216.92	189,477	2,422	605,761	312.79	399.83
Santa Catarina	1,326	2	23,470	56.50	8.52	54,125	970	7,164,788	7.55	13.54
Sergipe	14	1	6,244	2.24	16.02	98,206	2,932	2,298,696	42.72	127.55
São Paulo	5,799	25	231,287	25.07	10.81	147,728	3,475	45,919,049	3.22	7.57
Tocantins	437	0	4,481	97.52	0.00	170,806	2,720	1,572,866	108.60	172.93
Brazil	**23,054**	**108**	**747,336**	**30.85**	**14.45**	**4,147,794**	**126,960**	**210,147,125**	**19.74**	**60.41**

Source: DEPEN, Ministry of Justice and Public Safety (2020)

by the fact that it is much easier to test the inmates for coronavirus than the general population. Prison populations, besides being confined, are much smaller than those found in the cities where prisons are located, facilitating the process of testing suspected cases. Conversely, mortality rates due to COVID-19 are higher for the population when compared to the prison population (Table 4). On average for each group of 100,000 Brazilians, 60.45 lost their lives due to coronavirus until the 7th of September, whereas in the penitentiary system the mortality rate due to COVID-19 was 14.45/100,000 prisoners. Many factors explain this discrepancy, such as a much younger population behind bars (Carvalho et al., 2020). Also, inefficient mortality record systems inside prison units might explain why six states have not recorded deaths by COVID-19 until September 7th (Siqueira et al., 2020).

The proportion of confirmed cases and deaths by COVID-19 is different among Brazilian states. Noticeably, sixteen from 27 states have a higher rate of confirmed cases among inmates than in the population as a whole. It is worth highlighting the case of Sergipe, which has only 14 confirmed cases and a single death by coronavirus, standing in sharp contrast with the rest of the country.

Acre, Amapá and Rio de Janeiro have mortality rates higher than 30 inmates per 100 thousand, while Alagoas, Bahia, Pará, Piauí, Rio Grande do Norte and Tocantins have not recorded any deaths inside the prison system. Overall, mortality rates are lower among prisoners than the general population (14.45 *versus* 60.41 per 100 thousand, respectively). Roraima is an outlier, as this state not only contradicts the national trend, displaying higher mortality by COVID-19 among prisoners (216.82 deaths per 100 thousand inmates) (Graph 3), but also staggering death rates (Graph 4). Roraima has also the highest occupancy rate among Brazilian states, with an average of four inmates per vacancy, which could be the cause of such a high level of mortality due to COVID-19.

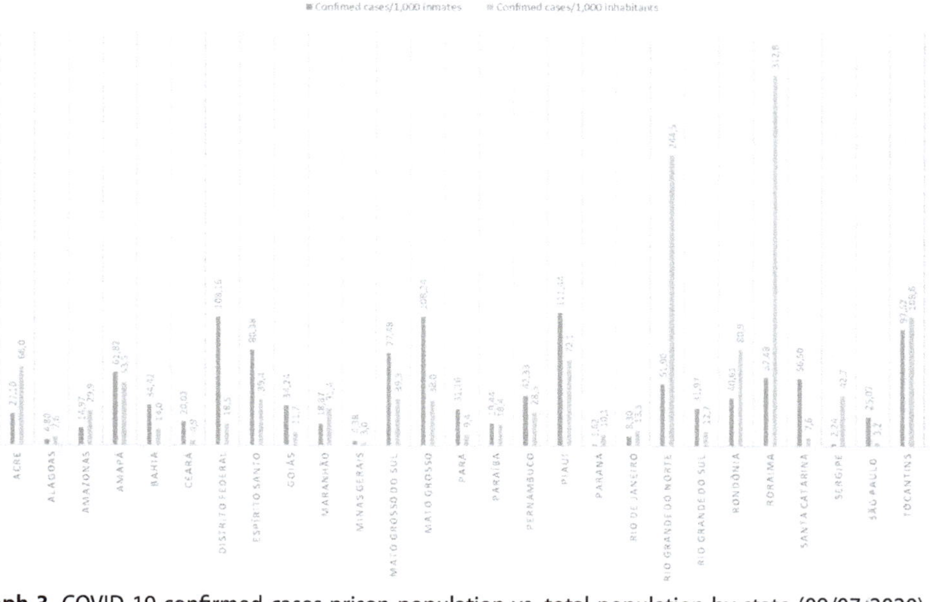

Graph 3. COVID-19 confirmed cases prison population vs. total population by state (09/07/2020). Sources: DEPEN, Ministry of Justice and Public Safety (2020) and Ministry of Health (2020)

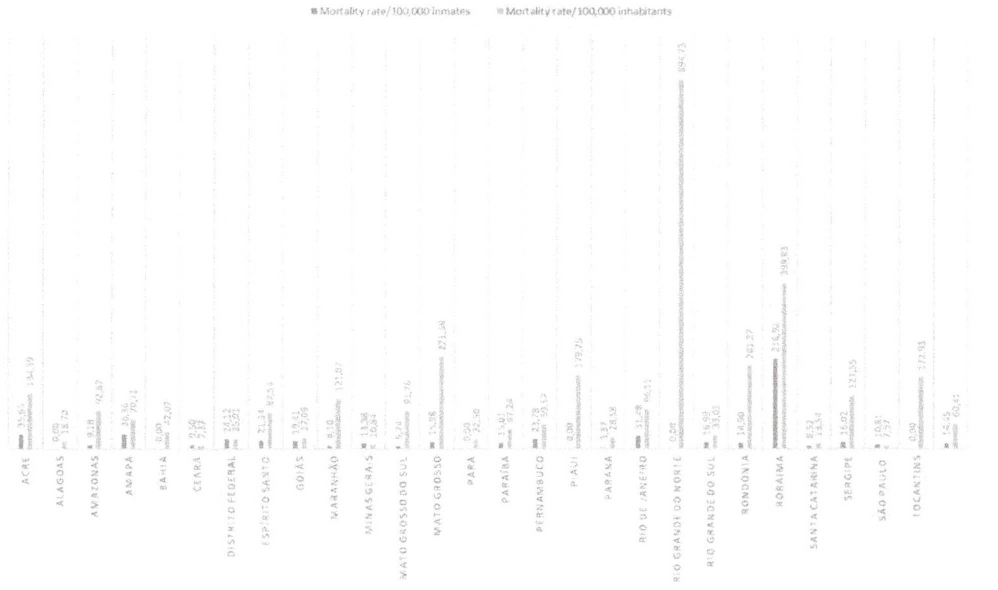

Graph 4. COVID-19 death cases prison population vs. total population by state (09/07/2020).
Sources: DEPEN, Ministry of Justice and Public Safety (2020) and Ministry of Health (2020)

Having identified national patterns and states' specificities, we turn our attention to the factors that explain why the incidence and mortality rates by COVID-19 vary across Brazilian state prison systems. We have two major sets of hypotheses. Table 1 displayed how the state prison systems have large discrepancies in terms of installed infrastructure and services provided. It is expected that better equipped and staffed prison systems are better prepared to face the pandemic and should have a lower number of COVID-19 cases and deaths. Table 3 demonstrated the vast array of preventive measures adopted by different state penitentiary systems to cope with the coronavirus pandemic. We assume that these measures have a dampening effect on the number of COVID-19 cases and deaths, although, they are poor representations of the penitentiary population, given the abysmal differences in infrastructure, quality of services, number of administrative and custody personnel across the state prison systems (Oliveira Andrade, 2020; Sánchez et al., 2020).

To measure the quality of the infrastructure, we used information related to the overall conditions of the penitentiary systems, including the overcrowding indicator, the number of prisons and jails, the number of pretrial detainees and the percentage of units managed by the private sector (together with NGOs). We also included the availability of designated facilities, such as classroom, library, workshop and health module and the presence of designated space for visitors and intimate visits. Finally, we added indicators related to the quality of health services provided, measured by the number of medical appointments inside and outside the unit and the number of laboratory tests. These numbers were made available through Infopen survey carried out in 2019 (DEPEN, 2019), and are presented in Table 5.

Table 5. List of dependent and independent variables.

Infra-structure Measures (data gathered from Depen, 12/2019)	Expected effects upon confirmed cases and deaths by COVID-19:	N	Minimum	Maximum	Mean	Std. Deviation
Overcrowding (number of inmates per vacancy)	+	27	1.23	3.99	1.94	.62
Number of penitentiary units (jails + prisons)	-	27	5	223	52.67	51.58
% of establishments not directly managed by the State	-	27	0.0	0.5	.06	.12
Number of provisional detainees	+	27	689	46,298	8242.89	9942.765
Number of releases per year	-	27	52	50,094	8248.11	11,925.61
Number of laboratory tests	-	27	339	153,103	14,289.93	28,679.80
Number of general medical appointments inside the unit	-	27	341	172,888	24,548.70	32,961.61
Number of medical appointments outside the unit	-	27	104	40,958	6205.41	9834.56
% of prison units with classroom	-	27	38.2%	100.0%	68.7%	19.0%
% of prison units with computer room	-	27	0.0%	53.8%	16.8%	13.3%
% of prison units with library	-	27	20.0%	100.0%	52.7%	24.2%
% of prison units with designated places for visitation	-	27	14.3%	100.0%	55.5%	23.5%
% of prison units with designated places for intimate visits	-	27	0.0%	85.7%	36.9%	24.7%
% of prison units without a designated health module	+	27	0.0%	69.3%	22.6%	20.5%
% of prison units without workshop	+	27	5.8%	89.3%	57.3%	19.6%
Preventing Measures (data gathered from Depen, 09/07/2020)						
% states adopting home prison	-	27	0.0%	100.0%	81.5%	39.6%
% states adopting daily cell asepsis	-	27	0.0%	100.0%	70.4%	46.5%
% states adopting increased sunbathing time	-	27	0.0%	100.0%	51.9%	50.9%
% states adopting suspension of Attorney Attendance	-	27	0.0%	100.0%	70.4%	46.5%
% states adopting suspension of transfers	-	27	0.0%	100.0%	81.5%	39.6%
% states adopting suspension of temporary exits	-	27	0.0%	100.0%	66.7%	48.0%
% states adopting isolation of prisoners over the age of 60/and those with chronic diseases	-	27	0.0%	100.0%	74.1%	44.7%
% states adopting isolation of symptomatic prisoners	-	27	0.0%	100.0%	81.5%	39.6%
Days without external visits	+	27	159	179	173.30	4.20
Dependent variables (data gathered from Depen, 09/07/2020)						
Number of deaths by COVID-19		27	27	0	25.0	4.0
Number of COVID-19 confirmed cases		27	27	14	5799.0	853.9

Source: DEPEN, Ministry of Justice and Public Safety (2020)

To measure the preventive measures adopted by each state, we created a series of dummy variables using September 7th, 2020 as reference date. Since all states have adopted the suspension of visits, we opted to include the number of days without external visits (Table 5).

To estimate the linear regression models, we used the forward stepwise method, which is widely applied to identify covariables in small datasets. According to Steyerberg et al., 1999, p. 935), "stepwise selection indicates covariables with a statistically significant effect, simultaneously adjusting for the other covariables in the regression model", which increases the overall explanatory power of the model. In the first step, we included all independent variables listed on Table 5.

Since the dependent variables were highly skewed, we normalized both transforming them into Z-scores. Then, as we had only 27 cases, the stepwise method selected the independent variables that better fitted the models. To assess the collinearity issues, tolerance, and variance inflation factor (VIF) were used. Based on Gabbidon et al. (2011), we used tolerances below.20 and VIF's above 10.00 as indicators of problems with multicollinearity. Results partially supported our hypotheses.

For the normalized number of confirmed COVID-19 cases, the OLS stepwise method generated a model with three independent variables and an adjusted R^2 of 0.499. Tolerance and VIF values indicated that multicollinearity was not an issue in this model. All predictors were associated with the infrastructure hypothesis. The number of medical appointments held at the prison facility and the number of laboratory tests by inmate were positively associated with the number of confirmed cases of coronavirus, indicating that prison facilities offering these services were more likely to record cases of the disease. Conversely, the percentage of prison establishments not directly managed by the State displayed a dampening impact upon the number of COVID-19 cases, suggesting that privately run prison units were either providing better sanitary conditions for inmates or failing to properly register and report cases (Table 6).

For the number of deaths, the OLS stepwise method generated a model composed of two independent variables, which taken together, generated an adjusted R^2 of 0.492. Again, tolerance and VIF values indicated that multicollinearity was not an issue in this model. All predictors were associated with the infrastructure hypothesis (Table 7). The number of pretrial detainees presented a positive linear relationship with the number of deaths from

Table 6. OLS regression coefficients – # of COVID-19 confirmed cases as the dependent variable.

	Unstandardized Coefficients		Correlations			Collinearity Statistics	
Variables in the model	B	SE	Zero-order	Partial	Part	Tolerance	VIF
(Constant)	269.14	280.07					
Number of medical appointments held at the prison facility	0.014**	0.005	0.52	0.51	0.40	0.938	1.066
% of establishments not directly managed by the State	−39.699**	12,221	−0.43	−0.56	−0.45	0.982	1.018
Number of laboratory tests by inmate	12.106*	4828	0.41	0.46	0.35	0.927	1.078

***p < 0.001. **p < 0.010. * $p < 0.050$
Adjusted R^2 0.499; F 9.635 ($p < 0.001$)

Table 7. OLS regression coefficients – # of deaths by COVID-19 as the dependent variable.

	Unstandardized Coefficients		Correlations			Collinearity Statistics	
Variables in the model	B	SE	Zero-order	Partial	Part	Tolerance	VIF
(Constant)	−0.646	1.427					
Number of pretrial detainees	0.001	0.000	0.669	0.719	0.708	0.971	1.029
% of prison units without educational facilities	0.080*	0.960	0.173	0.390	0.290	0.971	1029

***p < 0.001. **p < 0.010. * $p < 0.050$
Adjusted R^2 0.492; F 13.601 ($p < 0.001$)

COVID-19. The same effect was observed for the percentage of prison units without educational facilities.

The OLS models exclusively supported the prison infrastructure hypothesis, corroborating the thought that better-equipped and staffed prisons with health services are better prepared to face the pandemic, displaying lower numbers of COVID-19 confirmed and death cases. The preventive measures adopted by prison states were not included in any of the models, as they are statistically unrelated to the number of COVID-19-confirmed and death cases.

Discussion

This paper seeks to identify the chief factors behind the incidence of COVID-19 cases and deaths inside the Brazilian prison system. This is an important subject because the country has the third-largest penitentiary population behind bars, living in overcrowded conditions, and being exposed to high mortality rates (Souza, 2020). These adverse conditions are expected to worsen with the coronavirus crisis, as the spread of COVID-19 is facilitated by the lack of hygiene and social agglomeration, aspects impossible to avoid in overfull prison units (Oliveira Andrade, 2020).

To build context for the examination of the factors controlling the spread of COVID-19 in the Brazilian penitentiary system, we described the main policies and laws that came into force over the last 30 years. Restrictions on pre-trial detention and progression of prison regime (de Azevedo, 2017; Campos, 2014; Macaulay, 2002), along with the war on drugs (Campos & Alvarez, 2017; Grillo et al., 2011) contributed to the skyrocketing number of inmates (de Azevedo, 2017; Sinhoretto, 2018).

The rapid growth of the incarceration rates led to the construction of new prison units, which failed to alleviate overcrowding (Dias, 2017; Godoi et al., 2019). As a result, jails and prisons in Brazil lack basic living conditions, where hygiene products, uniforms, medicines, and even food are scarce (Gabriel et al., 2019). These precarious circumstances jeopardize the health of inmates (Franco-Paredes et al., 2020), making mortality rates inside correctional facilities higher than outside (Souza, 2020). The poor living conditions are eased by family members who fill the gaps left by the State, providing prisoners with basic needs (Silvestre, 2012, 2016). Visitors also bring news of family members and neighbors and information about the next hearing will take place (Godoi, 2015).

COVID-19 has changed this precarious equilibrium as visitation has been prohibited in all Brazilian prison units since April 2020. The suspension of external visits suppressed the flow of goods and news, which are essential for the survival of the inmates. Without the possibility of meeting the loved ones, inmates are left without news (which includes the progress of their criminal trials), food, beverages, medicines, etc. (FGV, 2020). Also, "the suspension of family visits exacerbates the inmates' feeling of isolation and insecurity, generating concern over the health and lives of family members" (Sánchez et al., 2020, p. 3). To make matters worse, the odds of psychic illnesses increase dramatically (Alcântara et al., 2018), along with the deterioration of preexisting illnesses, whose control depends on continuous use medication (Lermen et al., 2015), often not provided by the prison unit, but usually brought by family members (FGV, 2020). In the long term, the total suspension of family visits can significantly contribute to the increase of deaths due to COVID-19 (Siqueira et al., 2020).

However, the length of time since the suppression of external visits was not included in any of the OLS models, indicating that this change affects neither the number of deaths nor the number of confirmed cases of coronavirus. In addition to being inefficient to contain the spread of the virus, this measure substantially worsens life behind bars (Siqueira et al., 2020), as detainees are prevented from receiving the basic items they are in desperate need of (Carvalho et al., 2020). Family members are critical of this measure, seen as a means to offset the deteriorating living conditions inside the prison system. They report how the administrator of these facilities would be imposing a more repressive system, withdrawing rights such as sunbathing time, access to medicines and information regarding criminal trials (FGV, 2020).

Family members are not the sole outside visitors. Prison guards, managers, post officers, and food providers move in and out regularly increasing the risk of introducing coronavirus inside prisons and jails (Abraham et al., 2020). New inmates might also be a source of coronavirus. In this sense, it is interesting to note that the number of pretrial detainees increases the number of deaths by COVID-19. The linear regression model suggests that the release of pretrial detainees could be an effective measure in preventing coronavirus. Nevertheless, most Brazilian authorities refuse to adopt Recommendation 62 as it would lead to the release of powerful criminals (Siqueira et al., 2020). For some state governors, it might be better to have a larger number of deaths inside prison units, than losing the next election for setting free those seen as "dangerous detainees".

CNJ (2020) also recommended the release of detainees over 60 years of age and those with comorbidities. Still, the state penitentiary systems decided to house this subpopulation in designated spaces to prevent them from contamination. The OLS linear regression models demonstrate that this measure has no statistically significant effect upon COVID-19 cases and deaths. Given the overcrowding conditions in most prison units, it is virtually impossible to segregate detainees with any given profile. Again, it would be much better to simply release these inmates, preserving their lives.

The infrastructure variables explained the number of COVID-19-confirmed and death cases. The number of medical appointments held at the prison facility and the number of laboratory tests by inmate increase the number of cases, as contaminated individuals have the necessary means to be officially recorded. Conversely, the percentage of prison units managed by private institutions decreases the number of COVID-19 cases, raising the need for further research, as this outcome could be either a result of improved sanitary conditions and better infrastructure or the lack of comprehensive testing and reporting of cases.

It is also noteworthy that the number of pretrial detainees and the percentage of prison units without educational facilities increase the number of deaths by COVID-19. New inmates might be a source of coronavirus, and the lack of educational facilities indicate a precarious infrastructure and absence of information, preventing inmates from being educated not only about COVID-19 but also by other infectious diseases and prophylactic measures.

In short, the preventive measures adopted lack empirical evidence. Not a single one of them proved to be an effective predictor of COVID-19 cases and deaths. This unexpected result could be an outcome of the partial or mistaken adoption of these measures by Brazilian states, or the failure of the state authorities to recognize the specificities of the prison population and the non-transferability of several preventive measures adopted outside prison walls. In either case, these results have significant policy implications, calling for a research agenda on prophylactic measures and contamination by coronavirus within the Brazilian penitentiary system.

Final considerations

The Brazilian Penitentiary System is still unprepared to face the outbreak of COVID-19. The absence of a centralized national coordination, the resistance against early release polices, and the pressure for more severe punishments have made matters worse. The Ministry of Justice and Public Safety should press state authorities to adopt the following preventive measures to cope with the coronavirus crisis inside the penitentiary system.

First, the obligation to test every inmate, including asymptomatic ones. In Brazil, only the Federal District enforces a testing policy in order to prevent the spread to the virus. States such as Alagoas have recorded only 44 cases and not a single death, an unrealistic number considering the experience of other States. A testing initiative could solve the question whether "the elevated rate of positive tests is the result of increased spread or widespread testing" (Abraham et al., 2020, p. 783).

Second, every prison or jail should quarantine symptomatic inmates. Seven Brazilian states have neglected this measure in their contingence plans, while others are unable to implement it given the lack of prison vacancies. As overcrowding is ubiquitous, early releases could help creating designated cells for inmates with COVID-19 symptoms (Franco-Paredes et al., 2020). Instead of blocking this measure, the judicial authorities could use this opportunity to develop risk assessment tools for the release of inmates, especially pretrial detainees.[11] The development of such a tool could also improve the high-level of recidivism in the country.

Third, Brazil should put in force a policy banning admissions of new inmates into state prisons. Such a measure could release the pressure upon the growing penitentiary population, and the risk of coronavirus infection (Abraham et al., 2020). However, the path followed by public safety policies was exactly the opposite, as the number of pretrial detainees has been rising since the beginning of the pandemic (CNJ, 2020), increasing the number of deaths due to COVID-19 inside prisons and jails.

Lastly, the suspension of services (such as legal assistance) and external visitors (such as family), widely adopted across Brazilian state prison systems, should be replaced by less deleterious measures for prison life. Among the ones suggested are routine screening of those entering the prison facility (Matos, 2020); testing new inmates (Sánchez et al., 2020); and making the provision of hand sanitizers and the use of masks mandatory for detainees, prison guards, staff, visitors, and suppliers (FGV, 2020). In certain state penitentiary systems not even the daily asepsis of prison cells has been adopted, making it difficult to prevent the spread of coronavirus within the overcrowded institutions (Souza, 2020).

At this juncture, we would also like to discuss the limitations of this paper. It uses data released from DEPEN (2019, 2020), whose validity and reliability have been criticized (Siqueira et al., 2020). Given the common challenges faced by Brazilian prison units, we can assume that these issues are somewhat consistent, allowing comparisons between the 27 state prison systems. It is also important to note the lack of reliable information regarding the cause of deaths inside the prison system. Part of the deaths registered in connection with COVID-19 could have had different causes (such as respiratory problems or cardiovascular problems) (Sánchez et al., 2020); whereas, deaths officially connected to respiratory complications could be coronavirus-related (Carvalho et al., 2020). Nonetheless, as visitation is no longer allowed in detention facilities, DEPEN (2020) is the only source of information about the numbers of COVID-19 cases and deaths.

Second, given the absence of COVID-19 information available at the prison unit level, we used data aggregated by state. We recognize that this is not the optimum scale of analysis, as Brazilian states display internal differences related to their prison units. Also, we suggest the collection of primary data from correctional facilities on the socio-economic profile of detainees with and without coronavirus. These data would improve our understanding of the factors behind COVID-19 cases and deaths in Brazilian prisons and jails, as well as the characteristics of affected detainees.

Finally, we also expect that COVID-19 presents an opportunity "to question the utility of mass incarceration and to explore decarceration and the decades-long tough-on-crime laws, harsh sentencing, and accelerated incarceration which brought about today's era of mass incarceration" (Abraham et al., 2020, p. 789).

Notes

1. Available at: http://depen.gov.br/DEPEN/depen/sisdepen/infopen/bases-de-dados/bases-de-dados, accessed on September 7th.
2. Available at https://www.gov.br/depen/pt-br/assuntos/acoes-contra-pandemia/covid-19-painel-de-monitoramento-dos-sistemas-prisionais, accessed on September 7th.
3. See Henderson and Denison (1989) and Thayer (2002) for further details.
4. In the database provided by the Ministry of Justice and Public Safety, the number of detainees, vacancies, and services made available by inmates in each of these five federal penitentiaries could be aggregated at the state level. Also, the measures adopted to prevent COVID-19 are the same enforced by each Brazilian state. As a result, the federal penitentiaries are not going to be analyzed as a separate "system", but as part of the state system on where they are built.
5. It is important to note that LEP made a distinction between jails (designed to house provisional inmates) and prisons (designed to house the sentenced inmates). However, on a daily basis this distinction does not apply and several provisional detainees are housed in prisons and vice-versa (Darke, 2013). The overcrowding that affects the Brazilian penitentiary system does not allow a proper distinction on the use of vacancies available (Dias, 2017).
6. According to Mariner and Cavallaro (1998, p. 29), the prison regime progression in Brazil can be described as follows: "first, the sentencing judge should consider the defendant's individual circumstances in imposing the sentence. Thus, for example, the question of whether a prisoner is a recidivist or a first-time offender is relevant in deciding whether he is sentenced to a closed prison, to an open facility, or to community service. Second, the judge of penal execution should continually monitor the prisoner's case while he is imprisoned, adjusting the terms of sentence according to the prisoner's conduct. Normally, a prisoner who begins his sentence in a closed prison should, after he has served part of his sentence, be transferred to a semi-open facility and from there, after further time has passed, to an open facility, and finally to release into society. In sum, this view of incarceration sees it as a dynamic process, not simply a fixed term of years." It means that a detainee sentenced to 30 years of imprisonment should be held in closed regime for 10 years, then transferred to a semi-open regime for 10 years and finally released in a system similar to parole. The laws approved in the last 30 years changed this system, making these detainees serve most of their sentences in closed regime.
7. They are not granted a progression to semi open regime or open regime, having to spend most of their sentences in maximum security prisons.
8. Under terrible detention conditions, inmates are more prone to engage in illicit activities hoping to achieve a better life not only for them but also for their families (Biondi, 2016; Feltran, 2012).

9. According to Feltran (2012), Dias and Salla (2013), Biondi (2016), Manso and Dias (2017), and Duarte and de Araújo (2020) among others, increasing the number of people behind bars, the prison's situation became worse in the country. As a result, the discourse of the PCC that criminals should be aligned and tied up in a network to fight against the state (always referred to as the system) became even more convincing. The expansion of this network was carried out with the policies implemented by the Brazilian authorities. Usually, after a rebellion, a PCC's leader would be transferred to a different Brazilian state to reduce its influence in the system. The side effect was exactly what the authorities were aiming to contain. Once inside a new detention center, the leaders would introduce the slogan of this organization, promising better living conditions for inmates and their families. For those interested in engaging it, the PCC leaders would baptize several inmates, making them part of this criminal organization. This is how PCC spread all over the country. In 2005, PCC was present in approximately 90% of prison units in the state of São Paulo, as well as in most urban areas with detention facilities (Biondi & Marques, 2010). By the end of 2016, PCC has entrenched in most Brazilian states, except for Mato Grosso, Rio Grande do Sul and Rio de Janeiro (Manso & Dias, 2017). However, it is worth highlighting that PCC does not control the majority of jails and prisons in the country (Duarte & de Araújo, 2020).
10. According to the rebellion database that the Federal University of Minas Gerais is constructing throughout the news about the relationship between COVID-19 and riots inside the Brazilian penitentiary system. The consultation to this database was carried out on August 4th, 2020.
11. Brazil does not have a risk assessment tool for prisoner release, being up to the judges to decide on this issue based on the time served by the detainee and the inmate previous behavior.

Disclosure statement

No potential conflict of interest was reported by the author(s).

Funding

This work was supported by the Conselho Nacional de Desenvolvimento Científico e Tecnológico.

ORCID

Ludmila Ribeiro http://orcid.org/0000-0003-4304-2254
Alexandre M. A. Diniz http://orcid.org/0000-0002-5649-7736

References

Abraham, L. A., Brown, T. C., & Thomas, S. A. (2020). How COVID-19's disruption of the US correctional system provides an opportunity for decarceration. *American Journal of Criminal Justice*, *45*(4), 780–792. https://doi.org/10.1007/s12103-020-09537-1

Adorno, S. (2008). Políticas públicas de segurança e justiça penal. *Cadernos Adenauer*, *9*(4), 9–27. https://doi.org/10.15448/1984-7289.2015.1.20481

Alcântara, R. L. D. S., Sousa, C. P. C., & Silva, T. S. M. (2018). Infopen women of 2014 and 2018: Challenges for research in psychology. *Psicologia: Ciencia E Profissao*, *38*(special issue 2), 88. https://doi.org/10.1590/1982-3703000212154

Akiyama, M. J., Spaulding, A. C., & Rich, J. D. (2020). Flattening the curve for incarcerated populations—Covid-19 in jails and prisons. New England Journal of Medicine, 382(22), 2075–2077.

Beato Filho, C. C., Silveira, A. M., Ribeiro, L. M. L., Rocha, R. L. S., & Souza, R. L. (2020). Percepções Sociais sobre o Sistema Prisional Brasileiro: Um estudo quantitativo. *Revista Brasileira De Execução Penal, 1*(1), 279–305. http://rbepdepen.depen.gov.br/index.php/RBEP/article/view/139

Biondi, K. (2016). *Sharing this walk: An ethnography of prison life and the PCC in Brazil.* UNC Press Books.

Biondi, K., & Marques, A. (2010). Memória e historicidade em dois" comandos" prisionais. *Lua Nova: Revista De Cultura E Política*, São Paulo, *79*, 39–70. https://doi.org/10.1590/S0102-64452010000100004

Campos, M. D. S. (2014). Crime e Congresso Nacional: Uma análise da política criminal aprovada de 1989 a 2006. *Revista Brasileira De Ciência Política, 29*(15), 315–347. https://doi.org/10.1590/0103-3352201415011

Campos, M. D. S., & Alvarez, M. C. (2017). Pela metade: Implicações do dispositivo médico-criminal da "nova" Lei de Drogas na cidade de São Paulo. *Tempo Social, 29*(2), 45–74. https://doi.org/10.11606/0103-2070.ts.2017.127567

Carvalho, J. A. M. (2016). O tamanho da população brasileira e sua distribuição etária: Uma visão prospectiva. *Anais Da ABEP*, (VI), 37–66. http://www.abep.org.br/publicacoes/index.php/anais/article/view/432

Carvalho, S. G., Santos, I. M., & Dos Santos, A. B. S. (2020). *The pandemic in prison: Interventions and overisolation.* Ciência e Saúde Coletiva, *25*(9), 3493–3502.https://doi.org/10.1590/1413-81232020259.15682020

Cifali, A. C., & de Azevedo, R. (2017). Public security, criminal policy and sentencing in Brazil during the Lula and Dilma Governments, 2003-2014: Changes and continuities. *International Journal for Crime, Justice and Social Democracy, 6*(1), 146. https://doi.org/10.5204/ijcjsd.v6i1.392

CNJ. (2020). *CNJ renova Recomendação nº 62 por mais 90 dias e divulga novos dados.* Retrieved August 2, 2020, from https://www.cnj.jus.br/cnj-renova-recomendacao-n-62-por-mais-90-dias-e-divulga-novos-dados/

Costa, J. S. D., Silva, J. C. F. D., Brandão, E. S. C., & Bicalho, P. P. G. (2020). COVID-19 in the Brazilian prison system: From indifference as a policy to a death policy. *Psicologia & Sociedade, 32*(e020013), 1–9. http://dx.doi.org/10.1590/1807-0310/2020v32240218

Cruz, M. V. G. D., Souza, L. G. D., & Batitucci, E. C. (2013). Percurso recente da política penitenciária no Brasil: O caso de São Paulo. *Revista De Administração Pública, 47*(5), 1307–1325. https://doi.org/10.1590/S0034-76122013000500011

Darke, S. (2013). Inmate governance in Brazilian Prisons. *The Howard Journal of Criminal Justice, 52* (3), 272–284. https://doi.org/10.1111/hojo.12010

Darke, S. (2014). Managing without guards in a Brazilian police lockup. *Focaal - Journal of Global and Historical Anthropology, 68*, 55–67. https://papers.ssrn.com/sol3/papers.cfm?abstract_id=2368781

Darke, S., & Garces, C. (2017). Surviving in the new mass carceral zone. *Prison Service Journal, 229*, 2–9. https://papers.ssrn.com/sol3/papers.cfm?abstract_id=2893022

de Azevedo, R. G. (2017). Reformas da justiça penal no Brasil–a democratização inacabada. *Acta Sociológica, 72*, 43–69. https://doi.org/10.1016/j.acso.2016.12.001

DEPEN (2019). *Statistical information system of the Brazilian penitentiary system.* Retrieved August 2, 2020, from http://depen.gov.br/DEPEN/depen/sisdepen/infopen

DEPEN (2020). *World penitentiary systems - panel for consultation.* Retrieved august 2, 2020, from http://depen.gov.br/DEPEN/COVID-19-painel-de-monitoramento-dos-sistemas-prisionais

Dias, C. N. (2017). *Encarceramento, seletividade e opressão: A "crise carcerária" como projeto político.* Friedrich-Ebert-Stiftung (FES).

Dias, C. N., & Salla, F. (2013). Organized crime in Brazilian prisons: The example of the PCC. *International Journal of Criminology and Sociology, 2*, 397–408. https://www.lifescienceglobal.com/pms/index.php/ijcs/article/view/1459

Dias, C. N., & Salla, F. (2019). Violência e negociação na construção da ordem nas prisões: A experiência paulista. *Sociedade E Estado, 34*(2), 539–564. https://doi.org/10.1590/s0102-6992-201934020008

Duarte, T. L., & de Araújo, I. C. A. (2020). PCC em pauta: Narrativas jornalísticas sobre a expansão do grupo pelo Brasil. *Dilemas-Revista De Estudos De Conflito E Controle Social, 13*(2), 505–532. https://doi.org/10.17648/dilemas.v13n2.23020

Feltran, G. (2012). Governo que produz crime, crime que produz governo: O dispositivo de gestão do homicídio em São Paulo (1992–2011). *Revista Brasileira De Segurança Pública, 6*,(2), 232–255. http://revista.forumseguranca.org.br/index.php/rbsp/article/view/118

FGV. (2020). *Pandemia de COVID-19 e os familiares de presos no estado de São Paulo*. Fundação Getulio Vargas. Retrieved August 2, 2020, from https://www.impacto.blog.br/sem-categoria/sete-em-cada-dez-familiares-nao-tem-noticias-de-parente-encarcerado-na-pandemia/

Franco-Paredes, C., Jankousky, K., Schultz, J., Bernfeld, J., Cullen, K., Quan, N. G., Krsak, M., Henao-Martínez, A. F., Krsak, M., & Kon, S. (2020). COVID-19 in jails and prisons: A neglected infection in a marginalized population. *PLoS Neglected Tropical Diseases, 14*(6), e0008409. https://doi.org/10.1371/journal.pntd.0008409

Gabbidon, S. L., Higgins, G. E., & Martin, F. (2011). Moving through the faculty ranks: An exploratory study on the perceived importance of book publishing and publishing in peer-reviewed journals in criminology/criminal justice. *Journal of Criminal Justice Education, 22*(2), 165–180. https://doi.org/10.1080/10511253.2010.517767

Gabriel, A. C. G., Pinheiro, D. H. P., Fernandes, L. M. S., Wind, M. M., Ferreira, V. R., & Silva, C. T. X. (2019). Caos: O atual cenário da saúde prisional no Brasil. *RESU – Revista Educação Em Saúde: V7*, (suplemento 1). http://periodicos.unievangelica.edu.br/index.php/educacaoemsaude/article/view/3811

Godoi, R. (2015). Communicating vessels, penitentiary flows: Between inside and outside of the prisons in São Paulo. *Vivência: Revista De Antropologia, 1*(46), 93–105. https://periodicos.ufrn.br/vivencia/article/view/8777

Godoi, R., Araújo, F., & Mallart, F. (2019). ESPACIALIZANDO A PRISÃO: A conformação dos parques penitenciários em São Paulo e no Rio de Janeiro. *Novos Estudos CEBRAP, 38*(3), 591–611. https://doi.org/10.25091/S01013300201900030003

Goffman, E. (1958). Characteristics of total institutions. In *Symposium on preventive and social psychiatry* (pp. 43–84). US Government Printing Office.

Grillo, C. C., Policarpo, F., & Verissimo, M. (2011). A" dura" e o" desenrolo": Efeitos práticos da nova lei de drogas no Rio de Janeiro. *Revista De Sociologia E Política, 19*(40), 135–148. https://doi.org/10.1590/S0104-44782011000300010

Henderson, D. A., & Denison, D. R. (1989). Stepwise regression in social and psychological research. *Psychological Reports, 64*(1), 251–257. https://doi.org/10.2466/pr0.1989.64.1.251

IBGE. (2020). *Tábuas Completas de Mortalidade*. Retrieved August 2, 2020, from https://www.ibge.gov.br/estatisticas/sociais/populacao/9126-tabuas-completas-de-mortalidade.html?=&t=notas-tecnicas

JHC. (2020). *COVID-19 dashboard by the center for systems science and engineering (CSSE) at Johns Hopkins University (JHU)*. Retrieved august 2, 2020, from https://coronavirus.jhu.edu/map.html

Lermen, H. S., Gil, B. L., Cúnico, S. D., & de Jesus, L. O. (2015). Health in prison: Analysis of health social policies targeting the Brazilian prison population. *Physis, 25*(3), 905. https://doi.org/10.1590/S0103-73312015000300012

Lima, R. S. D., Bueno, S., & Mingardi, G. (2016). Estado, polícias e segurança pública no Brasil. *Revista Direito GV, 12*(1), 49–85. https://doi.org/10.1590/2317-6172201603

Macaulay, F. (2002). *Political and institutional challenges of reforming the Brazilian prison system* (Working Paper CBS-31-02). University of Oxford Centre for Brazilian Studies.

Madeira, L. M., & Rodrigues, A. B. (2015). Novas bases para as políticas públicas de segurança no Brasil a partir das práticas do governo federal no período 2003-2011. *Revista De Administração Pública-RAP, 49*(1), 3–21. https://doi.org/10.1590/0034-76121702

Manso, B. P., & Dias, C. N. (2017). PCC, sistema prisional e gestão do novo mundo do crime no Brasil. *Revista Brasileira De Segurança Pública, 11*, 2. https://revista.forumseguranca.org.br/index.php/rbsp/article/view/854/259

Mariner, J., & Cavallaro, J. (1998). *Behind bars in Brazil*. Human Rights Watch, *11*(2), 10–29.

Matos, M. A. D. (2020). New Coronavirus (SARS-CoV-2): Advances to flatten the curve the prison population. *Revista Da Sociedade Brasileira De Medicina Tropical*, *53*(53), 1–2. https://doi.org/10.1590/0037-8682-0219-2020

Oliveira Andrade, R. (2020). COVID-19: Prisons exposed in Brazil's crisis. *bmj*, (370), 1–2. https://doi.org/10.1136/bmj.m2884

Oliveira Carmo, H., & Oliveira Araújo, C. L. (2011). População idosa no sistema penitenciário: Um olhar por trás das grades. *Revista Kairós: Gerontologia*, *14*(4), 183–194. https://doi.org/10.23925/2176-901X.2011v14i4p183-194

Ortega, F., & Orsini, M. (2020). Governing COVID-19 without government in Brazil: Ignorance, neoliberal authoritarianism, and the collapse of public health leadership. *Global Public Health*, *15*(9), 1257–1277. https://doi.org/10.1080/17441692.2020.1795223

Rangel, F. M., & Bicalho, P. P. G. D. (2016). Superlotação das prisões brasileiras: Operador político da racionalidade contemporânea. *Estudos De Psicologia (Natal)*, *21*(4), 415–423. http://dx.doi.org/10.5935/1678-4669.20160040.

Ratton, J. L. (1996). *Violência e crime no Brasil contemporâneo: Homicídios e políticas de segurança pública nas décadas de 1980 e 1990*. Editora Cidade.

Ribeiro, L. M. L., & Lopes, A. G. (2018). Public safety policy in the state of Minas Gerais (2003-2016): Agenda problems and path dependence. *International Journal of Criminology and Sociology*, *7*, 121–134. https://doi.org/10.6000/1929-4409.2018.07.08

Ricard, J., & Medeiros, J. (2020). *Using misinformation as a political weapon: COVID-19 and Bolsonaro in Brazil. The Harvard Kennedy School Misinformation Review*. https://misinforeview.hks.harvard.edu/article/using-misinformation-as-a-political-weapon-covid-19-and-bolsonaro-in-brazil/

Sánchez, A., Simas, L., Diuana, V., & Larouze, B. (2020). COVID-19 in prisons: An impossible challenge for public health? *Cadernos De Saúde Pública*, *36*(5), e00083520. https://doi.org/10.1590/0102-311x00083520

Silvestre, G. (2012). *Dias de visita: Uma sociologia da punição e das prisões*. Alameda Casa Editorial.

Silvestre, G. (2016). Local consequences of the prison policies in state of São Paulo, Brazil: A case study of the town of Itirapina. *Crime, Law and Social Change*, *65*(3), 269–285. https://doi.org/10.1007/s10611-015-9583-5

Sinhoretto, J. (2018). Violência, controle do crime e racismo no brasil contemporâneo. *Novos Olhares Sociais*, *1*(2), 4–20. https://www3.ufrb.edu.br/ojs/index.php/novosolharessociais/article/view/451

Siqueira, I., Biondi, K., & Godói, R. (2020). Los efectos del coronavirus en las cárceles de Latinoamérica – sección Brasil. https://criminologialatam.wordpress.com/2020/06/12/efectos-del-covid-19-carceles-de-latino-america/

Souza, C. D. F. D. (2020). Brazilian Justice response to protect the prison population from COVID-19. *Revista Da Associação Médica Brasileira*, *66*(5), 577–579. https://doi.org/10.1590/1806-9282.66.5.577

Steyerberg, E. W., Eijkemans, M. J., & Habbema, J. D. F. (1999). Stepwise selection in small data sets: A simulation study of bias in logistic regression analysis. *Journal of Clinical Epidemiology*, *52*(10), 935–942. https://doi.org/10.1016/S0895-4356(99)00103-1

Templeton, G. F. (2011). A two-step approach for transforming continuous variables to normal: Implications and recommendations for IS research. *Communications of the Association for Information Systems*, *28*, Article 4. https://aisel.aisnet.org/cais/vol28/iss1/4

Thayer, J. D. (2002). *Stepwise regression as an exploratory data analysis procedure*. A paper presented at the annual meeting of the American Educational Research AssociationNew Orleans, Louisiana, April 2, 2002. https://eric.ed.gov/?id=ED464932

Williams, B., Ahalt, C., Cloud, D., Augustine, D., Rorvig, L., & Sears, D. (2020). Correctional facilities in the shadow of COVID-19: Unique challenges and proposed solutions. *Health Aff*, (10). https://www.healthaffairs.org/do/10.1377/hblog20200324.784502/full/

World Prison (2020). *World prison brief data*. Retrieved august 2, 2020, from https://www.prisonstudies.org/world-prison-brief-data

Assessing the Effects of COVID-19 in Prisons in the Northern Triangle of Central America

Wayne J. Pitts and Christopher S. Inkpen

ABSTRACT

This article examines the impact of COVID-19 on penitentiary systems in the Central American countries of Honduras, El Salvador, and Guatemala (the Northern Triangle). Despite similar conditions in terms of crowding, lack of personal protective equipment, and infrastructure deficiencies, the neighboring countries have implemented distinctly different approaches to managing their incarcerated populations. In Honduras, in recognition of the elevated risks to certain inmates, nearly 2,000 prisoners were released in the early stages of the contagion. In El Salvador, President Bukele capitalized on the COVID crisis to implement curfews and national lockdowns to ensure conditions approaching martial law, declaring extreme security steps to address gang violence, while claiming incarcerated gang leaders were behind the increased violence. In Guatemala, the President Giammattei, a medical doctor, recognized prisons as epicenters of focus for reducing transmission rates and quickly advanced plans to contain a much larger outbreak. Using data collected from public media sources and in-depth qualitative interviews with prison administrators and staff, we provide a descriptive overview of the COVID impacts in these countries and consider possible longer-term prison policy implications.

Prison health is public health

The association between prison systems and the spread of communicable diseases is well documented (Braun et al., 1989; Valway et al., 1991; Young et al., 2004). Incarcerated populations have been found to have disproportionately high prevalence rates of diseases, including co-occurrences of HIV, hepatitis, and tuberculosis (Dolan et al., 2016; Gough et al., 2010; Kinner et al., 2020). Research on the spread of blood-borne diseases in incarcerated populations often links the risk of transmission in prison or jail to a greater public health crisis (Macher, Kibble, & Wheeler, 2006; Sacchi et al., 2015). However, given the challenges of over-crowding, inadequate healthcare resources, and often unhygienic conditions, the spread of the SARS-CoV-2 virus and the resulting COVID-19 illness through prison systems represents a unique global challenge.

The pandemic has spread from a regional concern in December of 2019 to a global concern impacting all facets of life. Since then, human-to-human transmission of the virus numerous countries and territories worldwide. On March 11, the World Health Organization (WHO) declared the global outbreak a pandemic (WHO, 2020). Virus-screening and quarantining measures are being implemented at airports worldwide, as well as extensive travel restrictions.

Although the impacts of COVID-19 on the health of the general population are still being discovered, prison administrators in the Northern Triangle have attempted to situate their response to the pandemic into their general mandate. For example, one prison administrator discussed their response to COVID-19 as it fits into the general role of prison administration, which is, "to ensure care, custody, and control of the people in our facility . . .."

Given the logistical difficulties in maintaining social distancing and proper hygiene in a confined population, the COVID-19 pandemic has presented heretofore unseen challenges to prison administrators in their balancing of theses priorities. While the first COVID-19 diagnosis in the U.S. involving a detained person was announced on March 16, 2020, the rest of the world had already responded to the outbreak within their confined populations. Iran, for example, temporarily released 70,000 prisoners serving sentences of less than 5 years to reduce in-custody transmission (Akiyama et al., 2020; Al Jazeera, 2020). During Italy's well-documented crisis, failure to calm incarcerated populations led to widespread rioting (Amante, 2020). In the United States, the Federal Bureau of Prisons suspended visitation by community members, limited visits by legal representatives, and reduced facility transfers for incarcerated persons to control the spread of the virus. However, state facilities and local jails implemented interventions at varying levels, which led to outbreaks in corrections facilities (CDC, 2020; Marshall Project, 2020). Countries worldwide rushed to implement mitigating strategies aimed at taming the outbreak within their confined populations.

As the entire world grapples with the effects of COVID-19, prisons, jails, and other detention facilities may not be the first among the concerns that the public considers. Yet, these institutions allow us to consider the management of the outbreak from a micro-societal viewpoint that could offer important mitigation strategies for other settings. Because prison populations often reflect the disparities in health affecting groups that are disproportionately likely to be incarcerated, the illustrate how the pandemic can have different impacts across socioeconomic and racial lines. Racial minorities, persons with substance abuse and/or mental health disorders, persons living in poverty are also more likely to have comorbid health concerns (e.g., diabetes, hypertension, heart diseases). Other illnesses such as tuberculosis and Hepatitis-C, which are more common amongst prisoners, exacerbate complications due to COVID-19 infections and are also significant comorbid factors. Some researchers have argued that "multimorbidity" is common among the prison population which may cause earlier onset of COVID-19 symptoms and result in a higher proportion of more severe cases when compared with general population (Dolan et al., 2016; Kinner & Young, 2018).

In prison settings, communicable diseases have the potential to be transmitted between prisoners, by staff and visitors, between prisons through transfers, and by staff cross-deployment to and from the community. COVID-19 outbreaks in custodial settings are especially important for public health because an outbreak could quickly overwhelm prison health-care services. Furthermore, prisons are a vector for community transmission that will disproportionately impact marginalized communities. In other words, in situations where COVID-19 has already overrun a facility, released prisoners and inmate visitors could impact the most vulnerable communities by carrying the infections back home. The concerns about secure facilities, especially jails and prisons, should be embedded within the broader public health response. Controlling communicable infections and other public health concerns such as COVID-19, HIV and Hepatitis C, in correctional settings can have positive effects both in these settings and on surrounding communities (Akiyama et al., 2020).

Many jurisdictions worldwide have chosen to "decarcerate," or release as many people as possible, specifically those individuals who pose low risks of new violent criminal activity. Additionally, some prisons and jails have also released inmates with the highest medical risk profiles for disease, based on age and other preconditions that may make certain individuals at higher risk of infection (ABA, 2020). Similarly, law enforcement authorities in many areas were given broader discretion to avoid arresting certain types of offender, opting for civil citations, rather than arrest whenever possible (Dewan et al., 2020). The courts too, suspended some hearings and allowed longer continuances during the outbreak, and some sentences were downgraded to less restrictive confinement to contain transmission (Gershman & Tau, 2020). These mitigation efforts will help control the spread of the disease, thereby stabilizing the impact of the virus, and reducing the burden on the correctional health-care system as well as the broader community response.

This article considers the response and impact of COVID-19 on penitentiary systems in the Central American countries of Honduras, El Salvador, and Guatemala (the Northern Triangle). Despite similar conditions in terms of crowding, lack of personal protective equipment, and infrastructure deficiencies at the beginning of the crisis, the neighboring countries have implemented distinct approaches to managing their incarcerated populations.

Research methods

Beginning in mid-March through mid-September, 2020 our team collected relevant articles with any mention of COVID-19 related to jails, prisons, staff, or inmates in the Northern Triangle. Data were obtained from the public domain using Boolean searches via general and academic online search engines. Search parameters included newspaper articles, credible blogs, other government and non-government publications, and TV news reports produced in English or Spanish. The review of source relevancy included multiple reader reviews and regular coder reviews to discuss the findings with in-country colleagues, which helped to assess whether the contextual detail identified through these sources was consistent with observations on the ground.

In addition to the scan of local media, as the COVID-19 crisis continued, we developed two separate structured interview guides for prison administrators and prison line staff. Being sensitive to competing demands resulting from the pandemic, we recruited administrators and prison staff based on availability, starting with established contacts that were identified from ongoing investigations. Our recruitment strategy emphasized prison administrators, given that interviews with prison staff were often logistically infeasible due to workloads, availability, and difficulty in obtaining contact information. The research team collected a total of seven interviews with prison administrators, two in Honduras, two in Guatemala, and three in El Salvador. We also adapted the administrator instrument and interviewed an administrator from a non-governmental agency that works closely with the prison system in Guatemala. These interviews were conducted by cellphone and length and breadth varied considerably. At least two interviews lasted an hour or longer, while another was fewer than 10 min in duration. To confirm interview details, the research team also corresponded with interviewees and other relevant prison officials via e-mail including correspondence with law enforcement authorities, U.S. Embassy representatives, and other relevant actors in the region.

Pre-COVID overview of crime and incarceration in the Northern Triangle

The countries of the Northern Triangle are regularly introduced as being among the most violent in the world, with homicide rates well above global averages during the past 10 years.[1] In recent years however, intentional homicide rates in the three countries have been trending downward. See Figure 1.

These reductions in homicide rates are often attributed to improvements in policing investigations and more effective prosecution strategies which have resulted in a steadily increasing prison population rate (Byrne et al., 2015). See Figure 2.

Despite the continuous increase in incarceration rates, significant crime problems continue to plague all three countries. Data collected by the Latin American Public Opinion Project in each country over the past few years persistently show that the chief concerns for most citizens are the lack of economic opportunities and security matters (Raderstorf et al., 2017).

El Salvador

Despite its small land mass, El Salvador is one of the most densely populated countries in Central America (Central Intelligence Agency, 2020). President Nayib Bukele, former mayor of San Salvador, assumed office on June 1, 2019 and has achieved widespread

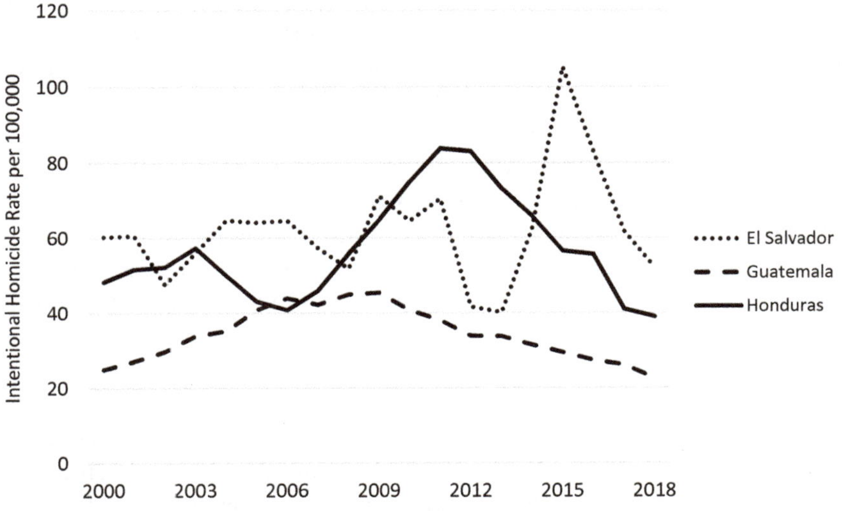

Figure 1. Annual homicide rates in the Northern Triangle, 2000–2018.

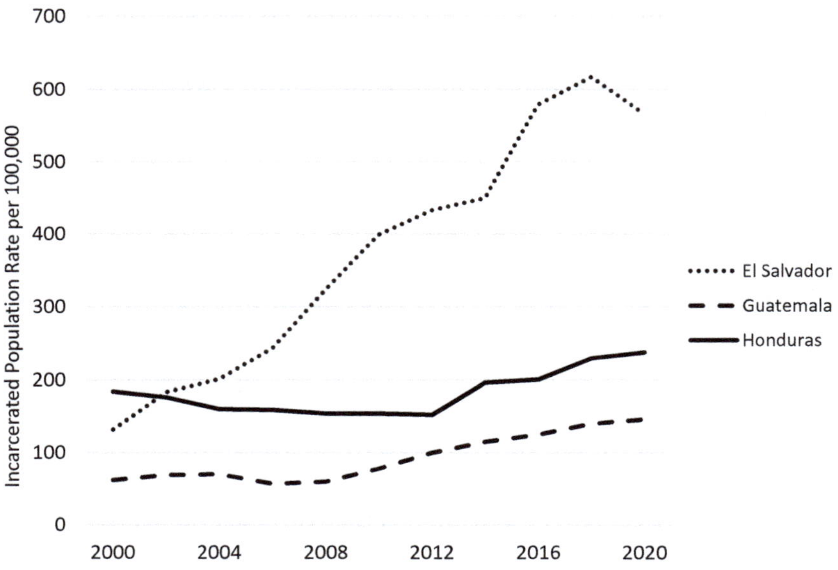

Figure 2. Annual Prison Population Rate in the Northern Triangle, 2000–2020*. *Prison rates presented for 2020 requires additional explanation. Data for all three countries are based on population estimates from the United Nations. El Salvador rate is calculated using August2020 population estimates of 6.48million. Guatemala data is from June2020 population estimate of 17.88million. Honduras rate is calculated using aSeptember2019 population estimate of 9.11million.

popularity for his active, and often strong-handed opposition to organized crime and gangs. Though generally favored by the American administration, President Bukele has shown a disquieting tendency to skirt democratic principles, including sending the military to take over the National Assembly on February 9, 2020, which led to public rebukes from the U.S government and international observers (The Washington Post, 2020). In a recent move that received considerable attention by U.S. lawmakers, Bukele enacted several modifications to the regulation of country's freedom of information act (*Ley de Access de la Información Pública – LAIP*) that essentially make it more difficult to obtain public information from government institutions (Urquilla & Escalante, 2020).

Six months after closing March 18 due to the coronavirus disease (COVID-19) pandemic, the El Salvador International Airport reopened on September 19. During the closure, the airport has only been operating cargo, repatriation, and other special flights. President Bukele announced that the second phase of economic reopening in El Salvador would be postponed as experts' assessments identified a continued rise in the number of confirmed COVID-19 cases. In El Salvador, the second phase reportedly allows public transportation, business services, manufacturers, and several industries and restaurants to resume operations, the third phase allowing for greater loosening of restrictions contingent on persistent decreases in reported cases. The Salvadoran government began the gradual process of reopening the economy on June 16 with the easing of some movement and business restrictions and the lifting of a 24/7 nationwide curfew. Certain business operations resumed, though businesses are still urged to allow employees to work from home if possible, and those which have resumed will be at a limited capacity. These industries included construction, textile, and electronic manufacturing business, cargo transport, medical and veterinary services for emergencies and appointments, restaurants and retail stores for delivery and take away services, government offices, and repair and maintenance services. Essential services such as supermarkets, pharmacies, banks, petrol stations, and home delivery food outlets, can continue to operate. Private transport can resume for employees returning to work. Taxis and ride-sharing services have also resumed operations. Individuals are required to wear face masks when leaving their residences. Schools, universities, and parks remain closed.

There are 24 prisons in El Salvador with a total inmate population that hovers just under 40,000 persons, approximately double the original design capacity.[2] Salvadoran prison authorities have provided regular updates regarding the number of confirmed and suspected cases of COVID-19 throughout the crisis, though reported counts have not been independently verified, and the availability and application of testing has been inconsistent. For example, the Ministry of Health offers snap shots of the situation that are seemingly in conflict with prison administrators' reports. On March 29, the government reported 108 confirmed COVID cases among inmates, adding that an additional 945 were suspected of having the virus. However, in the same report, one facility (*La Esperanza*) reported that 85 persons were screened and 34 were determined to be positive. The *La Esperanza* example leads to two observations: (1) the high rate of positive tests and (2) the limited number of actual tests. The highest numbers of suspected cases on March 29 were in San Vicente (297), Quetzaltepeque (135) and 58 in the psychiatric hospital of the prison system. Prison administrators pointed to prison custodial and administrative staff as leading to the spread of the disease in the prison system, as they rotate in and out of the facilities between shift changes. For example, in some facilities a prison doctor had been identified as the potential source of a COVID-19 outbreak within prisons (J. López, 2020). To highlight the logistic limitations of prisons in the country, one administrator indicated that lack of space required some inmates with confirmed cases of COVID-19 to be housed in the same areas as other inmates, increasing the likelihood of infection spread.

As of September 20, 2020, the government of El Salvador has reported 27,553 confirmed cases of COVID-19 with 812 deaths attributed to the virus (Worldometer.info, 2020). The Bukele administration's response to the COVID-19 crisis has received both acclaim and concern. On the one-hand, it was President Bukele who attracted worldwide attention when he announced very early stimulus incentives to undergird the Salvadoran economy when he suspended payments for basic services including water, electricity, and internet for 3 months in March 2020. Also, the administration recognized the urgency of addressing the COVID-19 crisis in jails and prisons very early in the outbreak, and on March 10, he ordered prison authorities to renew focus on "sanitary protocols to prevent Coronavirus in the prison population," (Human Rights Watch, 2020). However, a month later, in the midst of an extreme bout of violence with 77 homicides occurring between April 24–27, President Bukele announced that undisclosed intelligence sources had revealed that these murders had been ordered by incarcerated gang members operating from within the country's jails and prisons. The Bukele administration then took an aggressive stance against suspected gang members, issuing an open call to law enforcement to round up suspected gang members and place them in crowded and unsanitary conditions in the nation's jails and prisons. A statement released by Human Rights Watch (2020) reported,

> *In the face of the Covid-19 pandemic, prisons in El Salvador, as in other places, are a potential epicenter of an outbreak. This risk has been exacerbated by the new containment measures ordered by the Bukele government. Paradoxically, the heavy-handed speech that President Bukele uses in the face of the 77 murders of the last days, puts many more lives at risk for possible contagion, both inside and outside the detention centers.*

In photographs and videos released by the government during the weekend of April 25 and 26, thousands of detainees are seen often unclothed and left handcuffed on the floor inside the jails while the police searched their cells. Very few of the prisoners had masks and their positioning on the ground inhibited any social distancing measures. Reports from the media failed to highlight the importance of following public health guidelines inside prisons to prevent the spread of COVID-19 in the wider population.[3] Acting on suggestions that gang members were organizing murders on the outside, Bukele ordered severe restrictions, with some suspected gang members confined to their cells, often in total darkness and in extreme isolation in an attempt to control the use of hand signals and other types of inmate communication (BBC, 2020; Bukele, 2020). These aggressive measures taken by President Bukele are not new. This punitive response and "*mano dura*" (tough on crime) policies have been in place for decades in the country. They have proven to be an ineffective strategy to deal with gangs in and outside the prison as well as to reduce criminality in the country (Dudley, 2010).

Nationally, President Bukele issued the first, and most restrictive quarantine in Central America, even before there was a positive case of COVID-19 in the country. Many observers have openly questioned whether these his motivations were truly rooted in concerns about public health or if measures such as travel restrictions and curfews, nearing martial law in some instances, were intended to intensify the war on gangs and reduce criminal activities and homicide. Despite these seemingly strict measures, there is evidence to suggest that some of the practices implemented during the heavy-handed prison lockdown measures, such as housing members of competing gangs in common areas, may have been intentional efforts to fuel inter-gang conflicts (Council on Hemispheric Affairs, 2020).

Guatemala

President Giammattei, who assumed office on January 14, 2020, is both a medical doctor and the former director of the Guatemalan penitentiary system from 2006 to 2008 (Economist, 2020), designations which provide both an understanding of the threat of coronaviruses and the specific contexts and working conditions of prisons in Guatemala. Perhaps it is not surprising that he has been especially active, issuing regular press conferences and detailed policies and procedures regarding the pandemic, including prisons. On March 15, only 2 days after Guatemala confirmed its first positive case, the President suspended all family face-to-face visits with prisoners (Pitán, 2020). A day later, all visits from court authorities to prison were also suspended, following a suspected COVID-19 case was reported in Preventative Center in Zone 18, Guatemala City (though this suspected case was in fact negative).

The Guatemalan government declared a "state of calamity" to expand measures aimed at protecting the health and safety of all persons in Guatemala. Like a "state of emergency" in the United States, declaring a state of calamity allows the Guatemalan government to take exceptional measures to protect national security. The Giammattei administration implemented several restrictions to curb the spread of the COVID-19 pandemic, limiting travel to and from Guatemala on March 5 and suspending commercial flights less than two weeks later. A nationwide weekday and weekend nightly curfew remain in place as of July 2020, restricting all non-essential movement, with violations resulting in a fine or imprisonment. Outside of curfew hours, social distancing and mask-wearing are mandatory, with violations resulting in substantial fines. Nationwide travel restrictions remain in place and all land, sea, and air borders remain closed. Supermarkets, grocers, other markets, and other essential businesses are permitted to operate from 06:00 to 16:00. However, most public and private sectors are suspended, and shopping centers remain closed. The Giammattei administration also prohibited the consumption of alcohol in public areas, and the sale and purchase of alcohol is only allowed during limited hours. In light of the outbreak, public or religious gatherings have been banned and in-person schooling has been suspended. The Aurora International Airport in Guatemala City reopened on September 18, though curfews, some travel restrictions, social distancing, and mandatory mask use continue to be enforced. As of September 20, there are 85,444 confirmed cases of COVID-19 in Guatemala and 3,119 associated fatalities (Worldometer.info, 2020).

The Guatemala prison system is marked by persistent challenges and international efforts to support improvements have been hampered by government bureaucracy, weak political will, and limited budgets. One person interviewed for context on the Guatemalan prison system characterized it this way:

> *Due to corruption, there is considerable disorder in terms of infrastructure. The installations and general living conditions are unacceptable and, while crowding is over 300% capacity, there is apparently no intention to address the problems. In theory, there are documents to implement prison reform, but nothing has happened and there is no operational plan. This is an institution that must start over every day, addressing the same issues … we have to improvise a lot.*
>
> *The Guatemalan penitentiary system is an institution known for its functional deficiencies, especially in terms of the lack of training for prison personnel. There is no professional career track or institutional hierarchy like there is for the national police. Here correctional officers only receive three months of initial training. Technical staff and administrators learn on the job without any further training. Senior administrators rarely last more than a year before they are replaced.*

Upon this backdrop, the penitentiary system is working to control the spread of COVID-19 within its 21 prisons with roughly 15 outpatient physicians[4] serving just over 26,000 persons in custody, despite only being equipped originally to house approximately 6,800 inmates.

Over capacity since 1996, social distancing in prisons is near impossible and unsanitary conditions and access to healthcare are perpetual concerns (K. López, 2020). Concerned about the virus and lack of protective equipment, in some prisons such as *Pavoncito*, located in Fraijanes, inmates began to make cloth masks for their own use, manufacturing at least 3000 masks in the last two weeks of March. A spokesperson for the prison system was reported as saying, "[Inmates] are doing their best to take care of themselves because they are aware of how bad it would be if the virus is found in some prison," (K. López, 2020). A Guatemalan administrator interviewed in early September, confirmed this point sharing that adolescents in juvenile detention as well as male inmates imprisoned in *El Preventivo* in Zona 18 continue to sew masks for donations to community hospitals. Yet while prisoner labor is used to manufacture donated masks, prison administrators discuss shortages of masks and indicate that prisons continues to purchase masks for internal use, but also saying that procurement processes are not transparent.

According to media accounts, prison inmates were generally accepting of the restrictions set by the government early in the crisis, but some soon began to advocate for early-release, additional preventative measures, and expanded videoconferences capabilities for visitors. The government promised to consider using existing videoconferencing equipment available through the National Court System,[5,6] to allow inmates to visit with family and friends, if the visitation restrictions continued for longer than 1 month. However, by mid-August, all visitations continues to be suspended and the video-conferencing equipment is not available for use by prisoners, in large part due to logistical and procedural concerns, according to interviews with a current prison administrator and another professional who works closely with the administrative office of the courts.

On March 28, Guatemala's Attorney General for Human Rights filed a legal complaint before the Supreme Court of Justice against the Guatemalan Ministry of the Interior, the Ministry of Public Health, and the General Directorate of the Penitentiary System. The lawsuit argued that the government was not doing enough to guarantee prisoners access to hygiene products and medical care and that protocols to prevent the spread of the coronavirus in prisons were insufficient. A month later, the Commission for Citizen Protection, a recurring congressional subcommittee, provided recommendations to lawmakers on how to decongest the prisons to help avoid the spread of the coronavirus, which included alternatives to incarceration for pregnant women, terminally ill inmates, and persons over 60 years old. These measures would immediately impact about 2,000 of the most vulnerable incarcerated persons, though to date no specific reforms to the penal code have been instituted (González, 2020).

On May 28, the first prisoner testing positive for COVID-19 in Guatemala died. The inmate, who had been housed in the Male Prison in Zone 18 in the Guatemalan capital, had been interned in the prison infirmary for nearly a month before being transferred to a community hospital, where he died 4 days later. Tests administered after the patient had been transferred outside of the facility revealed the presence of the SARS-CoV-2 virus, and soon the Attorney General for Human Rights began to publicly speak out about the lack of testing available for inmates and prison employees along with delays in obtaining results (Chumil, 2020a; Cuevas, 2020). By early June, three prisons in Guatemala had further substantiated cases of coronavirus and definitive steps were underway to create a separate isolation unit with a capacity for housing nearly 500 inmates at the prison facility known as *Fraijanes* II. By June 24, the number of inmate fatalities increased to eight and 91 prisoners, out of 103 known cases systemwide, were housed and treated for confirmed COVID-19 infections at *Fraijanes II* (Álvarez, 2020). Fourteen correctional officers, five administrative workers, and three nurses had also tested positive.

By the end of July, more than 200 positive cases of COVID-19 infections have been confirmed with just over 20 inmates deceased within the prison system (Prensa Latina, 2020). Approximately half of all positive cases are found in the Male Preventative Prison in Zone 18 in Guatemala City and the second largest number of cases are in the Pavón Penal Farm in Fraijanes. In the same period, 1,000 fatalities were attributed to COVID-19, as the government continues to manage increasing concerns of viral spread. On August 7, 12 corrections officers in the same prison in Mazatenango tested positive for COVID-19. With no long-term isolation location available to house the infected guards, representatives from the national health system initially advised the patients to go home. The Ministry of Health followed-up with a thorough cleaning of the facility. The guards were ultimately housed in hotel rooms, paid by the government, where the correctional officers could avoid infecting their families or others in the community (Soto, 2020). However, according to an interview conducted with a high-level prison administrator conducted in early September, the actual number of positive infections among prisoners and guards is likely higher. The administrator shared,

> *the Ministry of Health no longer wants to assume responsibility for testing because of how long it takes to obtain results. For example, if they do a swab today, it will likely take 30 days to get the results. By that time, the person will either be fully recovered, in the hospital, or already dead. The only thing we can do is put suspected cases in quarantine.*

Now several months into the COVID crisis, Guatemala's resources, especially in the penitentiary system are stretched thin. In an August interview, a prison administrator shared that the daily operations are increasingly difficult to sustain. With family visits suspended, prisoners are no longer receiving care packages. Food costs are increasing daily. The administrator reported,

> *there are beans served for every meal, with maybe some eggs or a piece of sausage. Chicken is rare and the prisons are no longer able to provide beef or pork. It's a serious situation and it is getting worse.*

Perhaps more concerning is the fact that some prison staff have grown weary of the safety precautions and cultural differences that may affect compliance. According to a current administrator, "we have made site visits to some of the departments [areas outside of the capital] and of course, the people there are not wearing masks – that's how they live there. They have different coexistence rules that are difficult to understand for those who don't live there."

The recommendations submitted to Congress by the President's Commission for Citizen Protection in April resulted in a list of 520 inmates who had been screened and determined eligible for early release from prison based on their criminal profile, age, medical conditions, and conduct reports while in custody. Of these, 140 were approved for early release and the applications for the remaining 380 persons under consideration were still being processed (Chumil, 2020b). At least six bills were being considered by Congress in July to further reduce prison crowding including a new mediation law, revisions to criminal procedure laws, steps to improve electronic notification, a "minor quantities" law, opportunities to expand video hearings, among others (Chumil, 2020b). Thus, despite dealing with similar conditions to El Salvador, Guatemala's response included decarceral measures along with public attempts to mitigate the side effects of isolation for prisoners.

Honduras

On December 26, 2019, before COVID-19 commanded global attention, the Honduran branch of the Office of the United Nations High Commissioner for Human Rights (OHCHR) and the Inter-American Commission on Human Rights (IACHR) declared a State of Penitentiary Emergency in Honduras. The declaration followed extreme violence in three adult prisons and one juvenile facility in the month of December that led to more than 40 deaths, including four adolescents, and multiple serious injuries (Organization of American States, 2019). The OHCHR/IACHR declaration called for the demilitarization of the penitentiary system and renewed focus on ensuring human rights. Simultaneously, an executive decree on December 16 by two-term President Juan Orlando Hernandez announced a state of emergency in the National Prison System, which is a measure of volatility and internal capacity to ensure rule of law. Both conditions had been exacerbated by an overwhelmed penitentiary system comprised 25 facilities holding more than 22,000 persons in custody. A day later, the entire Honduran Penitentiary System was placed under the control of the military Armed Forces in coordination with the Inter-institutional Security Force.[7] Notably, the IACHR report indicated that, " ... overcrowding, lack of hygiene, and inadequate ventilation constitute a serious threat to the health of detainees. This ... (is), due to the increased risk of contagion of infectious diseases, such as tuberculosis" (IACHR, 2019, p. 149). Thus, conditions prior to the COVID-19 outbreak were already dangerously susceptible to the spread of disease.

In response to the ongoing COVID-19 pandemic, Honduran authorities have extended the nationwide daily curfew and stay-at-home order through August 2020, which limits movement at night and during the day, strictly detailing the requirements of essential activities. Although land and sea borders remain closed generally, open only for the transport of cargo goods and supplies, airports have opened at limited capacity as of mid-August 2020, though curfews and mandatory mask usage has now been extended at least through September 20. As of September 20, there have been 71,616 confirmed cases of COVID-19 in Honduras, and 2,184 associated fatalities (Worldometer.info, 2020).

The specific details of the impact of COVID-19 in prisons in Honduras have been far more challenging to ascertain due to a lack of government transparency. The first prisoner identified as COVID-19 positive in Honduras died on April 23. The details of the conditions of any interventions that may have been performed were not made public, and reports question the official timing of testing for COVID-19 (Ávila, 2020). The maximum-security prison, *El Pozo*, where this inmate was housed prior to his death, limited information regarding the situation. A month later, a second positive case was reported in the national prison in the *Tamara* prison, just outside of Tegucigalpa, and similarly limited the release of information about diagnostic testing, steps toward prevention, and intervention capacity.

In the early weeks of the COVID-19 crisis in Honduras the government made a concerted effort to explore opportunities to reduce crowding in prisons, especially among high-risk inmates. Interviews with prison administrators indicate that a list of high medical risk and elderly prisoners was created in May that included 2,424 names. An additional 1,240 inmates were identified whose preliminary period of preventative detention had expired and these prisoners were scheduled for release. On June 16, the Penitentiary system released 1,624 prisoners as part of the measures being implemented to prevent the spread of the coronavirus (Agencia EFE, 2020). Table 1 provides a summary of several indicators collected between April 23 and August 10 related to COVID-19. The number of tests conducted is not shown and thus a positivity rate cannot be calculated.

Interviews with Honduran National Prison administrators revealed that Honduran prisons are outdated and especially crowded and that the conditions are far from ideal, especially in terms of internal security processes and preparing inmates for reinsertion into the community. Essentially, rather than classifying inmates by risk level, they are instead

Table 1. Select indicators for COVID-19 in the Honduras Penitentiary System.

COVID-19 Statistics – Honduran Prison System[a]	
Positive PCR (swab) tests administered	1,121
Positive PCR tests (prisoners)	930
Positive PCR tests (operational and administrative staff)	161
Positive PCR tests (Healthcare workers)	30
Patients tested positive, presumed recovered	570
Suspected COVID cases in isolation	929
Substantiated and suspected COVID-19 deaths	33
Other deaths (not COVID related)	13
General hospitalizations	24
Hospitalizations due to COVID-19	5

[a]Source: Data provided by the Honduran Penitentiary System, April 23 to August 10, 2020.

housed by suspected gang-affiliation. Three large maximum-security prisons are set aside for *MS-13* and *Barrio-18* gang members and especially high-risk inmates, while the other facilities house individuals from other criminal organizations and other lower risk detainees. According administrators, the COVID-19 crisis has highlighted the fact that certain lower risk and special categories of inmates (i.e., pregnant women, women with children, elderly, and chronically ill persons), should be prioritized for early release. However, corrections professionals explained, "... we are only responsible to protect prisoners during their stay, the courts decide who gets in and gets out."

New intakes to corrections facilities are especially challenging since many prisoners are coming "straight off of the streets," officials shared, suggesting that, " ... we must assume these individuals have likely been exposed." Therefore, after a "rapid test" for the disease, these individuals are held in isolation, which may vary from 15 to 21 days, to determine if they have symptoms of the disease. Interviews with administrators suggest that this practice will likely be one of the permanent procedures that continues after this current crisis subsides. As a result of the pandemic, staff leave is restricted, and staff are only allowed to return home once a month. Upon their return, they also must submit to a screening and have a period of restricted duty before having contact with inmates or other staff. Honduran prison administrators lauded the prison healthcare system and the contributions of the International Red Cross saying that the strict isolation practices have been the key to controlling a much larger outbreak and can be attributed as a cause of a steady decrease in cases. Interviews with prison administrators instead suggest that while early attention on prisons suggested they might be a source of COVID-19 spread; attention is placed instead now on the unconfined population.

Yet in interviews, prison officials voiced concerns about the continued availability of personal protective equipment and other supplies, saying, "remember, this equipment is essentially disposable and must be constantly replaced, and we are using a lot! I would say that we are going to run out of hand gel, biosafety suits, medical supplies, tests, all the other biosafety equipment like masks and stuff ... " Interviews suggest that while staff have access to basic equipment, they are regularly forced to reuse disposable equipment. One official laments, " ... we are not a wealthy country. We do not have a bonanza of resources like other countries. Essentially, we depend on whatever the government can send us." In response to questions on logistics of purchase orders, one official noted, "The government is practically closed, and the economy is stagnant, there is no movement of capital. Each

Table 2. Shifts in routine prison activities due to COVID-19.

Routine prison activities	El Salvador	Guatemala	Honduras
Public reception services	↓	↓	↑
Prisoner communications (mail, telephone)	Ξ	↑	↑
Inmate injuries	↓	↓	↓
Prisoner work details	↓	↓	Ξ
Family visits	↓	↓	↓
Inmate transfers to other facilities	↓	↓	↓
Inmate housing transfers within the facility	↑	↑	Ξ
Prisoner access to showers	Ξ	Ξ	Ξ
Negative incident reports	Ξ	Ξ	Ξ
Sports/recreation time	Ξ	Ξ	Ξ
Social worker meetings	↓	↓	↓
Health clinic checkups	↓	↓	↑
Substance use programming	↓	Ξ	↓
In-person court appearances	↓	↓	↓
Injuries to staff	↓	Ξ	↓
Ability of inmates to file grievances	↓	Ξ	Ξ
Education/training activities	↓	↓	↓
Prisoner access to public spaces (dining)	Ξ	Ξ	↓
Intakes into the facility	Ξ	Ξ	↓
Discharges into the community	↓	↓	↑

Source: Interviews with national-level prison administrators
Key: Increased (↑), Decreased (↓), Remained the same (Ξ).

time we need to submit a purchase order; it gets more difficult to fulfill." He then added, "look, this pandemic affects us all, the inmates, the staff, the community. We face a greater risk of dying and we are all stressed out!"

As part of the interview, we asked the administrator to share how twenty specific activities, ordinarily associated with life on the inside, had been affected during the pandemic. Familiar with the entire Honduran prison system, his answers, as seen in Table 2, detail the logistical changes in prison activities in response to the COVID-19 pandemic.

Discussion

Prisons in the Northern Triangle suffer from several decades of humanitarian crisis, exacerbated by state abandonment, and a lack of financial and human resources. While intensive efforts to strengthen policing and prosecution efforts are increasing arrests and steadily elevating incarceration rates, the corrections system remains neglected, overcrowded, poorly staffed, and sorely mismanaged. The harshest critics argue prisons systems in the Northern Triangle are governed by a symbiotic balance of corrupt government officials and imprisoned organized crime interests. The result of these practices impedes efforts to improve security and strengthen democratic practices in the region. The government responses to COVID-19 further underscores these persistent issues and highlights the ongoing vulnerabilities to organized crime, politicians with right-leaning tendencies, and weak rule of law in these countries.

In 2017, Insight Crime, an important foundation dedicated to studying organized crime in Latin America, referred to prisons in the Northern Triangle as "powerful incubators for organized crime groups" (Dudley & Bargent, 2017). Their analysis accurately asserts that organized crime and gangs in these prisons thrive for a variety of reasons. Inadequate classification systems focus on gang affiliation as the most heavily weighted factor to determine placement in already overcrowded facilities. With few housing options, gang members are concentrated in common areas which strengthen recruitment strategies and promote even deeper integration of affiliates. Segregation and quarantining strategies to control the spread of COVID-19 have intensified this housing dilemma. Similarly, COVID-19 responses have exacerbated the strains felt by an underpaid, poorly trained prison staff who now face longer hours and added duties, reduced opportunities to visit with family, and increased occupational stress. These conditions are conducive to increased susceptibility to staff corruption. The already insufficient prison programming such as social worker case management activities, substance abuse interventions, educational and vocational training that existed before COVID-19, has largely been suspended, further increasing the available time, physical proximity, and lack of supervision that organized crime thrives on inside these prisons. Data tracking systems, notoriously weak and often unable to provide even basic daily headcounts of inmate populations, have further deteriorated during the current crises due to reduced staffing, fewer rotations and manned supervision stations, and less prison programming. Prisons are currently "suspended in time" due to COVID-19, as governments are distracted by other priorities. Finally, while the functions of prison gangs vary, COVID-19 has presented new deprivations, stemming mostly from reduced personal supplies normally delivered through family visitations, but also by increased demands for personal protection equipment. Criminal enterprises on the inside, fueled by corruption and fanned by government indifference and incompetence, are adjusting to meet these basic needs of prisoners in the short term.

Our worldwide experience in responding to natural disasters, humanitarian crises, and other pandemics should inform our current responses. While the worldwide epidemiological details of COVID-19 continue to emerge, global policymakers and prison administrators are now forced to deal with both the long-term impacts of the outbreak and the likelihood of the annual presence of the SARS-CoV-2 virus. Moreover, the lessons observed in this current crisis and the responses in prisons in Central America and around the world can provide important lessons to aid in better preparation for future pandemics. As evidenced by the current situation, pandemic preparedness is essential, and it is incumbent now to revisit and update prison policies and procedures.[8] These plans should include strategies on how to limit introduction, control spread once it is already in circulation, and treat patients once they are infected. Additionally, administrators must prepare for identifying correctional staff and vendors on an ongoing basis to isolate and separate them from spreading the virus internally. Prisons equipped with video-conferencing capability can alleviate some of the social isolation experienced by some prisoners through video visitations. This same technology is often used for prisoner meetings with attorneys and even electronic court hearings.

The longer-range effects of COVID-19 for prisons are more challenging to untangle. Pending prison reforms in all three countries could be deprioritized and possibly derailed altogether, as autocratic leaders seek to use this opening to strengthen harsh responses to crime and criminals and reduce transparency. On the other hand, this crisis may help draw attention to the security vulnerabilities and the ongoing erosion of rule of law that is occurring within this important branch of the criminal justice system. The overarching economic impact of the pandemic, while not yet fully projected, is likely to be detrimental to the woefully inadequate tax base and corresponding budgets that would be required to implement the remodeling and new construction required to address prison crowding in the Northern Triangle. Similarly, it seems unlikely that prison reform, including hiring more qualified and vetted prison staff, better training, improved human resource practices, upgraded classification, implementation of prison management best practices, etc., will be prioritized by governments seeking to retore normalcy once this crisis subsides.

The COVID-19 pandemic has illustrated the challenging conditions under which many prisons normally operate, highlighting the inadequate preparation required to curtail a spreading disease, and the logistical limitations associated with a lack of funding and overcrowding. As evidenced in this report, the Northern Triangle countries of El Salvador, Guatemala, and Honduras face similar conditions that limit their ability to respond to the health crisis. El Salvador, initially viewed as a regional bellwether in taking a strict response to limit the spread of the virus, has not extended these preventative measures to prisons, instead prioritizing limiting gang violence thought to originate from the prison system. In comparison, Guatemala has begun processes to decarcerate prisoners who pose a low risk to public safety but present a high risk for infection and fatality due to COVID-19. The Honduran prison systems face similar challenges, including substantial gang-related prison violence, but limited transparency has made the official Honduran response opaque. Despite facing similar challenges to the national prison systems and dealing with the influence of prison-based gangs, this report suggests that the Northern Triangle countries have responded quite differently. Further reporting along with verified accounts of testing, treatment, and mortality rates will be required to assess the full extent of the impact of the COVID-19 on the prison systems in the Northern Triangle.

Notes

1. See the UNODC 2019 Global Study on Homicide for a comprehensive exploration of this complex phenomenon and an updated dataset of cross-national data. Available at https://www.unodc.org/unodc/en/data-and-analysis/global-study-on-homicide.html [Accessed on 18 September 2020].
2. Details on the number of facilities, inmate population, and the distribution by status fluctuate frequently. Updated monthly, the University of London, Institute for Crime & Justice Policy Research maintains the World Prison Brief (2020) database. See http://www.prisonstudies.org/world-prison-brief.
3. On April 29, The BBC World News released shocking images of some of the especially harsh treatment of prisoners in El Salvador. See https://www.youtube.com/watch?v=nqcPD2pmxJw.
4. Sources regarding the number of physicians are conflicting and range between 13–16 individuals. Based on personal conversations, the discrepancy seems to be rooted in whether some physicians are currently available to treat patients. Five prison doctors are reportedly in high-risk categories, presumably because of their ages and/or preexisting medical conditions.
5. Known in Spanish as the *Organismo Judicial (OJ)*. This video conferencing equipment was donated to Guatemala through the Security and Justice Program, coordinated by the United States Agency for International Development (USAID and the Department of State, Bureau of International Narcotics and Law Enforcement (INL); These are available in El Preventivo, Cantel in Quetzaltenango, El Boquerón in Santa Rosa, El Infiernito in Escuintla and Fraijanes II in Guatemala.
6. These are available in El Preventivo, Cantel in Quetzaltenango, El Boquerón in Santa Rosa, El Infiernito in Escuintla and Fraijanes II in Guatemala.
7. In Spanish this refers to the, *Fuerza de Seguridad Interinstitucional (Fusina)*. This measure was taken on December 17, 2019 after the murder of the former director of the prison known as "*El Pozo*," who had been suspended from his post after an inmate was murdered inside that prison.
8. This pandemic call to action is not novel. See Maruschak et al. (2009).

Disclosure statement

No potential conflict of interest was reported by the author(s).

References

ABA. (2020, April 3). *COVID-19 and the compassionate release of the elderly, infirm or high risk.* American Bar Association, Civil Rights & Social Justice (CRSJ). COVID –19 Webinar Series. https://www.americanbar.org/groups/crsj/events_cle/program-archive/covid-compassionate-release/

Agencia EFE. (2020, June 16). Más de 1.600 presos liberados en Honduras por el COVID-19, que deja 322 muertos. *Agencia EFE.* https://www.efe.com/efe/america/sociedad/mas-de-1-600-presos-liberados-en-honduras-por-el-covid-19-que-deja-322-muertos/20000013-4273187

Akiyama, M. J., Spaulding, A. C., & Rich, J. D. (2020). Flattening the curve for incarcerated populations — Covid-19 in jails and prisons. *New England Journal of Medicine, 382*(22), 2075–2077. https://doi.org/10.1056/NEJMp2005687

Álvarez, N. (2020, June 24). COVID-19: Presidios reporta 103 casos positivos en reos y nueve fallecimientos. *Publinews.* https://www.publinews.gt/gt/noticias/2020/06/24/covid-19-sistema-penitenciario-casos-reos.html

Al Jazeera. (2020, March 10). UN urges Iran to free political prisoners amid coronavirus spread. *Al Jazeera.* https://www.aljazeera.com/news/2020/03/urges-iran-free-political-prisoners-coronavirus-spread-200310184750920.html

Amante, A. (2020, March 10). Death toll rises from Italy's coronavirus prison riots. *Reuters.* https://www.reuters.com/article/us-health-coronavirus-italy-prisons/death-toll-rises-from-italys-coronavirus-prison-riots-idUSKBN20X2DG

Ávila, J. (2020, May 25). Prisiones de Honduras: El reino de precariedad, violencia y militarismo al que llegó la pandemia. *No Ficción.* https://www.no-ficcion.com/project/prisiones-honduras-pandemia

BBC. (2020, April 28). *El Salvador gangs: 'No ray of sunlight for inmates'.* British Broadcasting Corporation. https://web.archive.org/web/20200429231027/https://www.bbc.com/news/world-latin-america-52454519

Braun, M. M., Truman, B. I., Maguire, B., DiFerndinando, G. T., Wormser, G., Broaddus, R., & Morse, D. L. (1989). Increasing incidence of tuberculosis in a prison inmate population. *Journal of the American Medica Association, 261*(3), 393–397. https://doi.org/10.1001/jama.1989.03420030067031

Bukele, N., [@nayibbukele]. (2020, April 27). *Justo el día siguiente, comenzaron los homicidios. Pero ¿de qué sirve sellar las celdas si eso no evitará que el ...* [Tweet]. Twitter.com. https://twitter.com/nayibbukele/status/1254979105264730112

Byrne, J., Pattavina, A., & Taxman, F. (2015). International trends in prison upsizing and downsizing: In search of evidence of a global rehabilitation revolution. *Victims and Offenders: An International Journal of Evidence-based Research, Policy, and Practice, 10*(4), 420–451. https://doi.org/10.1080/15564886.2015.1078186

CDC. (2020, May 15). *COVID-19 in correctional and detention facilities — United States, February–April 2020* (Morbidity and mortality weekly report). Centers for Disease Control and Prevention. https://www.cdc.gov/mmwr/volumes/69/wr/mm6919e1.htm

Central Intelligence Agency. (2020). El Salvador. In *In the world factbook.* https://www.cia.gov/library/publications/the-world-factbook/geos/es.html

Chumil, K. (2020a, June 8). El coronavirus llegó a tres centros carcelarios de Guatemala. *La Prensa Libre.* https://www.prensalibre.com/guatemala/justicia/el-coronavirus-llego-a-tres-centros-carcelarios-de-guatemala/

Chumil, K. (2020b, July 4). Liberan a 140 reos de forma temprana durante la pandemia. *Prensa Libre.* https://www.prensalibre.com/guatemala/justicia/liberan-a-140-reos-de-forma-temprana-durante-la-pandemia/

Council on Hemispheric Affairs. (2020, May 11). *El Salvador: Bukele's heavy-handed response to COVID-19 pandemic violates human rights*. https://www.coha.org/el-salvador-bukeles-heavy-handed-response-to-covid-19-pandemic-violates-human-rights/

Cuevas, D. (2020, June 10).*Coronavirus: Expertos consideran necesario ampliar pruebas en cárceles con casos positivos*. Prensa Libre. https://www.prensalibre.com/guatemala/justicia/coronavirus-expertos-consideran-necesario-ampliar-pruebas-en-carceles-con-casos-positivos/

Dewan, S., Swales, V., & Vigdor, N. (2020, March 22). Police tread lightly as pandemic spreads. *New York Times*. https://www.nytimes.com/2020/03/22/us/coronavirus-police.html.

Dolan, K., Wirtz, A. L., Moazen, B., Ndeffo-mbah, M., Galvani, A., Kinner, S. A., Courtney, R., McKee, M., Amon, J. J., Maher, L., Hellard, M., Beyrer, C., & Altice, F. L. (2016). Global burden of HIV, viral hepatitis, and tuberculosis in prisoners and detainees. *The Lancet*, *388*(10049), 1089–1102. https://doi.org/10.1016/S0140-6736(16)30466-4

Dudley, S. (2010). How 'mano dura' is strengthening gangs. *Insight Crime*. https://www.insightcrime.org/investigations/how-mano-dura-is-strengthening-gangs/

Dudley, S., & Bargent, J. (2017, January 19). The prison dilemma: Latin America's incubators of organized crime. *InSight Crime*. https://www.insightcrime.org/investigations/prison-dilemma-latin-america-incubators-organized-crime/

Economist. (2020, January 9). Guatemala's new president Alejandro Giammattei, outlines his plans. *The Economist*. https://www.economist.com/the-americas/2020/01/09/guatemalas-new-president-alejandro-giammattei-outlines-his-plans

Gershman, J., & Tau, B. (2020, March 17). Coronavirus disrupts U.S. court system. *Wall Street Journal*. https://www.wsj.com/articles/coronavirus-disrupts-u-s-court-system-11584445222

González, A. (2020, April 27). Buscan descongestionar cárceles para evitar contagio de Covid-19. *La República*. https://republica.gt/2020/04/27/descongestionar-carcel-covid-19/

Gough, E., Hempf, M. C., Graham, L., Manzanero, M., Hook, E. W., Bartolucci, A., & Chamot. E. (2010). HIV and Hepatitis B and C incidence rates in US correctional populations and high risk groups: A systematic review and meta-analysis. *BMC Public Health*, 10, 1–14. Retrieved July 29, 2020, from https://bmcpublichealth.biomedcentral.com/articles/10.1186/1471-2458-10-777

Human Rights Watch. (2020, April 29). El Salvador: Trato inhumano a reclusos en centros penitenciarios. *Human Rights Watch*. https://www.hrw.org/es/news/2020/04/30/el-salvador-trato-inhumano-reclusos-en-centros-penitenciarios

IACHR. (2019, August 27). *Human rights situation in Honduras*. http://www.oas.org/en/iachr/reports/country.asp

Kinner, S. A., & Young, J. T. (2018). Understanding and improving the health of people who experience incarceration: An overview and synthesis. *Epidemiologic Reviews*, *40*(1), 4–11. https://doi.org/10.1093/epirev/mxx018

Kinner, S. A., Young, J. T., Snow, K., Southalan, L., Lopez-Acuña, D., Ferreira-Borges, C., & O'Moore, E. (2020). Prisons and custodial settings are part of a comprehensive response to COVID-19. *Lancet*, *5*(10226), 188–189. https://doi.org/10.1016/S2468-2667(20)30058-X

López, J. (2020, May 29). Contagio masivo en cárceles: 108 reos positivos de COVID-19 y 945 casos sospechosos. *ElSalvador.com*. https://www.elsalvador.com/noticias/nacional/covid-19-coronavirus-reo-internos-centros-penales-carcel/718867/2020/

López, K. (2020, March 31). Qué pasa en las cárceles con el coronavirus (donde el distanciamiento social no existe). *Nómada*. https://nomada.gt/pais/actualidad/que-pasa-en-las-carceles-con-el-coronavirus-donde-el-distanciamiento-social-no-existe/

Macher, A., Kibble, D., & Wheeler, D. (2006). HIV transmission in correctional facility. *Emerging Infectious Diseases*, *12*(4), 669–671. https://doi.org/10.3201/eid1204.050484

Marshall Project. (2020, August 14). *A state-by-state look at coronavirus in prisons*. https://www.themarshallproject.org/2020/05/01/a-state-by-state-look-at-coronavirus-in-prisons

Maruschak, L. M., Sabol, W. J., Potter, R. H., Reid, L. C., & Cramer, E. W. (2009). Pandemic influenza and jail facilities and populations. *American Journal of Public Health*, *99*(S2), S339–S344. https://doi.org/10.2105/AJPH.2009.175174

Organization of American States. (2019, December 26). *IACHR, OHCHR urge the state of honduras to protect the lives and integrity of individuals held in penitentiary and juvenile detention facilities*, *following the declaration of a state of penitentiary emergency in the country.* http://www.oas.org/en/iachr/media_center/PReleases/2019/334.asp

Pitán, E. (2020, March 18). Coronavirus: Personas que lleven comida a reos deben usar mascarillas para minimizar riesgo en cárceles. *Prensa Libre.* https://www.prensalibre.com/guatemala/justicia/prohiben-visitas-a-25-mil-600-reclusos-por-riesgo-de-contagio-masivo-de-covid-19/

Prensa Latina. (2020, July 25). Fallece por la Covid-19 otro reo en cárcel de Guatemala. *La Prensa Latina.* https://www.prensa-latina.cu/index.php?o=rn&id=384561&SEO=fallece-por-la-covid-19-otro-reo-en-carcel-de-guatemala

Raderstorf, B., Wilson, C. J., Zechmeister, E. J., & Camilleri. (2017). *Beneath the violence: How insecurity shapes daily life and emigration in Central America.* Latin American Public Opinion Project and the Inter-American Dialogue. https://www.thedialogue.org/wp-content/uploads/2017/10/Crime-Avoidance-Report-FINAL-ONLINE.pdf

Sacchi, Flávia P. C., Praça, R. M., Tatara, M. B., Simonsen, V., Ferrazoli, L., Croda, M. G., Suffys, P. N., Ko, A. I., Andrews, J. R., & Croda, J. (2015). Prisons as reservoir for community transmission of tuberculosis, Brazil. *Emerging Infectious Diseases, 21*(3), 452–455. https://doi.org/10.3201/eid2103.140896

Soto, C. (2020, August 7). 12 guardias de presidios dan positivo a COVID-19 en cárcel de Mazatenango. *CRN Noticias.* https://crnnoticias.com/12-guardias-de-presidios-dan-positivo-a-covid-19-en-carcel-de-mazatenango/

Urquilla, K., & Escalante, D. (2020, September 10). Bukele entorpece acceso de ciudadanos a obtener información pública. *El Diario de Hoy.* https://www.elsalvador.com/eldiariodehoy/ley-de-acceso-a-la-informacion-publica-nayib-bukele-iaip/751733/2020/

Valway, S. E., Richards, S. B., Kovacovich, J., Greifinger, R. B., Crawford, J. T., & Dooley, S. W. (1991). Outbreak of multi-drug-resistant tuberculosis in a New York state prison. *American Journal of Epidemiology, 140*(2), 113–122. https://doi.org/10.1093/oxfordjournals.aje.a117222

Washington Post. (2020, February 12). The Salvadoran president alarmingly violates democratic norms, Editorial Board. *The Washington Post.* https://www.washingtonpost.com/opinions/global-opinions/the-salvadoran-president-alarmingly-violates-democratic-norms/2020/02/12/dffbe720-4d01-11ea-bf44-f5043eb3918a_story.html

WHO. (2020, March 15). *Preparedness, prevention and control of COVID-19 in prisons and places of detention.* World Health Organization Regional Office for Europe, 2020. https://www.euro.who.int/__data/assets/pdf_file/0019/434026/Preparedness-prevention-and-control-of-COVID-19-in-prisons.pdf?ua=1

World Prison Brief. (2020). *World Prison Brief.* University of London, Institute for Crime & Justice Policy Research. http://www.prisonstudies.org/world-prison-brief

Worldometer.info. (2020, August 11). *Worldometer.* https://www.worldometers.info/coronavirus/

Young, L. C., Dwyer, D. E., Harris, M., Guse, Z., Noel, V., & Levy, M. H. (2004). Summer outbreak of respiratory disease in an Australian prison due to influenza A/Fujian/411/2002 (H3N2)-like virus. *Epidemiology & Infection, 133*(1), 107–113. https://doi.org/10.1017/S0950268804003243

Responding to COVID-19 in Latin American Prisons: The Cases of Argentina, Chile, Colombia, and Mexico

Lina Marmolejo, Daniela Barberi, Marcelo Bergman, Olga Espinoza, and Gustavo Fondevila

ABSTRACT

The purpose of this paper is to identify and analyze how prison systems in Argentina, Chile, Colombia, and Mexico respond to the coronavirus disease (COVID-19). It explores the challenges these institutions face, the actions taken, the beneficiaries from such measures, and their immediate effect. We argue that governments and prison authorities struggle to put in place comprehensive measures to prevent and control the spread of COVID-19 within these institutions and that more concrete and swift actions are needed to address the magnitude and the consequences of the pandemic. This paper uses both primary and secondary data to describe the current prison situation and analyze institutional responses to the COVID-19 pandemic in these countries.

Introduction

The COVID-19 pandemic hit Latin American prisons in the midst of a decades-long crisis of mass incarceration, endemic overcrowding, violence, and lack of access to basic needs and services, including health care. Latin America as a region houses 12% of the world's total prison population (1.2 million, Walmsley, 2018). Moreover, the incarceration rate in the region has doubled from 118.8 to 241 per 100,000 inhabitants since 2000. This is one of the highest incarceration rates in the world, compared to the global average of 145 incarcerated individuals per 100,000 inhabitants (Bergman, 2018; Vilalta & Fondevila, 2019; Walmsley, 2018).

The rapid growth of the prison population is causing many institutions to operate on an average of 60% over bed capacity (Limoncelli et al., 2020). Overcrowding, poor hygiene, substandard living conditions, limited access to basic goods, insufficient health-care services, and lack of funding are common features of prisons in Latin America (Bergman, 2018; Carranza, 2009; Dammert & Zuñiga, 2008; Darke & Karam, 2016; United Nations Development Program [UNDP], 2013). These conditions make prisons vulnerable settings for outbreaks of significant illnesses and infectious diseases like COVID-19 (Kinner et al., 2020; Montoya-Barthelemy et al., 2020). It is virtually impossible for people in prison to practice social distance and maintain basic hygiene to prevent the spread of the coronavirus. For these reasons, Latin American governments must concern themselves with the virus' presence in unsanitary prisons as a part of their efforts to address the pandemic within the larger community.

In this paper, we conduct a comparative analysis of how the COVID-19 pandemic has impacted prison systems in Argentina, Chile, Colombia, and Mexico and discuss governments' responses to address this health crisis. Our analyses focus on three core questions: How has the global pandemic affected the daily life of people inside prisons? How have these four countries responded and managed the pandemic inside prisons? What are the lessons learned from the variety of responses to the pandemic? In addition to addressing these questions, we consider the implications of COVID-19 for future preparedness in Latin American prisons.

We begin by providing an overview of the objectives and data sources used in this research. Then, we examine the current situation of COVID-19 in prisons in the four countries of study. In the third section, we describe the measures taken by correctional authorities to control the virus by releasing incarcerated individuals, reducing new admission to prisons, and implementing mitigation actions inside correctional facilities. Lastly, we conclude by comparing actions taken by governments and discussing opportunities for policy change and future research.

The current study

The current study examines the COVID-19 outbreak in the corrections systems of four countries: Argentina, Chile, Colombia, and Mexico. These countries are among the top 10 Latin American countries with the highest prison population (Institute for Crime and Justice Policy Research [ICPR], 2019; see Table 1).

The study relies on three sources of information. The first source includes available databases, public and nonpublic reports from NGOs, governments, international organizations, and newspaper articles that discuss the response of prison systems to the pandemic.

The second source uses quantitative data collected from all Latin American countries,[1] except El Salvador, through an online survey. The regional survey includes both centralized (i.e., a single national correctional system), and decentralized correctional systems in the region. For the former group of countries (i.e., Argentina, Brazil, and Mexico), the survey counted in the federal prison system and one key state prison system.[2] The online survey was designed and implemented by one of the authors of this paper in collaboration with the Center for Latin American

Table 1. Top 10 Latin American countries with the highest prison population (2018–2020).

	Country	Correctional system	Number of prisons	Total prison pop.	Prison pop. rate (per 100,000 inhabitants)
1	Brazil	Decentralized	2,608	755,274	357
2	Mexico	Decentralized	342	198,384	158
3	Colombia	Centralized	132	109,034	217
4	Argentina	Decentralized	308	103,209	230
5	Peru	Centralized	69	96,870	292
6	Venezuela	Centralized	58	57,096	178
7	Chile	Centralized	113	39,584	214
8	Ecuador	Centralized	52	39,251	224
9	El Salvador	Centralized	25	38,114	590
10	Guatemala	Centralized	21	26,160	146

Source: ICPR (2019).

Studies on Insecurity and Violence (Centro de Estudios Latinoamericanos sobre Inseguridad y Violencia, CELIV), and the Latin American Society of Criminology (Sociedad de Criminología Latinoamericana, SOCLA). The goal of the survey was to gather information about the initial responses of Latin American correctional systems to COVID-19 and its impact on incarcerated individuals and prison staff. The survey instrument consisted of 58 questions, mostly in closed-ended format, and divided into five thematic areas: 1) general information and data about the correctional system, 2) measures taken by correctional authorities to protect the prison population during the pandemic, 3) measures taken by each system to protect the correctional staff during the pandemic, 4) the incidence of COVID-19 within the system, and 5) possible justice reforms to help control the pandemic. The link to the online survey, using google forms, was distributed by e-mail to 31 Latin American prison scholars[3] on April 26, 2020. They collected data from official sources and when such information was unavailable, informants relied on personal reports from high-rank prison officials or from secondary sources such as the media or reports from NGOs. Data collection ended on June 1, 2020, and CELIV received responses from 27 prison systems representing 18 Latin American countries. The survey covered prison systems that house more than 90% of Latin American inmates (see Bergman et al., 2020 for survey details).

Lastly, the third source analyzes four semi-structured interviews with prison scholars and practitioners from Argentina, Chile, and Colombia. The interview instrument focused on: 1) a general overview of prisons in each country, 2) the incidence of COVID-19 in the prison system, 3) measures taken by each country to deal with the pandemic in correctional facilities, and 4) interviewees' perceptions of the potential short-, medium- and long-term impact of COVID-19 in the prison system. Interviews were conducted online, by one of the authors of this paper, each interview lasted approximately 25 minutes and was voluntary.

We caution the reader that our review and analysis are preliminary, as the pandemic situation is constantly evolving within each prison and country. In addition, our ability to document the situation varied across countries due to availability and reliability of the data.[4]

COVID-19 and prisons in Latin America

Even before COVID-19, Latin American prisons were facing a serious crisis that the pandemic has exacerbated. While the situation varies from country to country, they share several characteristics: mass incarceration, endemic overcrowding, high levels of pretrial detention, poor infrastructure, scarcity of financial and human resources, shortage of basic goods and services, and increasing recidivism (Bergman, 2018; Carranza, 2009; Dammert & Zuñiga, 2008; Darke & Karam, 2016; UNDP, 2013). These structural conditions of confinement illustrate that correctional systems are ill-equipped and unprepared to respond accurately and effectively to a worldwide health crisis such as the COVID-19 and at the same time protect the fundamental rights of incarcerated people.

At the time of writing this article, Latin America is the region with the most confirmed coronavirus cases globally, surpassing the combined infections of the United States and Canada, and accounting for more than a quarter of global cases (Desantis & Leira, 2020). The group of countries under analysis are among the top 10 countries with the highest count of cases in the region, along with Brazil, Bolivia, Dominican Republic, Guatemala, Ecuador, and Peru (Horwitz et al., 2020).

The first case of coronavirus was confirmed in Mexico, on February 28, 2020. Shortly after that, COVID-19 landed in Argentina and Chile on March 3, 2020, and in Colombia on March 6, 2020. Since then, cases have grown exponentially. As of September 7, 2020, there were more than two million confirmed cases of COVID-19 in the countries under study (see Table 2). The country with the most reported positive cases is Colombia with 671,848 cases (Ministerio de Salud de Colombia, Reportes diarios sobre el Coronavirus, 2020), followed by Mexico (637,509, Gobierno de Mexico, 2020), Chile (425, 541, Ministerio de Salud de Chile, Cifras oficiales sobre el Coronavirus, 2020) and Argentina (268,574, Ministerio de Salud de Argentina, Reportes diarios sobre el Coronavirus, 2020).

Data from correctional authorities indicate that the first documented case of COVID-19 in prisons was reported on March 29, 2020, in Chile. By September 7, 2020, there were over 6,620 reported cases of coronavirus inside prisons, among a total of 450,211 incarcerated people in the four countries under study. In other words, this is equivalent to 1,470 cases per 100,000 prisoners, which is close to two times higher than the national case rate of 810 cases per 100,000 people. Table 2 summarizes the dates and number of coronavirus cases in the general population and inside prisons.

The country with the highest number of COVID-19 cases and deaths in prisons is Mexico, with 3,055 infections (87% inmates and 13% correctional staff) and 285 deaths (79% inmates and 21% staff) (Asistencia Legal por los Derechos Humanos [AsiLegal], 2020). It is followed by Chile with 3,043 positive coronavirus cases (57% are inmates and 43% correctional staff) and 15 deaths (87% inmates and 13% staff) in prisons (Gendarmería de Chile, 2020a). Colombia reports 2,374 positive cases of COVID-19 (94% inmates and 6% staff) in 51 correctional facilities (Instituto Nacional Penitenciario y Carcelario [INPEC], 2020a). Lastly, Argentina's prisons report the lowest number of confirmed cases of COVID-19. At the federal level, 350 positive cases and 12 deaths have been reported (SPF, 2020). At the state level, each prison authority is responsible for reporting data on the pandemic. The Buenos Aires province prison system reported in early August the first seven cases of coronavirus. However, this information is unreliable as this low level of contagion is unlikely in one of the largest and overcrowded state prison system in the country.

In sum, available data suggest that the rate of COVID-19 cases in prisons is higher than national rates in most countries under analysis. However, it is important to recognize that correctional systems in the region often lack adequate information systems to gather and report systematic data (UNDP, 2013). Thus, data availability and reliability, as well as, limited testing constitute a challenge to estimate the real magnitude of the pandemic outbreak inside prisons.

Table 2. Reported cases of COVID-19 in general population and in prisons.

	General population			Prison population				
						Number of Cases*		
	Total population	Date of first case	Number of cases*	Total Prison population	Date of first case	Prison residents	Staff	Deaths
Argentina	44,938,712	March 3	268,574	103,209	April 19	350	N/A	12
Chile	18,952,035	March 3	425,541	39,584	March 29	1,745	1,298	15
Colombia	50,339,443	March 6	671,848	109,034	April 10	2,221	153	70
Mexico	132,829,000	February 28	637,509	198,384	March 31	2,654	401	285
Total	247,059,190		2,003,472	450,211		6,970	1,852	382

*Cases reported as of September 8, 2020. Sources: Coronavirus cases in general population: Ministerio de Salud Argentina, Chile, Colombia and Gobierno de Mexico. Coronavirus in prisons: Argentina (SPF, 2020); Chile (Gendarmería de Chile, 2020a); Colombia (INPEC, 2020a); Mexico (AsiLegal, 2020). Total prison population: ICPR (2019).

Responses and measures to address COVID-19 in prisons

The World Health Organization issued guidelines to address, prevent and control COVID-19 inside prisons and other detention centers (World Health Organization [WHO], 2020). In addition, several agencies from the United Nations system issued joint statements and guidance notes on the impact of COVID-19 on human rights (United Nations Office on Drugs and Crime [UNODC], 2020; Inter-American Commission on Human Rights [IACHR], 2020). These institutions urged governments to take measures to minimize the risk of contagion within prisons and to safeguard the rights of prisoners. Specifically, they state that governments must take actions to reduce overcrowding, guarantee the health, safety, and dignity of incarcerated people, ensure the continuity of access to health services, and respect human rights. Most of these guidelines can be grouped into three broad categories.

The first category involves *prison releases* to reduce prison population and prevent and control the spread of COVID-19. Examples include granting parole to people nearly the end of their sentences who committed low-level offenses, providing early release to individuals serving short sentences for nonviolent offenses, releasing vulnerable individuals (e.g., elderly inmates, pregnant women, women with children, and individuals with chronic diseases). In addition, they recommended providing alternatives to detention for people waiting for trial and implementing special mechanisms such as commutations, pardons, or suspension of sentences. Second, international organizations suggest to *limit new prison admissions*. Criminal justice systems are encouraged to consider reducing arrests, particularly for low-level offenses, set lower bail amounts, postpone the enforcement of sentences of up to 6 months, and convert sentences into fines. The third type of recommendations relates to *prevention and mitigation actions inside prisons* to manage the spread of COVID-19. These actions include temporary limitations on movement or visits, increase cleaning, infection control, testing, access to hygiene products, personal protective equipment, health care, and medical isolation of suspected cases.

Based on these categories, the following section identifies key characteristics of correctional systems pre-pandemic and details the actions taken by the four countries under study to prevent and control the spread of coronavirus in prisons.

Prison releases

While conditions and circumstances of prison releases differ in each country, this measure is being implemented under the premise that early release is a suitable humanitarian act for some incarcerated individuals. Data from the regional survey show that most countries focused their releases on the elderly, people with mental and physical underlying medical conditions, pregnant women, women with children, and prisoners associated with non-violent, non-serious, nonsexual offenders (Bergman et al., 2020). Most countries struggle in conducting early releases that can make a meaningful contribution in reducing the prison population and alleviate the negative impacts of overcrowding. Results from the regional survey show that between March and June 2020, five out of the 26 prison systems included in the survey released less than 1% of their prison population and nine released between 1% and 5% (Bergman et al., 2020). Table 3 summarizes prison releases due to COVID-19 in the four countries under study.

Table 3. Releases from prison to prevent and control the spread of COVID-19*.

	House arrest	Probation	Parole	Exceptional mechanisms**	Other	Releases (% prison population)
Argentina – Federal Prison System	735	84	242		841	Approx. 13%
Argentina – Buenos Aires Province Prison System	800					Approx. 2%
Chile	2,489	1,591		1,860		Approx. 14%
Colombia	20,910			889		Approx. 20%
Mexico – Federal Prison System				None		
Mexico – Mexico State Prison System			2,583			Approx. 2%
Mexico – Other States			1,135			

*Data reported for Argentina and Chile as of June 1, 2020. For Mexico and Colombia as of July 15, 2020.
**Exceptional mechanisms include: amnesties, pardons and commutations.

Argentina

The incarceration rate in Argentina doubled between 2000 and 2019, from 102 to 230 incarcerated individuals per 100,000 inhabitants (ICPR, 2019). This increase resulted in occupancy levels that surpass official capacity. In 2019, the Argentinian federal prison system housed close to 14,000 incarcerated people (15% of the total prison population in the country) and operated 13% above its official bed capacity. At the state level, the Buenos Aires province prison system gathered over 49,000 people or 45% of the national prison population. The overcrowding rate was 71% (Centro de Estudios Legales y Sociales [CELS], 2020).

Most people in Argentinian prisons are young males, incarcerated for the first time, and serving short sentences for low-level offenses. In 2018, 95% of the total prison population were male, mostly adults between 25 and 44 years of age (62%) and first-time offenders (74%) (Sistema Nacional de Estadísticas sobre Ejecución de la Pena [SNEEP], 2018). In the Federal prison system, 28% of sentenced individuals were serving time for low-level drug-related offenses, and another 36% for property crimes. In the Buenos Aires prison system, 30% of people are in prison for theft and 11% for low-level drug crimes (CELS, 2020). Pretrial detainees account for almost half of the total prison population, 54% at the federal level and 49% in the Buenos Aires province (CELS, 2020).

The coronavirus pandemic increased the need to reduce the prison population to avoid an outbreak of the virus and a collapse of health systems inside and outside prisons. In April 2020, the Criminal Court of Appeals under the framework of a collective habeas corpus decided to grant house arrest to people considered to be at risk of contracting the virus and those arrested for the commission of low-level offenses. This measure benefited approximately 735 incarcerated individuals in federal prisons, which represents less than 2% of the prison population (Procuración Penitenciaria de la Nación [PPN], 2020). However, a month later this decision was revoked by the provincial Supreme Court of Justice, mainly in response to critics and opposition from citizens and politicians to prisoner releases. Ultimately, those cases were re-channeled to be dealt on a case-by-case basis and be resolved by judges of first instance (Bergman et al., 2020). Other early releases at the federal level have happened between mid-March and the end of May through probation, parole, or other mechanisms, benefiting 1,167 people in prison (PPN, 2020).

Releases made at the federal level have contributed to reduce overcapacity from 13% to 2% (CELS, 2020). While this new situation represents an improvement, it does not mean that prisons are better equipped to deal with the virus. The deficits in terms of living conditions, health care, food, and shelter are still critical and remain far from meeting human rights standards. At the end of April, there were riots in one of the federal prisons, where inmates requested access to sanitary products to combat the virus and demanded better infrastructure. Currently, there are no individual cells, but community pavilions inwhich more than 100 people live (Angulo, 2020).

Any effort to decongest prisons is also needed at the state level. In the Buenos Aires province, there have been close to 800 releases directly attributed to COVID-19. This is not a very significant number as it represents 1.6% of the prison population of this jurisdiction (Bergman et al., 2020). Although the Buenos Aires province prison system reported a reduction of 3,500 people between December 2019 and May 2020, it is unclear whether this reduction was due to early releases in the face of COVID-19 or other measures (CELS, 2020).

Chile

Since 2010 the incarceration rate in Chile has substantially dropped. From 320 inmates per 100,000 inhabitants to 215 in 2019 (ICPR, 2019). While there is no conclusive empirical evidence to explain the cause of this decline, a contributing factor was the measures taken by the government to address prison overcrowding after the dramatic San Miguel prison fire of 2010 where 81 people died (Tamayo, 2016). These included legislation to increase the use of alternatives to incarceration through the expansion of the catalog of non-custodial sanctions to include probation with intense supervision, parole, community service orders, and expulsion of foreigners. In addition to procedural reforms to grant parole that reduced bureaucracy in the decision-making process (Salinero & Morales, 2019; Godoy, 2016; Wilenmann, 2020).

In 2018, the majority of people in Chilean prisons were young males (88.8%) between the ages of 18 and 19 (43%) and 30 to 39 (33%). More than half (61.4%) were first time offenders and of those who were convicted, 58% were serving ten-year sentences or shorter (Gendarmería de Chile, 2018a, 2018b). Pretrial detainees account for 31.7% of the total prison population (ICPR, 2019).

In the face of COVID-19, the Chilean government took advantage of non-custodial sentences, already in place in the country to reduce its prison population (e.g., probation, parole, house arrest, suspended sentences, electronic monitoring, and work release). Between March and June 2020, probation was granted to 1,591 sentenced inmates (Gendarmería de Chile, 2020c) and 2,489 pretrial detainees with vulnerable health conditions were released under house arrest or other pretrial options (Defensoría Penal Pública, 2020). Also, a Presidential pardon benefited 1,860 sentenced people (280 in probation and 1,580 in prison) who were vulnerable to contracting COVID-19 and who were serving sentences for nonviolent offenses (Gendarmería de Chile, 2020c). There have been approximately 5,660 releases which represent close to 14% of the country's total prison population.

However, not every incarcerated individual is willing to accept early release, particularly those coming from and returning to marginalized communities. For instance, over 100 prisoners did not accept the President's pardon in response to the pandemic and opted to remain in prison. They expressed that in prison they have access to a secure job, shelter, food, and a salary to help their families, which might not be available in the community (Reyes, 2020). In many countries of the region, prison systems offer few options to support prisoner reentry and facilitate the reintegration process (Bergman, 2018), as in Chile, where there are two main post-release programs with capacity for a thousand people. However, the demand for such services originates from more than 28,000 people being released from prison (Morales et al., 2018).

Colombia

In 2019, the incarceration rate in Colombia was 217 inmates per 100,000 inhabitants and the occupancy rate was 135%. Pretrial detainees account for 33% of the total prison population (INPEC, 2019). As in other countries under analysis, people in prison are mostly young males (92.9%), around 39% of them are between the ages of 18 and 29 and another 31% between 30 and 39 years of age (INPEC, 2019). Incarcerated people are mostly serving short sentences, less than 10 years (59%), and for nonviolent offenses such as theft (15%), conspiracy to commit a crime (13%), and low-level drug-related offenses (13%). About 14% of the prison population is serving time for homicide, 13% traffic, or possession of firearms, 9% sexual offenses, and 23% for other crimes (INPEC, 2019).

Violent riots in several Colombian prisons pushed the National Government to take measures to deal with the pandemic inside prisons. On March 21, 2020, there were 13 simultaneous riots in prisons around the country that resulted in the death of 23 incarcerated individuals and over 80 officers and inmates injured (Bergman et al., 2020; Colectivo de Estudios de Drogas y Derecho [CEED], 2020). Prisoners expressed their outrage at the lack of response from the government to prevent and control the pandemic inside prison facilities. In mid-April 2020, the Ministry of Justice published Decree 546 granting release, under temporary house arrest, to vulnerable populations (e.g., elderly, pregnant women, women with kids, individuals with chronic diseases). Prison authorities estimated that this action could benefit 4,000 incarcerated people. However, between its publication and until mid-July 2020, only 889 individuals have been released under this measure. These releases represent less than 1% of the total prison population (INPEC, 2020b). This low level of releases can be explained by the extensive list of exceptions and limitations of the Decree 546. For instance, it excludes those serving sentences for nonviolent crimes such as theft (Ministerio de Justicia, 2020), which represents 15% of the total prison population. These restrictions constitute a limitation to its effectiveness in reducing overcrowding and in offering protective measures for the prison population (Hernandez, 2020). An additional group of 20,910 individuals have been released from prison under ordinary law since the end of March. This represents almost 18% of the total prison population (INPEC, 2020b). This group of people include individuals who were ordinarily granted house arrest or received their freedom because of other ordinary reasons such as completing or exceeding their pretrial detention.

Mexico

Mexico's incarceration rate registered a clear decline since 2014, from 214 inmates per 100,000 inhabitants to 158 in 2018 (Instituto Nacional de Estadística y Geografía [INEGI], 2019; ICPR, 2019). This reduction can be explained, among other reasons, by the switch from an inquisitorial to an adversarial justice system that emphasized the presumption of innocence and the use of alternatives to incarceration for misdemeanor crimes (World Justice Project [WJP], 2018). The federal prison system reduced its occupancy rate to half of its operating capacity in 2017 (INEGI, 2019). At the state level, occupancy rates also decreased from 127% in 2011 to 103% in 2017. However, there are still state prisons with high concentrations of prisoners, such as Nayarit (573 inmates per 100,00 inhabitants), Baja California (378), Sonora (367), Durango (329) and Mexico City (323) (INEGI, 2019).

Close to 14.5% of the total prison population are held in federal prisons, and 85.5% at state prison facilities. In total, the majority of the people in prison are males (94% of the total prison population), between the ages of 18 and 29 (32.4%) and are first time offenders (73.9%) (INEGI, 2019). Pre-trial detainees account for 34.6% of the population, while 65.4% have confirmed sentences: the majority for robbery (32.7%), homicide (17.9%), rape (8.4), drug dealing (5.9%), and 28.2% for a variety of other crimes (INEGI, 2019).

In September 2019, the President proposed an Amnesty Law as a measure to decongest prisons. Its rationale was that a large number of prisoners, especially first-time offenders, have been incarcerated because they committed crimes prompted by circumstances of extreme poverty and vulnerability (e.g., abortion, theft, political riots, treason, simple drug possession and low-level property offenses; Diario Oficial de la Federación [DOF], 2020). The Senate approved the bill in April 2020, in the midst of the pandemic furthering its rationale to mitigate the spread of coronavirus in prisons. The government estimated that this measure could benefit 1,589 people in prison, which represents about 7% of the total federal prison population (Angel, 2020). Although this measure seemed appropriate, it was flawed and it was implemented at a slow pace. First, the amnesty was restricted to prisoners in federal prison system, which does not suffer from extreme overcrowding and holds less than one-fifth of the total prison population in the country. Second, the crimes under the bill are not generally prosecuted at a federal level but at the state level (Órgano Administrativo de Prevención y Readaptación Social del Gobierno Federal [OADPRS], 2020). Third, the bill mandates that all potential cases for release should be reviewed and approved by an Amnesty Commission, that was formally established on June 18, 2020. At the time of writing this article, no releases have been made under the Amnesty Law. Currently, none of the states have declared a similar amnesty, but most have accelerated releases through ordinary mechanisms. As of July 15, 2020, approximately 3,718 individuals have been released on parole (AsiLegal, 2020) which represents 2% of the prison population at the state level. As shown above, and similar to Argentina, the real challenge of reducing prison population and preventing the spread of the pandemic in Mexico, lies at the state level.

Limiting new prison admissions

Equally important to prison releases are the measures taken by other criminal justice agencies to decongest correctional facilities, especially those related to reducing arrests and diverting pretrial detainees from prison. However, these actions have been limited and, in some cases, have caused negative collateral consequences. For example, in Argentina and Colombia restricting new entries to prisons has created overcrowding in temporary detention facilities. Simply moving the imminent threat of contagion and spread of the virus from the corrections system to police stations.

Argentina

According to the Secretary of Security and based on partial national crime statistics, the number of thefts, assaults and drug-related crimes decreased by more than 25% during the first months of the strict national lockdown, imposed in March after the first confirmed cases of coronavirus, then slowly began to increase after the month of June, 2020 (Bajaron los delitos por cuarentena, dijo Frederic, 2020). A recent report for the Buenos Aires province suggests that criminal homicide investigations initiated between March 20 until June 25, 2020 declined 6% and theft investigations declined 37% when compared to the same time period in 2019 (Ministerio Público Provincia de Buenos Aires, Fuero Criminal y Correccional, IPP Iniciadas por Bien Jurídico Protegido Periodo 20 de Marzo al 25 de Junio años 2019 y 2020). These reductions in crime and in investigations have impacted new prison admissions since arrests substantially diminished. In addition, to reduce new prison admissions, arrested individuals were sent to temporary detention centers at police stations not suited to house large numbers of people for long periods of time. By the end of July 2020, close to 5,000 people were housed in these detention centers, causing overcrowding, and increasing contagion.

Chile

While the government of Chile has taken specific actions to reduce the prison population, other measures might be threatening such efforts. For instance, the government recently passed a bill modifying the Penal Code to increase sanctions for crimes against public health (including prison sentences from 61 days to 3 or 5 years). These crimes include violations of stay at home orders, or the nonobservance of sanitary rules in place due to the pandemic (Londoño, 2020). Arresting and detaining people who do not comply with quarantine and lockdowns puts them at greater risk of contagion. Alternatively, enforcement could be done through citations, fines and fees, or community service orders.

Colombia

One of the measures to prevent COVID-19 contagion focused on stopping new prison admissions. The booking facilities and the police stations in the country collapsed with this prohibition. Policymakers highlighted that what it seemed as steps in the right direction to decongest prisons, with the release of more than 20,000 individuals, was undermined by the crowding of police stations holding at least 12,000 people (Reyes, 2020). This means that even if there is a reduction of overcrowding in the correctional system, the problem moved from this system to the police stations. Also, measures taken by the Colombian police have not directly targeted the reduction of arrests or prison intakes. Instead, they focused on protecting police officials by providing biosecurity elements and limiting the number of officers on the field (Ministerio de Defensa, 2020).

Mexico

Information on judicial measures that aimed at alleviating pressure on the correctional system is scarce. At the federal level, the Ministry of Interior called on federal and local congresses, as well as on the Executive and Judicial branches, to not use the criminal law to confront the health emergency. This means desisting from criminally pursuing individuals for not complying with lockdown orders. Additionally, courts adopted informal measures to manage the pandemic. For example, the Mexico City Supreme Court of Justice reported the suspension of 1,788 transfers of sentenced individuals to prison and 1,537 transfers of defendants to court through the use of videoconferencing during the pandemic emergency (Tribunal Superior de Justicia arranca programa justicia virtual ante COVID-19, 2020).

Lastly, it is not clear if any measures have been put in place by police departments at the federal, state, and municipal level to reduce arrests of minor offenses and avoid increasing the number of people in prisons. The only known action coming from the police relates to ensuring the safety of its personnel by providing biosecurity equipment and by exempting at-risk police officers from service in the field (Despliegan militares en Ciudad de Mexico tras retirar policias por COVID-19, 2020).

Prevention and mitigation actions inside prisons

Results from the regional survey show that Latin American prison authorities have mainly locked down prisons and restricted contact between incarcerated people and the outside world as a mechanism to deal with the pandemic (Bergman et al., 2020). Ninety-six percent of prison systems included in the survey, limited visits, 52% curtailed work, and 90% restricted educational activities. These measures have increased tensions and violence, as more than half of the surveyed prison systems experienced violence inside prisons (Bergman et al., 2020). Restrictions have also put people in prison at greater risks of deprivation, since they heavily depend on relatives to provide food, hygiene products, clothes, and other basic goods. Governments have failed to implement other critical measures such as ensuring mass testing for people behind bars, providing protecting equipment for inmates and prison staff, and guaranteeing access to health-care services. Table 4 summarizes information on these measures in the countries under study.

Argentina

The Federal system and the Buenos Aires Province prison system have put in place several measures to prevent the spread of the coronavirus inside its facilities. First, educational and work programs were suspended. This measure is estimated to impact over half (57%) of incarcerated people who regularly participate in educational activities or work inside prisons (Bergman et al., 2014). Second, all in-person visits were temporarily restricted. This measure affects 74% of the total prison population who frequently received family visits and 40% of prisoners who received conjugal visits (Bergman et al., 2014). Incarcerated individuals and families reacted negatively against this action because people in prison rely on family and friends to have better access to food and basic goods. An inmate survey in Argentinian prisons showed that 85% of respondents depended on their families to access basic goods such as food and clothes and 35% to have access to medications (Bergman et al., 2014). As a safeguard to supplement the loss of in-person visits, the judiciary authorized the possession and use of cell phone devices inside prisons, despite its prohibition stipulated in prison regulations. Videocalls and videoconferences have allowed people to keep contact with families and lawyers. However, it is still unclear what procedures were put in place to facilitate access to cell phones, how often people are able to communicate with their families and at what cost if any. No safeguards were identified to enable family members to continue to provide food and other supplies.

Prison authorities also restricted movement within prisons, and transfers to and between prisons. Including the number of professional staff (e.g., psychologist, social workers, health workers, etc.) entering the facilities. This measure reduced access to health care which was already a scarce service for people in prison. For instance, the inmate survey showed that more than half (55.5%) of incarcerated people reported being ill during their incarceration,

Table 4. Measures taken inside prisons to prevent and control the spread of COVID-19.

	Prevention measures							Identifying, assessing, and controlling cases			
	Suspension of educational activities	Suspension of work activities	Restriction on-site prison visits	Restriction on staff per unit	Restriction of transfer btw prisons	Vaccination campaign against influenza	Educational campaigns	Clinical controls for at-risk groups	Testing incarcerated individuals and staff	Health kits/PPE for incarcerated individuals and staff	Designated area for isolation
Argentina – Federal Prison System	x	x	x	x	x			x	x	x	x
Argentina – Buenos Aires Province Prison System	x	x	x	x				x		x	x
Chile	x	x	x	x		x	x	x	x		x
Colombia	x	x	x	x	x		x		x	x	x
Mexico – Federal Prison System	x	x	x				x		x		x
Mexico State Prison System	x		x	x	x				x		x

and one-third did not receive medical attention (Bergman et al., 2014). Lastly, efforts to provide testing to people in prison have been limited. As of early August 2020, less than 4% of the total population at the federal prison system had been tested (SPF, 2020).

Chile

The Chilean correctional system restricted in-person visits, suspended educational and work activities, and designated spaces inside the prison for medical isolation. Additionally, prison authorities conducted preventative information campaigns about the contagion of COVID-19 and implemented a massive vaccination campaign against the influenza for prison residents and staff (Gendarmería de Chile, 2020a). It is still unclear if and how the last two measures contributed to prevent the spread of the virus inside prisons.

Respondents to our interviews view these institutional responses undesirably as they can "accentuate the dramatic situation inside prison, especially in terms of subsistence. While these [measures] are taken to protect the inmate, they can also aggravate and make the prison experience more complex." As in Argentina, 84% of Chilean prisoners receive food and other basic goods from family members. In a recent inmate survey, 95% of respondents reported that the institution provided them with a mattress, but other basic goods (e.g., sheets, clothing, shoes, toilet paper, soap, toothpaste) are provided by family members (Sánchez & Piñol, 2015). In order to compensate for the lack of in-person visits, alternative methods were provided by prison authorities to maintain contact with families and lawyers. Cellphones and other technological tools were allowed inside prison facilities to have video calls. Additionally, family members were allowed to continue to deliver food and other goods, without entering the prisons, and on specific dates and times established by prison authorities (Gendarmería de Chile, 2020b).

However, prison authorities have failed to provide mass testing for people in prison (Colegio Médicos de Chile, 2020). Close to 5,792 COVID-19 tests have been conducted incorrectional facilities, of those, half were used for staff and the other half for incarcerated individuals. This measure benefited only 7.2% of people in prison and more than 14.3% of prison staff (Rochow & Mateo, 2020). Limited availability of testing for people in prison means that infections and deaths among this population can be much higher than reported. This situation reflects both the lack of resources of correctional institutions as well as the low priority of prisons and prisoners for governments and politicians.

Colombia

The Colombian correctional system took very similar measures to the other countries under study. These included restricting all in-person visits, limiting the number of non-essential staff or individuals that work in the facilities, and the suspension of all educational and work activities. These actions impacted the daily lives of approximately 81% of the prison population who work or study (INPEC, 2020b).

In addition, the correctional administration put in place strict sanitary protocols to protect both staff and inmates, including the distribution of personal protective equipment and hygiene products, and establishing regular cleaning and disinfecting procedures in the prisons and jails (Medidas complementarias al plan de contención del COVID-19 en centros penitenciarios y carcelarios del país, 2020). However, reports from people in prison suggest that access to protective equipment through the prison administration is still very limited. For this reason, inmates organized themselves to buy or to request from family members face masks, hand sanitizers, and cleaning products (¿Como se vive la pandemia en la cárcel la Picota? Un preso lo cuenta, 2020). Inmates have also pressured correctional authorities to ease the restrictions on movement and on visits for doctors and nurses to be able to access health services inside prison. Prison administration was already deficient in guaranteeing health care for incarcerated people and COVID-19 only aggravated this situation. A recent study found that, prior to the pandemic, 78% of the people who enter a prison will get ill, of which 9% reported that they were never assigned a medical appointment and 32% mentioned that it took 1 month to see a doctor (Riaño & Mora, 2019).

Moreover, respondents to our interviews expressed concern over overcrowding facilities and the "continuous challenge of ensuring social distancing and quarantine spaces." While the prison administration designated special accommodation sectors for those who contracted COVID-19, it is unclear how and under what conditions people are being isolated (e.g., ventilation, access to toilets, water, medicine, sanitary items, and contact with health professionals and the outside world). Inmates from La Picota, one of the largest prisons in Colombia, operating at 53% over capacity, report that isolation is partial due to the limited space available and infected people are kept in places where there is high traffic of people (¿Como se vive la pandemia en la cárcel la Picota? Un preso lo cuenta, 2020).

Mexico

At a federal level, in March 2020, the Ministry of Health approved a protocol for dealing with COVID-19 inside prisons. It established a mechanism for early detection, isolation, identification of severity, and policies for the evacuation of the seriously ill (Secretaría de Seguridad y Protección Ciudadana [SSPC], 2020). This measure solely applied to federal prisons and not to more than 300 state prisons. As a result, measures by federal prison authorities have taken the form of prohibiting or limiting in-person visits. Federal prisons have approximately 3,500 visitors a day (e.g., lawyers, employees, suppliers) of which approximately 400 are family members (SSPC, 2020).

State prisons have taken alternative approaches to in-person visits. Some have reduced the frequency of visits by half, from four weekends to two weekends per month, and have implemented sanitary protocols to monitor and detect symptoms of visitors before entering the facilities. Others, allowed families and visitors to leave food, clothing, and personal hygiene products in a special distribution area outside prison facilities. In addition, prisons have restricted movement of people and staff inside the facilities, as well as suspended work and/or educational activities. These actions impact the daily lives of close to 51% of the prison population estimated to perform some occupational activity and 29% who either study or participates in some form of training (INEGI, 2019).

A window for bold action

Efforts from correctional systems have fallen short in their response to the pandemic. Under the three groups of measures analyzed, governments and correctional systems have limited themselves to adopt the easiest and least demanding actions to alleviate overcrowding, improve sanitation conditions of prisoners, and provide access to goods and health-care services. This section examines opportunities and obstacles for more comprehensive and decisive actions in the face of the pandemic.

Prison releases

There is international consensus that to confront the pandemic, prison decongestion is an urgent matter. One route, undoubtedly controversial and difficult, is to reduce the prison population through releases. Our analysis shows that the number of releases vary across the region and the four countries under study. In general, most Latin American countries have released less than 5% of their prison population (Bergman et al., 2020). In particular, Colombia has released the highest percentage of prisoners since the start of the COVID-19 pandemic, with approximately 20% of its total prison population. On the other side, Mexico, the country with the largest prison population has released only 2% of its total prison population. In Argentina, close to 2% of the prison population has been released from the Buenos Aires province prison system, while close to 13% have been released from federal prisons. Chile has released close to 14% of its prison population. Worldwide prison releases account for approximately 639,000 people or merely 5.8% of the global prison population (Penal Reform International [PRI], 2020). Chile, Colombia, and the Argentine federal system seem to be over the regional and global average but way below the releases in other countries in the world. For example, Iran and Turkey have released large numbers of inmates accounting for 35% of their total prison population (PRI, 2020; Pakes, 2020).

These efforts are steps in the right direction, but more needs to be done to have a real impact on crowded prisons. There are concrete opportunities to increase the number of releases, which until now have mostly focused on incarcerated people at risk of contracting COVID-19. For instance, the release of people on pretrial detention, who significantly contribute to prison overcrowding. Pretrial detainees make up one-third or more of the prison population in most of the countries under analysis. Detainees are often housed in the same facilities as sentenced inmates and spend long periods of time, usually years, in detention before trial (Bergman, 2018; Schönteich, 2014; UNDP, 2013). It is also important to recognize that most of them are held in prison under charges for low-level offenses, such as theft and nonviolent drug-related offenses. Thus, governments, prison authorities, and the judiciary should prioritize reviewing the cases of people held in prison unnecessarily while awaiting for trial as a way to help decongest prisons. For example, in Colombia, there are close to 65,000 people in prison waiting for trial on charges related to low-level crimes such as conspiracy to commit a crime (17%), drug-related offenses (13%), and theft (12%) (INPEC, 2019). In Argentina, people in pretrial detention account for 49% of the Buenos Aires prison system and most are in custody for low-level crimes involving theft and drug-related offenses (CELS, 2020).

Second, the use of alternatives to incarceration that allows individuals to serve their sentences and seek treatment in the community is another avenue to reduce incarceration and recidivism rates (Byrne et al., 1992; Morris & Tonry, 1990; Taxman, 2012). However, with the exception of Chile, the availability and use of these alternatives in the countries under study are very limited. Governments have mostly relied on the use of prison as the sole form of punishment rather than using it as a measure of last resort. The current public health crisis provides a unique opportunity to drive reforms in the way punishment is delivered. Alternatives to incarceration can allow governments to protect both public health and public safety at the same time. However, there is an associated risk with implementing such practices. Notably, widening the net of State social control (Cohen, 1979) through punitive and intensive supervision that instead of preventing incarceration can increase it (Klingele, 2013; Phelps, 2013). Governments should ensure that alternatives are conceived and implemented in a way that promote greater emphasis on social support to help formerly incarcerated people with their needs rather than on creating additional burdens (Durnescu, 2011; Payne & Gainey, 1998), or on emphasizing penal control (Rhine & Taxman, 2017). Providing the necessary dosage of state supervision and increasing opportunities for treatment and support in the community (Byrne et al., 2015; Georgiou, 2014; Hyatt & Barnes, 2014) are key elements in ensuring successful reintegration.

It is important to emphasize that releasing people from prison while maintaining public health and public safety conditions is easier said than done. To begin with, governments face numerous obstacles and challenges while embarking on such unpopular endeavors. Inevitably, the decision to release inmates under extraordinary circumstances requires strong political will from policymakers. Even if releases and community corrections are a cost-effective alternative to incarceration, such measures are not usually welcomed by the Latin American citizenry that is used to a tough-on-crime, penal populism discourse and commonly favors harsh prison sentences (Iturralde, 2019; Latin America Public Opinion Project [LAPOP], 2019; Müller, 2012). Moreover, policymakers might be reluctant to apply these measures due to negative media coverage that can portrait judicial lenience and highlight sensationalist accounts of crimes committed by those released under special conditions. Thus, media can further exacerbate the fear of crime and encourage public opinion support for tougher laws to punish crime (Bonner, 2018). For example, public protests took place in Buenos Aires against the releases of incarcerated individuals under house arrest due to fear of crime and spread of the virus in the community (Cacerolazo: Fuerte protesta contra la excarcelación de presos, 2020). Respondents to our interviews coincide that "there was a strong negative social reaction to releases from prison, which ultimately limited their implementation. But what they [the citizenry] do not realize is that at some point people in prison are going to return to the community. If they are at greater risk of becoming ill inside, they will be spreading the coronavirus in the outside [community]."

Another challenge relates to the lack of reliable and easily accessible prison data (UNDP, 2013). In the wake of the pandemic crisis, these deficiencies have become more notorious. There is scare information on the number of COVID-19 confirmed cases, on people in isolation, recovered patients, or tests performed. There are also limited disaggregated data by gender, age, or prison institution. The lack of reliable data represents an obstacle for evidence-informed decision-making that can result in negligence, corruption, and opacity in the process of releasing people from prison and the provision of health care and access to goods. For instance, respondents to our interviews highlighted this challenge, "we need to improve data collection, academia and universities should support governments in this effort."

Prevention and mitigation actions inside prisons

Governments and prison authorities in all countries under study opted for quick and easy fixes to deal with the pandemic by locking down prisons and restricting contact between incarcerated people and the outside world (i.e., limiting visitation, suspending educational and work activities, and reducing the in-person presence of health professionals, therapists, and social workers in prison). At the same time, they refrained to take major measures to actually decrease the transmission and contagion of the virus. They have failed to provide mass testing, guarantee unlimited and free access to personal protective equipment, implement clinical controls, and warrant access to health personnel for the at-risk groups. It is still unclear for how long restrictive measures will be in place and what their long-term consequences will be. But at first sight, they have increased conflicts and exacerbated the utterly poor living conditions of inmates.

Suspending in-person visits is particularly troublesome in Latin American prisons. First, incarcerated individuals in the countries under study receive visits frequently, as they depend on relatives to provide food, clothes, hygiene products, and other basic goods during imprisonment that are not supplied by prison authorities. Overcrowding, harsh prison conditions, lack of programming, and limited access to basic goods can aggravate material deprivations that can later lead to misconduct and violence (Byrne et al., 2008; Steiner et al., 2014; Sykes, 1958). As seen above, the pandemic has brought situations of violence in prisons in several countries. If in times of "normality" prisons represent spaces of violence, COVID-19 has worsened these risks and further exposed the fragility of the prison population. In the short term, correctional management must take concrete actions to provide alternative ways in which people in prison can access their basic goods and can attend programs. In fact, Chile and Mexico are allowing relatives to deliver goods in prison at specific times and places. In the long term, prison authorities have the opportunity to revamp prison conditions and push for additional resources to guarantee access to basic goods and services to prison residents. It was not possible to identify alternative strategies to provide prison rehabilitation programs to inmates during the pandemic.

Second, lack of meaningful contact with family members can further hinder the strength of social bonds while in prison, which has been found to be a key element in the process of rehabilitation and reintegration (Bales & Mears, 2008; Casey et al., 2020; Duwe & Clark, 2013; Mitchell et al., 2016). The Province of Buenos Aires, Chile, and Colombia has facilitated communication through video conferencing, but with the massive interest from inmates and loved ones, this strategy has already resulted in significant scheduling delays. Again, prison authorities should set limits to measures restricting contact with the outside world and find ways to resume in-person visits in open-air spaces that can provide a safe environment for visitors and prison residents.

Finally, prison authorities are legally obliged to guarantee the same quality of health for incarcerated individuals, as the rest of the citizens, as established by international treaties and covenants. However, as seen above, all prison systems in the countries under analysis have great deficiencies in guaranteeing a universal right to health for persons deprived of liberty. COVID-19 has exacerbated these deficiencies and has shown that health care in prison is not equipped to deal with the threat of this infectious disease. Thus, the pandemic brings an important opportunity to revamp health services, as well as prison conditions for health reasons in ways that otherwise would be politically impossible to carry out.

Future research

COVID-19 is eliciting enormous opportunities for correctional research and for researchers from the Global North to learn from more dramatic prison experiences in Latin American countries. First, it is necessary to examine the politics and economics of decision-making processes about prison population levels and prison conditions. Second, it is important to explore the long-term effects of restrictive measures for incarcerated people, their families, and the prison environment. Third, governments, prison authorities, and scholars have a strategic opportunity to strengthen mechanisms to collect reliable prison data. Fourth, it is important to further study the perspectives and experiences of inmates during COVID-19, whose voices are often absent from policy discussions. Lastly, community corrections constitute a key area of research to better understand the criminal justice system response to the pandemic.

Conclusion

While there is great variability across Latin American prisons, we examined the critical situation of these institutions in Argentina, Chile, Colombia, and Mexico when facing COVID-19. This study provided a detailed description of the actions and measures taken by government officials in each of these countries to slow the spread of COVID-19 inside prisons. We argued that while government officials have undertaken efforts to implement guidance from international agencies (e.g., WHO, UNODC, IACHR) these measures have not been enough to alleviate overcrowding, to improve prison conditions, to strengthen the prisons' health system or to stop the rapid spread of the disease. On the contrary, in many instances, these actions have increased the burdens of incarceration because the deprivations and vulnerabilities of people in prison have been accentuated. More needs to be done and there is a bold opportunity to rethink the use of imprisonment, and to implement the necessary actions to enact policy change.

Notes

1. Argentina, Belize, Bolivia, Brasil, Chile, Colombia, Costa Rica, Ecuador, Guatemala, Honduras, Nicaragua, Mexico, Panama, Paraguay, Peru, Republica Dominicana, Uruguay and Venezuela.
2. For the case of Mexico, we focus on the Mexican federal prison system and the State of Mexico (which is the most populous state and where Mexico City is located). Similarly, in Argentina, we focus on the federal and the Buenos Aires Province prison systems (one or the largest state and where the capital of the country is located).
3. There was one local informant per prison system. Informants were selected by the leaders of the survey based on academic or public service trajectory. All informants are scholars specialized in correctional issues.
4. In general, data on COVID-19 (e.g., confirmed cases and deaths in the community and in correctional systems, as well as, prison releases) is scattered across multiple sources, it is often not publicly available or regularly updated. In particular, data from state-level prison systems in Mexico and Argentina was difficult to gather. We report the most up-to-date information that we were able to collect until the manuscript was submitted for publication.

Acknowledgments

We would like to thank all the local correctional practitioners and scholars who helped the authors gather accurate and recent information about responses to COVID-19 in each country. We are also thankful for the anonymous reviewers and the journal editors for their valuable suggestions and thoughtful feedback on this article.

Disclosure statement

The author(s) declared no potential conflicts of interest with respect to the research, authorship, and/or publication of this article.

Funding

The author(s) received no financial support for the research, authorship, and/or publication of this article.

ORCID

Lina Marmolejo http://orcid.org/0000-0002-2841-2627
Daniela Barberi http://orcid.org/0000-0002-8427-4134
Olga Espinoza http://orcid.org/0000-0002-4447-991X
Gustavo Fondevila http://orcid.org/0000-0003-4818-0584

References

¿Como se vive la pandemia en la cárcel la Picota? Un preso lo cuenta. (2020, July 3). *El Tiempo*. https://www.eltiempo.com/bocas/coronavirus-colombia-hoy-asi-se-vive-la-pandemia-en-la-carcel-la-picota-entrevista-511826

Angel, A. (2020, April 28). *Ley de Amnistía solo sacará de la cárcel a 7% de presos y las liberaciones tardarían meses*. Animal Político. https://www.animalpolitico.com/2020/04/ley-de-amnistia-impacto-presos-liberaciones/

Angulo, M. (2020, April 29). Coronavirus en Argentina: Por un doble efecto, ya no hay sobrepoblación en las cárceles federales. Infobae. https://www.infobae.com/sociedad/2020/04/29/coronavirus-en-argentina-por-un-doble-efecto-ya-no-hay-sobrepoblacion-en-las-carceles-federales/

Asistencia Legal por los Derechos Humanos (AsiLegal). (2020, July 1). *Mapa Penitenciario COVID-19*. https://asilegal.org.mx/

Bajaron los delitos por cuarentena, dijo Frederic. (2020, July 7). *BAENegocios*. https://www.baenegocios.com/politica/Bajaron-los-delitos-por-la-cuarentena-dijo-Frederic-20200716-0109.html

Bales, W. D., & Mears, D. P. (2008). Inmate social ties and the transition to society: Does visitation reduce recidivism? *Journal of Research in Crime and Delinquency*, *45*(3), 287–321. https://doi.org/10.1177/0022427808317574

Bergman, M. (2018). *More money, more crime: Prosperity and rising crime in Latin America*. Oxford University Press.

Bergman, M., Cafferata, F., & Ambrogi, J. (2020). *The effects of coronavirus in prisons in Latin America. Center for Latin American Studies on Insecurity and Violence (CELIV)*. Universidad Tres de Febrero. Argentina. https://criminologialatam.wordpress.com/2020/06/12/efectos-del-covid-19-carceles-de-latino-america/

Bergman, M., Massello, D., & Arias, Y. C. (2014). *Delito, marginalidad y desempeño institucional en la Argentina: Resultados de la encuesta de presos condenados. Center for Latin American Studies on Insecurity and Violence (CELIV)*. Universidad Nacional 3 de Febrero.

Bonner, M. D. (2018). Media and punitive populism in Argentina and Chile. *Bulletin of Latin American Research, Journal of the Society for Latin American Studies, 37*(3), 275–290. https://doi.org/10.1111/blar.12744

Byrne, J. M., Hummer, D. C., & Taxman, F. S. (2008). *The culture of prison violence*. Pearson/Allyn and Bacon.

Byrne, J. M., Lurigio, A. J., & Petersilia, J. (Eds.). (1992). *Smart sentencing: The emergence of intermediate sanctions*. Sage Publications.

Byrne, J. M., Pattavina, A., & Taxman, F. S. (2015). International trends in prison upsizing and downsizing: In search of evidence of a global rehabilitation revolution. *Victims and Offenders: An International Journal of Evidence-based Research, Policy and Practice, 10*(4), 420–451. https://doi.org/10.1080/15564886.2015.1078186

Cacerolazo: Fuerte protesta contra la excarcelación de presos. (2020, April 30). *La Nación.* https://www.lanacion.com.ar/politica/cacerolazo-hoy-a-que-hora-es-protesta-nid2360230

Carranza, E. (2009). *Cárcel y Justicia Penal en América Latina y el Caribe.* Instituto Latinoamericano de las Naciones Unidas para la Prevención del Delito y Tratamiento del Delincuente (ILANUD). Siglo XXI editores.

Casey, W. M., Copp, J. E., & Bales, W. D. (2020). Releases from a local jail: The impact of visitation on recidivism. *Criminal Justice Policy Review,* 088740342091948. https://doi.org/10.1177/0887403420919480

Centro de Estudios Legales y Sociales (CELS). (2020). *COVID-19 y Sobrepoblación Carcelaria.* https://www.cels.org.ar/web/wp-content/uploads/2020/05/coronavirus-y-carceles.pdf

Cohen, S. (1979). The punitive city: Notes on the dispersal of social control. *Contemporary Crises, 3* (4), 339–363. https://doi.org/10.1007/BF00729115

Colectivo de Estudios de Drogas y Derecho (CEED). (2020). *Del Miedo a la Acción. Aliviar el Hacinamiento Carcelario: Salvar Vidas en Tiempos de COVID.* De Justicia (Editores). https://www.dejusticia.org/wp-content/uploads/2020/07/DMAA-2-CEDD-Nuevo2.pdf

Colegio Médicos de Chile. (2020). *Visita al Centro de Detención Preventiva Santiago Sur (Ex Penitenciaria) en el contexto de Pandemia Coronavirus COVID-19 en el marco de los Derechos Humanos.* Departamento Nacional de Derechos Humanos. http://www.colegiomedico.cl/wp-content/uploads/2020/03/INFORME-VISITA-DDHH-CDP-PTE-ALTO-2-ABRIL-2020_compressed.pdf

Dammert, L., & Zuñiga, L. (2008). *La cárcel: Problemas y desafíos para las Américas.* Facultad Latinoamericana de Ciencias Sociales (FLACSO).

Darke, S., & Karam, M. L. (2016). Latin American prisons. In Y. Jewkes, B. Crewe, & J. Bennett (Eds.), *Handbook on prisons* (pp. 460–474). Routledge.

Defensoría Penal Pública. (2020). *Discurso de Cuenta Pública del Defensor Nacional.* http://www.dpp.cl/resources/upload/files/documento/f3409870c30c2f3d7a5f0336dec284b5.pdf

Desantis, D., & Leira, J. (2020, July 26). *Latin America leads world in coronavirus cases, Reuters count shows.* Reuters. https://www.reuters.com/article/us-health-coronavirus-latin-america/latin-america-leads-world-in-coronavirus-cases-reuters-count-shows-idUSKCN24R0JL?emci=9d70c11e-02d0-ea11-9b05-00155d03bda0&emdi=dbf92327-03d0-ea11-9b05-00155d03bda0&ceid=4606001

Despliegan militares en Ciudad de Mexico tras retirar policias por COVID-19. (2020, April 14). *Agencia EFE.* https://www.efe.com/efe/america/mexico/despliegan-militares-en-ciudad-de-mexico-tras-retirar-a-policias-por-covid-19/50000545-4221294

Diario Oficial de la Federación (DOF). (2020). Secretaría de Gobernación. https://www.dof.gob.mx/nota_detalle.php?codigo=5592105&fecha=22/04/2020

Durnescu, I. (2011). Pains of Probation: Effective practice and human rights. *International Journal of Offender and Therapy and Comparative Criminology, 55*(4), 530–545. https://doi.org/10.1177/0306624X10369489

Duwe, G., & Clark, V. (2013). Blessed be the social tie that binds: The effects of prison visitation on of-fender recidivism. *Criminal Justice Policy Review, 24*(3), 271–296. https://doi.org/10.1177/0887403411429724

Salinero, S., & Morales, A. M. (2019). Las penas alternativas a la cárcel en Chile. Un análisis desde su evolución histórica. *Revista de derecho (Valparaíso),* (52), 255–292. https://doi.org/10.4067/S0718-68512019005000304

Gendarmería de Chile. (2018a). *Compendio Estadístico Penitenciario 2018.* Gendarmería de Chile, Ministerio de Justicia y Derechos Humanos, Gobierno de Chile. https://html.gendarmeria.gob.cl/doc/estadisticas/Compendio_Estadistico_Penitenciario_2018.pdf

Gendarmería de Chile. (2018b, April). *Presentación institucional en Mesa de Instituto de Estudios Judiciales*. [Power Point]. Gendarmería de Chile, Ministerio de Justicia y Derechos Humanos, Gobierno de Chile.

Gendarmería de Chile. (2020a). *Reporte diario de contagios y proceso de vacunación*. Gendarmería de Chile, Ministerio de Justicia y Derechos Humanos, Gobierno de Chile. https://www.gendarmeria.gob.cl/apisitio.gendarmeria.gob.cl/Api/SitioGendarmeria/informacion_covid_PDF?id_covidPDF=441

Gendarmería de Chile. (2020b). *Plan de Acción de Gendarmería para enfrenta al Coronavirus*. Gendarmería de Chile, Ministerio de Justicia y Derechos Humanos, Gobierno de Chile. https://www.gendarmeria.gob.cl/corona2020.html

Gendarmería de Chile. (2020c). *Comunicado de prensa, 6 de junio*. Gendarmería de Chile, Ministerio de Justicia y Derechos Humanos, Gobierno de Chile. https://www.gendarmeria.gob.cl/corona.html

Georgiou, G. (2014). Does increased post-release supervision of criminal offenders reduce recidivism? Evidence from a statewide quasi-experiment. *International Review of Law and Economics*, *37*, 221–243. https://doi.org/10.1016/j.irle.2013.12.001

Gobierno de Mexico. (2020). *COVID-19 en México*. https://coronavirus.gob.mx/datos/

Godoy, A. (2016). Ley No.20.603 sobre penal sustitutivas y mixtas: Revisión crítica de la historia de la ley y del acuerdo político legislativo que le dio origen. *Derecho y Justicia*, *6*, 29–69. https://doi.org/10.29344/07196377.6.1406

Hernandez, J. S. (2020, June 1). *Solicitamos a la Corte Consitucional ampliar el decreto de excarcelación elimando algunos apartados incostitucionales*. DeJusticia. https://www.dejusticia.org/solicitamos-a-la-corte-constitucional-ampliar-el-decreto-de-excarcelacion-eliminando-algunos-apartados-inconstitucionales/

Horwitz, L., Nagovitch, P., Sonneland, H., & Zissis, C. (2020, August 5). *The coronavirus in Latin America*. Americas Society Council of the Americas. https://www.as-coa.org/articles/coronavirus-latin-america

Hyatt, J., & Barnes, G. (2014). An experimental evaluation of the impact of intensive supervision the recidivism of high-risk probationers. *Crime and Delinquency*, *63*(1), 3–38. https://doi.org/10.1177/0011128714555757

Institute for Crime and Justice Policy Research (ICPR). (2019). *World prison brief*. Online Database. https://www.prisonstudies.org/world-prison-brief-data

Instituto Nacional de Estadística y Geografía (INEGI). (2019). *Censo Nacional de Gobierno, Seguridad Pública y Sistemas Penitenciarios Estatales*. https://www.inegi.org.mx/contenidos/programas/cngspspe/2019/doc/cngspspe_2019_resultados.pdf

Instituto Nacional Penitenciario y Carcelario (INPEC). (2019). *Informe Estadístico Población Reclusa a Cargo del INPEC No.12*. Oficina Asesora de Planeación, Grupo Estadística. https://www.inpec.gov.co/documents/20143/767956/INFORME+ESTADISTICO+DICIEMBRE.pdf/60c6810d-fb87-c7a2-b099-dff6bb6cca46?download=true

Instituto Nacional Penitenciario y Carcelario (INPEC). (2020a). *Situación actual de COVID-19*. Oficina Asesora de Planeación - Grupo Estadística, Instituto Nacional Penitenciario (INPEC), Ministerio de Justicia y del Derecho. https://www.inpec.gov.co/en/covid-19-establecimientos-inpec

Instituto Nacional Penitenciario y Carcelario (INPEC). (2020b). *Informe Estadístico No 2, Población privada de la libertad*. Ministerio de Justicia y el Derecho.

Inter-American Commission on Human Rights (IACHR). (2020). *The IACHR urges states to guarantee the health and integrity of persons deprived of liberty and their families in the face of the COVID-19 pandemic*. Organization of American States (OAS). https://www.oas.org/en/iachr/media_center/PReleases/2020/066.asp

Iturralde, M. (2019). Neoliberalism and its impact on Latin American crime control fields. *Theoretical Criminology*, *23*(4), 471–490. https://doi.org/10.1177/1362480618756362

Kinner, S. A., Young, Y. T., Snow, K., Southalan, L., Lopez-Acuña, D., Ferreira-Borges, C., & Moore, E. (2020). Prisons and custodial settings are part of a comprehensive response to COVID-19. *The Lancet Public Health*, *5*(4), e188–e189. https://doi.org/10.1016/S2468-667(20)30058-X

Klingele, C. (2013). Rethinking the use of community supervision. *Journal of Criminal Law and Criminology, 103*(4), 1015–1070. https://search-proquest-com.mutex.gmu.edu/docview/1494725057?accountid=14541

Latin America Public Opinion Project (LAPOP). (2019). *Support for harsher criminal punishment is greater among the young, the insecure, victims, and those with low trust in the police. Insight series #140*. Vanderbilt University. https://www.vanderbilt.edu/lapop/insights/IO940en.pdf

Limoncelli, K., Mellow, J., & Na, C. (2020). Determinants of intercountry prison incarceration rates and overcrowding in Latin America and the caribbean. *International Criminal Justice Review, 2*(1), 1–20. https://doi.org/10.1177/1057567719830530

Londoño, F. (2020). *¿Responsabilidad penal para los infractores de la cuarentena? Revisión crítica de los arts.* 318 y 318 bis del Código Penal (nueva ley nº 21.240): más micro que macro. www.criminaljusticenetwork.eu

Medidas complementarias al plan de contención del COVID-19 en centros penitenciarios y carcelarios del país. (2020, March 13). *Presidencia de la República*. https://id.presidencia.gov.co/Paginas/prensa/2020/Medidas-complementarias-al-plan-de-contencion-del-COVID-19-en-centros-penitenciarios-y-carcelarios-del-pais-200313.aspx

Ministerio de Defensa. (2020, April). *Circular 007 de 2020*. Ministerio de Defensa Nacional, Policía Nacional, Dirección General. https://www.policia.gov.co/sites/default/files/descargables/circular_no_007.pdf

Ministerio de Justicia. (2020, March). *Resolución 1144 de 22 de Marzo de 2020*. Ministerio de Justicia y del Derecho, Instituto Nacional Penitenciario yCarcelario (INPEC). http://www.suin-juriscol.gov.co/viewDocument.asp?ruta=Resolucion/30038994

Ministerio de Salud de Argentina, Reportes diarios sobre el Coronavirus. (2020). Reportes diarios de Coronavirus. https://www.sadi.org.ar/rss/item/1218-informe-diario-ministerio-de-salud-de-la-nacion-12-07-2020

Ministerio de Salud de Chile, Cifras oficiales sobre el Coronavirus. (2020). Ministerio de Salud de Chile. https://www.gob.cl/coronavirus/cifrasoficiales/

Ministerio de Salud de Colombia, Reportes diarios sobre el Coronavirus. (2020). Ministerio de Salud de Colombia. https://www.minsalud.gov.co/salud/publica/PET/Paginas/Covid-19_copia.aspx

Ministerio Público Provincia de Buenos Aires, Fuero Criminal y Correccional, IPP Iniciadas por Bien Jurídico Protegido Periodo 20 de Marzo al 25 de Junio años 2019 y 2020. (2020). Ministerio Público Provincia de Buenos Aires. https://www.mpba.gov.ar/files/content/ASPO%20-%20IPP%20FCC%20bien%20juridico%20protegido.pdf

Mitchell, M. M., Spooner, K., Jia, D., & Zhang, Y. (2016). The effect of prison visitation on reentry success: A meta-analysis. *Journal of Criminal Justice, 47*, 74–83. https://doi.org/10.1016/j.jcrimjus.2016.07.006

Montoya-Barthelemy, A. G., Lee, C. D., Cundiff, D. R., & Smith, E. B. (2020). COVID-19 and the correctional environment: The American prisons as a focal point for public health. *American Journal of Preventive Medicine, 58*(6), 888–891. https://doi.org/10.1016/j.amepre.2020.04.001

Morales, A. M., Pantoja, R., Piñol, D., & Sanchez, M. (2018). *Una Propuesta de Modelo Integral de Reinserción Social para Infractores de Ley*. Fundación Paz Ciudadana. http://www.cesc.uchile.cl/Modelo_ReinsercionSocial_CESC_FPC.pdf

Morris, N., & Tonry, M. (1990). *Between prison and probation. Intermediate punishments in a rational sentencing system*. Oxford University Press.

Müller, M. M. (2012). The rise of the penal state in Latin America. *Contemporary Justice Review, 15* (1), 57–76. https://doi.org/10.1080/10282580.2011.590282

Órgano Administrativo de Prevención y Readaptación Social del Gobierno Federal (OADPRS). (2020). Secretaría de Seguridad y Protección Ciudadana, Gobierno de Mexico. https://www.gob.mx/prevencionyreadaptacion

Pakes, F. (2020, April 20). Coronavirus: Why swathes of prisoners are being released in the world's most punitive states. The conversation. https://www.infobae.com/sociedad/2020/04/29/coronavirus-en-argentina-por-un-doble-efecto-ya-no-hay-sobrepoblacion-en-las-carceles-federales/

Payne, B., & Gainey, R. (1998). A qualitative assessment of the pains experienced on electronic monitoring. *International Journal of Offender Therapy and Comparative Criminology, 42*(2), 149–163. https://doi.org/10.1177/0306624X9804200207

Penal Reform International (PRI). (2020). *Coronavirus: Preventing harm and human rights violations in criminal justice systems.* https://cdn.penalreform.org/wp-content/uploads/2020/07/Coronavirus-briefing-July-2020.pdf

Phelps, M. (2013). The paradox of probation: Community supervision in the age of mass incarceration. *Law & Policy, 35*(1), 52–80. https://doi.org/10.1111/lapo.12002

Procuración Penitenciaria de la Nación (PPN). (2020). *La situación de la población privada de libertad ante la emergencia sanitaria por COVID-19.* Procuración Penitenciara de la Nación, Dirección General de Protección de Derechos Humanos, Observatorio de Cárceles Federales. https://www.ppn.gov.ar/pdf/boletines/ReporteestadisticoPPLCOVID19-3.pdf

Reyes, C. (2020, April 27). *No quieren salir de la cárcel: Más de 100 reos rechazan indulto para abandonar penales por coronavirus.* La Tercera. https://www.latercera.com/la-tercera-pm/noticia/no-quieren-salir-de-la-carcel-mas-de-100-reos-rechazan-indulto-para-abandonar-penales-por-coronavirus/PNUDTSGGORBB7FZMUDJQPLCSMQ/

Reyes, Y. (2020, July 14). *Hacinamiento carcelario y cuarentena.* El Espectador. https://main-elespectador-caracoltv.content.pugpig.com/2020/07/13/hacinamiento-carcelario-y-cuarentena-2/pugpig_index.html

Rhine, E., & Taxman, F. (2017). American exceptionalism in community supervision: A comparative analysis of probation in the United States, Scotland and Sweden. In K. Reitz (Ed.), *American exceptionalism in crime and punishment* (pp. 67–409). Oxford University Press.

Riaño, A. C., & Mora, S. L. C. (2019). Morbilidad en un centro penitenciario de Colombia. *Revista Facultad Ciencias De La Salud: Universidad Del Cauca, 21*(1), 16–22. https://dialnet.unirioja.es/descarga/articulo/7075876.pdf

Rochow, D., & Mateo, M. (2020, June 16). *La realidad de las cárceles en pandemia y la falta de información pública.* El Mostrador. https://www.elmostrador.cl/destacado/2020/06/26/la-realidad-de-las-carceles-en-pandemia-y-la-falta-de-informacion-publica/

Sánchez, M., & Piñol, D. (2015). *Condiciones de vida en los centros de privación de libertad en Chile.* Centro de Estudios en Seguridad Ciudadana (CESC). Universidad de Chile. https://www.cesc.uchile.cl/docs/CESC_condiciones_centros_privacion.pdf

Schönteich, M. (2014). *Presumption of guilt: The global overuse of pretrial detention.* Open Society Institute.

Secretaría de Seguridad y Protección Ciudadana (SSPC). (2020). *Protocolo de actuación para la atención de COVID-19 al interior de Centros Federales de Reinserción Social (CEFERESOS).* https://coronavirus.gob.mx/wp-content/uploads/2020/04/Protocolo_De_Actuacion_COVID-19_CEFERESOS.pdf

Sistema Nacional de Estadisticas sobre Ejecución de la Pena [SNEEP]. (2018). *nforme Anual. Ministerio de Justicia y Derechos Humanos.* https://www.argentina.gob.ar/sites/default/files/informe_sneep_argentina_2018.pdf

Sistema Penitenciario Federal (SPF). (2020). *Reporte diario de COVID-19.* Sistema Penitenciario Federal, Ministerio de Justicia de la Nación. http://www.spf.gob.ar/www/covid_diario/catcms/164/Reporte-diario-COVID-19

Steiner, B., Butler, H., & Ellison, J. (2014). Causes and correlates of prison inmate misconduct: A systematic review of the evidence. *Journal of Criminal Justice, 42*(6), 462–470. https://doi.org/10.1016/j.jcrimjus.2014.08.001

Sykes, G. M. (1958). *The society of captives: A study of a maximum security prison.* Princeton University Press.

Tamayo, T. (2016). *Incendio en la Torre 5. Las 81 muertes que Gendarmería quiere olvidar.* Ediciones B Chile.

Taxman, F. S. (2012). Probation, intermediate sanctions, and community-based corrections. In J. Petersilia & K. Reitz (Eds.), *Oxford handbook of sentencing and corrections* (pp. 363–385). Oxford University Press. https://doi.org/10.1093/oxfordhb/9780199730148.013.0015

Tribunal Superior de Justicia arranca programa justicia virtual ante COVID-19. (2020, June 9). *El Universal*. https://www.eluniversal.com.mx/metropoli/cdmx/tsj-arranca-programa-justicia-virtual-ante-covid-19

United Nations Development Program (UNDP). (2013). *Citizen security with a human face: Evidence and proposals for Latin America*. Regional Human Development Report 2013-2014.

United Nations Office on Drugs and Crime (UNODC). (2020). *UNODC, WHO, UNAIDS and OHCHR joint statement on COVID-19 in prisons and other closed settings*. World Health Organization (WHO). https://www.who.int/news-room/detail/13-05-2020-unodc-who-unaids-and-ohchr-joint-statement-on-covid-19-in-prisons-and-other-closed-settings

Vilalta, C., & Fondevila, G. (2019). *Prison populism in Latin America: Reviewing the dynamics of prison population growth. Igarape institute*. Strategic Note 32. https://igarape.org.br/en/prison-populism-in-the-americas/

Walmsley, R. (2018). *World prison population list* (12th ed.). Institute for Criminal Policy Research. https://www.prisonstudies.org/sites/default/files/resources/downloads/wppl_12.pdf

Wilenmann, J. (2020). Neoliberal politics and state modernization in Chilean penal evolution. *Punishment and Society*, *22*(3), 259–280. https://doi.org/10.1177/1462474519882974

World Health Organization (WHO). (2020). *Preparedness, prevention and control of COVID-19 in prisons and other places of detention*. World Health Organization (WHO), Regional Office for Europe, Copenhagen, Denmark. https://www.euro.who.int/__data/assets/pdf_file/0019/434026/Preparedness-prevention-and-control-of-COVID-19-in-prisons.pdf?ua=1

World Justice Project (WJP). (2018). *Mexico's new criminal justice system: Substantial progress and persistent challenges*. https://worldjusticeproject.org/sites/default/files/documents/WJP-NewJusticeSystemMexico_.pdf

Women Providing and Men Free Riding: Work, Visits and Gender Roles in Mexican Prisons

Carolina Agoff, Sveinung Sandberg, and Gustavo Fondevila

ABSTRACT

Facing the Covid-19 pandemic, prisons in Mexico City prohibited visits. This sparked clearly gendered protests: male prison inmates complained that the restrictions left them without resources to deal with prison shortages, while women complained that it prevented them from sending resources to their families. Based on data from life story interviews conducted before the pandemic, we explore visits, prison work, and gendered child-rearing practices in Mexican prisons. We argue that incarcerated mothers adopt a provider role in prison, in contrast to incarcerated fathers, who abandon this traditionally masculine fatherhood role. Suspension of visits thus have distinctly gendered consequences.

Introduction

On February 27, 2020, the first person infected with Covid-19 was reported in Mexico City. The man, who had traveled from Italy, was admitted to the City's National Institute of Respiratory Diseases (INER).[1] Three weeks later, on March 20, 2020, quarantine began with the official suspension of school activities.[2] One month later there were already 131 confirmed cases and 4 deaths. At the start of the pandemic, the criminal justice system implemented a 4-phase protocol for prisons: prevention, early case identification and isolation, identification of disease severity, and evacuation.[3] Within a few days, 20 suspected Covid-cases were detected in prisons, leading to the implementation of stricter measures. Among these, and most importantly, was the suspension of family visits.[4] With an average of 10,000 daily visits to state prisons (including suppliers, lawyers, family members, etc.), this was a significant interruption of prison life. It also raised concerns for unrest as in 2009, when visits were suspended during the AH1N1 influenza epidemic, riots had broken out in 5 prisons.

Indeed, to date, there have been a series of protests over the suspension of visits in Mexican prisons, with significant differences between the complaints emanating from the male prison inmates and the female ones. The suspension of visits affected both populations, but in men's prisons, inmates complained that they had lost access to resources supplied during visits, while women protested that the lack of visits meant that they had no way of providing their families (and especially children) with the resources they were able to generate in prison. We will argue, and demonstrate, that these differences in protest motivations reveal highly gendered child-caring and child-rearing practices, as well as important gendered differences in prison work and prisoner roles in Mexico.

Historically, women prisoners have received less attention in criminological studies than men (Greer, 2000; Pollock, 2002). In recent years, however, a growing body of literature has compared the adjustment of incarcerated men and women (Jiang & Winfree, 2006, p. 33). In this paper, we use literature on gendered prisonization processes to understand work, visits, and child-rearing practices within Mexican prisons. We explain the difference in the objections to the Covid-19 measures with the help of life story interviews conducted before the outbreak of the pandemic. We suggest that women with children adopt a traditionally masculine provider role in prison, by sending money to their families and children, while in contrast, male prisoners abandon this conventional provider role and receive money and other goods from their families.

Mexican prisons, Covid-19 and visits

On April 11, prison authorities in Mexico confirmed the first six cases of Covid-19 in the country's prisons: five in the Penitentiary and Social Reintegration Center of Cuautitlán (State of Mexico), and one in the Center for Social Reintegration in Mérida (Yucatán). The outbreak in the Cuautitlán prison was particularly concerning, as it is one of the most overcrowded prisons in the country.

On April 22, Congress approved an amnesty law[5] for those sentenced or prosecuted, at the federal level, for the crimes of abortion, homicide due to kinship, crimes against health, simple robbery, sedition, and finally for any crime committed by indigenous people who were sentenced without the presence of interpreters or defense attorneys with knowledge of their language or culture. Although the amnesty aimed to relieve pressure on the penitentiaries, in reality, it was relatively ineffectual as it only applied to 7% of the total population of 43,255 inmates in federal prisons, which also only have 52.47% occupancy (Censo Nacional de Gobierno, Seguridad Pública y Sistema Penitenciario Estatales [CNGSPSPE], 2019). Although, on average, state prisons are not overcrowded (with 93.57% occupancy – capacity of 216,237 and 202,337 prisoners), 110 of the 297 prisons do show levels of overcrowding, reaching a peak of 472% in Chalco and 433% in Lerma (both in the State of Mexico). There was no amnesty at the state level, although some states accelerated the release of prisoners who were in the last stages of their sentences. For example, in Mexico City, the Judicial Power released 78 prisoners on humanitarian grounds in April,[6] and another 250 prisoners[7] were released by May.

In March, another measure was taken with the publication of the Action Protocol for the Care of Covid-19[8] in federal centers. States later published their own protocols that included basic recommendations such as implementing information campaigns, reinforcing sanitary measures, having an isolation area for possible cases, tightening health surveillance to detect cases, and considering restrictions on family visits. A third preventative measure was the restriction on or suspension of visits to social reintegration centers. At the federal level, the visiting system was not modified, but the vast majority of States adopted some type of measure, which included: a) restricting the number/days of visits (respecting social distancing); b) restricting contact (although visitors could leave food or objects for their relatives); or c) total suspension of visits. The latter was applied in April to the highest risk prisons, such as the Cuautitlán prison (State of Mexico),[9] where 23 inmates were found to have coronavirus symptoms. Four of these cases were later confirmed and 19 inmates were transferred to Neza Norte suspected of being infected, which had been set up as a hospital to serve prisoners with Covid-19. The suspension of visits was later extended to other prisons and states, such as Guanajuato and Veracruz.[10]

In this study we are particularly interested in the consequences of the restrictions on visits for the prison population. There are different types of visits: family, intimate, family inter-prison units and visits from children in the charge of some welfare institution. It is calculated that on average, 3,500 people per day pass through federal prisons, a number that increases on holidays (Protocolo de actuación para la atención de Covid-19 al interior de Centros Federales de Reinserción Social [PAACEFERESOS], 2020). Suspension of visits is not a trivial measure as visits are not only prisoners' emotional connection with their loved ones, but also a source of economic and material resources. Visitors in Mexico bring a range of items to the prisons: food, water, clothing, hygiene items, materials for making crafts, money, and so on. This is particularly important given the serious deficiencies in the provision of basic commodities in Mexican prisons. According to *Diagnóstico Nacional de Supervisión Penitenciaria* ("National Diagnostic of Penitentiary Supervision" – DNSP, 2019b) of the National Human Rights Commission (CNDH), state penitentiary centers have: insufficient personnel (72.68%), insufficient work and training activities (66.84%), poor material conditions, insufficient equipment and hygiene in the dormitory areas (62.84%), and a deficiency of health services (32.79%) (DNSP, 2019b).

Some of these deficiencies are covered by families when visiting, and "70% of the inmates depend entirely on supplies and resources provided by their relatives, from personal hygiene items to money to pay other prisoners to guarantee their well-being".[11] With the suspension of visits, prisoners lost access to resources and faced a much more expensive and inaccessible black market. For example, shortages and drastic price increases were reported for cleaning products.[12] In many Mexican prisons, inmates are responsible for cleaning their own cells, and for acquiring the necessary equipment to do so. During epidemics, basic hygiene becomes especially important, but also more difficult due to the lack or cost of soap and other cleaning equipment.

The prison population in Mexico is relatively young (32% are between 18 and 29 years of age and 35.3% are between 29 and 39), with basic levels of education (72.1%), economic dependents at the time of arrest (70.3%), or dependent children (64.1%). There are usually more than 5 prisoners per cell (51.1%) and inmates often do not receive even the most basic items from the prison system. For example, only very few report receiving clothing (25%), blankets (21%), footwear (8.9%) and personal hygiene items (7.6%). The prison population therefore depends on work inside the prisons or on visits to obtain these resources (Encuesta Nacional de Población Privada de la Libertad [ENPOL], 2016). The lack of basic commodities during incarceration is generally problematic, but becomes even more critical when visits are suspended, as occurred during the coronavirus pandemic.

The suspension of visits thus significantly impacts the quality of life of prisoners and regularly causes protests by inmates and their families. The National Human Rights Commission (CNDH) designed and implemented the "National Monitoring Mechanism for Covid-19 in Penitentiary Centers"[13] that detected "the existence of acts and/or events of protest, riots, and other expressions of violence"[14] in the country's prisons. On April 15, the first incident was reported in the Cuautitlán prison (Edomex), with prisoners refusing to return to their cells after recess in protest against the cancellation of family visits. Outside the prison, a group of family members protested for the same reason, and clashed with approximately 200 riot police.[15] These protests began to spread to other penitentiary centers, such as Barrientos, in Tlalnepantla; Chiconautla in Ecatepec, Neza Bordo in Nezahualcóyotl, Huitzilingo in Chalco, Molino de Flores in Texcoco, Tepachico in Otumba, and Zumpango".[16]

Women, work and children in Mexican prisons

Women represent only 4.6% of the total prison population (ENPOL, 2016). According to prison statistical information (INEGI, 2019, p. 54), prisoners perform the following formal jobs: basic level teachers (599), operators of construction elements, equipment and electrical installations (774), painters, designers, artistic draftsmen, sculptors and set designers (3,706), *maquiladora*[17] workers (10,844), cleaners (17,025), artisans (52,894) and others *maquila.* (22,646). Within this spectrum, women are assigned gendered kitchen tasks, laundry, weaving, sewing, and crafts (Luna et al., 2003). In addition, there are countless informal jobs that prisoners undertake, ranging from washing other prisoners' clothes, bringing water and cooking, to writing love letters for other inmates (Ríos Miranda, 2014).

This context of deprivation and formal or informal jobs is particularly difficult for incarcerated women because most of them are mothers: 89.1% of women in prison have dependent children compared to 62.9% of men (ENPOL, 2016). In most cases they do not have a spouse who shares responsibility for their children. In Mexico, the age limit for minors to remain with their mothers in reclusion is set at three, and women can only have two children living with them at any given time. Men do not have these rights. This is indicative of the highly gendered organizational logic of prisons, which for example, only provides infrastructure for children in women's prisons, and programs of physical exercise (Britton, 1997) or sport (Baumer & Meek, 2018) in men's prisons. The penitentiary system have highly gendered expectations of prisoners and thereby conveys a strong gender message. For men, exercising responsible paternity, including involvement in childcare, thus implies confronting a prison apparatus that reinforces traditional gender roles.

Conditions for children who live with their mothers in prison are precarious: they do not have their own bed (they sleep with their mother), they share cells with other inmates, and they are not provided with food, diapers or clothing. Mothers remain responsible for meeting these needs, in whatever way they can afford. Occasionally charitable organizations help inmates through donations (Diagnóstico Nacional de Supervisión Penitenciaria, 2019a). Because minors are not allowed to remain in the prisons beyond the age of 3, they are subsequently taken care of by relatives. Most of the women who live with children in prison have other children who have been left with female family members, such as grandmothers, aunts, or sisters. In the event that women do not have the support of partners or family to take care of their children, the criminal justice administration chooses an institution that will.

Children in prison represent a great challenge for penitentiary institutions (Palomar, 2007) as there is normally no special budget for child support. Prisons thus need to adjust their budget (when a new minor enters) to cover the extra food service: breakfast, lunch and dinner. However, milk, diapers, blankets, clothing and footwear, as well as hygiene items, remain the responsibility of the incarcerated mothers. Prisons are also not equipped with reserved areas for pregnant women or single mothers and the children who live with them, nor do they have special staff members to care for or monitor the comprehensive development of the children. The only exclusive space for the care of minors are the Child Development Centers (Cendi), but not all women's prisons have such a center. Furthermore, facilities (classrooms and furniture), teaching resources and staff are insufficient to attend to the 618 minors who live with their mothers in prisons in Mexico City (ENPOL, 2016). There is also a lack of specialized personnel such as pediatric doctors, social workers, psychologists and child psychiatrists.

Gender and imprisonment

According to Zingraff (1980, p. 275) and Kruttschnitt et al. (2000, p. 681), literature on the gendered prisonization process offers two classic models for explaining responses to the deprivations of imprisonment. The functionalist tradition understands the adaptation of behavior to prison as a reaction to the coercion of the penitentiary institution (Sykes, 1958; Wilson, 1968), while the importation tradition focuses on experiences prior to confinement and the subcultures outside of prison to understand prisoners adaptive behavior (Irwin, 1970). Since the 1960s, both models have explained gendered differences in adaptation to prison (for example, Ward & Kassebaum, 1965). These results were later confirmed by other similar studies, such as that of Giallombardo (1966) and Hefferman (1972), and more recently, those of Alarid (1997). In contemporary research these models have been integrated, with the understanding that gender is not a "monolithic experience nor an inflexible identity". They have also increasingly acknowledged the diversity in men and women's experiences in prison (Kruttschnitt et al., 2000, p. 683). For example, there are many in-prison factors (overcrowding, violence, confinement, length of sentence, etc.) as well as out-prison factors (age, race, economic level, etc.) that influence gendered responses to imprisonment.

Gendered responses to imprisonment can be seen in relation to other inmates and to the family outside of prison (especially children). Men for example, generally tend to "cut loose" from family relationships, while women strive to maintain these ties as best they can (Hart, 1995; Pollock, 2002). Most studies indicate that there is a fundamental gender difference in the way that imprisoned parents relate to their children. Jiang and Winfree (2006, p. 37), state that "incarcerated fathers rarely exhibit concern about their children´s fate", perhaps because they know that the children's mothers or family will take care of them. Women seem to be more aware of the emotional harm caused to their children by their imprisonment, and acknowledge that their imprisonment is a burden on families already struggling with limited resources (Dodge & Pogrebin, 2001). Incarcerated women for example, typically feel frustration and guilt over not being able to take care of their children (Bloom & Chesney-Lind, 2000).

The main concern of many women prisoners is the fate of their children's, reporting that it is "the hardest part of doing time" (Kruttschnitt et al., 2000, p. 711), while men rarely report such feelings (but see Sandberg et al., 2020). Separation from children is painful for men too, but they are usually able to discharge their role as provider to the mother (if she is not imprisoned) or to her family, whereas this is more difficult for women who were single-parents before their incarceration (Datesman & Cales, 1983, p. 142). These gender differences in inmates' relationships with their children are reflected in prison visits. According to

Hairston (1990, p. 26), fathers receive far fewer visits from their children than mothers do. Women get more visits from children and grandmothers, while more "wives and girlfriends" are coming to see the men (Pollock, 2002, p. 111). Arguably, lack of contact with children affects men and women differently, and for imprisoned mothers, the loss of their children is one of the greatest stressors of their life in prison (Harris, 1993, p. 53).

In this study, we explore life story interviews conducted with incarcerated mothers and fathers in Mexican prisons before the coronavirus pandemic, to better understand the impact of the suspension of visits in these penitentiaries. We argue that the restrictions imposed may have affected not only the visits that serve to diminish the "pains of imprisonment" (Sykes, 1958), but also prisoners' (especially women's) opportunities for parenting while in prison. The measures taken in Mexican prisons to avoid the spread of Covid-19 highlight some important gender differences and parenting roles between imprisoned mothers and fathers in Mexico. Our study suggests that Covid-19 measures may have very different consequences for women and men in prison, as well as for their families and children.

Materials and method

Data in this study are from life story interviews with incarcerated fathers and mothers in two Mexico City prisons. The interviews formed part of a larger qualitative research project with the overall goal of investigating imprisonment and life-trajectories of Mexican offenders. In total, 24 inmates (12 women and 12 men) were interviewed between January and July of 2019. The interviews were conducted before the pandemic. They inform this study by opening up for understanding the background for the gendered protests to the visits restriction introduced during the Covid-19 crisis. Interviews contextualize what male and female prison inmates may experience in the face of restrictions and explain the gendered challenges of the pandemic for imprisoned parents in Mexican prisons.

Interviews were repeated, on average 3 interviews per inmate, with each session lasting approximately 2 hours. The interviews were conducted in rooms used for workshops, without the presence of guards and at a time chosen by the respondents. A group consisting of a coordinator and an interviewer requested authorization from prison unit directors to interview the prisoners. Participants were contacted through purposeful sampling (Patton, 1990) and selected based on the criteria of being mothers or fathers, but otherwise representing a variety of crimes, convictions and ages. Respondents were explained the objectives of the study, informed consent was obtained and strict confidentiality was maintained. Four of the inmates contacted had no interest in participating.

Participants in this study vary in age, income, and education, but all had children, and all were born in Mexico or were Mexican nationals. They were convicted prisoners and had been in prison for at least one year, for a variety of crimes. The interviews were semi-structured and organized as life story interviews (Atkinson, 1998), covering participants' lives from childhood to the present. The flexible research design and repeated interviews allowed participants to emphasize the topics most important to them. Family relations was one such topic, particularly their relationship with their own children. We obtained extensive data on parenting roles and practices, from both before and during their time in prison. Another important topic was prison conditions and the work they did while in prison. An interviewer audio recorded the interviews (with participants' permission) and then transcribed them. During transcription, we removed identifying information such as their names (the ones provided below are aliases) and the particularities of their crime as well as other identifying information.

Data analysis

Data collected in interviews were analyzed by an interdisciplinary group of researchers. We used thematic analysis and constant comparison to identify primary analytic themes, and transcripts were entered into ATLAS.ti (version 2008) to facilitate data management. The categories were produced in two iterative data coding and analysis processes: first identifying a set of emergent categories, and then developing the final themes for this paper. The categories for the initial coding scheme were inductively drawn from the interviews and then refined through peer discussions of key themes concepts identified in the research literature about for example, life-course criminology and parenting roles in prison. Thus, categories were both data-driven and theoretically informed. In this initial analysis we coded broadly for a variety of categories, such as "care-taker", "relationship to children before prison", "relationship to children in prison", "work in prison", " violence in prison", " prison conditions" and others (a total of 16 codes). The initial coding of data was done before the Covid-19 pandemic, and included a wide variety of categories that might be potentially interesting later on in the research process. The second stage of coding took place after Covid-19 and involved rereading and recoding interviews and initial categories for the analysis and argument in this paper; most importantly "visits and deficiencies in Mexican prisons", "work in prison" and "gendered expectations for parenting while in prison".

Relationship to children was important in all interviews, more abstractly for men (Sandberg et al., forthcoming) and in more practical terms for women (Sandberg et al., 2020). Women also tended to speak more extensively about their children. The emphasis on children in the interviews with women probably reflects the importance of motherhood for women, including or maybe especially, for marginalized women (Grundetjern, 2018). It is also possible that this was influenced by gender dynamics in the interviews. Interviews were conducted by a 48-year-old woman with extensive experience in interviewing people at risk (prisoners, street children, victimized women, etc). Relationships with children, and family relations more generally, might have been a "natural" emphasis in these conversations. In all cases, respondents were given the opportunity to express themselves freely on the issues raised in the interviews. Only interpretations were included that the research team coincided on, assuming a certain "truth by agreement" in the analysis. The interviewer also checked the interpretations to ensure that they represented what had been expressed by the respondents and to identify any gaps that needed to be addressed. In some cases, a triangulation with other sources of data was done to either support our interpretations, or to account for alternative explanations.

The study has 24 interviews, and the standard limitations of qualitative methods (e.g., selection bias, random results). The positionality of the interviewer (women in her forties) might have toned down "macho" and "street-wise" identities in interviews, and self-selection to participate might have left out participants with particular experiences or characteristics (but only four rejected to participate). The qualitative study design, was purposive, and has important strengths that were particularly important for this research:

Repeated life story interviews give time for participants to reflect on their life between interviews, for an interviewer to prepare follow-up questions, and for both to get to know each other better than in one-time interviews. Building trust between interviewer and interviewee is pivotal, especially when themes include highly stigmatized practices such as child rearing under difficult circumstances. Prisoners parenting and relationship to family is also complex, with nuances and subtleties that cannot be captured in surveys or through other research designs. Repeated qualitative interviews are therefore especially suitable to explore the different gendered consequences of coronavirus measures in Mexican prisons, especially regarding the possible consequences of the suspension of visits.

Results

In the qualitative analysis below, we analyze gendered parental responses to imprisonment. Particularly the gendered forms of confronting prison deficiencies in Mexico City, in relation to the family (work and visits); the greater restrictions imposed as a result of Covid-19 (prohibition on visits); and the gendered effects of these restrictions. We begin by describing prison deficiencies and the role of visits for the prisoners in this study. We then provide an overview of the types of work available in prison in order to cover these deficiencies. Finally, we turn to our main argument, which is a suggestion that imprisoned men and women spend the income generated from prison work differently, and that visits fulfill different roles for them.

Visits and deficiencies in Mexican prisons

In the overcrowded and under-resourced conditions of state and municipal prisons, restricting visits means much more than losing the sociability of affection and community ties (Fuller, 1993). In Mexico, inmates receive money or objects through visits that are not provided by the prison system. The incarcerated mothers and fathers in this study all said that they did not get their basic needs covered by the prison. Elsa, for example, emphasized that "soap and bleach is the basic thing you should buy here". Reference was seldom made to luxuries, but rather, to necessities and small things that make life in prison a little easier:

Gabriela: Here if you don't work, you don't die of hunger, but you need more things. They give food, right? But you need sanitary napkins, shampoo, toothpaste, a brush.

Benito: To have my soap, my razor, because I also bathe. Then the food they give here they give you tea, but without sugar, you have to buy your sugar, they give you food, but without salt.

Typically, family members provide toiletries and food, or the money for inmates to buy these products themselves. Inmates in Mexican prisons need either the support from family or prison work to cover their basic needs, as there are many deficiencies.

María: They say it is the most expensive hotel and really it is the most expensive hotel. Everything costs money, even toilet paper, for everything you have to give money. You want to go to court in sneakers, you have to pay for shoelaces. A blanket to avoid being cold costs ten pesos. You want to rent a frying pan; it costs ten pesos. You want to listen to music, you must pay, you want to watch TV you must pay.

Ignacio: It is more expensive to live in prison. I pay here to use the phone, for soda, for the "support" of prison guards (bribes), coffee, bread, all that. I have been spending a minimum of 70, 80 pesos a day.

In Mexican prisons, everything must be paid for, from basic necessities to more luxury goods or bribes, for example, paying the guards to take prisoners to the doctor. However, even with money, it can be difficult, due to the scarcity of basic goods inside prison:

Cristina: About two months ago there was an epidemic of lice and I with my long hair, said "oops, oops, oops". Then I went out to cry at one of the visitors and I said 'forgive me, but the truth is that I don't want to have lice, please "help me". They brought me a gift and I gave them money. I'm not sorry saying "you know what, I wash your clothes, but give me soap, because I stink like a dead dog", I don't feel sorry.

Cristina did not feel the need to apologize for begging for help, since supplies in prison were so limited. This is a commonly used strategy in non-pandemic times. In some cases, when inmates do not have money, they use other means to get what they need. For example, in the absence of financial support from relatives, they may enlist the help of other inmates. But such help comes at a cost, often in an exchange of favors or services in a gift economy (Mauss, 1970), or even from begging. Talking about a companion, Dolores explained how a mother with a child met their needs:

Dolores: Since she entered, she lost contact with her daughter's father and does not have the support of her family; for this reason, in order to obtain some income, she sells sweets and cigarettes to the visitors, while her daughter asks for money from the relatives of the inmates who come on visiting days.

Women seem to face particular difficulties instead. Not only do they have extra costs, but men appear to get more help from their families. Many men, for example, emphasized that they did not only eat *rancho* (food from the prison service), which was of poor quality, but got their mothers to bring them food in prison.

Daniel: Every Saturday and Sunday, my mom brings me food for the week.

Interviewer: And where do you keep it?

Daniel: In some refrigerators.

Interviewer: And how much is the rent?

Daniel: About 5 pesos, per day.

The incarcerated men admitted that they would not starve with the food provided by the prison, but pointed out that getting extra food supplies increased their health and well-being. Such patterns were not a particular or unique adaption to prison life (Wilson, 1968), but rather, an importation of gender patterns established prior to imprisonment and reproduced in the deprivation conditions of prison. The men continue to take the role of "children" (of their mothers), despite the fact that they were adults and had their own children (Datesman & Cales, 1983). For example, Antonio, an incarcerated father who had been in prison for 20 years, said: *"My mother leaves me food on Sundays and the other days*

I eat "rancho". Such statements highlight the role that mothers play in the lives of their sons in Mexico, a role that seems to be reinforced when men go to prison.

Braulio: Here in jail your wife, your dad, your brothers, your children can leave you, but your mom is never going to leave you. She's always at the foot of the canyon, always(...) At first, she made weekly visits, maybe the first few months, but afterward they faded out a little (...) I told my mom when I started working in prison, "look I'm already working, don't worry, if you want to come every 15–20 days, it's ok".

This pattern of mothers looking after their sons in prison, often more than they support their daughters, is deeply rooted in gender inequality and patriarchal cultures. It has severe and problematic consequences for incarcerated women, especially for those with children.

In the meager conditions of Mexican prisons, women also have greater needs than men. In addition to items needed by both (food, clothing, soap), there are a range of women-specific products (sanitary towels, tampons, contraceptives). Furthermore, when mothers live with their children in prison, they must also cover the extra expenses that this entails (diapers, special food, etc.). These gender specific needs generally go unnoticed by the prison system due to the low female prison population. In Mexico City, as elsewhere in Mexico, prisons tend to be organized administratively, according to the needs of men (Azaola & José, 1996; Briseño, 2006; Giacomello, 2013). This is made worse by the patriarchal society outside of prison, and its highly differentiated expectations of men and women concerning children. Following these gendered patterns, prisons authorities expects women to fulfill a specific gender role (to take care of their children) that is not demanded of the men. Prison thus not only reproduce external social conditions of gender, but also reinforce them.

Work in prison

In state prisons, authorities allow some form of work, making it possible for prisoners to make an income while being incarcerated. This is not an opportunity for all prisoners, since it is part of a system of privileges and punishments implemented by the institution (Montoya, 2015, p. 190), but some inmates for example, get irregular jobs in the textile They are possibly the most privileged and often feel lucky to receive a salary, despite poor working conditions and worker exploitation:

Cristina: I worked making boxes (...) and many of them do not pay even the minimum salary.

Interviewer: And how many hours of work?

Cristina: It was from 8 in the morning to 6 in the afternoon, they gave me 80 pesos. They did not pay me daily, they gave it to me at the end of the week, it's really nothing.

Another form of work approved by the prison authorities allows mothers with children to offer various services on visiting days (four days a week). They assist by carrying bags or offering chairs to visitors, they act as waitresses for which they earn tips, rent blankets for visitors to sit on the floor, and offer products such as sweets, cigarettes or snacks for their companions' visitors ("basking"). All these represent a welcome opportunity to earn money:

Bety: I work here in the big room, "basking", carrying the bags to the bedrooms and as a waitress.

Gabriela: Blankets are for everything where there is a wall to sit; obviously who pays for the blanket is the one with the most resources, right? Because they can charge it at 10, at 15 to 30 pesos for one.

The women have to be assigned to "basking" by prison authorities, and women with children are prioritized. This illustrates how the institution expects women with children to assume a provider role, while not expecting the same of the men. Other work is also available to those inmates with the necessary resources. An informal, but accepted, job in prison is trading all kinds of commodities, with the supply often coming from family members during visiting hours:

Verónica: I sell telephone cards, I sell underwear. I have a girl who helps me. So, I have the merchandise on Sunday, I deliver and they pay me. The same Sunday I run out of merchandise.

Xochitl: Yes, I do thank my mother very much, because it was always like that and she brought me ice, juices, water, in winter she brought coffee, tea, hot food, also fruit. She is always seeing what I need, and what I don't need can be sold here. So, thanks to her I have something to help myself.

By providing commodities that can be sold within the prison, supportive family networks are important for the welfare of inmates. Differences between being in prison and outside (where family networks are also crucial) are therefore less notable in Mexico than in prison systems where inmates can rely on getting their basic needs covered by the prison authorities. However, in some cases, the supply of goods to be sold in prison comes from trading companies, cooperating with inmates and using prison visiting hours to expand their business:

Francisco: Right now, my means of providing for myself is by selling bread and coffee. The days I sell the most are Monday, Tuesday and Saturday, to visitors. In fact, with that sale sometimes I even support myself for the week, because in here, very little sells, here the prices have to be very cheap, for people who have few resources.

Interviewer: And where do you get it from?

Francisco: Outside, there is a trading company, which is the one that monopolizes the distribution of all supplies within the prison. So, you have to do it, from the catalog they teach you, bring me so many pieces of these.

Prisoners can also sell products that are produced in the various workshops. These training workshops reflect a social reintegration ideology, according to which inmates can learn a useful trade for when they obtain their freedom. The workshops are typically gendered, and those offered to women often refer to "styling" (nails, eyelashes, hairdressing), cooking, or making boxes and bags. Dora for example, said that "here we have a chocolate course, though right now I'm learning how to do nails and make stuffed animals". Again, family networks and visiting hours play an important role. Families can, for example, receive the products made by the inmates and sell them outside of prison:

Irma: In the workshops that they give us here, we're taught how to work with rhinestones, with raffia, nail beauty, I say all that I like, that is to say, I can get it all from here, because I have really worked here and my husband has sold it and with what we have, we have come out ahead, we have sold boats, boxes, bags and thank God everything is sold by us.

Men also attend workshops to generate income within the prison in order to cover the deficiencies of the prison system. (These workshops were also suspended due to the pandemic, exacerbating the men's dependence on their families.) Some of these are similar to those of women, such as workshops where they learn certain crafts and produce goods that they can later sell:

José: There are workshops to learn how to make monkeys with papier mâché, or dolls with soap, make lamps, notebooks, woven or paper handbags.

Interviewer: Where do they sell this?

José: Here during the visits. But very few people come. The ones who buy the most are the lawyers.

While there may be opportunities to produce goods in prison, the market for selling these is generally limited, so it is hardly a lucrative business.

Those prisoners who do not receive money from their relatives or from products sold inside the prison, and who do not have access to more formal jobs or workshops, can offer services to other prisoners who are able to afford them. These services include, for example, cleaning, doing laundry, or cooking:

Gabriela: I have always washed other people's clothes, doing chores, I have washed blankets and I have scrubbed.

Cristina: There are people who want me to wash their clothes or to clean them, they don't give me money, they give me toilet paper, soap, shampoo and with that my basic needs are met.

Hilario: An inmate next to me was about 29, 30 years old, already older than me (...) I was his servant, I was the one who did his things, washed his clothes, his sneakers; he had money (...) I charged the phones. Then he would give me 100, 150, 200, give me shoes, clothes, etc.

These kinds of jobs are considered to be the lowest rung in the hierarchy of prison work, reflecting work hierarchies elsewhere (Duffy, 2007). Being someone's servant, washing their clothes, making their bed and so on, is regarded as lowly work both within and outside prison. Obviously, these types of jobs are more easily accepted by women than men, as, once again, they reproduce external standards of gender.

The incarcerated mothers and fathers in this study work hard to compensate for the lack of basic goods in prison, and sometimes to make money to send to family and children on the outside. They do a variety of work while in prison. They may hold more formal jobs, such as in a textile *maquila*, or have particular positions such as offering services to visitors; participate in a vibrant internal prison market with goods purchased from outside or provided by family members; sell products produced in a wide variety of workshops; or offer services to other prisoners who have more money. This is sometimes an economy based on the use of money, but just as often, it is a complex gift or exchange economy.

Whatever form the market exchanges take, it is crucial for the welfare of the prisoners, and sometimes for that of their families outside of prison as well.

Gendered expectations for parenting while in prison

Both women and men have many expenses while in prison, but as there is a greater social expectation for women to look after their children, their expenses were often higher than those of men. Social expectations of mothering appear to exert such a strong influence on social identity and self-image (Rich, 1986), that regardless of their circumstances, these imprisoned Mexican mothers seem to make every effort to fulfil these expectations and feel guilty if they are unable to (Bloom & Chesney-Lind, 2000). One incarcerated mother, who live with her son in prison, said that she worked hard to:

Gabriela: (...) be able to pay for my and my son's expenses here. I have a visit every six months, but even when they come, they don't bring me anything, right? There are many girls who have visitors bringing them things, but I don't. For my son, the burden of the things I need for him now is lighter, but at the beginning, I had to pay 350 pesos every night for milk and diapers. And besides, I had to pay for water, soap, bleach, toothpaste, toilet paper, sanitary towels, yogurt, porridge, carrots, vegetables, and so on.

In a prison system where inmates' basic needs are not covered, and conditions are generally skewed toward men so that women must also cover the expenses of their children living with them, there is a lot of pressure to find ways to make money. The mothers in this study also talked about the difficulties of providing for their children outside of prison.

Elsa: Three thousand pesos. I save money to send home and the rest to pay what I owed. I gave money to my mom and the rest I kept. Actually, of all that money I just keep 100 pesos for myself.

Semiri: There are girls who obviously have money and they don't get their hands dirty, so I come in there, I get them dirty for them. They pay me for that and I live on that, thank God, it's not a lot of money but at least I have something to give to my mom and my son.

The profits obtained from working in the textile *maquilas*, in workshops, or from selling goods or services in prison often allow women to provide for their family outside the prison, although even so, their families were sometimes still not satisfied (Sandberg et al., 2020, p. 9). Such expectations can be demanding and earning money while imprisoned is not easy. Nevertheless, in general, being able to provide for their children and family was a source of great pride for the incarcerated women. Their effort to cover their children's needs, despite imprisonment, became a source of identity and a way to recover their self-esteem. This attitude allowed them to position themselves with a new strength: despite committing a crime and their imprisonment, they could still be good mothers. (The Covid-19 restrictions have hindered this ability to be "good mothers" from prison).

Gabriela: I was very proud of myself, because my mom came, right, I gave her 500 pesos from the work that I have done here. I said to her: you can have it; you are going to need it after your operation. "Those days when you are not going to be able to work, you are going to need money. I told her: don't worry, I will not run out of food here, don't worry about that. You have taken care of my daughters, you have been with me, and I earned this money with the sweat of my brow".

From the interviews in this study, it appears that imprisoned Mexican women are expected to continuously support their children, both outside and inside prison. Men, on the other hand, seem to leave the responsibility of their children's care to mothers and families outside of prison. This was illustrated in the Covid –19 protests. While men were unhappy about their loss of access to resources, women complained that they were unable to help their children.

The incarcerated fathers often asked their families for help in taking care of their children in addition to the support for themselves. For example, one father of five, relied entirely on his family's support:

Daniel: The first thing that helped me a lot was the support of my family. My parents, my brothers, all are those who have been aware of my children, what they lack, what they need, because it is not easy to give them money, there are very, very low wages here.

Another father, who had been in prison for 11 years, admitted to never having worked while inside. He was supported by his family (mother and sister), while his wife provided for his children:

Hector: My family helps me, they bring me my things, everything they can to help. My mom is already 80 years old or older and comes to visit me and brings me my things

Interviewer: Have you never done a job that paid for it?

Hector: No

Interviewer: Didn't you have that need?

Hector: No, thank God no, my sisters are professionals. I have a sister who is single and she is the strong one, she is the one who contributes almost everything, my mom helps me. My wife works for the children, I cannot demand more of her.

He had never considered working to support his children, like most of the mothers do (Jiang & Winfree, 2006). There seems to be less pride and self-esteem associated with being a provider for men than for women, and it did not seem to be an important source of identity. Instead, the fathers highlighted the emotional connection to their children (Sandberg et al., forthcoming). In fact, rather than taking on their economic responsibilities as fathers, it appears relatively easy for the men to assume the role of victims that are in need of help from their families. (The Covid-19 measures have impacted the opportunities prisoners families have to provide such care).

Another inmate, Augusto, said that the mother of his children and some neighbors came to visit him weekly, and he benefited from what they brought him: "So they are the ones who see me and bring me food, money, cards, I need nothing". Augusto even accepts support from the mother of his children, who also took care of them.

Most men count on family and relatives to provide for their children while they are in prison. The men's stories of work in prison mainly emphasize their concern for paying their own expenses. One father for example, when asked about the work he did in prison, assumed that the money he made would go toward his own expenses:

Interviewer: And who covers your expenses or how do you cover them?

Braulio: Well, selling crafts, sweets.

Interviewer: What crafts do you work on?

Braulio: Paintings, embossments.

Interviewer: And where do you sell them?

Braulio: Well, to visitors or family or acquaintances. So, that's how I pay my expenses.

In contrast with almost all the mothers, only three of the fathers in this study spoke about wanting to provide for their children from prison, and only two actually contributed, sporadically, to their children's expenses.

Juan: At the beginning when Laura was born and then José came, I tried to give them as much as I could, and I always bought them shoes, things, so that they did not have to look for it on the street. I said "what can I give my family, money to eat, walking shoes, clothes". I can't buy it here, but I try to support them with something.

Mario: I have been able to buy shoes for my daughter, I already bought a lamp for my son too. I mean, I also gave him money for his sneakers. Now it's only small expenses, but in prison, it is difficult to get (...) Before I used to spend the money on myself, that is, how much or how little I earned always focused on me and me. But not now, I have passed on from that, if my children enjoy it, it gives me a satisfaction, a totally different one from the one I had when I spent everything on myself.

These were the exception however, as generally, the men seemed less concerned with providing for their children than the women inmates. The men appeared to be able to rely on more support and help from family members than the women could. The women, in contrast, were expected to continue supporting their children even during their imprisonment, and the pandemic highlights how the institution makes no attempt to break these gender stereotypes. While the men in this study seemed to expect to support their children outside prison, in accordance with the traditional role of men as providers (Marks & Palkovitz, 2004), such expectations appear to be put on hold while they are in prison.

Discussion

Our data indicate the same gendered response in relation to the family outside of prison, and especially to children, as the literature on gendered prisonization indicates: When imprisoned, men break or put family relationships on hold, while women do their best to maintain these (Hart, 1995; Pollock, 2002). We further this research, by arguing that women prisoners, at least in this study from a Mexico City, prison seem to adopt a provider role for their children. This is made possible by the extensive formal and informal jobs available in many of these prisons. In addition to working to cover their own needs, which are not provided by the criminal justice authorities, they send money to their relatives to cover the costs of raising their children. Although our results are only explorative, and further and more systematic research is necessary, the opposite seems to be the case for men. Most of the men in this study work in prisons to fund their own needs, and if they struggle to cover these needs, they can often rely on help from their families. This gendered pattern is mirrored in the protests following the coronavirus measures in Mexican prisons: men complained of being cut off from access to goods brought to them by visitors, while women complained that the measure prevented them from sending resources to their families. In this way, the coronavirus crisis simply exacerbated prior differences in roles assumed by men and women regarding the care of children in prison.

Following the importation model on the processes of gendered prisonization, experiences prior to confinement are pivotal to understanding what happens while in prison (Irwin, 1970). The Mexican context for example, is crucial for understanding family dynamics: it is a society based on familism and Marianism identities, which essentially mean placing the family ahead of individual interests (Ingoldsby, 1991; Ruiz & Ransford, 2012). However, gender inequality serves to reinforce and uphold traditional gender norms and expectations, leaving women vulnerable in a gendered hierarchy of familism. Thus, in extreme situations such as incarceration, it tends to be women who assume full responsibility for their children. Prison reproduces these differentiated conceptions of gender, and these have been exacerbated by the Covid-19 crisis. As seen above, the prison infrastructure and administrative apparatus tend to orient organizational structures in such a way that they preserve traditional gender roles (sport, maternity, etc). For marginalized Mexican women, raising a child is an interchangeable responsibility between women of the extended family, which continues even during incarceration (Sandberg et al., 2020). Men, on the other hand, seem to be able to disregard their financial responsibility when incarcerated, and instead hang on to their fatherhood through stories of their dreams to be emotionally supportive and caring fathers, especially after their release (Sandberg et al., forthcoming).

Prison visits in Mexico entail the exchange of goods, money and access to basic supplies. Importantly, and as opposed to prisons in many other countries, the flow does not only go in one direction: it is an economy, formal, informal and illegal, from which prisoners' families and children can also benefit. Visits form part of a complex apparatus for the circulation of goods and services, and provide a veritable market. These are not markets governed by formal rules and regulations, but rather, complex networks of exchanges that resemble the laws that govern informal commerce, exchange- and gift economies. Prison visits thus reveal the "porous" nature of prison walls, and the agency and creativity that emerge in order to meet the basic needs of both prisoners and their families outside.

This crucial system of exchange has been temporarily stopped following the implementation of coronavirus pandemic measures. Suspensions of visits come with a huge cost for prisoners and their families, with devastating effects on the gendered informal economy. Rather than breaking the circle of familism, they reinforce connections based on traditional conceptions of gender. In countries such as Mexico, with an under-funded prison system, and large informal and formal economies in prison, banning visits not only carries emotional costs (Carlson & Cervera, 1991), but also some highly practical ones. Although justified by the pandemic, the ban on visits has further worsened the welfare and quality of life of prisoners dependent on support to cover their basic needs. It also creates great difficulties for families and children who depend on the economic support generated by work in prison. The gender patterns highlighted by the Covid-19 pandemic, points to fundamental societal and prison problems in Mexico, and possibly elsewhere in Latin

America. They also reveal the vulnerabilities and risks of a penitentiary system that relies on prison visits to feed the internal and external prison economies.

Notes

1. https://www.forbes.com.mx/confirman-el-primer-caso-de-coronavirus-covid-19-en-mexico/.
2. https://www.marca.com/claro-mx/trending/2020/03/31/5e82a827268e3e515c8b45b0.html.
3. https://www.eleconomista.com.mx/politica/Presentan-protocolo-de-actuacion-para-centros-penitenciarios-de-la-CDMX-por-Covid-19-20200318-0073.html.
4. https://www.jornada.com.mx/2020/03/19/capital/028n3cap.
5. https://www.dof.gob.mx/nota_detalle.php?codigo=5592105&fecha=22/04/2020.
6. https://www.elfinanciero.com.mx/cdmx/liberan-a-78-reos-para-reducir-riesgo-de-contagios-por-coronavirus-en-prisiones-de-la-cdmx.
7. https://www.animalpolitico.com/2020/05/cdmx-liberacion-personas-carcel/.
8. https://coronavirus.gob.mx/wp-content/uploads/2020/04/Protocolo_De_Actuacion_COVID-19_CEFERESOS.pdf.
9. https://www.jornada.com.mx/ultimas/estados/2020/04/14/gobierno-de-edomex-suspende-las-visitas-a-las-carceles-por-el-covid-19-3849.html.
10. https://www.animalpolitico.com/2020/03/visitas-restringen-estados-carceles-covid-coronavirus/.
11. https://www.animalpolitico.com/2020/04/carceles-covid-19-distancia-insumos/.
12. https://www.sandiegouniontribune.com/en-espanol/noticias/story/2020-04-27/covid-19-y-car celes-latinoamericanas-un-coctel-explosivo.
13. https://www.cndh.org.mx/documento/la-cndh-manifiesta-su-preocupacion-por-el-indice-de-letalidad-en-las-prisiones-del-pais.
14. https://www.forbes.com.mx/noticias-suman-395-contagios-de-covid-19-en-prisiones/.
15. https://www.animalpolitico.com/2020/04/rina-penal-cuautitlan-edomex-reos-custodios-covid -19/.
16. https://www.elsoldetoluca.com.mx/local/protestan-afuera-de-los-penales-piden-atender -a-enfermos-y-prevenir-contagios-de-covid-19-5088060.html.
17. Work in industries, usually factories, that allows these to be largely duty free and tariff-free.

Disclosure statement

No potential conflict of interest was reported by the author(s).

ORCID

Gustavo Fondevila http://orcid.org/0000-0003-4818-0584

References

Alarid, L. F. (1997). Female inmate subcultures. In J. W. Marquart, & J. R. Sorensen (Eds)., *Correctional contexts: Contemporary and classical readings* (pp. 134–139). Roxbury.

Atkinson, R. (1998). *The life story interview*. Sage.

Azaola, E., & José, C. (1996). *Las mujeres olvidadas. Un estudio sobre la situación de las cárceles de mujeres en la República Mexicana*. Colegio de México.

Baumer, H., & Meek, R. (2018). Sporting masculinities in prison. In M. Maycock & K. Hunt (Eds.), *New perspectives on prison masculinities* (pp. 197–221). Springer.

Bloom, B., & Chesney-Lind, M. (2000). Women in prison: Vengeful equity. In RoslynMuraskin (Ed.), *It's a crime: Women and justice* (pp. 183–204). Prentice Hall.

Briseño. (2006). *Garantizando los derechos humanos de las mujeres en reclusión*. Instituto Nacional de las Mujeres y Programa de las Naciones Unidas para el Desarrollo.
Britton, D. M. (1997). Gendered organizational logic: Policy and practice in men's and women's prisons. *Gender & Society*, *11*(6), 796–818. https://doi.org/10.1177/089124397011006005
Carlson, B. E., & Cervera, N. (1991). Inmates and their families: Conjugal visits, family contact, and family functioning. *Criminal Justice and Behavior*, *18*(3), 318–331. https://doi.org/10.1177/0093854891018003005
Censo Nacional de Gobierno, Seguridad Pública y Sistema Penitenciario Estatales (CNGSPSPE). (2019). INEGI. https://www.inegi.org.mx/programas/cngspspe/2019/
Censo Nacional de Sistema Penitenciario Federal. (2019). INEGI. https://www.inegi.org.mx/programas/cnspef/2019/
Datesman, S. K., & Cales, G. L. (1983). I'm still the same mommy": Maintaining the mother/child relationship in prison. *The Prison Journal*, *63*(2), 142–154. https://doi.org/10.1177/003288558306300212
Diagnóstico Nacional de Supervisión Penitenciaria. (2019a). CNDH. https://www.cndh.org.mx/web/diagnostico-nacional-de-supervision-penitenciaria
Diagnóstico Nacional de Supervisión Penitenciaria (DNSP). (2019b). CNDH. https://www.cndh.org.mx/sites/all/doc/sistemas/DNSP/DNSP_2019.pdf
Dodge, M., & Pogrebin, M. R. (2001). Collateral costs of imprisonment for women: Complications of reintegration. *The Prison Journal*, *81*(1), 42–54. https://doi.org/10.1177/0032885501081001004
Duffy, M. (2007). Doing the dirty work: Gender, race, and reproductive labor in historical perspective. *Gender & Society*, *21*(3), 313–336. https://doi.org/10.1177/0891243207300764
Encuesta Nacional de Población Privada de la Libertad (ENPOL). (2016). INEGI. https://www.inegi.org.mx/programas/enpol/2016/En números (2017) http://www.cdeunodc.inegi.org.mx/unodc/wp-content/uploads/2018/01/en_numeros2.pdf
Fuller, L. G. (1993). Visitors to women's prisons in California: An exploratory study. *Fed. Probation*, *57*, 41–47. https://heinonline.org/HOL/LandingPage?handle=hein.journals/fedpro57&div=64&id=&page=
Giacomello, C. (2013). *Género, drogas y prisión*. Tirant lo Blanch.
Giallombardo, R. (1966). Social roles in a prison for women. *Social Problems*, *13*(3), 268–288. https://doi.org/10.2307/799254
Greer, K. R. (2000). The changing nature of interpersonal relationships in a women's prison. *The Prison Journal*, *80*(4), 442–468. https://doi.org/10.1177/0032885500080004009
Grundetjern, H. (2018). Negotiating motherhood: Variations of maternal identities among women in the illegal drug economy. *Gender & Society*, *32*(3), 395–416. https://doi.org/10.1177/0891243218759006
Hairston, C. F. (1990). Men in prison: Family characteristics and parenting views. *Journal of Offender Counseling Services Rehabilitation*, *14*(1), 23–30. https://doi.org/10.1300/J264v14n01_03
Harris, J. W. (1993). Comparison of stressors among female vs. male inmates. *Journal of Offender Rehabilitation*, *19*(1–2), 43–56. https://doi.org/10.1300/J076v19n01_03
Hart, C. B. (1995). A primer in prison research. *Journal of Contemporary Criminal Justice*, *11*(3), 165–176. https://doi.org/10.1177/104398629501100302
Hefferman, E. (1972). *Making 11 in prison: The square, the cool and the life*. John Wiley & Sons.
Ingoldsby, B. (1991). The Latin American family: Familism vs. machismo. *Journal of Comparative Family Studies*, *22*(1), 57–62. https://doi.org/10.3138/jcfs.22.1.57
Irwin, J. (1970). *The Felon*. Prentice Hall.
Jiang, S., & Winfree, L. T., Jr. (2006). Social support, gender, and inmate adjustment to prison life: Insights from a national sample. *The Prison Journal*, *86*(1), 32–55. https://doi.org/10.1177%2F0032885505283876
Kruttschnitt, C., Gartner, R., & Miller, A. (2000). Doing her own time? Women's responses to prison in the context of the old and the new penology. *Criminology*, *38*(3), 681–718. https://doi.org/10.1111/j.1745-9125.2000.tb00903.x
Luna, H. A., Cisneros, J. L., & Ornelas, A. R. M. (2003). *La condición del trabajo de la mujer en prisión*. UAM. http://www2.izt.uam.mx/sotraem/Documentos/Documentos/Amet2003/templates/res/tema%2015/ALMA%20MARIN.pdf

Marks, L., & Palkovitz, R. (2004). American fatherhood types: The good, the bad, and the uninterested. *Fathering: A Journal of Theory, Research and Practice about Men as Fathers*, *2*(2), 113–129. https://doi.org/10.3149/fth.0202.113

Mauss, M. (1970). *The gift: Forms and functions of exchange in Archaic Societies*. Cohen & West.

Montoya, V. (2015). *Maternidad en prisión: Patrones de interacción de madres reclusas e hijos(as) menores que viven con ellas en el Centro Femenil de Readaptación Social Santa Martha Acatitla* [Tesis doctoral]. Universidad Nacional Autónoma de México (UNAM).

Palomar, C. (2007). *Maternidad en prisión*. Universidad de Guadalajara.

Patton, M. Q. (1990). *Qualitative evaluation and research methods*. Sage.

Pollock, J. M. (2002). *Women, crime, and prison*. Wadsworth.

Protocolo de actuación para la atención de Covid-19 al interior de Centros Federales de Reinserción Social (PAACEFERESOS). (2020). Ministry of Health. https://coronavirus.gob.mx/wp-content/uploads/2020/04/Protocolo_De_Actuacion_COVID-19_CEFERESOS.pdf

Rich, A. (1986). *Nacemos de Mujer*. Cátedra.

Ríos Miranda, A. (2014). Los mundos imaginados de la precariedad global: La prisión en la ciudad de México. *Nueva antropología*, *27*(81), 149–180. http://www.scielo.org.mx/scielo.php?script=sci_arttext&pid=S0185-06362014000200008&lng=es&tlng=es.

Ruiz, M., & Ransford, H. (2012). Latino elders reframing *familismo*: Implications for health and caregiving support. *Journal of Cultural Diversity*, 19(2), 50–57. PMID: 22924203.

Sandberg, S., Agoff, C., & Fondevila, G. (2020). Doing marginalized motherhood: Identities and practices among incarcerated women in Mexico. *International Journal for Crime, Justice and Social Democracy*, advance online publication. https://doi.org/10.5204/ijcjsd.v10i1.1538

Sandberg, S., Agoff, C., & Fondevila, G. (forthcoming). Stories of the 'Good Father': The role of fatherhood among incarcerated men in Mexico. *Punishment & Society*. https://doi.org/10.1177/1462474520969822

Sykes, G. E. (1958). *The society of captives*. Princeton University Press.

Ward, D. A., & Kassebaum, G. G. (1965). *Women's prison, sex and social structure*. Aldine.

Wilson, T. P. (1968). Patterns of management and adaptations to organizational roles: A study of prison inmates. *American Journal of Sociology*, *74*(2), 146–157. https://doi.org/10.1086/224617

Zingraff, M. T. (1980). Inmate assimilation: A comparison of male and female delinquents. *Criminal Justice and Behavior*, *7*(3), 275–292. https://doi.org/10.1177/009385488000700303

Europe Regional Overview and Reports from Spain, Portugal, Italy, Germany, Russia, Romania, Sweden, and the United Kingdom

The Impact of COVID-19 Outbreaks in the Prisons, Jails, and Community Corrections Systems Throughout Europe

Sabrina S. Rapisarda and James M. Byrne

ABSTRACT

This article documents country-level differences in the extent of COVID-19 outbreaks in corrections systems across the European region. Variations in the timing, duration, and intensity of front-end, in-prison, and back-end mitigation strategies are also identified. We conclude by providing a preliminary assessment of the effectiveness of these mitigation strategies, particularly in those countries that combined transparency and proactive, early release mechanisms.

Introduction and overview

Prisons are key settings for communicable diseases due to the greater prevalence of health issues, such as hypertension, diabetes, asthma, substance–use disorders and mental health issues among inmates, relative to community settings, in addition to environmental factors including unavoidable close contact, over-crowding, poor ventilation, and limited access to health care services (WEPHREN, 2020; World Health Organization: Regional Office for Europe, 2020). Once infected, inmates, staff, and visitors can rapidly transmit communicable diseases such as COVID-19 throughout prisons. Due to the contagious nature of the virus, COVID-19 can easily transfer from community and staff members to inmates, and can also spread between prisons through staff transfers and employment crossing. Consequently, correctional settings are an important part of the public-health response to COVID-19. While responses to COVID-19 have differed and continue to differ in correctional settings across and within regions and countries, there is value in investigating trends regarding the impact of COVID-19 within prison systems at the global scale to illuminate and compile the most effective responses to the virus thus far. Due to increased risk of spreading COVID-19 in large prison systems, the response to the threat of the virus is critically important.

COVID-19 outbreaks in European prisons

Europe accounts for 10 of the 50 largest prison systems in the world (see Table 1), including the Russian Federation, Turkey, the United Kingdom (England and Whales), Poland, France, Germany, Spain, Italy, Ukraine, and Belarus (World Prison Brief, 2020). On January 1, 2020, there were 1,390,683 inmates in the Council of Europe member states'

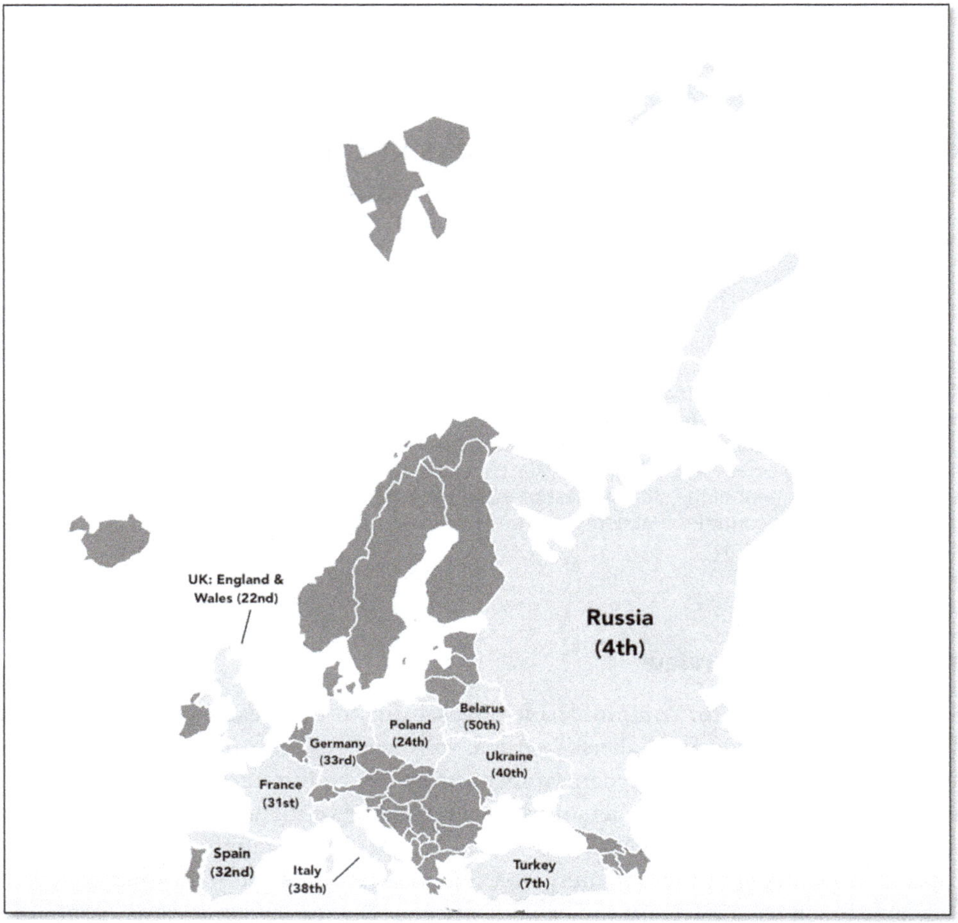

Figure 1. Europe's largest prison systems. The labeled countries in Figure 1 are among the top 50 largest prison systems globally and represent the ten largest prison systems in Europe. Among the 50 largest prison systems, the Russian Federation is placed fourth, Turkey is seventh, the UK (England and Whales) is 22nd, Poland is 24th, France is 31st, Spain is 32nd, Germany is 33rd, Italy is 38th, Ukraine is 40th, and Belarus is 50th (World Prison Brief, 2020). **Notes.* Portions of the United Kingdom that are represented in the top 50 largest prison systems are limited to England and Whales (excluding Northern Ireland and Scotland). The rankings for European countries within the top 50 largest prison systems are based on current data between February 14 and August 28, 2020. For purposes of categorization, the Russian Federation is included as part of Europe; however, it should be noted that the Russian Federation is a transcontinental country spanning from Europe into Asia.

46 correctional institutions (Aebi & Tiago, 2020).[1] Aebi and Tiago (2020) found the approximate incarceration rate across European prisons, as of January 1, 2020, to be 106 inmates per 100,000 individuals. By April 20, 2020, the incarcerated population rate remained at 106 inmates per 100,000 individuals, implying that the rate had remained stable during the early stages of the pandemic. This situation has changed in more recent months, due to front-end and back-end mitigation strategies designed to reduce the spread of COVID-19 in prisons and jails.

Table 1. Europe's largest prison systems in the world's top 50.

Rank	Global Region	Country	Prison Population	Date of Most Recent Report
4	Europe/Asia	Russian Federation	496,791	August 2020
7	Europe/Asia	Turkey	281,094	July 2020
22	Northern Europe	UK: England and Wales	79,433	August 2020
24	Central and Eastern Europe	Poland	69,375	July 2020
31	Western Europe	France	58,695	July 2020
32	Southern Europe	Spain	58,642	February 2020
33	Western Europe	Germany	57,600	June 2020
38	Southern Europe	Italy	53,619	July 2020
40	Central and Eastern Europe	Ukraine	52,609	April 2020
50	Central and Eastern Europe	Belarus	32,500	October 2018

Notes. All data were extracted from the World Prison Brief database (2020).

The majority of European countries have reported outbreaks among inmates,[2] staff, or both, (Aebi & Tiago, 2020).[3] Based on data provided by the Council of Europe on April 15, 2020, there does not appear to be a clear association between prison population size or geographic location and the outbreak of COVID-19 cases among inmates, staff, or both. However, on April 22, 2020, EUROPRIS reported that countries within the European Union whose general population was highly impacted by COVID-19 (e.g., Spain and Italy), were the same countries that reported the highest number of cases among inmates and/or staff.[4]

Mitigation strategies used in European countries

We have highlighted the front-end, in-prison, and back-end mitigation strategies for five of the European countries in the top 50 largest prison systems globally (see Table 2). Romania, Portugal, and Sweden are also included in Table 2 and are examined in more depth in the country-level reports in this volume (see Durnescu, Redondo Illescas et al., and Lindström et al., this volume, respectively). According to the Council of Europe (2020), the initial response from the vast majority of countries in Europe, Sweden aside, was to emulate the community's response to COVID-19: to place the prisons on lockdown, suspending visitation rights and confining inmates to very little movement away from their cells. However, contrary to containing inmates through a lockdown approach, in April, the European Committee for the Prevention of Torture (CPT) of the Council of Europe urged all member states to apply alternative practices to detention, whenever possible and without discrimination, to combat COVID-19. To establish recommended practices such as social distancing as a means of prevention and intervention (i.e., to contain the spread of the virus, once detected)—and to comply with the CPT's request to divert imprisonment as a sanction, some prison systems in countries across Europe released (and have continued to release) inmates to varying degrees. For example, in a preventative effort to reduce the size of prison populations and to alleviate overcrowding, some European countries/regions including Norway, Denmark, Ireland, Italy, France, the United Kingdom (Northern Ireland), Portugal, and Turkey reported the release of inmates between January and April[5] (Aebi & Tiago, 2020).

Turkey, for instance, preventatively released approximately 35% of its prison population ($N = 281{,}094$) into the community,[6] thus accounting for the largest total number of inmates released from prisons in Europe as of April (Aebi & Tiago, 2020; Kuru, 2020). About half of

Table 2. A comparison of mitigation strategies used in European prisons and jails.

Country (Rank)	Front-End	Within-Prison	Back-End
Russian Federation (4th)	Suspension of in-person court hearings (in some cases); suspension of visitation (in some regions); reduction in the use of pretrial detention; preventive screening of prison staff and visitors before admission to facility	Lockdowns (quarantining); aggressive testing; daily preventive sanitation and disinfection; mask-wearing by prison staff and visitors; isolation of infected inmates; rotations of 14 consecutive days on and off work among prison staff; newly admitted inmates in isolation for 20 days prior to assimilation with the general prison population	None
United Kingdom (22nd)	Temporary suspension of visits; suspended educational programs and non-essential work; halted interprison transfers; movement from courts to prison effectively stopped (court hearings were held remotely by video and by phone); lockdown of facilities with only essential staff permitted access to facilities	Establishment of hand-washing stations and adequate soap and cleaning supplies; distribution of personal protective equipment (PPE) to staff; routine testing of prison officers; isolated confinement of inmates for social distancing purposes; movement from prisons to courts effectively stopped (court hearings were held remotely by video and by phone)	Early release of some inmates (if deemed necessary); addition of temporary accommodations across prisons; implementation of a "cohorting" strategy
Spain (32nd)	Suspension of visitation but free telephone and video-conferencing with families and attorneys; use of pre-trial and sentencing alternatives; electronic monitoring; decline in the number of offenders remanded to prison by courts during the pandemic (50% decrease between early 2020 and the same time period in 2019)	All external communications and all leave exits suspended except for reasons of force or extreme necessity; prohibition of access to prisons of any person (volunteers, collaborating entities, etc.) who are not part of the prison staff, unless their work inside was considered essential; suspension of teaching activity and production workshops; suspension of inmate transfers, except for health or judicial reasons; authorization for the inmates to stay voluntarily in their cells; staggering of mealtimes in dining areas; communication of mitigation efforts to inmates; provision of PPE to inmates and staff	Extensive release to community (an increase of over 400% of the number of offenders on home confinement)
Germany (33rd)	Courts limited their work and mainly dealt only with cases of alleged offenders being sent to pre-trial detention, reducing new prison admissions; elimination of incarcerations for non-payment of fines; restricted visits by suspending all visits with personal contact; implementation of video telephone calls	Provision of masks, hygiene products, and other PPE to inmates; establishment of quarantine areas in facilities; restriction of inmates to cells for more hours per day; suspension of activities such as work, reentry programs, and recreation	Early release or non-execution of short-term prison sentence since March (i.e., Germany's prison occupancy level has decreased from 83.3% to 78.7% between March and September 2020)

(Continued)

Table 2. (Continued).

Country (Rank)	Front-End	Within-Prison	Back-End
Italy (38th)	Restricted access into and out of prison facilities; substitution of phone calls or other available technology in lieu of in-person visits with relatives or third parties (other than defense lawyers)	Temporary suspension of treatment programs that involved participation from persons in the local community; curtailment of work-related activities serving the facilities that involve persons coming in from outside; extended release time for those already out on leave	Eligible persons with 18 months or less of their sentence to serve remainder of sentence at home or at other private health care facilities; expanded use of electronic monitoring for those released to the community; measures resulted in a decrease of nearly 10% of the incarcerated population
Romania (70th)	Restriction of new intakes during the first weeks of the pandemic; court hearings through video-conferencing or rescheduling upcoming hearings	Certain penitentiary units were specially designated to serve as quarantine units; monitoring and isolating of those inmates who, after an epidemiological screening, had symptoms of coronavirus infection and/or were new to a facility; reducing staff who come into contact with inmates by 30% (those staff remained home while accomplishing professional tasks); psychological services provided only in critical situations; informational campaigns for inmates; disinfection of accommodation-based areas	None
Portugal (88th)	Temporary suspension of visitation; restriction on outside goods coming into facilities	Creation of specific facilities for COVID-positive inmates; quarantine of new inmates coming into facilities; suspension of transfers between facilities other than in cases of security; work activities with external entities and leisure activities suspended; reassignment and differentiation of inmates' daily routines to try to separate, as much as possible, inmates considered most vulnerable (e.g., aged over 60 years, with immunosuppression or chronic disease such as respiratory ailments, hypertension, or diabetics); increased testing and monitoring of staff and inmates	Partial pardoning of sentences for those whose sentences were less than two years, age 65 years and older, having mental or physical diseases, or with degrees of autonomy that are incompatible with life in prison ($N = 1,289$)
Sweden (117th)	Cancellation of furloughs and visitation	Isolation and quarantine of new intakes; minimizing the size of the custodial and treatment staff; use of PPE by staff; elimination of face-to-face contact in probation and parole when possible; no-charge phone calls to compensate inmates for the loss of visitation and furlough and as a way to maintain the treatment plans of many inmates who need prosocial contacts as a part of their rehabilitation; communication with inmates to keep them informed of safety protocols	None

Note. See country-level articles in this volume for more detail regarding the variability in European countries' mitigation strategies to address COVID-19 within their prison systems.

these inmates were released temporarily and will remain released until as late as November 2020 (Kuru, 2020). In April, Turkey's parliament paved the path for countries in similar situations by developing and implementing legislation that would allow for the release of large numbers of inmates to mitigate the negative impact of public health emergencies such as the COVID-19 pandemic (Kuru, 2020).

The patterns that have emerged early on in the pandemic in Europe insinuate that traditionally less punitive countries, such Norway, Iceland, and Denmark, and countries whose general populations were burdened by a larger number of infections and/or characterized by large prison populations (e.g., Turkey, France, Italy, and Spain), were more inclined to adopt the preventative, back-end approach of releasing inmates in response to the threat of COVID-19 in prison settings.

According to the European Organization of Prison and Correctional Services (EUROPRIS, 2020), some jurisdictions released inmates by replacing short and nearly expired (longer-term) sentences with release, in addition to replacing pre-trial detention with non-custodial measures such as home detention (in homes, in health care centers, or in half-way homes/supervised apartments). Other inmates were required to report to supervising officers regularly (sometimes supported with electronic monitoring) through phone calls, video calls, and/or alcohol meters. While the majority of jurisdictions banned the transport of inmates between prisons to contain individual prison populations, some reinstated the travel of small groups between prisons on a limited basis to alleviate large prison population sizes in areas of need (EUROPRIS, 2020).

Other European countries, including Finland, the Netherlands, Sweden, Romania, Scotland, the United Kingdom (England and Wales), Poland, Czech Republic, and the Russian Federation, also experienced prison population reductions[7]; however, these countries did not actively facilitate this process through the proactive release of inmates (Aebi & Tiago, 2020). One potential explanation for the decline of these inmate populations, despite the lack of proactive release, is that although inmates may have been released at the same rates as usual, there were fewer opportunities and locations to commit new crimes due to societal lockdowns and, therefore, fewer opportunities to be arrested and prosecuted for those crimes. Moreover, jurisdictions have been postponing prison sentences because judiciaries in most countries have also postponed the adjudication of criminal cases (EUROPRIS, 2020). Regardless of the mechanism by which prison population sizes have decreased, increased space within prisons is more conducive to the isolation of infected inmates and distancing among non-infected inmates (e.g., one inmate per cell), thus, reducing the likelihood of viral transmission.

Banning and/or limiting in-person visitations between loved ones and inmates, in theory, reduces the likelihood of transmission via visitors to inmates and/or to staff. However, doing so does not mitigate the contraction of COVID-19 among prison workers that enter facilities every day. To address this potential issue, jurisdictions in Europe have required that prison staff who manifest symptoms of COVID-19, have chronic illnesses or health susceptibilities, are 60 years or older, and/or are pregnant, must stay home (EUROPRIS, 2020). Some countries have also temporarily suspended vacation days, canceled group trainings, and/or are working at a reduced staff size. Staff in most countries are required to wear a mask, protective clothing, and other protective gear (EUROPRIS, 2020).

Concluding comments

The governments of European countries, with a few notable exceptions, appear to be more transparent in their acknowledgment of the extent of the COVID-19 outbreaks in their prisons and jails than the governments of other global regions, most notably Asia. Many of these same governments have moved proactively to reduce the potential spread of outbreaks in prison by aggressively downsizing their prison and jail populations. There has been no documented crime increase linked to the utilization of these front-end and back-end release strategies at this point in the pandemic (Redondo Illesces et al., this volume). There appear to be two important lessons from a review of the country-level reports of how the problem was defined and how prison-population-reduction strategies were developed, namely, (1) be transparent about the nature and extent of the problem, and (2) be proactive in reducing prison and jail populations.

Notes

1. The total number of inmates reflects only member states that provided data on both January 1 and April 15, 2020.
2. The Romanian prison system reports that no inmate has contracted COVID-19 in its prisons during the first several months of the pandemic, but we are skeptical of this claim. See the country-specific review in this volume for more detail.
3. Bosnia and Herzegovina, Bulgaria, Georgia, Iceland, Latvia, Lithuania, Malta, Montenegro, and North Macedonia reported no outbreaks between January and April (Aebi & Tiago, 2020).
4. For example, Spain reported that 46 inmates and 238 staff members tested positive while Italy reported 37 infections among inmates and 163 among staff members.
5. Other countries/regions that released inmates between January 1 and April 20 as a tactic to prevent the spread of COVID-19 included Monaco, Iceland, Slovenia, Andorra, Cyprus, Luxembourg, Armenia, Spain (Catalonia, state administration, and total), the Republic of Serbia, Albania, and Azerbaijan.
6. Turkey has the second largest prison population among all European countries and holds seventh place globally (World Prison Brief, 2020).
7. Other countries/regions that have achieved prison-population reductions, but not through the active release of inmates, included Lichtenstein, Bosnia and Herzegovina, Croatia, Austria, North Macedonia, Greece, Bulgaria, Malta, Moldova, Hungary, Montenegro, Latvia, Estonia, Slovak Republic, Lithuania, and Georgia.

Disclosure statement

No potential conflict of interest was reported by the author(s).

References

Aebi, M. F., & Tiago, M. M. (2020). *Prisons and prisoners in Europe in pandemic times: An evaluation of the short-term impact of the COVID-19 on prison populations*. Council of Europe. http://wp.unil.ch/space/files/2020/06/Prisons-and-the-COVID-19_200617_FINAL.pdf

European Committee for the Prevention of Torture and Inhuman or Degrading Treatment or Punishment (CPT). (2020, March 20). *Statement of principles relating to the treatment of persons deprived of their liberty in the context of the coronavirus disease (COVID-19) pandemic*. Council of Europe. https://rm.coe.int/09000016809e3a34

Kuru, T. A. (2020, April 23). *Turkey releasing murderers – But not political opponents – From prison amid coronavirus pandemic.* The Conversation. https://theconversation.com/turkey-releasing-murderers-but-notpolitical-opponents-from-prison-amid-coronavirus-pandemic-136466

Overview of European prison services' responses to the COVID-19 crisis. (2020, April 20). EUROPRIS. https://www.europris.org/wp-content/uploads/2020/06/Overview-COVID-update-22-April.pdf

Preparedness, prevention and control of COVID-19 in prisons and other places of detention: Interim guidance. (2020, March 15). World Health Organization: Regional Office for Europe. https://www.euro.who.int/__data/assets/pdf_file/0019/434026/Preparedness-prevention-and-control-of-COVID-19-in-prisons.pdf?ua=1

WEPHREN. (2020, July 21). *COVID-19.* The Global Health Network. https://wephren.tghn.org/covid-19-prisons-and-places-detention/

World Prison Brief. (2020, August). *World prison brief data.* Institute for Crime & Justice Policy Research (ICPR). https://www.prisonstudies.org/world-prison-brief-data

The Impact of Covid-19 on Prisons and Penal Policy in Germany

Frieder Dünkel

ABSTRACT

In Germany, the situation of prisons before the outbreak of the Covid-19-pandemic was quite relaxed as the prison population was in decline and overcrowding not a problem. However, there was a special problem with fine defaulters, who comprise about 10% of the daily adult German prison population. Short-term prisoners in general are a problem resulting in a large influx of possibly infected people. Since March 2020 all German Federal states stopped (or reduced) incarcerating fine defaulters and some states went further, not executing prison sentences of up to one or even up to three years. The prison population dropped from about 77 per 100,000 inhabitants to 67. Prison conditions, however, worsened because of restricted contacts of prisoners with the outside world. On the other side, access to internet communication was introduced in order to compensate the lockdown of personal visits and of prison leaves. Since June some of the restrictions were repealed, as the pandemic was under control and almost no infections were observed for prisoners. Visits and prison leaves gradually are allowed again in a limited way. Further crime policy considerations to abolish or reduce fine default and other short-term imprisonment are discussed.

Introduction: the general situation in German prisons

Germany has operated as a Federal Republic since 1949. After the break of the East German wall and the transition of East Germany to a democratic society in 1990, West- and East-Germany were re-unified. With few exceptions, the legal system of West Germany was taken over for the whole country. The legislative competence for criminal law, criminal procedural law and penitentiary law was at the power of the central German Federal, not federal state level.[1] In 2006, a reform of the Constitution (*Grundgesetz*) changed legislative competencies for penitentiary law to the federal state level. Therefore between 2007 and 2015 the 16 federal states all had to pass substantive prison legislation (for the execution of prison sentences for adults, juvenile prison laws for 14–25-years old juveniles and young adults, pre-trial detention laws and laws for the execution of preventive detention, an indeterminate security and treatment measure for dangerous offenders).

The general sentencing policy in Germany is rather moderate and stable. Even at a time of increased violent crimes during the 1990s and early 2000s, there was a stable distribution of sanctions of about 82% of sentences against adults over 18 being fines (based on the so-called day-fine system), 12% being suspended sentences (probation) and 6% unconditional prison sentences. The average length of unconditional prison sentences is about two years. There is no evidence for a punitive turn in sentencing, although the legally provided penalties for violent and sexual crimes were slightly increased (see Dünkel, 2019).

Germany in February 2020 had an average prison population of 63,852 inmates, 13,137 in pre-trial detention (29.8%).[2] 45,062 served a prison sentence in prisons for adults, of them 4,773 (= 9.4%) were serving a substitute prison sentence because of not having paid a fine (fine defaulters).

At the end of February 2020, 47,855 out of 63,851 prisoners were accommodated in single cells (75.0%), 15,996 (= 25.0%) in communal cells (see below Figure 3) (mostly only with one other inmate).

According to the data collected by the International Center for Prison Studies in London (Birkbeck University)[3] for September 2019, Germany had the same prison population of 63,851 inmates as at the end of February 2020, which represented a prison population rate of 77 per 100,000 inhabitants. The prison population rate since 2004 (96 per 100,000) has declined by about 20%, and was stable since 2013,[4] although there had been fears that the refugee crisis of 2015 would contribute to an increase of the prison population. The world prison brief data for March 2020 reported a prison population rate of 71. The absolute numbers of prisoners further declined to 55,525 by the end of June, which would mean a prison population rate of 67, which – internationally compared – is exceptionally low (see Dünkel, 2017).

Despite considerable regional disparities, the downward trend is more or less uniform for all 16 federal states (see Figure 1). A particular big drop of the prison population can be observed in the federal states of Hamburg (since 2003) and Berlin (since 2009), which had a considerably higher-than-average prison population before (see for some explanations Dünkel, 2018).

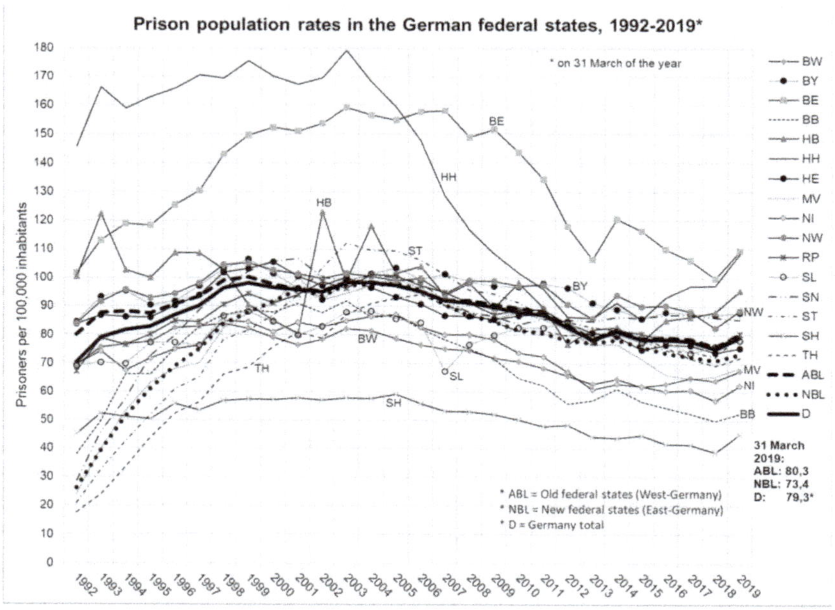

Figure 1. Prison population rates in the German federal states, 1992-2019*

The occupancy level at the end of February 2020 was 90%, which means that overcrowding (apart from a few closed prisons) generally was not a problem in Germany. Figure 2 reveals that in 2019 the general occupancy rate with 90% was identical, only in the federal state of Baden-Württemberg it was over 100%.

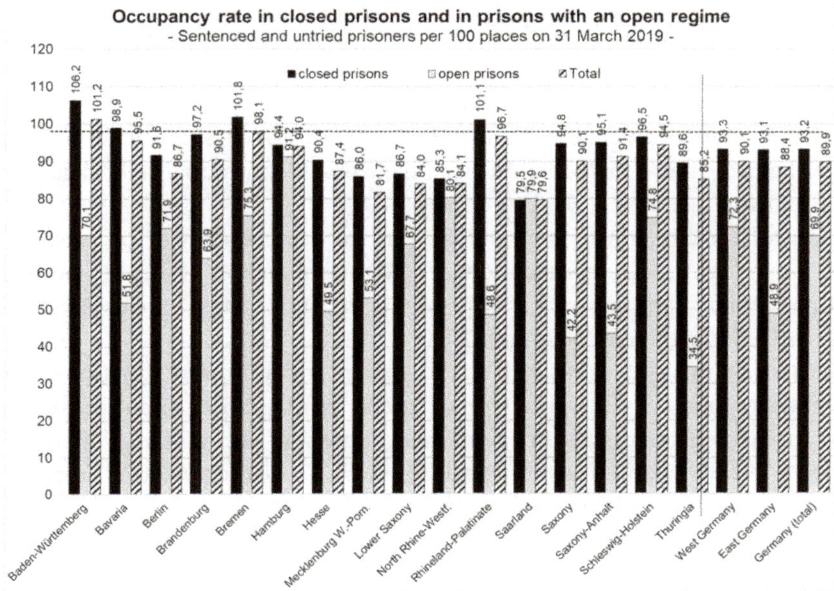

Figure 2. Occupancy rate in closed prisons and in prisons with an open regime -Sentenced and untried prisoners per 100 places on 31 March 2019-

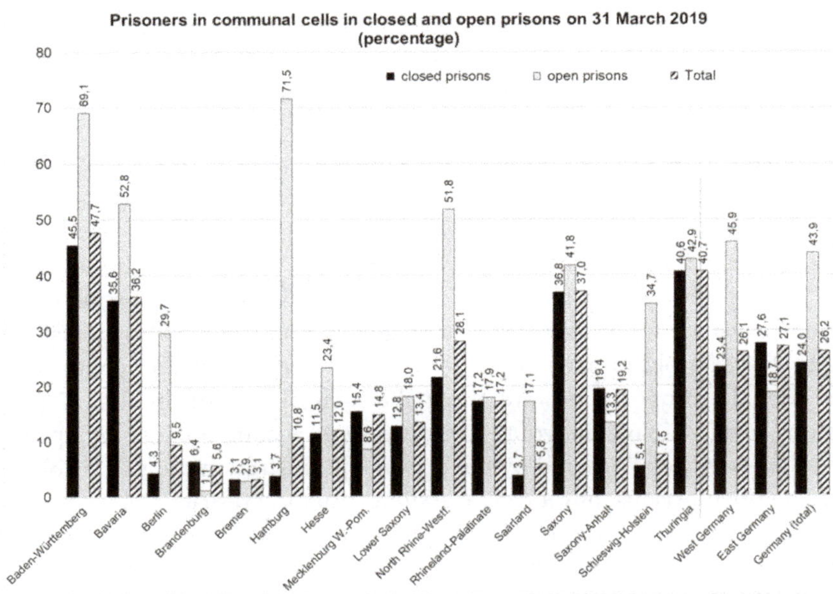

Figure 3. Prisoners in communal cells in closed and open prisons on 31 March 2019 (Percentage)

The situation has further calmed down due to the release and non-execution of short-term prison sentences since March 2020 with an occupancy level of 83.3%. At the end of June 2020, the occupancy rate was only 76.0%. Therefore, at the moment, overcrowding – even in the somehow problematic regions before the pandemic's outbreak (see Figure 2) – is no problem all over Germany.

One infection risk derives from accommodating too many prisoners in small and hygienically problematic accommodation. In Germany, prisoners in principle have a right to be accommodated in a single cell at night. This legal requirement is not totally met in all federal states and prisons. At the end of February 2020 75% of all prisoners (pre-trial and sentenced) were accommodated in single cells (47,855 out of 63,851) and 25% in communal cells (a year before, in March 2019: 74% in single, 26% in communal cells), again with large regional disparities (see Figure 3).

One month later after the prison population had decreased by 4,364 prisoners, which resulted from releases or non-execution of short-term prison sentences because of the Covid-19 pandemic. The proportion of prisoners accommodated in single cells increased from 75% to 77.5% at the end of March 2020.

The German prison system (as well as the system of community sanctions) is based on the rehabilitative goal or the principle of social reintegration (*Resozialisierung*). It is enshrined in substantive penal and penitentiary law and recognized with regard to the prison system by the Federal Constitutional Court (FCC) as a constitutional principle based on the prisoners' right of preserving human dignity (Art. 1 of the Constitution, *Grundgesetz*) and the principle of the social welfare state (Art. 20 of the Constitution, see Morgenstern, 2016; Pruin, 2019: 150f.).

The principle of social reintegration requires a system of a graduated relaxation of the prison system including regular prison leaves and the transfer to open prisons at least in the last stage of executing prison sentences (Dünkel & Rössner, 2001: 327 ff.; Dünkel, 2018: 428 ff.). As a consequence of this orientation to reentry programmes, per day several thousands of sentenced prisoners are on temporary leaves (at the end of February 2020: 2,847, i.e. 5.6% of the population of 50,675 sentenced prisoners). The proportion of temporary absent prisoners dropped at the end of March to 1,761 and at the end of June to 1,776, i.e. 3.7% and accordingly 4.0% of all sentenced prisoners.[5] The impact of the pandemic with restricting prison leaves is quite visible by these statistical data.

Another pillar of the orientation to social reintegration is the transfer to open prisons, which are defined as facilities without physical hindrances to prevent escape (i. e. there are no walls nor grilled windows). The principle of a graduated opening of prisons is based on trusting prisoners, who naturally are selected according to their dangerousness and risks of escape.[6] At the end of February 2020, 15.0% of the 45,062 prisoners serving a prison sentence in prisons for adults, were accommodated in an open facility, against 8.8% of the 3.557 14- to 24-years-old inmates serving a youth prison sentence in youth prisons. End of March 2020 the proportions were about the same: 14.9% of the 42,177 prisoners in adult prisons, against 8.6% in youth prisons, were accommodated in open prisons.[7] Therefore, the restrictions ordered by the prison administration are not visible as regards the transfer to open prisons, but it can be assumed that the restrictions concerning prison leaves that are typically concentrated on prisoners in open facilities during the main period of the pandemic has also influenced the practice in open facilities.

Sentencing and execution of sentences-policies before and after the pandemic and the impact on prison population rates

The following findings about changes of executing prison sentences and of prison policies with regards to the Corona crisis are based on a research undertaken by Christine Morgenstern of the Department of Criminology in Greifswald (also: Trinity College, Dublin) in March and further inquiries in June/July by the author of this paper.

As mentioned before, Germany is a federal state with 16 states ("Länder") having all their individual Prison Laws. Therefore, we had to explore the (sometimes) different approaches in the 16 federal states' prison legislation and practice. The sentencing practice of the courts is based on the (uniform) Federal Criminal Code. Regional disparities in sentencing practices are well-known. During the pandemic the courts were limited in their work and mainly dealt only with cases of alleged offenders being sent to pre-trial detention. Therefore, the influx of new admissions to prisons was reduced partly because of the fewer convictions during March to June 2020. Exact numbers are not yet available, but the prison statistics about admissions give some indication of the dimension: In February 2020 7,799 new incomers (*Erstaufnahmen im Strafvollzug*) were registered, whereas in March 2020 the statistics counted only 5,470, and in June 4,216 admissions to prisons (minus 45.9%).

One research question to the federal state prison administrations was if prisoners were released and which forms of prison sentences are not executed due to Covid-19 in order to diminish the risk of prisoners being infected. The results are unanimous insofar as all federal states declared to have stopped to order convicts to serve **fine default sentences** and most states released prisoners serving fine default sentences at the beginning of the crisis in March 2020. The reduction of the daily prison population serving fine-default prison sentences is clearly visible since March 2020. The absolute numbers of the daily fine default population dropped by 72% between February and June 2020, the proportion with regards to the prison population of adult offenders from 10.6% to 5.8% at the end of March (see Table 1) and further to 3.5% in June (= minus 67%).

Although all federal states had declared that fine default sentences would be not be executed, this policy until end of March was implemented in a rather reluctant way in

Table 1. Fine defaulters in the adult prison system in Germany (absolute numbers at the end of the month).

2019	Prisoners serving a prison sentence in prisons for adults	Of them: Fine default sentences	Percentage of prisoners in adult prisons
March	46.477	4.861	10,5
April	45.917	4.546	9,9
May	46.008	4.549	9,9
June	45.687	4.482	9,8
September	45.244	4.616	10,2
December	43.760	4.122	9,4
Average 2019	45.417,75	4.569,5	10,1%
2020			
January	44.720	4.664	10,4
February.	45.062	4.773	10,6
March	42.177	2.447	5,8
April	39,528	1,553	3.9
May	38,595	1,312	3.4
June	38,154	1,333	3.5

Bavaria, Lower Saxony and Saxony-Anhalt. In North Rhine-Westphalia, the decrease was under the average as well. In contrast, in Baden-Württemberg, Berlin, Hamburg and Mecklenburg-Western Pomerania the fine default population dropped by 75% or more (see Table 2).

With the end of some restrictions of the lockdown since May 2020 outside prisons, some prison administrations started to slow down the non-execution of fine default sentences. However, all federal states kept their policy of non-executing these short terms of imprisonment, in particular Berlin, Brandenburg and Mecklenburg-Wester Pomerania. They kept only those fine defaulters in prison who in addition had to serve another prison sentence. Only a few federal states not only postponed the execution of fine default sentences, but also granted an amnesty with regards to the fines imposed originally (see e. g. Berlin).

Some Federal states went even beyond the non-execution of fine-default sentences by not executing prison sentences of up to 6 months (Baden-Württemberg, Bavaria), 12 months (Lower Saxony, North Rhine-Westphalia) or even up to 3 years (Berlin, Hamburg, Saxony).[8] Hamburg did not start to execute prison sentences of up to 3 years and interrupted the execution of sentences of up to 18 months. In some federal states, a decisive policy decision is unclear, but apparently, some states did not decide to release other short-term prisoners than fine defaulters. Different levels of occupancy rates and problems of overcrowding cannot explain the differences between e.g., Berlin and Bavaria, but a more or less punitive climate in penal and prison policy, which traditionally is more severe in Bavaria and more relaxed in Berlin.

The prison administration has not much influence on an early release after half or two thirds of the prison sentence (it is a decision of the Court for the Execution of Sentences, see §§ 57, 57a Penal Code, 88, 89 Juvenile Justice Act).[9] If the statements of the prison administration concerning the decision of an early release have changed in favor of granting more such releases during March and the following months in 2020 is unclear. The absolute numbers of releases after having served two thirds of the prison sentence between January

Table 2. Fine defaulters in German prisons for adults before and during the Covid-19-pandemic in comparison of the federal states (absolute numbers at the end of the month).

Federal state	10/31 2019	2/28 2020	3/31 2020	4/30 2020	5/31 2020	6/30 2020	Change February-March 2020 (Index 2/2020 = 100)	Change February-June 2020 (Index 2/2020 = 100)
Baden-Württemberg	564	543	128	88	82	125	23.6	23.0
Bavaria	667	650	555	350	268	248	85.4	38.2
Berlin	271	325	87	37	29	29	26.8	8.9
Brandenburg	156	175	22	15	14	23	12.6	13.1
Bremen	47	53	28	14	13	13	52.8	24.5
Hamburg	116	118	29	16	19	43	24.6	36.4
Hesse	388	391	166	94	92	92	42.5	23.5
Mecklenburg-Western Pomerania	105	78	17	14	8	13	21.8	16.7
Lower Saxony	346	358	289	178	135	125	80.7	34.9
North Rhine-Westphalia	1.092	1.089	688	472	394	378	63.2	34.6
Rhineland-Palatinate	192	206	91	67	63	44	44.2	21.4
Saarland	34	35	19	12	8	13	54.3	37.1
Saxony	279	336	105	54	58	71	31.3	21.1
Saxony-Anhalt	168	205	154	101	78	60	75.1	29.3
Schleswig-Holstein	90	78	24	11	18	19	30.8	24.4
Thuringia	123	133	45	30	33	37	33.8	27.8
Germany (total)	4.598	4.773	2.447	1,553	1,312	1,333	51.3	29.0

and March 2020 increased from 421 to 498,[10] but a similar increase could be observed in the same period in 2019 as well. Therefore, there is no statistical evidence indicating some causal relationship, at least not yet.

Measures of the prison administration to protect prisoners from being infected

All 16 prison administrations of the federal states in March 2020 took immediate actions for the protection of inmates as well as of staff members in prisons. At the beginning, there was a shortage of masks and hygiene materials, but by about mid-April this problem was solved. Due to the further reduction of the numbers of prisoners and of admissions to prisons all prisons disposed of prison capacities to establish quarantine areas and also to accommodate new prisoners in these areas for about up two weeks.

Other measures aimed to reduce the influx of new prisoners by the non-execution of in particular short-term prison sentences have been dealt with above.[11]

Covid-19 infections in prisons

From March to End of July, only a few prisoners and staff members have been infected. Infected prisoners immediately have been separated in quarantine, no prisoner died because or in combination with the Covid-19-virus. Although complete data for all federal states are missing, the largest federal state, North Rhine-Westphalia, reported on 16 July 2020 that 11 prisoners had been infected, all have recovered. With regard to a total prison population of 15,307 in March 2020, this means a percentage of 0.07%. As far as data are available, most other federal states have registered less than 10 infections of prisoners and thus were practically not affected by the pandemic. In Bavaria, 13 prisoners and 28 staff members were infected by mid-May (average prison population in March 2020: 11,416, i.e. the infection rate was about 0.1%, in Berlin only two prisoners and in the small state of Saarland none.

The general policy is not to isolate the whole group of inmates, but only the ones who are positively tested with the virus.

As to infections of prison staff members, again North Rhine-Westphalia was reporting that 35 staff members were infected since the outbreak of Covid-19, 32 of them are recovered.

In general one can say that the German prison administrations were very successful in keeping Covid-19 outside of prisons.

Contacts with the outside world for prisoners during the pandemic

All Federal states have restricted visits by suspending all visits with personal contact. Some prisons dispose of visitors' facilities with cutoff wheels (*Trennscheibe*, where prisoners can see their visitors, but are separated by a plexi-glass window). Some prisons have introduced such facilities. Visits of lawyers, particularly in pre-trial detention, are not restricted, but if possible also executed by cutoff wheels.

Most Federal states have introduced some compensatory measures such as video telephone calls (Skype etc.), but it is unclear if the compensation is more than a symbolic one for a few cases. A very positive example is that already before the appearance of the pandemic the state of

Lower Saxony had introduced individual cell phones in each of the priosners' cells, which allows them to have phone calls every day withe their relatives and friends. In open prisons prisoners were and are now allowed to use mobile phones. The regular amount of visits is between 2 and 4 hours per month and additional visits for family members and children.

In closed prisons, prison leaves have been stopped (day leaves of several hours and long-term leaves of several days). Also in open prison regimes similar restrictions have been introduced on the one hand, but also long-term leaves of two weeks or more (in some state jurisdictions up to 6 months long-term leaves are possible) are granted, but this concerns probably only a few individual cases. The lockdown of granting prison leaves and work release schemes in closed prisons negatively impacts the efforts for preparing release and of a systematic transition management. One of the key factors of social reintegration in the German prison system is the early preparation for relesase and contacts between the prison and aftercare services which aim at a system of through care as established in several Federal states such as Mecklenburg-Western Pomerania or North Rhine-Westpalia (see Pruin, 2019; Dünkel & Weber, 2019). This underlines the necessity of further going ("reduction-sit") crime policy considerations laid down at the end of the paper in order to minimize the negative impacts of the Corona crisis in prisons.

Since June in North Rhine-Westphalia prisoners are allowed to receive visits from one relative and in addition from their children. Similar regulations and relaxation of the lockdown measures are visible also in the other federal states. However, the plexi-glass window mentioned above is getting the regular form for visits.

The impact of Covid-19 in daily prison life: activities (work, reentry programmes, sports etc.)

Other common activities (work, recreational activities) partly have been reduced, In case working facilities were closed the prisoners in consequence did not receive work remuneration. Instead of about 200–300 € earnings they received only a pocket money of about 40 €. Some Federal states, however, increased the pocket money up to 70% of the regular remuneration (e.g. Lower Saxony). In particular in pre-trial detention the situation is hard and can mean that prisoners are locked up for up to 23 hours per day in their cells. In prisons for sentenced offenders the time of joint activities with co-inmates has also been reduced, in particular team sports activities such as soccer. On the other hand, other sports activities were expanded (jogging, small group activities etc.). The prison administrations try to find a balance between necessary restrictions and calming down prisoners' anger at them by providing compensatory activities.

With regard to the very low infection rates, work activities since June/July are widely taking place in the regular form under considering the Corona protection measures such as wearing masks and keeping distance.

The positive side of the pandemic crisis: what could be kept for further developing prison conditions and the working situation of staff members?

The pandemic had not only a negative impact on prison regimes and daily life in prison. Some of the new forms of communication via internet (Skype and other internet-based communication systems) have been proved manageable without increased security problems. Such communication forms have also been used for court hearings (on pre-trial detention or early release). One should use the experiences with these forms of communication also in the future. Allowing prisoners skype or similar communication is in line with the aim to protect family life and to intensify relations with partners, children and friends.

As to working conditions for staff members, another good experience was allowing homework, at least for some administrative work, naturally not supervision tasks.

The pandemic has resulted in an interruption of executing short-term imprisonment, which – because of its detrimental effects on social re-integration (see Dünkel, 2020) and its negative impact on the prison management (with high numbers of incoming and released prisoners) – is a principally desirable development. We should, however, not just come back to reinstall the same situation as before the pandemic after the lockdown will be ceased, but think of creating possibilities to replace short-term imprisonment by alternative modes of executing prison sentences. In countries, such as Finland, Austria, England and Wales, Lithuania, the Netherlands, Scotland, Spain or Switzerland short prison terms or a short remainder of long-term sentences can be served under probationary supervision, by doing community service work in the community or by serving a specific term under electronic house arrest (see Dünkel & Weber, 2019: 408 ff.). In Finland – and most other countries mentioned – with sentences up to six months, there is a de facto forward of (early) release. The decision is made by the prison administration, i.e. the prison director. Introducing alternative forms of executing short prison terms can reduce the prison population considerably. It really replaces imprisonment and no other alternative sanctions (addressing the problem of net-widening).

For the moment an amnesty for offenders, whose execution of a short-term prison sentence was interrupted would be a feasible solution (see for a positive example insofar the practice in Berlin mentioned above; see also Feest, 2020: 120f.; in North-Rhine Westphalia sentences of a maximum of slightly more than 4 months), as it is a particular high burden to serve a short prison term maybe after a year, when the offender e. g. has shown his or her social integration into work and family life.

Changes in criminal and penitentiary laws and perspectives for a reductionist penal policy

The debate in Germany goes in two directions: Do we need reforms in Criminal and Penitentiary Law, for example, to criminalize noncompliance with pandemic induced restrictions? Should penitentiary laws ease the restrictions practiced during the pandemic? On the other hand, a debate raises concerns against the incarceration policy toward short-term imprisonment.

As to General Criminal Law (*Strafgesetzbuch, StGB*): No changes concerning the Corona-crisis are envisaged. Noncompliance with contact restrictions is not a punishable offense (there is also no demand for it), but it can result in an administrative fine and the amount of these fines have been increased in the last days (August 2020) after some collective events with people not wearing masks or celebrating parties without keeping sufficient distance. These fines can never end in substitute prison sentences.

As to Penitentiary Laws: No changes on that level are discussed, yet, all restrictions are based the existing prison legislation and on directives of the prison administration.

There is, however, a debate starting to what extend these restrictions are justifiable and probably court decisions will be released in the near future. Restrictions of visits and other contacts with the outside world may infringe substantive Penitentiary Law and also constitutional human rights of prisoners and their families. The prison administrations have recently reacted to these discussions by lowering the restrictions and expanding relaxations of the prison regimes.

The general crime policy question raised (mainly) by academics is: Should we not use the pandemic as a reminder that we incarcerate people who should not be in prison and instead could be sanctioned in the community? In Germany, the large number of fine defaulters is certainly an issue and the pressure of the left and green political parties increases. As in other European countries, fine default imprisonment could be widely avoided by alternative forms of executing fines and replacing them by community service or by abolishing fine default imprisonment at all by transferring the execution to civil law agencies (see Dünkel, 2019 with further references).

Many academics also take the opportunity to remind the decriminalization of soft drugs and of the possession for use of all drugs as well as of petty property offenses, which for recidivists may result in prison sentences (Dünkel, 2019, 2020; Harrendorf, 2020; Mohr, 2020). Germany has the largest proportion of short-term prisoners in Europe (see Dünkel, 2017: 642f.), mainly because of the fine default problem, but also because of many short-term prison sentences (although a law reform in 1969 wanted to ban them, see Dünkel, 2019). Therefore, the need of further reforms of criminal law and the criminal sanctions system is evident (Mohr, 2020).

Notes

1. See for the development of the German prison system Dünkel and Rössner (2001), Dünkel (2018).
2. The statistical data on the prison population and the distribution of inmates in comparison of the federal states are taken from *Statistisches Bundesamt* (Ed.). Rechtspflege. Bestand der Gefangenen und Verwahrten in den deutschen Justizvollzugsanstalten nach ihrer Unterbringung auf Haftplätzen des geschlossenen und offenen Vollzugs (monthly statistics on prisoners in closed and open prison facilities), https://www.destatis.de.
3. See world prison brief: http://www.prisonstudies.org/info/worldbrief/wpb_stats.php (last access: 16 August 2020).
4. See for the German development in comparison to other European jurisdictions Dünkel (2017).
5. The absolute numbers of sentenced prisoners were 42,195 at the end of March and 45,715 at the end of June 2020.
6. It does not mean that only low-risk offenders are granted to serve their sentence in open prisons. Also medium- and high-risk offenders – at least in the very last stages of the execution of prison sentences –, should have the right to be transferred to open prisons in order to alleviate the transition process from closed prisons to an open environment and the after-care situation, see for that Dünkel in Dünkel, Jesse, Pruin, & von der Wense (2016): 91 ff.
7. At the end of June 2020 the proportion of prisoners accommodated in open prisons for adults was 14.1% and in youth prisons 8.2%, which underlines the statement that the pandemic had no visible impact on the strategy of furthering the reentry of prisoners by a graduated release and the transfer to open prisons. However, further statistical analysis is needed on the question of differential effects and on which offender groups were preferably selected.
8. North Rhine-Westphalia in the response to a Parliamentary Inquiry declared that prisoners who served a fine default or prison sentence of up to 18 months that ended between 20 March and 31 July 2020 had been released by interrupting the execution of the sentence according to §

455a Criminal Procedure Act (for organizational reasons). In total 1,051 prisoners were released, which corresponds to 9.7% of the North Rhine-Westphalian prison population in March 2020, see Parliamentary printed matter, *Landtags-Drucksache* 17/3468 of 8 June 2020.

9. See for the legal requirements in Germany and in comparison to other European jurisdictions Dünkel (2015); Dünkel and Weber (2019).
10. The absolute numbers remained on this relatively high level also in April to June 2020 (498, 506, and 471), leaving open the question of a pandemic induced more favorable early release policy.
11. Unfortunately, Germany does not report the measures taken against Covid-19 infections and other changes in prison life during the pandemic to the internet-platform Europris, although the Federal Ministry of Justice is a member of Europris, see https://www.europris.org.

Disclosure statement

No potential conflict of interest was reported by the author(s).

References

Dünkel, F. (2015). Mandatory release versus discretionary release – A comparative approach. In M. Herzog-Evans (Ed.), *Offender-release and supervision: The role of courts and the use of discretion* (pp. 167–192). Wolf Legal Publishers.

Dünkel, F. (2017). European penology: The rise and fall of prison population rates in Europe in times of migrant crises and terrorism. *European Journal of Criminology*, *14*(6), 629–653. https://doi.org/10.1177/1477370817733961

Dünkel, F. (2018). Strafvollzug. In D. Hermann & A. Pöge (Eds.), *Kriminalsoziologie. Handbuch für Wissenschaft und Praxis* (pp. 399–438). Nomos Verlag.

Dünkel, F. (2019). Reforms of the criminal sanctions system in Germany – achievements and unresolved problems. *Juridica International* (Estonia), *28*, 37–48. Internet https://doi.org/10.12697/JI.2019.28.05

Dünkel, F., Jesse, J., Pruin, I., & von der Wense, M., (Eds.). (2016). *European treatment, transition management, and re-integration of high-risk offenders*. Forum Verlag Godesberg.

Dünkel, F. (2020). Short-term imprisonment and the „reductionist" approach. In K. Beyens, (Ed.), *Liber amicorum for Sonja Snacken*. Free University of Brussels. (forthcoming).

Dünkel, F., & Rössner, D. (2001). Germany. In D. van Zyl Smit & F. Dünkel (Eds.), *Imprisonment today and tomorrow – International perspectives on prisoners' rights and prison conditions* (2nd ed., pp. 288–350). Kluwer.

Dünkel, F., & Weber, J. (2019). (Early) release, probation and collateral consequences (directives) after release. Legal conditions and practice. In F. Dünkel, I. Pruin, A. Storgaard, & J. Weber (Eds.), *Prisoner resettlement in Europe* (pp. 403–434). Routledge.

Feest, J. (2020). Corona und Knast – Ein Zwischenbericht. *Neue Kriminalpolitik*, *32*(2), S. 113–122. https://doi.org/10.5771/0934-9200-2020-2-113

Harrendorf, S. (2020). Plädoyer für eine umfassende Entkriminalisierung des Umgangs mit Betäubungsmitteln zum Eigenkonsum. In K. Drenkhahn, B. Geng, J. Grzywa-Holten, S. Harrendorf, C. Morgenstern, & I. Pruin (Eds.), *Kriminologie und Kriminalpolitik im Dienste der Menschenwürde. Festschrift für Frieder Dünkel zum 70. Geburtstag* (pp. 351–379). Forum Verlag Godesberg.

Mohr, N. (2020). *Die Entwicklung des Sanktionenrechts im deutschen Strafrecht – Bestandsaufnahme und Reformvorschläge*. Forum Verlag Godesberg.

Morgenstern, C. (2016). "Der Resozialisierungsgrundsatz". Social reintegration as the dominant narrative for community punishment in Germany? In G. Robinson & F. McNeill (Eds.), *Community punishment. European perspectives* (pp. 72–94). Routledge.

Pruin, I. (2019). Prisoner resettlement in Germany. In F. Dünkel, I. Pruin, A. Storgaard, & J. Weber (Eds.), *Prisoner resettlement in Europe* (pp. 150–166). Routledge.

Fears of COVID-19 Contagion and the Italian Prison System Response

April Pattavina and Michael J. Palmieri

ABSTRACT
Italy was the first country outside of Asia to deal with a major COVID-19 outbreak. The first cases dated back to January 31, 2020, when two Chinese tourists visiting Rome tested positive for the virus. As the number of infections surged over the next few weeks, the world watched as Italy faced the grim reality of the dangers associated with the virus and how the nation struggled to contain it. By mid-March, the entire country was in lock down. This article chronicles the impact of the virus on incarcerated persons and the ways in which the government reacted to several prison riots that took place in response to crowded prisons, the COVID-19 outbreak, and the initial lock down measures put in place. In the concluding section, the impact of Italy's mitigation strategy on the problems of (1) prison crowding, (2) prison violence, and (3) prisoner and staff health is assessed.

Introduction: Covid-19 in Italy

Italy was the first country outside of Asia to deal with a major COVID-19 virus outbreak. The timeline began on January 31, 2020, when two Chinese tourists visiting Rome tested positive for the virus (Harlan & Pitrelli, 2020). The following week, a man who repatriated from Wuhan China, the place believed to be the epicenter of the virus, was confirmed as the third case (Za & Bastianello, 2020). Soon after, the government declared a six month state of emergency to try and contain the virus and was the first country to ban direct flights from China ("Italy Suspends All China Flights," 2020). Unfortunately, the international travel restriction did little to stop the internal spread of the virus.

The first instance of community transmission and death involved a 78-year-old man from the Veneto region in northern Italy reported on February 21, 2020 (Harlan & Pitrelli, 2020). The next day, the Prime Minister ordered a targeted lockdown of 50,000 in northern regions of Lombardy and Veneto. By March 8, with 5,900 confirmed cases, Italy extended the lockdown to include 16 million people in the Northern provinces (Harlan & Pitrelli, 2020). No travel was allowed in these areas unless for verifiable work-related activities, emergencies, or health reasons ("Coronovirus: Northern Italy Quarantines 16 Million", 2020). Schools, museums, theaters, and sporting events were closed for the entire country. People were told to stay at home as much as possible and a social distance of one meter was mandated (Kington & Sage, 2020). By mid-March the lockdown expanded nation-wide, and all commercial activity except supermarkets and pharmacies was halted ("Coronavirus: Italy Extends Emergency Measures", 2020).

Infections continued to surge over the next few weeks and the world watched in real time as Italy faced the grim reality of the health perils posed by the virus and how the nation struggled to contain it. On March 19, Italy reported 3,405 COVID-19 related deaths and surpassed China as the country with the largest number deaths due to the virus (Alberti et al., 2020). The government moved to the next stage in the lockdown, and the new measures included some of the most drastic steps taken by a modern democracy (Harlan & Morris, 2020). The police were given authority to stop and ask people the reasons why they were trying to leave or enter certain areas. Those needing to travel for work or health reasons were required to produce a written declaration of necessity (Sylvers & Legorano, 2020). Those who broke quarantine could face fines or a jail term ("Coronavirus: Northern Italy Quarantines 16 Million", 2020). By the end of March, the Italian military was officially called to enforce the quarantine and the Italian police were allowed to use surveillance drones to monitor the movement of citizens (Meisenzahl, 2020).

A brief overview of the Italian prison system: crowding and Covid-19

There are 189 adult prisons in Italy; over 60,000 individuals were held in these prisons as of February 2020. Significant numbers of inmates are pretrial detainees (32.4%) and foreign prisoners (32.7%) (Institute for Crime & Justice Policy Research, 2020). Twenty five percent of the inmates are over the age of 50, the second highest rate in Europe (Antigone, 2020). Figure 1 displays the average prison operating capacity by region in 2019. Nationwide, the regional average was 119% capacity, but some individual facilities were reported to be as high as reaching a Pre-COVID-19 capacity of 194.7%, making Italy among the most overcrowded prison systems in Europe (Antigone, 2020). At of the end of February 2020 Italy had a prison capacity of 50,931 and a prison population of 61,230 (Bunham, 2020).

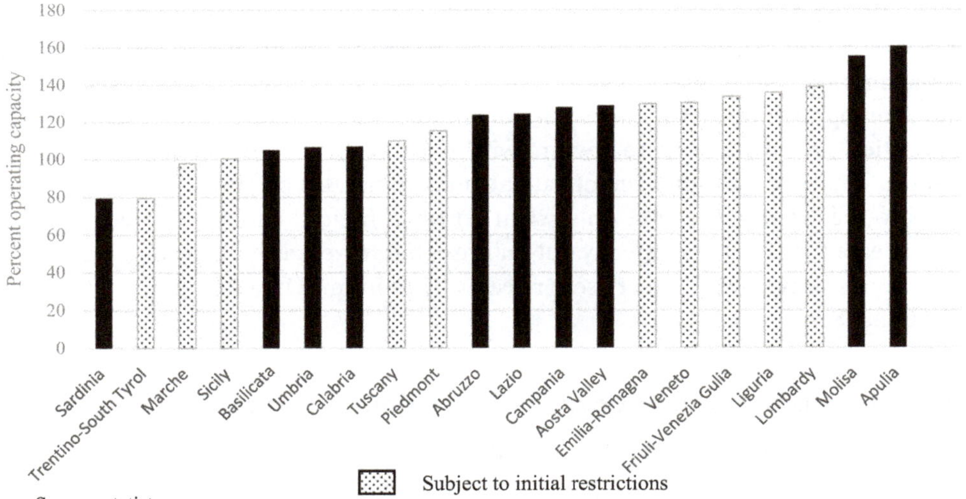

Source: statista.com

Figure 1. Italian prison operating capacity by region in 2019.

Overcrowding was of concern because the recommended precautions against coronavirus spread such as quarantines, social distancing, and sanitation were difficult to implement under such conditions (Raghavan & Loveluck, 2020). Like many countries, the Italian prison system had been struggling with overcrowding in many of its facilities in recent years. For example, in 2013, the European Court of Human Rights demanded that Italy take steps to alleviate overcrowding. Complainants in the *Torreggiani and Others V. Italy* human rights case heard by the court alleged that three inmates were being held in a 9 square meter cell designed for one person allowing each only 3 square meters of personal space. There were also complaints about a lack of hot water and inadequate lighting in the cells (European Court of Human Rights Registrar, 2020). Recommendations made by the court to alleviate crowding included reducing pretrial detention and making greater use of alternatives to prison sentences, but any progress made to reduce incarceration levels appears to have been short lived. In 2012, the year before the case, the imprisonment rate was 110 per 100,000 and decreased to 88 in 2014, but by 2018 the rate increased back up to 99 (Institute for Crime & Justice Policy Research, 2020), fueled in part by an increase in sentence length over the last ten years with 27% lasting more than 10 years (Antigone, 2020).

Prison-based mitigation strategies

The Justice Ministry's immediate plan to prevent COVID-19 contagion was to restrict access into and out of prison facilities. Starting at the end of February, initial restrictions on access to prisons applied to people coming to work in facilities from communities with high numbers of infections, located mainly in northern Italy (European Organisation of Prison and Correctional Services.org, 2020). Inmate transfers out of prisons located in highly affected areas, called "red zones", were also suspended. In Figure 1 the northern regions are highlighted and in all but two of the regions the operating capacity was at or greater than 100%. As infections continued to rise at alarming levels throughout the country, the restrictions were soon extended to the entire penal system and additional measures were established to prevent the spread in prisons.

The additional restrictions promulgated by the Italian government included the temporary suspension of treatment programs that involved participation from people in the local community, the curtailment of work related activities serving the facilities that involve people coming in from outside, and the substitution of in person visits with relatives or third parties other than defense lawyers with phone calls or other available technology. Video conferencing and other remote attendance would also be available for incarcerated persons to receive hearings, but only when possible. Judicial authorities were advised to extend release time for those already out on leave, but temporarily suspend the granting of prison bonus leaves and supervised releases (European Organisation of Prison and Correctional Services.org, 2020).

The links between crowding, Covid-19, mitigation strategies, and prison violence

In the early stages of the Covid-19 outbreak in Italy's prisons, prisoner advocacy groups warned that inmates were growing increasingly anxious about their vulnerability to the virus given the crowded conditions in which they were living and the lack of information about the virus (Winfeld, 2020). Fears about infection, combined with restrictions on family visits and the anxiety about the possibility of having to endure even longer delays in already burdened court system, escalated tensions to the point where violent protests broke out in 24 prisons throughout Italy in early March that involved an estimated 6,000 inmates (Roberts, 2020). The unrest led to 13 deaths among detainees and 59 injured guards. The prisoner deaths were attributed to overdoses that happened after detainees raided prison pharmacies (Bunham, 2020).

One of the largest riots happened at the Modena prison. Six inmates died after they broke into the prison infirmary and overdosed on methadone, which is used to treat opioid dependence (Winfeld, 2020). Inmates set mattresses on fire and took two guards hostage during an escape attempt. They were stopped by the riot police, but enough physical damage had been done to the prison to require the relocation of inmates to temporary facilities. Inmates from other prisons also started fires. Flames from a mattress fire in Pavia prison could be seen from more than half a mile away and led to the evacuation of part of the facility (Nadeau, 2020).

Riots in several prisons resulted in dozens of escapes. From Foggia prison about 50 inmates escaped and from Rebibbia around 30 inmates broke out (Winfeld, 2020). Most were apprehended a short time after their escape (Nadeau, 2020). In the San Vittore prison in Milan, prisoners waived a sheet to the outside with "Indulto" (Italian for pardon) painted on it. Prosecutors responded by going up on the roof to listen to complaints about overcrowding and demands for better treatment. According to one prosecutor's account, the prison was holding 1,200 inmates in the facility that was originally designed to house 700 inmates (Winfeld, 2020). Inmate-rights groups launched complaints about the lack of testing inside prisons across the country and that the low number of confirmed cases among the incarcerated was not reflective of the current situation (Nadeau, 2020). The penitentiary police union was also going public with concerns about the lack of sufficient support from the government to prevent the spread of the virus or to manage anxious, angry inmates (Winfeld, 2020).

By mid-March the Italian government announced further measures intended to relieve overcrowding, support workers, and implement protocols for the handling of infected persons (European Organisation of Prison and Correctional Services.org, 2020). To relieve overcrowding, eligible persons who had 18 months or less of their sentence to serve would be released to home detention or other private healthcare facilities. Those excluded from eligibility were persons imprisoned for mafia related crimes, terrorism, kidnapping for ransom, international drug trafficking, domestic violence, habitual offenders, and the inmates who participated in the recent prison riots. Those with more than 6 of 18 months to serve in home confinement would be subject to electronic monitoring. These strategies had a significant impact on the level of crowding in Italy's prisons. The Counsel of Europe (2020) reported that Italy released 9.4% of its prison population during the height of the outbreak, largely resulting from the early release decree and by the end of June was operating at 106% capacity with a population of 53,579 (Institute for Crime & Justice Policy Research, 2020).

In addition to inmate-focused mitigation strategies, the Italian government also adopted measures to protect prison staff. Support for prison officers came in the form of an increase in the 2020 budget to pay for overtime, the addition of 1,100 new penitentiary police agents, and access to protective equipment. Specific protocols relating to the testing and treatment of infected inmates as well as those with potential exposure were further established by the

Ministry of Health to prevent the spread. Some prisoners were enlisted to help produce much needed protective equipment. In one facility where inmates had been producing sheets and pillowcases for all Italian prisons, shifted to producing surgical masks that would be distributed first to staff, then to prisoners, and last to others with reasons to be at the prisons ("Coronavirus, Contagions in San Vittore." 2020).

COVID-19 in Italian prisons

In early March 2020, Covid-19 infections had been detected in four prisons ("Coronavirus, Contagions in San Vittore", 2020). Prison staff and human rights monitors had been warning of an impending public health emergency given the poor living conditions in many of the prisons. Recognizing the potential for Covid-19 outbreaks in prisons, the guarantor of prisoners representing the Municipality of Milan filed a complaint with the Public Prosecutor about reported ill treatment of inmates in a local prison. The complaint referenced reports from several sources which convinced the guarantor to request that the government formally investigate the allegations of mistreatment and conduct inspections of the facility ("Coronavirus, Contagions in San Vittore.", 2020).

On April 2, 2020 the first prisoner died of Covid-19 (Cingoliani et al., 2020). By mid-May, 137 inmates tested positive for the coronavirus and four had died. Penitentiary staff were also affected, with 202 testing positive (Povoledo & Bubola, 2020) leading to the death of two officers and two doctors (Antigone, 2020).

What works? Assessing the short-term impact of the Italian model

The World Health Organization praised the approach established by the Italian health professionals to prevent contagion in prisons and suggested their efforts serve as a model for others to follow (World Health Organization, 2020). Much of the praise centered on the fact that since 2008 tasks and duties relevant to inmate healthcare were under the auspices of the Ministry of Health rather than the Ministry of Justice. Confidence in the ability of the Ministry of Health to oversee the administration of healthcare in prisons led some healthcare professionals to claim that prisons were the preferable location to house potentially infected inmates since the prison is where they were more likely to receive necessary healthcare and keep the virus contained (Malta et al., 2020).

Other Italian health experts have voiced skepticism about the ability of legislative measures to limit the spread of the virus given the structural and situational circumstances unique to the prison environment. Camposeragna (2020) reported that the commitment to adequate healthcare in prisons is lacking given that there are no provisions by the Health Ministry that guarantee health services offered in prisons would be the same as those offered to the community, a stark reality expressed in the (pre-COVID-19) 1 to 315 ratio of doctors to inmates, an estimate far below the ratio 1 to 200 required by law.

Cingoliani et al. (2020) claim that legislative dictates do not sufficiently support containment efforts including social distancing, voluntary isolation for suspected cases, and health care for positive cases given current prison conditions. They further argued that the lack of a plan to conduct large scale testing of the inmate population would render primary and secondary prevention efforts futile. Given the difficulty of restricting the close inter-personal contacts that inevitably occur in crowded prison settings and the legislative failure to provide valid measures to reduce the risk of infection in such environments, they concluded that the only concrete alternative to control the spread was to significantly reduce the number of prisoners.

Concluding comments: the past as prologue to long term prison reform

Italy had recently experimented with a large-scale pardon of prisoners in 2006 to relieve crowding. In July of that year, the government implemented an unanticipated collective pardon of those with a sentence of less than three years resulting in the release of about 37% of the total prison population. The pardon was followed by substantial increases in crime in the 2006–2008 period (Drago et al., 2017). Intense media coverage of crime right up to the next election in 2008, along with public opinion attributing the crime increase to the pardon, and by extension the ruling party, proved costly to the incumbent party in the 2008 election cycle (Drago et al., 2017).

Concerns about potential political fall-out from the 2020 dictate to release inmates to prevent Covid-19 contagion have also been reported. The left leaning government currently in power can't afford to appear soft on crime (Roberts, 2020), especially since the far right opposition party is presumed to be more capable of managing the crime problem (Drago et al., 2017). These concerns came to fruition when it was reported that although the early release decree in response to COVID-19 excluded inmates housed in maximum security and persons convicted of mafia related crimes, hundreds of offenders sentenced for mafia type offenses managed to get judicial approval for early release after officials decided they would also consider early release for those whose age and health conditions made them susceptible to COVID-19 dangers ("Hundreds of Mafia Members Leave Prison", 2020).

Specific public attention focused on requests for release by mafia bosses who had originally been sentenced under article 41-bis of the Italian penal code, which included physical isolation and the suspension of privileges specifically for this group of serious offenders in an effort crack down on the decades old serious problem with mafia related crime (Povoledo & Bubola, 2020). Although ineligible for early release under the decree, a number of Mafioso managed to get judicial approval for release because their advanced age or health conditions made them especially vulnerable to the virus – even though the isolation requirement under 41-bis had already kept them segregated from the general prison population and less likely to get infected. The release of several high-profile elderly mafia bosses sparked public outrage that led to the resignation of a top prison official (Taylor, 2020). Judicial authorities subsequently revoked the house arrest of at least one Mafioso and put the cases of other released mobsters under review (Povoledo & Bubola, 2020).

The COVID-19 pandemic continues to unfold across the world and the Italian experience with containment will continue to evolve. As of this writing, there have been 251,713 reported infections and 35, 225 deaths in Italy (Worldometers, August 12, 2020). Italy's experience as one of the first modern democracies to deal with a major COVID-19 virus outbreak does offer some noteworthy insights into the philosophy about the role that prisons play in modern society. Indeed, some underlying assumptions about the purpose of incarceration were fundamentally challenged in the face of a highly contagious and deadly virus for which traditional health, justice, and penal institutions were ill prepared to manage.

Italy's initial response to prevent contagion was to curtail movement into and out of prisons, effectively seeking to disconnect prison facilities from the community and isolate prisoners. While a main goal of incarceration is incapacitation where prisoners are kept separate from the rest of society for public safety, the prison, as an institution, is closely connected to the community through the people that work there, the family members who visit, and the prisoners who will eventually return home. In the face of a highly infectious virus such as COVID-19, it is naive to think that prisons can be quickly and effectively isolated without consequence. The fear of infection, further isolation from family and community, and the slowing of procedural justice in Italy's initial response created anxiety and anger that erupted into riots.

The second assumption challenged by the COVID-19 crisis has to do with the view that many hold of prisons as places of punishment and retribution and how those perceptions work to limit prisoner's rights and the level of health care governments were willing to provide in the interests of virus containment. Cingoliani et al. (2020) remind us that the Italian constitution dictates that in depriving persons of their freedom, "there must be full respect of their rights to health, life, and personal integrity" (p. 3). The curtailment of prisoner's rights in the interest of common good, in this case the prevention of COVID-19 contagion, implies that they too would be entitled to reasonable protections to prevent infection. However, prisoners are unlikely to benefit from protections because crowded prisons conditions make it impossible to effectively implement even basic prevention measures, such as social distancing or isolation for suspected cases. This imbalance in prisoner rights vs. health will be perpetuated if the Italian government remains unwilling to engage in long term, sustainable solutions to reduce crowding. Such issues are not new to the discourse on prison reform, but the pandemic certainly exposed the long term physical neglect of prisons and revealed the health, political and justice challenges that Italy and other countries face in meeting prison needs that will be necessary to manage infectious disease outbreaks in the future.

Disclosure statement

No potential conflict of interest was reported by the author(s).

References

Alberti, M., Ruotolo, N., DiDonato, V., & John, T. (2020, March 19). Italy surpasses China in number of coronavirus deaths. Cable News Network (CNN). https://www.cnn.com/2020/03/19/europe/italy-death-toll-intl/index.html

Antigone. (2020). *Prison at the Time of Coronavirus. Antigone's XVI report on prison conditions.* http://www.antigone.it/news/antigone-news/3301-il-carcere-al-tempo-delQ7coronavirus-xvi-rapporto-diantigone-sulle-condizioni-di-detenzione

Bunham, F. (2020, March 20). Wider steps needed to protect prisoners health in Italy. Human Rights Watch. https://www.hrw.org/news/2020/03/20/wider-steps-needed-protect-prisoners-health-italy

Camposeragna, A. (2020). Another effect of CoVid-19: Turning the lights on the Italian prison situation. *Recenti Progressi in Medicina*, *111*(5), 287–289. https://doi.org/10.1701/3366.33407

Cingoliani, M., Caraceni, L., Cannovo, N., & Piergiorgio, F. (2020). The COVID-19 epidemic and the prison system in Italy. *Journal of Correctional Health Care*, 1–8. https://doi.org/10.1177/1078345820929733

"Coronavirus, Contagions in San Vittore, Pavia and Voghera. The guarantor reports possible mistreatment at opera". (2020, March 20). La Repubblica. https://milano.repubblica.it/cronaca/2020/03/17/news/coronavirus_a_san_vittore_contagiato_un_detenuto_positivi_anche_a_voghera_pavia_e_due_medici_del_penitenziario_di_brescia-251552567/?ref=RHPPTP-BH-I251519435-C12-P6-S1.8-T2

"Coronavirus: Italy extends emergency measures nationwide". (2020, March 10). British Broadcasting Corporation (BBC). https://www.bbc.com/news/world-europe-51810673

"Coronavirus: Northern Italy quarantines 16 million people". (2020, March 8). British Broadcasting Corporation (BBC). https://www.bbc.com/news/world-middle-east-51787238

Counsel of Europe, Strasbourg. (2020, June 18). *Promoting more humane and socially effective penal sanctions.* Retrieved August 1, 2020, from https://www.coe.int/en/web/prison/home/-/asset_publisher/ky2olXXXogcx/content/sanctions-and-measures-without-deprivation-of-liberty-increasingly-used-in-europe-new-survey

Drago, F., Galbiati, R., & Sobbrio, F. (2017). *The political cost of being soft on crime: Evidence from a natural experiment.* IZA Discussion Papers, No. 10858. Institute of Labor Economics (IZA.

European Court of Human Rights Registrar. (2020, August 1). The Court calls on Italy to resolve the structural problem of overcrowding in prisons, which is incompatible with the Convention. *European Court of Human Rights.* https://www.radicali.it/sites/default/files/Chamber%20judgment%20Torreggiani%20and%20Others%20v.%20Italy%2008.01.2013-1.pdf

Europis.org. (2020, March 19). *Italy – provisions to fight the COVID-19 contagion in prisons.* Justice Programme of the European Union. Retrieved August 10, 2020, from https://www.europris.org/wp-content/uploads/2020/03/ITALY-provision-against-contagion-COVID-19-update-19-March-2020.pdf

Harlan, C., & Morris, L. (2020, March 12). Italy ramps up coronavirus lockdown, Merkel warns virus could infect two-thirds of Germany. *The Washington Post.* (https://www.washingtonpost.com/world/europe/merkel-coronavirus-germany/2020/03/11/e276252a-6399-11ea-8a8e-5c5336b32760_story.html)

Harlan, C., & Pitrelli, S. A. (2020, March 20). How coronavirus overwhelmed Italy, with more than 4,000 deaths in one month. *The Washington Post.* https://www.washingtonpost.com/world/europe/italy-coronavirus-deaths/2020/03/20/4a385552-6a20-11ea-b199-3a9799c54512_story.html

"Hundreds of Mafia members leave prison under Italy's lockdown". (2020, May 8). The Local. https://www.thelocal.it/20200508/hundreds-of-mafia-members-leave-prison-under-italys-lockdown

"Italy suspends all China flights as coronavirus cases confirmed in Rome". (2020, January 31). The Local. https://www.thelocal.it/20200131/italy-suspends-all-china-flights-after-coronavirus-cases-confirmed-in-rome/

Kington, T., & Sage, A. (2020, March 3). Italians told to stand a metre apart as coronavirus death toll exceeds 50. The Times. https://www.thetimes.co.uk/article/italians-told-to-stand-a-metre-apart-as-death-toll-exceeds-50-2f8nx3p9p

Malta, G., Zerbo, S., & Argo, A. (2020). The risk of the 'prison-emptying' effect in Italy due to the Covid-19 pandemic. *Medico-Legal Journal, 88*(2), 103–104. https://doi.org/10.1177/0025817220923697

Meisenzahl, M. (2020, April 1). Italian police are using drones to track down citizens who violate one of the strictest coronavirus lockdowns in Europe. *Business Insider.* https://www.businessinsider.com/coronavirus-italian-police-monitoring-lockdown-with-drones-2020-3

Nadeau, B. L. (2020,March 9). Italy in flames in Coronavirus lockdown riot among cut off inmates. *Daily Beast.* https://www.thedailybeast.com/six-inmates-dead-scores-escape-as-prisoners-riot-across-italy-after-visitor-restrictions-over-coronavirus

Povoledo, E., & Bubola, E. (2020, May 13). In Italy, some fear the virus is a get out of jail card for Mafiosi. *The New York Times.* https://www.nytimes.com/2020/05/13/world/europe/coronavirus-italy-mafia.html

Raghavan, S., & Loveluck, L. (2020 March 26). How the coronavirus is igniting riots, releases and crackdowns in world's prisons. *The Washington Post.* https://www.washingtonpost.com/world/how-coronavirus-is-igniting-riots-releases-and-crackdowns-in-the-worlds-prisons/2020/03/25/6ca94494-6aba-11ea-b199-3a9799c54512_story.html

Roberts, H. (2020, March 31). In Italy's overcrowded prisons, fear of Coronavirus. Politico. https://www.politico.eu/article/in-italys-overcrowded-prisons-fear-of-coronavirus

Statista.com. (2020). Statista Research Department. Retrieved August 1, 2020, from https://www.statista.com/statistics/575343/prison-population-and-capacity-by-region-italy/

Sylvers, E., & Legorano, G. (2020, March 12). Italy hardens nationwide quarantine. *The Wall Street Journal*. https://www.wsj.com/articles/italy-hardens-nationwide-quarantine-11583962093

Taylor, L. (2020, May 8) Coronavirus crisis causes almost 400 members of the mafia to be released from jail in Italy. EuroWeekly. https://www.euroweeklynews.com/2020/05/08/coronavirus-crisis-causes-almost-400-members-of-the-mafia-to-be-released-from-jail-in-italy/

Winfeld, N. (2020, March, 9). *Prison riots hit Italy amid virus; 6 die in overdose*. Associated Press, https://apnews.com/217a48a672070530363efa459a5f71f0

World Health Organization. (2020, May 28). *Experience of health professionals, police staff and prisoners in Italy informs WHO COVID-19 guidelines for prisons*. https://www.euro.who.int/en/countries/italy/news/news/2020/5/experience-of-health-professionals,-police-staff-and-prisoners-in-italy-informs-who-covid-19-guidelines-for-prisons

Institute for Crime & Justice Policy Research. (2020). *World prison brief*. Birkbeck, University of London. Retrieved August 10, 2020, from https://www.prisonstudies.org/country/italy

Za, V., & Bastianello, R. (2020, February, 22) Italy's coronavirus outbreak infects 51 people, kills two. Reuters. https://www.reuters.com/article/us-china-health-italy/italys-coronavirus-outbreak-infects-51-people-kills-two-idUSKCN20G0CQ

An Examination of The Romanian Prison System During The COVID-19 pandemic. Are "Zero Cases" Possible?

Ioan Durnescu and Ioana Morar

ABSTRACT

In spite of all the measures taken during the past decades, the Romanian prison system is still considered overcrowded by European standards (111% above rated capacity in June 2020). However, very much against the trend set by other European jurisdictions, Romania did not opt for an early release scheme to fight COVID-19. Instead, the government took steps to strengthen its internal mechanisms to ensure safe interactions between staff and inmates, between inmates themselves, and between inmates and the outside world.

This paper explains why that was the only option on the table for the Romanian authorities and then provides a preliminary assessment of the consequences of this strategic decision. Overall, with no known case of infected prisoners, while serving their sentence inside the penitentiary system, it seems that the route taken by the Romanian prison authorities was an effective one, at least in terms of minimizing the outbreak of Covid-19 in the prison system. At least so far ... However, the legal, psychological, and experiential consequences of these strict medico-carceral measures for the prisoners and their families remain to be explored.

The European context of the COVID-19 outbreak

Wuhan Municipal Health Commission in China reported the first COVID-19 cases in December 2019. On the 1st of January 2020, the World Health Organization (WHO) created the Incident Management Support Team placing the organization on an emergency footing for addressing the outbreak.[1] By February 2020, the virus had spread across most of China, and outbreaks were reported in 28 other countries. The first three cases detected in Europe were in France on the 24th of January 2020, but the situation had developed rapidly with a large outbreak identified in Northern Italy, with the transmission in several municipalities (e.g., Lombardy, Veneto and Emilia Romagna). The reports of these Covid-19 outbreaks continued, and by March 2020, there were already 4,250 cases and 113 deaths in Europe (Spiteri et al., 2020). Due to the steep increase in the number of infections and the wide number of countries and territories affected, WHO declared a global pandemic, COVID-19, on the 11th of March 2020.[2]

As the spread of the virus in detention centers is facilitated by prison overcrowding and poor sanitary conditions, the UN High Commissioner for Human Rights, Michelle Bachelet, urged the governments in March 2020 "not to forget" individuals behind bars.

In her speech, she recited that under the international human rights law, the States (i.e. countries) have an obligation to prevent threats to public health and protect those under its care. In this respect, she suggested that governments should work quickly to reduce the number of prisoners in custody, especially those particularly vulnerable to COVID-19 (e.g., older prisoners, those who are at risk due to underlying health problems, etc.) and also "low-risk" offenders who could be released without threatening community safety. She also cautioned that any restrictions on visits should be introduced in a transparent way and communicated clearly. These restrictions should be accompanied by alternative methods of communication, such as extending videoconferencing, more phone calls with family members and permitting e-mail. Most of these key recommendations were included in a joint document adopted by the Office of the UN High Commissioner for Human Rights and World Health Organization, titled: *Interim Guidance. COVID-19: Focus on persons deprived of their liberty (2020).*

It should come as no surprise that prison overcrowding has exacerbated the problem in many countries. According to a review by Aebi and Tiago (2020) for the Council of Europe, eleven European countries were facing some degree of prison overcrowding in April 2020, with rates higher than 100 inmates per 100 places: Slovenia, Austria, Czech Republic, Serbia, France, Italy, Cyprus, Hungary, Greece, Romania, and Turkey. Some countries moved quickly in the early stages of the pandemic to address the overcrowding problem. For example, in the case of Slovenia, although the prison system was overcrowded at the beginning of 2020, the level of crowding was reduced significantly by April 2020. This was possible due to the fact that Slovenia released 16% of its inmates as a preventive measure related to COVID-19.

Other countries appeared to move in the opposite direction during this initial review period. Sweden, for example, took a different route and passed from 99 to 102 inmates per 100 places. It is important to mention here that Sweden is the only country in EU that did not introduce a lockdown.

Apart from Slovenia, there were also several other countries that released some demographic of inmates as a preventive measure related to COVID-19, including Monaco, Iceland, Norway, Andorra, Denmark, Cyprus, UK, Ireland, Luxembourg, Italy, Armenia, France, Spain, Portugal, Serbia, Albania, Azerbaijan and Turkey. According to Aebi and Tiago (2020), a total of about 128,000 inmates were released in 20 European countries as a preventive measure to reduce the spread of COVID-19. By far the largest number of prisoners was released from Turkey (N = 102,944 or 35.3% of the prison population). A significant proportion of prisoners were also released in Spain (Catalonia) – 17%, Cyprus – 15.9%, Slovenia – 15.9%, Portugal – 14.8%, France – 14.4%, Norway – 13.3%, Italy – 9.4%, and the UK – 7.8%. Different penal vehicles or prison modalities were used to ensure the release of prisoners, including: (1) reducing the sentences of certain categories of inmates (France), (2) temporary release and transferring pre-trial inmates to alternative locations (UK), (3) early release with electronic monitoring for those with less than 18 months to serve, and deferral of the sentence for health reasons or semi-freedom (Italy) (AGENFOR, 2020).

Countries have used different measures to avoid or postpone new entries into prisons, such as postponement in commencing prison sentences (Czech Republic, Sweden, Finland, and Norway) or suspended entries into the prison system (Denmark). As highlighted in the AGENFOR (2020) report and by Aebi and Tiago

(2020), in many European jurisdictions, the prison population has decreased or remained stable due to a confluence of front-end and back-end factors, including a decrease in crime rates and criminal justice activity due to the pandemic, and the release of prisoners as a preventive measure to reduce the spread of COVID-19. An example that illustrates the effects of both front-end and back-end factors in Italy reporting 146,762 crimes nationwide in March of 2019, while only reporting 52,596 crimes in March of 2020, which translates to a 66.6% decrease in crime at the national level over the course of 1 year (AGENFOR, 2020).

The Romanian context of the COVID-19 crisis

With almost 110 inmates per 100 spaces, Romania was one of the eleven countries with a prison population exceeding its capacity at the beginning of 2020. Due to overcrowding and responses from other countries in similar situations, one might expect that Romania, too, would release inmates prematurely; however, this was not the case. Instead, due to internal factors, Romania relied on other health and safety measures that decreased direct contact between inmates and the outside world. Although it may be difficult to believe, there have been zero cases of COVID-19 inside Romania's penitentiary system, apart from seven inmates who were transferred from the police preventive detention centers. This reality may seem overly positive in a context in which the number of COVID-19 cases in Romania's general population continues to rise every day, and the penitentiary system is overcrowded and in poor material condition. However, in the next sections, we will describe the context, measures, and outcomes of the Romanian approach toward fighting the spread of COVID-19 inside its penitentiary system.

Romania's prison system has been the subject of international review and criticism for over a decade. As it was mentioned in several SPACE I reports (Council of Europe), reports published by the Committee for Prevention of Torture (CPT reports, hereinafter) and, as of late, in a pilot decision of the European Court of Human Rights (ECHR)[3] against Romania, the penitentiary system was affected by structural dysfunction due to severe overcrowding and poor material conditions of detention. Consequently, ECHR recommended that the Romanian Government reduce overcrowding, improve material conditions within detention centers, and introduce effective preventative and compensatory remedies, such as allowing a judge to respond either prior to, or after, the rights of a prisoner were breached.

In order to respond to these international pressures, the Romanian Government together with the Parliament adopted several measures in the last decade. Two of the most significant measures affecting the prison population, specifically, include a new Penal Code and an introduction of the compensatory remedy law. The new Penal Code was adopted in 2009 (Law no. 286/2009) and instituted on the 1st of February 2014. The main changes brought forth by this new regulation were an expansion of the community sanctions and measures (alternatives to detention), different minimum and maximum sentences for some offenses, and a different approach to juvenile offenders (providing educational, rather than punitive measures). The application of this new Penal Code has led to a significant decrease in the prison population since 2012 (see Graph 1).

Theoretically, reducing overcrowding should lead to improvement of material conditions within detention centers. The process of reducing the prison population was sustained by several other administrative measures, such as the creation of new

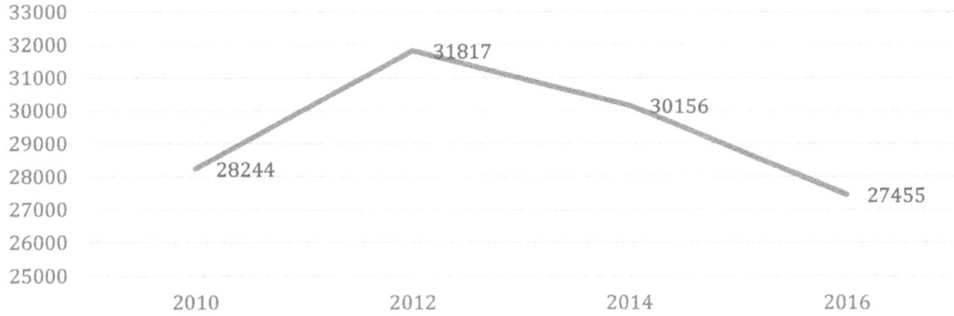

Graph 1. "Number of inmates in Romanian prisons between 2010–2016. Source: World Prison Brief (https://www.prisonstudies.org/country/romania)

detention facilities (i.e., 672 new detention centers were created in 2016 and 170 in 2017). Significant steps were also made toward building two new prisons – P47 Berceni and P48 Unguriu. It was hoped that by reducing crowding and improving the quality/capacity of the prison system, better outcomes would be reported. In 2017 Parliament also adopted Law no. 169/2017 on the compensatory remedy, which codified that for every 30 days served in sub-standard conditions, the prisoners were entitled to a reduction of 6 days from their sentences. Although there are no rigorous studies on this matter, official data from the National Administration of Penitentiaries states that 23,518 inmates benefitted from this measure between 2017 and 2019. This was not the intention of the law – to release inmates prematurely – but emerged as a main effect of implementing such a law (see Graph 2).

It can be inferred that the decrease in the prison population was a cumulative effect of the New Penal Code, the compensatory remedy law, and other measures such as discouragement of the use of pre-trial detention, a more predictable practice around conditional release, and more. Another practice worth mentioning here is the Credit system,[4] which ensures that inmates participate in rehabilitative activities and provides a clear, transparent, and motivational system of appraisal (Morar, 2019; Morar et al., 2019). Following a few tragic incidents in 2018, where heinous crimes were committed by inmates released prematurely,[5] on the basis of the compensatory remedy law, the Romanian Parliament enacted a cancelation law – Law no. 240/2019 on the abrogation/repeal of the compensatory remedy law. Pressure from the public was so strong that public protests were organized in opposition of this law.

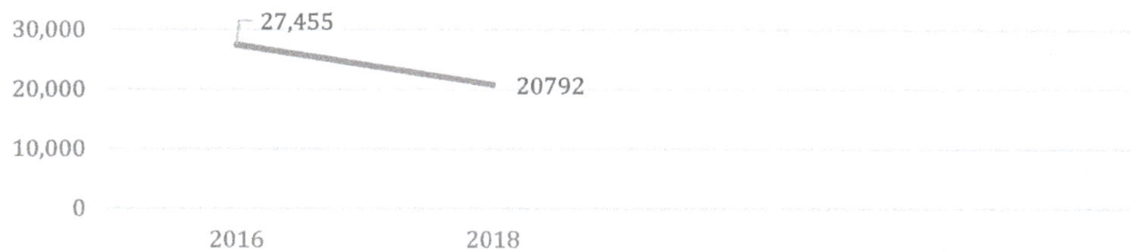

Graph 2. Change in the number of prisoners in Romanian prisons after adopting the compensatory remedy law. Source: World Prison Brief (https://www.prisonstudies.org/country/romania)

Prison administration's response during the first months of the pandemic

Preparatory measures

At the beginning of the COVID-19 crisis (at the end of February 2020), the National Administration of Penitentiaries developed and implemented a strategic plan for mitigating the problem in Romania's prison system: *Planned measures to prevent the spread of COVID-19 among staff and inmates* the plan included: (1) general prevention measures, (2) intervention measures – specific to inmates extradited from areas with high epidemiological risk of COVID-19, and (3) crisis intervention measures.

To implement the plan, a technical-medical support group was established within the National Administration of Penitentiaries (NAP hereinafter), in charge of monitoring and enforcing measures to prevent and counter the epidemic. As a first measure to protect the health of staff and inmates, contact between the prison population and potential sources of infection were limited. Two types of prisoners were targeted for these measures: the general prison population and those transferred from prison systems abroad. One of the first measures for the general prison population was to reduce or suspend some of the activities taking place outside the detention areas. For those extradited to Romania from other European states (e.g., Italy, Spain, and the UK), the accommodation of medical monitoring for a span of 14 days was implemented. Certain penitentiary units were specially designated for implementing quarantine in such circumstances. At the same time, measures were taken in the detention areas to carefully monitor the health condition of all inmates who had returned from prison furlough, within a 14-day follow-up period. Moreover, the administration identified possible new capacities for quarantine, monitoring, or isolating of those inmates who, after an epidemiological screening, would turn out to have symptoms specific to the new coronavirus infection. In order to ensure careful monitoring of the persons in medical isolation, [technological] solutions through [the PMSweb application, or prisoner information system,] were established to [designate] detention rooms for the sole purpose of isolation.

In order to reduce the movement of inmates, the administration requested the High Court of Cassation and Justice, the Appeal Courts, Regional Courts and First Instance Courts to analyze the possibility of hearing the inmates through videoconferencing or rescheduling upcoming hearings. At the very beginning of the emergency state, as an additional measure to maintain continuity of activities and to prevent the spread of Coronavirus, it had been decided that 30% of staff was to remain home while accomplishing professional tasks. Those from operative, medical, or psychosocial intervention sectors were exceptions to this rule. This measure was in place only during the emergency state, and other organizational measures regarding the schedule of the staff were put in place progressively (e.g., programming and partition scheduling).

During the state of emergency

On the 16th of March 2020, the *Presidential Decree no. 195/16.03.2020 declaring a state of emergency in Romania* was published in the Official Gazette of Romania. Annex 1 of this document included the first emergency measures to be applied within the criminal justice system, having a direct impact on the execution of sentences and of measures involving deprivation of liberty. Following the emergency state, the *Measures plan for the penitentiary system upon the declaration of the state of emergency in Romania* was established and applied to the entire prison system. In this document, instructions were provided for the implementation of social distancing measures, limiting of contact between prison officers and inmates, and granting online communications. All inmate-involved activities, including sports, were reconfigured to ensure that large groupings and interactions of inmates were limited. Moreover, access to the detention portions of penitentiaries was limited to staff members that were responsible for surveilling, monitoring, and protecting the units. Additional, protective measures were adopted to ensure that inmates were safe while in contact with treatment providers and administrative staff (National Administration of Penitentiaries [NAP], 2020a).

Treatment measures in Romanian prisons

From a treatment point of view, greater attention was paid toward informing inmates about the need to prevent the spread of COVID-19 and to understand the specific and necessary measures being implemented. Thus, information campaigns for inmates were carried out in penitentiary units, with distribution of informational materials (flyers and posters) and periodically producing and broadcasting announcements through the prisons' closed-circuit radio and TV systems. Individual counseling (educational, social, and psychological) activities were carried out in order to raise awareness and acceptance of strict hygiene measures, while also sanitizing and disinfecting accommodation spaces and other areas where transmission of the virus was more likely, including social reintegration spaces, all with the universal goal of limiting the spread of the virus in mind. In terms of social reintegration initiatives, the following activities were conducted with priority:

- schooling
- professional/vocational
- volunteering
- radio-TV studios were used intensively to broadcast information of interest and importance to inmates
- psychological assistance was only provided in risk circumstances (NAP, 2020a)

Inmate contact between prisons was temporarily halted, as well as group-based activities among inmates. When possible, group-based activities were replaced with individual activities.

Inmates were thoroughly informed about the measures ordered as a result of the state of emergency declared in Romania. In particular, treatment staff members were instructed to carry out individual sessions with certain categories of inmates, in order to monitor their states of mind. To comply with the right of inmates to be informed, the penitentiary units took measures to ensure inmates had access to public TV programs and were allowed to produce and broadcast from the internal radio-TV studio. Most of the educational, moral, and religious-based activities were transferred online to compensate for the lack of direct contact activities (NAP, 2020a).

In accordance with the provisions of Article 47 of the *Presidential Decree no. 195/ 16.03.2020 declaring the state of emergency in Romania*, inmates' rights to receive visits, conjugal visits,[6] goods through the visiting sector, or prison furlough were temporarily

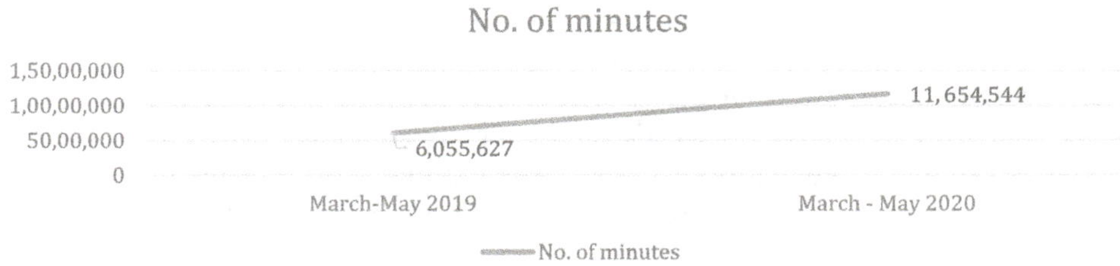

Graph 3. Romanian prisoners telephone usage (in minutes) in 2019 and 2020 (between the months of March & May).

suspended. However, in order to maintain a connection with the outside world, both the duration and number of telephone conversations for inmates within the maximum-security regime were increased from 3 to 5 calls per day and to a maximum duration of 45 minutes per day. The duration and number of telephone conversations for inmates in closed, semi-open, open, and temporary regimes or for those who had not yet been included in a certain regime, were increased to a maximum of 75 minutes per day. Between the periods of March and May of 2019 and 2020, Romanian prisons experienced a near 100% increase in the total number of minutes spent making calls (see Graph 3). Regarding online communications, inmates increased their usage by 98% during this same time period.

During the state of emergency, NAP requested for the operators providing voice services to temporarily reduce the price of phone calls, in addition to assistance in developing this infrastructure. Depending on their priorities and characteristics of each penitentiary unit, each service provider operated under different discounts. While it is difficult to place a specific number on the discount amounts inmates are receiving to make calls, a significant difference can be inferred because of the vast increase in minutes inmates have spent making phone calls. Moreover, the right of inmates to have online conversations, regardless of their disciplinary status or frequency of contact with family, was allocated according to each prison regime's guidelines (Decree no. 195/16.03.2020; NAP, 2020a). Inmates also have the opportunity to communicate with the prison administration daily, in order to inform them about any potential breaches of their rights or abuses. The same applies to contact with the judge supervising the deprivation of liberty.[7]

Health and economic measures in Romanian prisons

The National Administration of Penitentiaries has ensured the necessary, additional funds for purchasing medical supplies and disinfectants. Moreover, with assistance from different institutions and business sectors (e.g., the Ministry of Health, Ministry of Home Affairs – Department for Emergency Situations, Unifarm National Company, and other providers), NAP obtained materials in order to ensure there were stocks of masks, gloves, disposable protective equipment, medical supplies, and disinfectants. A special system of monitoring the stock of essential medical supplies was put into place. Three times per week medical supplies (respiratory protective masks, medical gloves, impermeable suits, shoe covers, coats, medical face shields, and others) and disinfectants (for hands, floors, other surfaces, nebulizers, and others) are numbered and allocated at the national level, according to need. Guidelines were established for supplying the medical materials and disinfectants to prison officers. According to these guidelines, the supplies were allocated to prison staff based on their role and functions and also on the frequency of contact with the prisoners. All prison staff workers were informed of these guidelines (NAP, 2020a).

Steps have been taken with all business operators serving inside the prison to ensure adequate supplies and maintain realistic, and even discounted, prices for products like fruits, vegetables, and hygiene products. Special arrangements were made for the rental of spaces within the prison system in order to ensure significant discounts for inmates.

Medical measures in Romanian prisons

Considering the need to play an active role in combatting the spread of COVID-9, the penitentiary administration established certain isolation areas in five units, intended for inmates considered to be infected with COVID-19. Thus, the following spaces within the prison system have been temporarily converted to quarantining, monitoring, and isolation areas for potentially infected inmates:

- Bucuresti-Jilava Penitentiary-Hospital: 35 beds for isolation
- Aiud Penitentiary: 20 beds
- Poarta Albă Penitentiary-Hospital: 30 beds
- Drobeta Turnu Severin Penitentiary: 40 beds
- Baia Mare Penitentiary: 42 beds

Moreover, under the Order of the Minister of Health,[8] the Hospital Penitentiary of Bucharest – Jilava was designated as a medical unit to carry out special assessment procedures for COVID-19, housing 31 beds for patients that tested positive for COVID-19. At the same time, two hospital penitentiaries were provided with anesthesia and intensive care divisions/departments (ro. ATI). As there were only seven imported COVID-19 cases within correctional settings over the course of the pandemic, these capacities were not overcrowded.

To ensure that units acquired enough medical supplies and protective equipment, the hospital penitentiaries were tasked with planning and purchasing all supplies and equipment necessary for their own use, but also for penitentiaries under their medical coordination Special guidelines were adopted to instruct the hospital penitentiaries on how to perform these extra duties. Instituted on the 14th of May, 2020, inmates leaving detention areas were required to wear personal protective equipment in the form of a face mask or face shield.[9] Since the beginning of the pandemic in Romania, there have been measures taken to enhance the epidemiological triage of both staff and inmates, physical distancing protocol, and disinfection practices.[10] Equipment has been provided by the penitentiary administration free of charge.

Specialized medical staff were responsible for tending to inmates that were suspected of having COVID-19. Two doctors specializing in anesthesia and intensive care and one doctor specializing in infectious diseases were appointed to oversee the medical situation among inmates. Special protocols were established to ensure an effective cooperation with public health authorities. All suspected cases of COVID-19 were to be reported to county public health departments, and depending on the nature and severity of the situation, the National Single Service for Emergency Calls may be contacted via 112.

In alignment with guidelines from the Ministry of Health and National Committee for Special Emergency Situations, NAP has adopted special practices regarding the optimal (and efficient) use and rationing of protective equipment. Training on how to properly use protective equipment, how to put on, wear, remove, and replace masks, and more was offered to non-medical staff as well. In this respect, informational materials (e.g., videos) regarding effective health and hygiene measures were also created and provided.

On the 14th of April, 2020 Presidential Decree no. 240 was issued ordering an *extension of the state of emergency in Romania*; thus, all transfers[11] between penitentiary units must be approved by the Medical Supervisory Directorate (NAP, 2020b). Moreover, from an operative point of view, some hospital penitentiaries were prioritized over others and therefore a transfer of material resources was essential. The Hospital Penitentiary of Bucharest-Jilava is now deemed as the medical unit responsible for carrying out priority actions for monitoring, treatment, and care of critical patients, with emerging and reemerging infections (AP-IER/RE), according to the Ministry of Health.[12]

In designing these measures, the National Administration of Penitentiaries was guided by the regulations strongly suggested by the European Committee for the Prevention of Torture and Inhuman or Degrading Treatment or Punishment (CPT) for managing inmates in the current epidemiological context. The 10 principles recommended by CPT (2020a)[13] were translated and communicated to all prison staff throughout the country.

Number of prisoners during the pandemic

Graph 4 further illustrates that Romania's strategy to manage the pandemic in prisons was not to release prisoners, but rather to contain them in safer conditions by ensuring that the virus did not infiltrate in the first place. During the first half of 2019 and 2020, released inmate totals were comparable.

While a closer look at Graph 4 may demonstrate a slightly lower number of inmates being released in 2020 as compared to 2019, a viable explanation can be offered: the total number of prisoners existing within Romania's prisons was smaller in 2020 than 2019, thus less prisoners were released.

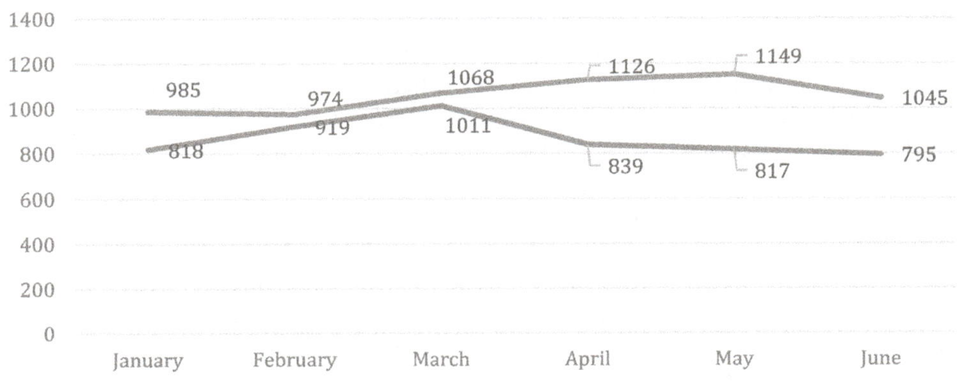

Graph 4. Number of prisoners released in the first 6 months – outputs 2019–2020.

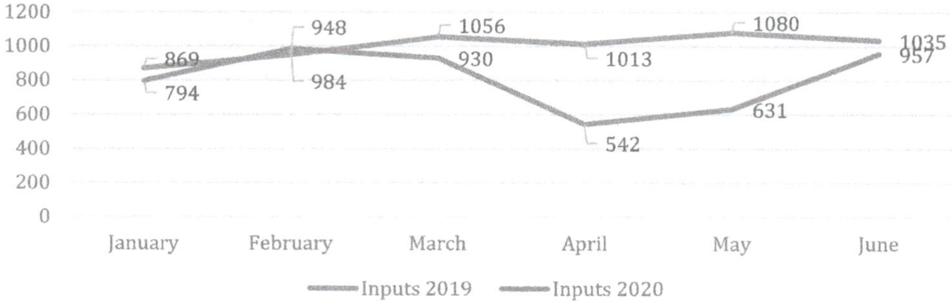

Graph 5. Number of new prisoners in the first six months 2019–2020.

A different dynamic can be observed in terms of inmates entering Romanian prisons in 2020. Graph 5 demonstrates that the number of newly-admitted prisoners in March and April of 2020 was significantly lower than during the same time period in 2019. Potential explanations for this difference are: (1) Romania experiencing a decrease in crime rates due to the pandemic as well as (2) slowing of the Romanian judicial system, which was also under emergency regulations. Unfortunately, official data regarding crime rates and sentencing are not yet available, but will likely be available nearer the end of 2020. However, it can be safely assumed that as the courts were experiencing lockdowns, less people were convicted and sentenced during this period of time.

Outcomes of Romanian strategies to combat COVID-19

The first COVID-19 case in Romania was reported on the 26th of February, 2020 in a 20-year-old in Gorj County after having had contact with an Italian man. In spite of all the measures taken by Ministry of Health and Ministry of Home Affairs, within 2 months, at least 10,000 people were reported as infected with COVID-19. The number of deaths within this same time period, an N of 601, was also alarming. According to the Strategic Communication Group,[14] by the 31st of August, 2020 as many as 87,540 people were infected with COVID-19 in Romania, of which 37,869 were declared as having recovered and 3,621 deaths were reported. The remaining cases were considered asymptomatic, and 7,447 persons were still in hospitals (506 of them in intensive care units). The death rate during this time was estimated to be 4.8%.

To date, 1,802,946 tests have been administered within the general population of about 19 million people. Testing is usually conducted when symptoms are reported or upon the request of individuals. In the latter case, testing comes at a cost. In the former, tests are covered by social and health insurance. Depending on the number of tests run each day, the proportion of positive cases falls near 10%. In other words, if on a given day 1,000 tests were administered, approximately 100 cases would be COVID-19 positive.

According to official data provided by the Romanian National Administration of Penitentiaries, since the beginning of the pandemic through the 31st of August, there have been 148 confirmed cases of COVID-19 among prison staff workers in Romanian penitentiaries. Of these confirmed cases, 147 were hospitalized for at least 24–48 hours. While writing this paper, a prison staff worker came into contact with the virus outside the penitentiary system, was reported as testing positive, and has since died.

Due to the restrictive preventive measures taken by the penitentiary administration described above during this same period, none of the prisoners have tested positive for COVID-19 while serving their sentence in the Romanian penitentiary system. However, as noted above, it is important to mention that during this period, seven cases of COVID-19 were confirmed before being transferred from the Pre-Trial Arrest and Detention Centers of the Ministry of Home Affairs. These individuals were promptly placed in the Penitentiary Hospital of Bucuresti-Jilava until recovered.

Testing for both staff and inmates are performed based on the case definitions and testing methodologies elaborated by the National Institute of Public Health for all Romanian citizens. Therefore, the tests are performed by authorized institutions based on symptoms and/or contact with infected persons.[15] No mass testing has been performed either inside or outside the penitentiary system. Based on the criteria mentioned above – symptoms and contact – 529 tests were administered for inmates in the first eight months of 2020. These tests were performed on those inmates who presented some symptoms or were in contact with people known to be infected by COVID-19. All of the tests performed on the prisoners yielded negative results. Some tested individuals underwent a second round of testing to better account for and exclude false-positive, false-negative, or inconclusive test results. There are no detailed data currently available on how many inmates yielded false-positive, false-negative, or inconclusive test results. Tests and testing procedures for inmates and prison staff emulate the national health authorities': real-time polymerase chain reaction (PCR).

The death rates confirmed in the Romanian penitentiary system for the first eight months of 2020 similarly reflected those recorded in the first 8 months in previous years: 65 in 2017, 73 in 2018, 47 in 2019 and 65 in 2020. The 27% increase in deaths from 2019 to 2020 require further investigation. Upon initial review, most of these deaths were attributed to different illnesses (51 in the first eight months of 2020, 40 in the same period of 2019). For instance, eight prisoners died in the first eight months of 2020 due to respiratory-related illnesses (compared to six in 2017). It is worth noting that a consequence of a lack of mass testing may allow for some infected prisoners to go undetected. In cases as such, it is likely that they may contribute to the increase in prisoner deaths reported in 2020, hence further investigation is required.

Discussion

As demonstrated consistently across the literature, prison population sizes are often a direct product of political decision-making (Boone et al., 2019; Hough et al., 2003). In Romania, when the political decision was made to decrease the prison population total, the Government and the Parliament together employed the most effective tool to do so – changing the Penal Code. The same end result was achieved when initially adopting the compensatory remedy law, though a decrease in this case can be more aptly described as a side effect or unintended consequence. The primary objective of that law was to provide a form of compensation to those serving their sentence in substandard conditions. However, due to the commission of heinous crimes by the hands of those benefiting from this law (e.g., rape, homicide, etc.), the public actively demanded that this law be abrogated. Due to the recency of abrogation (occurring in the second half of 2019), the moral climate in Romania was not conducive to a solution such as preventive release, despite the presence of a global pandemic and prisons still battling overcrowding. It is very likely that the public reaction to such a plan would have been aggressively opposed. Small declines in the number of prisoners can be mainly attributed to the overall decrease in crime rates and limited judicial activity during the state of emergency in Romania.

Instead of preventive release, Romanian authorities focused on socio-medical measures that drastically reduced the interaction between inmates and the outside world. To compensate for the lack of visits, prison leaves, work release and so on, the penitentiary administration put into action technologies that facilitated remote and online meetings and access to information. Considering the fact that there have been no infections among inmates through August 2020 (except in the seven imported cases), it can be assumed that, from a health-oriented point of view, the administration plan was an effective one. Thus, in response to the title's question, the answer is "yes."

We are aware that this picture may look overly positive. This was the reason we have tried to provide the reader with as many details as possible about the social and medical measures included in the Romanian penitentiary plan to fight the spread of COVID-19. It is worth mentioning here that the medical protocols applied in the penitentiary system are the same as the ones applied to the general public. The testing methodologies elaborated by the National Institute of Public Health has informed the testing process for all Romanian citizens and include the same two criteria: previous contact with an infected person and/or the presence of symptoms. The only difference is that the penitentiary administration has no capacity to organize testing upon personal demand of inmates, which is the case for non-incarcerated citizens. However, the situation is closely monitored by state agencies (e.g., national health agencies, penitentiary inspections, etc.), non-governmental organizations (e.g., Apador-CH[16]) and the National Preventive Mechanisms established within the Ombudsman Office. Therefore, it is an impressive feat for the penitentiary system to keep the prison population COVID-19 free, despite that reported cases in the general public has been rising continuously for the last four weeks[17] and the penitentiary system is still overcrowded (111% as of June 2020).

What seems to have had a great influence on this somewhat surprising outcome of zero COVID-19 cases among inmates, is the dramatic reduction in direct interactions between inmates and the outside world from very early on in Romania's response to the pandemic, while also considering the context of multidisciplinary measures taken by the prison administration. As noted above, all prisoners' transfers, visits, leaves, external work activities, and so on were drastically reduced during the state of emergency. They were compensated with increased online communication, more phone calls, and counseling. However, considering the legal, psychological, and experiential costs of these strict medico-carceral measures for both the inmates and their families will be important to investigate moving forward. For instance, working plays an important role in the conditional release mechanism in Romanian prisons. Thus, it will be important to assess to what extent the lack of work opportunities impacted the length of prison sentences. We hope that future research will shed more light on how penitentiaries have adapted to extreme crises, the intended and unintended consequences of implementing specific mitigations strategies, and how these adaptations affect prisoners and their families.

Notes

1. WHO Timeline – COVID-19. https://www.who.int/news-room/detail/27-04-2020-who-timeline—covid-19.
2. WHO announces COVID-19 outbreak a pandemic. https://www.euro.who.int/en/health-topics/health-emergencies/coronavirus-covid-19/news/news/2020/3/who-announces-covid-19-outbreak-a-pandemic.
3. Rezmives and others v. Romania (25th of April, 2017). http://hudoc.echr.coe.int/eng?i=001-173351.
4. Decision no. 443/2016 of the General Director of the National Administration of Penitentiaries on the approval of the Working procedure for giving rewards based on the Credit system for the participation in educational programs and activities, psychological and social assistance programs and activities, lucrative activities, as well as participation in the prevention of risk situations, published in the Romanian Official Gazette no. 427 from 07 June 2016.
5. See summary: https://www.nineoclock.ro/2019/01/16/compensatory-remedy-law-and-its-effects-theme-of-tough-debate-in-society-president-demands-from-govt-in-depth-analysis-solutions-jusmin-toader-we-are-analyzing-the-consequences-of-deeds-committ/.
6. Also known as an "intimate visit," is a visit that allows partners to spend a few hours together in a special cell.
7. According to the law, a special judge (a supervising judge of the deprivation of liberty) is appointed in every prison to observe the prisoner's rights. S/he is independent from the prison administration and his/her decisions regarding prisoner's rights are compulsory for the prison administration.
8. Order of the Minister of Health no. 489/2020 from March 23, 2020 *on the approval of the administration, financing and implementation of priority actions for monitoring, treatment and care of the critical patients, with emerging and reemerging infections (AP-IE/RE).*
9. According to the *Measures plan for the penitentiary system, at the cessation of the state of emergency*, approved by the decision of the general director of the National Administration of Penitentiaries no. 446/14.05.2020.
10. *Measures plan for the penitentiary system at the establishment of the state of emergency in the territory of Romania*, approved by decision of the general director of the National Administration of Penitentiaries.
11. According to the *Measures plan for the penitentiary system, upon the extension of the state of emergency in Romania*, approved by decision of the general director of the National Administration of Penitentiaries.
12. Order of the Minister of Health no. 489 from March 23, 2020 *on the approval of the administration, financing and implementation of priority actions for monitoring, treatment and care of the critical patients, with emerging and reemerging infections (AP-IER/RE).*
13. https://rm.coe.int/16809cfa4b Statement of principles relating to the treatment of persons deprived of their liberty in the context of the Coronavirus disease (COVID-19) pandemic.

    See also: https://rm.coe.int/16809ef566 for a follow-up statement regarding the situation of persons deprived of their liberty in the context of the ongoing COVID-19 pandemic.
14. Group for Strategic Communication is an official body established within the Ministry of Home Affairs to communicate the official data regarding the pandemic in Romania. More can

be found at https://www.mai.gov.ro/informare-covid-19-grupul-de-comunicare-strategica-1-septembrie-ora-13-00/.

15. Appointed according to the Order no. 377/2017 from March 30, 2017 from the Ministry of Health *on the approval of the technical standards for the achievement of the national public health programs for 2017 and 2018*, with subsequent amendments and additions.
16. Apador-CH made an inquiry on the COVID-19 situation in the Romanian prisons for the first three months of the pandemic and come up with the same conclusions. The report will be briefly available on the organization website: https://www.apador.org/en/.
17. A number of 1,298 new persons tested positive on the 2nd of September, compared with 1,053 new positive cases on the 1st of September. The number of positive tests depends on the total of tests performed but the overall trend now has been increasing. Source: https://stirioficiale.ro/informatii.

Acknowledgments

The authors are deeply grateful to the National Administration of Penitentiaries/Romania for all the data that was provided to support this paper.

Disclosure statement

No potential conflict of interest was reported by the author(s).

ORCID

Ioan Durnescu http://orcid.org/0000-0002-5631-7926

References

Aebi, M. F., & Tiago, M. M. (2020). *Prisons and prisoners in Europe in pandemic times: An evaluation of the short-term impact of the COVID-19 on prison population*. Council of Europe. http://wp.unil.ch/space/files/2020/06/Prisons-and-the-COVID-19_200617_FINAL.pdf

AGENFOR. (2020). *Prisons towards phase 3: Risks and challenges*. https://www.agenformedia.com/publication/prisons-phase-3/

Boone, M., Pakes, F., & Wingerden, S. (2019). Explaining the collapse of the prison population in the Netherlands. *European Journal of Criminology*. SAGE. https://doi.org/10.1177/1477370819896220

CPT. (2020a). *Statement of principles relating to the treatment of persons deprived of their liberty in the context of the coronavirus disease (COVID-19) pandemic*. Council of Europe. https://rm.coe.int/16809cfa4b

CPT. (2020b). *Follow-up statement regarding the situation of persons deprived of their liberty in the context of the ongoing COVID-19 pandemic*. Council of Europe. https://rm.coe.int/16809ef566

Decree no. 195 of March 16th, 2020 on the establishment of the state of emergency in the territory of Romania, Published in the Official Gazette no. 212 of March 16th, 2020.

Hough, M., Jacobson, J., & Millie, A. (2003). *The decision to imprison: Key findings* (Law and Criminology. Research Report). Prison Reform Trust. https://research.edgehill.ac.uk/en/publications/the-decision-to-imprison-key-findings-2

Morar, I. (2019). *Dysfunctional cognitive schemas emphasized in the hetero-aggression of the anti-social individual. Testing the impact of an application for the penitentiary environment* [PhD thesis]. University of Bucharest.

Morar, I., Motiuk, L. L., & Keown, L.-A. (2019). Characteristics of offenders participating in the Romanian prison service credit system. *European Journal for Crime, Criminal Law and Criminal Justice*, *27*(3), 242–259. https://doi.org/10.1163/15718174-02703004

National Administration of Penitentiaries (2020a). *The decision of the general director of the National Administration of Penitentiaries no. 381/16.03.2020 for the approval of the Plan of measures for the penitentiary system, at the establishment of the state of emergency in the territory of Romania* (internal document).

National Administration of Penitentiaries. (2020b). *The decision of the general director of the National Administration of Penitentiaries no. 419/15.04.2020 for the approval of the Plan of measures for the penitentiary system, upon the extension of the state of emergency in the territory of Romania* (internal document).

Spiteri, G., Fielding, J., Diercke, M., & Ciancio, B. C. (2020). First cases of coronavirus disease 2019 (COVID-19) in the WHO European region, 24 January to 21 February 2020. *Euro Surveill*, *25*(9). https://www.researchgate.net/publication/339730023_First_cases_of_coronavirus_disease_2019_COVID-19_in_the_WHO_European_Region_24_January_to_21_February_2020/citations

The Penitentiary System of Russia during the COVID-19 Pandemic: A Global Challenge and Initial Results

Sergei Ovchinnikov

ABSTRACT

This article describes the nature and extent of Covid-19 outbreaks in Russia's penitentiary system. It includes an examination of the features and effectiveness of applied measures to prevent and control the spread of COVID-19 among employees of Russian penitentiaries and persons who are in custody or serving a prison term (i.e. all detained inmates). The article also provides a comparative legal analysis that allows one to judge the extent of the spread of a new coronavirus infection in Russia, and in penitentiary institutions across Europe. The article concludes with an assessment of whether these short-term mitigation strategies will serve as a harbinger of long term reforms in Russia's penitentiary system.

Introduction: the European context of Covid-19

The Globalization of the modern world constantly forces us to analyze the possible consequences of threats to humanity. Today we see that danger is posed not only by man-made disasters such as climate change, but also by the global spread of a viral infection.

The large-scale spread of the novel Coronavirus has changed the daily life of populations in many countries. State authorities have been forced to apply extreme measures to protect public interests, limiting the individual rights and freedoms of citizens. Restrictive measures have also been taken to ensure that penitentiaries, where inmates are held, have proper sanitation and epidemiological states. Russia is no exception among the list of countries that have introduced special measures aimed at preventing the spread of the new Coronavirus.

While investigating the functioning aspects of criminal justice systems during the COVID-19 pandemic, general European trends in the spread of Coronavirus should be noted. Analyzing data from the World Health Organization, we see that the top leaders of infected populations in Europe (as of August 13, 2020) are Russia with 907,758 positive cases, Spain with 376,864, the United Kingdom with 313,798, Italy with 252,235, Turkey at 245,635, Germany with 221.977, France at 209,365, Ukraine with 86,140, Sweden with 83,852, and Belgium at 75,647 (World Health Organization, 2020). The total number of cases of COVID-19 among these ten countries amounts to almost three quarters of COVID-19 cases in all European states. At the same time, there is a significant difference in the proportion of deaths experienced by those who tested positive for COVID-19. The largest rate can be observed in San Marino where 1,238 individuals per 1 million of the country's population experienced death due to COVID-19. This is followed by Belgium with 854 deaths per 1 million, Spain with 611, the United Kingdom with 608, Italy with 583, Sweden with 571, France with 465, the Netherlands with 360, and Ireland with 359. The mortality rate among people diagnosed with Coronavirus in Russia amounts to 105 cases per 1 million of the country's population (Worldometer, 2020).

Analysis of the data presented in the EUROPRIS reports allows us to observe a similar picture among European penitentiaries. Here, however, it should be noted that not all countries provided data. Regardless, the data presented allows us to assess the trends in the spread of Coronavirus. Based on the available data, we can say that the dynamic of mortality among penitentiary staff differs from the mortality of inmates held in the same penitentiary (Graph 1) (Europris, 2020).

As can be seen in Graph 1, significant differences are noticeable in the dynamic and number of infected individuals. From March 31 to April 20, there is a sharp increase in penitentiary workers who have been diagnosed with COVID-19. It is during this period that the largest number of infected employees is observed in countries such as Spain (304 staff members), Italy (163 staff members) and Belgium (49 staff). Following this, due to the restrictive and preventive measures adopted, there is a stable downward trend in the number of infected employees, which has continued to date.

At the same time, the dynamic and number of infections among inmates held in European penitentiaries have a progressive growth trend throughout the entire period of observation. While the number of positive COVID-19 cases begins to decrease among staff members after peaking on April 20, the number of inmate cases has not stabilized and continues to increase. The largest number of COVID-19 cases among persons held in penitentiaries, as of July 1, 2020, is observed in Italy (132 inmates), Sweden (125 inmates), Spain (76 inmates), France (35 inmates) and the Netherlands (20 inmates) (Europris, 2020).

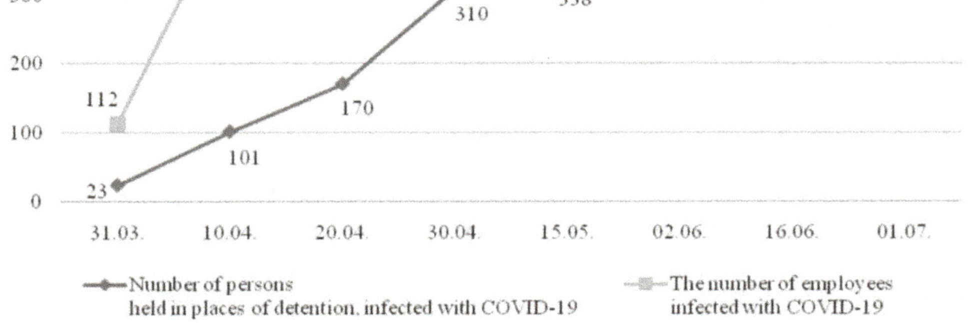

Graph 1. Number of employees and persons held in prisons in European countries infected with COVID-19.

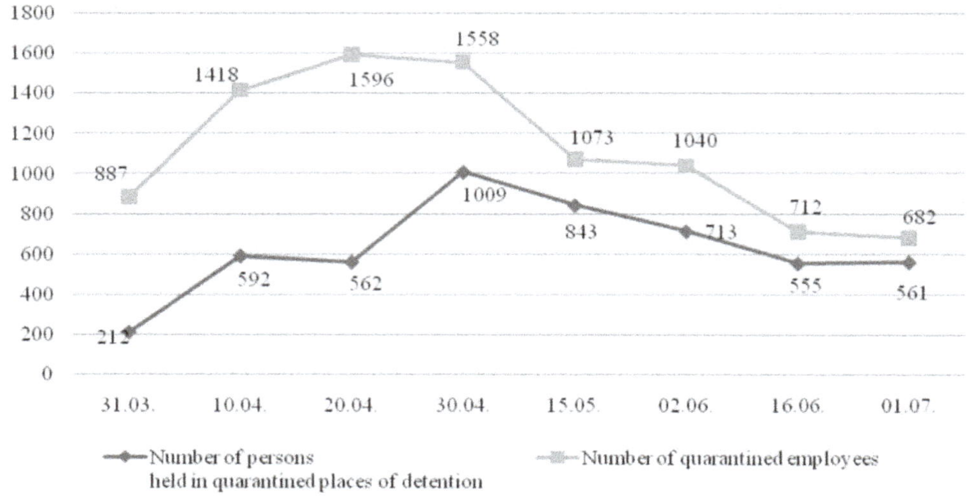

Graph 2. Number of employees and persons held in penitentiaries of European countries, isolated for medical reasons with suspected COVID-19 and contact persons.

We can observe a slightly different dynamic in the number of people isolated with suspicion of having symptoms of COVID-19 and people who have come into contact with others who have been diagnosed with a Coronavirus infection. Thus, the peak values for this indicator fall on April 20, among employees and on April 30 among persons held in the penitentiaries (Graph 2). At the same time, there is a similar trend in the number of isolated individuals among both employees and inmates. The number of employees at certain times exceeded the number of inmates who were quarantined by almost three times. It should be noted that the largest number of penitentiary employees who were sent to quarantine is observed (as of April 20, 2020) in Spain (1107 employees), Austria (250 employees), Poland (68 employees) and France (312 employees). The largest number of inmates, for which quarantine measures were taken, is noted (as of April 30, 2020) in Spain (510 inmates), Croatia (138 inmates), France (127 inmates), Poland (59 inmates), and Austria (43 inmates) (Europris, 2020).

The lowest statistics presented in this article regards COVID-19 related deaths of employees and inmates of which COVID-19 was detected. However, the data presented in Graph 3 again indicate an excess in the number of victims of COVID-19 among penitentiary employees. According to EUROPRIS, Spain, Italy and France provided information about deceased employees for which COVID-19 was detected.

Covid-19 outbreaks in Russia's penitentiary system

In order to understand the context of research, a few words should be said about the structure and current state of the Russian penitentiary system. In accordance with Article 16 of the Criminal Executive Code of the Russian Federation, the structure of the penal system includes criminal executive inspectorates that enforce criminal penalties and measures of a criminal legal nature that are not related to the isolation of convicts from society, such as house arrest, suspended sentences, compulsory labor, correctional labor, and restriction of freedom.

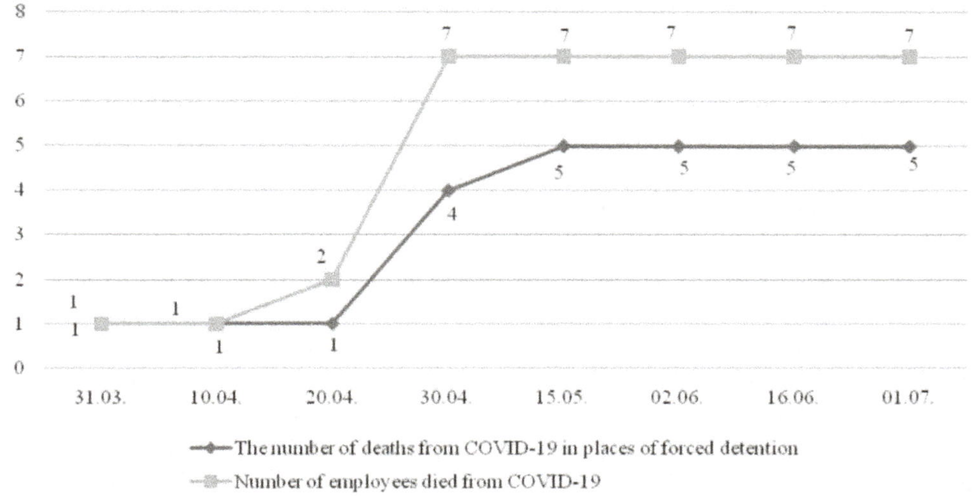

Graph 3. Number of deceased employees and persons held in penitentiaries in European countries diagnosed with COVID-19.

Currently, there are 81 criminal executive inspectorates and 1,348 branches in the penitentiary system of Russia, accounting for 451,376 people sentenced to punishments unrelated to the isolation of convicts from society and 7,788 people suspected and (or) accused of committing crimes under house arrest (Federal Penitentiary Service of Russia, 2020a).

Criminal punishment in the form of forced labor is carried out by correctional centers. As of August 1, 2020, there are 17 correctional centers and 70 isolated sections, functioning as correctional centers, in which 5,437 convicts of forced labor are registered (Federal Penitentiary Service of Russia, 2020a). (*Data on Covid-19 outbreaks among inmates sentenced to forced labor are not yet available*) Punishment in the form of imprisonment for a specified period and life imprisonment is enforced by correctional institutions. According to part 9 of Article 6 of the Criminal Executive Code of the Russian Federation, deprivation of liberty is executed by correctional institutions such as colony-settlements, educational colonies for minors, medical correctional institutions, correctional colonies of general, strict or special regimes,[1] or prisons.

As of August 1, 2020, 496,791 individuals were held in various institutions of the Russian penitentiary system, including:

- 389,450 people were serving sentences in 684 correctional colonies, including:
  - 111 colonies-settlements with 29,506 inmates serving their sentences;
  - 7 correctional colonies for those sentenced to life imprisonment and persons for whom the death penalty by way of pardon was replaced by imprisonment with 1,994 inmates serving their sentences;
  - 8 prisons with 1,173 inmates serving their sentences;
  - 22 educational colonies for minors with 991 inmates housed.

Currently, 40,111 women are held in penitentiaries in Russia, including:

- 30,873 individuals in correctional colonies, medical correctional institutions, medical institutions, and 9,238 in pre-trial detention centers.

The women's colonies have 13 orphanages with 384 children. Those accused of committing criminal offenses who have been selected to serve a form of detention as a preventative measure, are to be held in pre-trial detention centers. At present, 105,177 individuals are being held in 209 pre-trial detention centers and 92 facilities functioning as pre-trial detention centers in colonies.

After reviewing the underpinnings of the Russian penitentiary system, it can be stated that the penitentiary employees and persons held in penitentiary institutions can be classified within a vulnerable category for which the risk of contracting Coronavirus is very high. In fact, as of August 4, 2020, 187,294 laboratory tests were carried out to detect Coronavirus, including 116,844 tests in the laboratories of the penal system. Since introducing restrictive measures, 3,526 laboratory-confirmed cases of Coronavirus have been registered among the penitentiary staff, of which, 2,457 have recovered. Since the beginning of April 2020, 1,224 laboratory-confirmed cases have been identified among inmates, of which 933 have recovered.

The largest number of identified cases among inmates in the Central Federal District was 233. In the Ural Federal District, there were 111 confirmed cases. At the same time, in 28 regions, there have been no cases among inmates (Federal Penitentiary Service of Russia, 2020b). While looking at employees, the picture is different. Only 3 regions reported no cases of COVID-19 among employees. This confirms the general European trend that we discussed above. In European countries, the number of COVID-19 cases is also higher among prison staff than among inmates.

Mitigation strategies utilized in Russia

In order to prevent the spread of Coronavirus in certain regions of Russia, special, restrictive measures were taken. Thus, a regime of special conditions was introduced in pre-trial detention centers in 15 regions.[2] In addition, quarantines were announced in individual penitentiary institutions in 48 regions. In those regions where the situation stabilized, quarantine measures in institutions were loosened. As of August 4, 2020, the quarantine regime was maintained in individual penitentiary institutions in 29 regions (Federal Penitentiary Service of Russia, 2020b).

Along with the adoption of quarantine measures, the regional authorities made extensive use of preventive sanitary and anti-epidemic measures. For example, a mask regime was introduced in penitentiary institutions. Employees and visitors are required to comply with it. When visiting penitentiary institutions, visitors undergo thermometry. At all facilities, disinfection measures are carried out daily with the use of disinfectants and bactericidal irradiators. In addition, a sanitation day is held in all penitentiary institutions once a week.

The existing bacteriological and immunological laboratories were also redesigned to detect such diseases as tuberculosis and HIV infections, and to work to identify the COVID-19 virus, where diagnostics and testing of persons with symptoms of Coronavirus is carried out. Patients with clinical symptoms are immediately isolated in medical institutions and medical-sanitary units. The sewing of medical masks was organized in 303 penitentiary institutions. Today, on average, about 2 million medical masks are produced in penitentiary institutions per day.

Undoubtedly, the main threat that still remains is the introduction of the virus into penitentiary institutions from the outside. Therefore, when employees enter, they must undergo a medical examination and thermometry. Since the beginning of the epidemic, a number of restrictions have been introduced, including being on duty in some regions. Employees go on duty for 14 days without the opportunity to leave the institution during this entire period in order to exclude any contacts from outside. For citizens newly admitted to penitentiary institutions, the quarantine period was extended to 20 days, considering the fact that the development of the disease has a period of undetectability. All vehicles entering the premises of penitentiaries are sanitized with disinfectants at specially equipped areas.

Another potential source of infection is the transport of prisoners to courts. While it may be possible to ensure the separation of inmates in pre-trial detention centers, this is likely not the case in court rooms. Therefore, a number of regions began to use video conferencing when considering cases in courts. Also, control over the receiving parcels and transmissions was strengthened. Currently, employees are receiving parcels while using personal protective equipment. Premises for receiving parcels are equipped with bactericidal irradiators. In addition, employees conduct disinfection processing of packages and also disinfect the air in the room and surfaces of parcels with open-type bactericidal irradiators.

Dispensers with skin antiseptics were installed in the reception rooms of penitentiaries. Wet cleaning of premises (using detergents and disinfectants) is carried out at least 2 times a day.

As noted above, in order to prevent the spread of Coronavirus in penitentiaries, a number of restrictive measures were taken. From March 16, 2020 and until further instruction is provided, the provision of long and short-term visits was suspended in some regions. However, at the moment, depending on the epidemiological situation in these regions, restrictive measures have been gradually lifted. In some institutions, short-term and long-term visits have been granted.

Short-term visits with relatives and other persons are carried out through glass in compliance with the requirements of individual protection. During the period of imposed restrictions, regarding primarily communication with relatives and close persons, measures of a compensatory nature were and continue to be applied. Thus, in accordance with current legislation, inmates can communicate with their relatives by telephone and using stationary video communication without restrictions. It should be noted that currently about 8,500 telephones have been installed in the institutions of the Russian penitentiary system, through which inmates make more than 8 million calls annually, as well as 514 video terminals, supporting more than 45,000 video calls a year.

Attempts were also made to decongest penitentiaries, which is necessary to reduce contact between inmates. In order to reduce the number of persons held in pre-trial detention centers, the leadership of the Federal Penitentiary Service of Russia appealed to the Supreme Court of the Russian Federation with a request to order the courts not to use a preventive measure in the form of detention for persons suspected or accused of committing crimes of small to medium severity, but rather, to apply alternative measures not related to isolation from society (Rosbusinessconsulting, 2020).

Since the introduction of urgent measures to prevent the spread of Coronavirus, through land checkpoints to foreign states (in fulfillment by the Russian Federation of international legal obligations on extradition), 90 people have been transferred, and 31 people have been admitted to Russia. The extradition of persons on the international wanted list took place with 8 states, such as the Republic of Belarus, Kazakhstan, Ukraine, Azerbaijan, Georgia, Poland, South Ossetia, and China. At the same time, all extradited persons were examined for the presence of COVID-19 before being sent from Russia (Federal Penitentiary Service of Russia, 2020b).

It also became necessary to introduce measures to limit visits to penitentiaries by representatives of public organizations. The admission of lawyers is carried out using personal protective equipment and with negotiations through protective glass. In addition, despite the implementation of complex sanitary and anti-epidemic measures, including restrictive measures, since March 16, members of public monitoring commissions have visited the institutions of the Russian penitentiary system 202 times. Also, remote consideration of appeals by e-mail from inmates and their relatives was organized. Such visits revealed excessive restrictions on, and violations of, the rights of inmates such as daily walks and receival of parcels from relatives (Russia Today, 2020).

In summary, we can note the presence of pan-European trends in the dynamic and number of cases of COVID-19 among the penitentiary employees and inmates. In this case, the most vulnerable population is the penitentiary staff. Also, in order to prevent the spread of Coronavirus in penitentiaries, a set of measures was taken to isolate persons with COVID-19 symptoms. Additional measures were introduced to sanitize premises and use personal protective equipment. Furthermore, restrictions were imposed on visits to penitentiaries and control over incoming parcels was strengthened.

Concluding comments

It is important to assess the impact of specific mitigation strategies taken in combatting COVID-19 on the number of infected inmates to gauge the effectiveness of such strategies on desired outcomes (i.e., to reduce the number of positive cases among inmates). However, in Russia at present, we have not observed any significant changes in the number of infected inmates (i.e., a reduction of positive COVID-19 cases among inmates), despite implementing a wide range of mitigation tactics. One explanation for this lack of significant change is that the strategies implemented were both short-term and local in nature. While significant positive impacts of Russia's responses to COVID-19 in its penitentiary system have not yet been observed, it should also be noted that Russia has not experienced any major COVID-19 hotspots among inmates within its penitentiaries. Therefore, implying that current mitigation strategies being implemented in response to COVID-19 may not only show more promising impacts in the long-term, but may also be aiding in the prevention of inmate hot spots within penitentiaries to date. Continued monitoring of the state of Russian penitentiaries will be useful and essential for subsequent analysis of the long-term effects of mitigation strategies on the prevalence of COVID-19 cases among inmates.

Notes

1. According to article 58 of the Criminal Code of the Russian Federation, depending on the severity of the crime committed and other circumstances, convicts may be assigned to serve imprisonment in correctional colonies of general, strict or special regime. For example,

individuals committed serious crime, are held in a general regime colony, while those committed especially serious crime performing dangerous recidivism, are held in a special regime colony. Those sentenced to life imprisonment are also held in that type of colonies.

2. In accordance with Article 85 of the Criminal Executive Code of the Russian Federation, in cases of natural disaster, the imposition of a state of emergency or martial law in the area where penitentiary is located, and in other emergency circumstances, a regime of special conditions may be introduced in penitentiary. During the period of the special conditions regime in penitentiary, the exercise of certain rights of convicted may be suspended.

Disclosure statement

No potential conflict of interest was reported by the author(s).

ORCID

Sergei Ovchinnikov http://orcid.org/0000-0001-8942-0244

References

Europris. (2020). *EuroPris feedback collection from the European mailing group*. http://www.europris.org/covid-19-prevention-measures-in-european-prisons/

Federal Penitentiary Service of Russia. (2020a). *Brief characteristic of the criminal executive system*. http://fsin.gov.ru/structure/inspector/iao/statistika/

Federal Penitentiary Service of Russia. (2020b). *Interview of the deputy director of the fps of Russia Alexander Khabarov to the information agency «TASS»*. http://fsin.gov.ru/news/index.php?ELEMENT_ID=512204

Rosbusinessconsulting. (2020, April 19). *FSIN asked not to arrest for minor crimes because of the virus*. http://www.rbc.ru/society/18/04/2020/5e9ae92c9a79477104514365

Russia Today. (2020, May 14). *The public monitoring commission of Moscow reported on the reduction in the number of walks in a number of pre-trial detention centers*. http://russian.rt.com/russia/news/746528-sizo-moskvy-progulki-sokraschenie-onk

World Health Organization. (2020). *WHO coronavirus disease (COVID-19) dashboard*. http://covid19.who.int

Worldometer. (2020). *Reported cases and deaths by Country, territory, or conveyance*. http://www.worldometers.info/coronavirus/#countries

Corrections and Crime in Spain and Portugal during the Covid-19 Pandemic: Impact, Prevention and Lessons for the Future

Santiago Redondo, Rui Abrunhosa Gonçalves, Javier Nistal, Carlos Soler,
José Semedo Moreira, Joana Andrade, and Antonio Andrés-Pueyo

ABSTRACT

This paper analyzes the impact that the Covid-19 pandemic has had on corrections and crime in the southern region of Europe formed by Spain and Portugal. The main mechanisms of transmission of Covid-19 are the physical proximity between people and the fact of sharing eventually infected targets. In prisons and other correctional contexts people live in close proximity and share the same facilities. As a result, the correctional context has proven to be a critical "hot spot" for the transmission of the Covid-19 pandemic in inmates and correctional staff. First, the magnitude of the infection and their associated health and psychosocial problems (prison incidents, social isolation…) are described. Second, the main sanitary, social, and correctional measures applied to prevent contagion and their related damages are presented (lockdown, use of communication technologies with families, etc.). Third, it is analyzed whether there has been a relationship between the confinement caused by the pandemic and the crime rates observed in Spain and Portugal during this same period. Finally, from the impact in corrections of pandemic and the actions taken to fight it, several important lessons are derived for the future improvement of correctional systems.

Wisdom calls to you like someone shouting;
understanding raises her voice.
(Proverbs, 8.1)

Introduction

The year 2020 is likely to go down in history as a dark and fateful year, in which millions of people were infected, and hundreds of thousands became ill and died. There is a terrible historical background to analogous situations (Afonso, 2020; Wade, 2020). In the year 1349, the Black Death killed half of the European population. In 1520 smallpox devastated the American continent and wiped out 60–90% of the indigenous populations. A century ago, in 1918, the Spanish Flu killed almost 50 million people in the western world. Just over three decades ago, the AIDS pandemic was fatal to thousands of people in all countries and contexts

(Wade, 2020). Due to its priority transmission by unprotected sex and drug use with contaminated syringes, it had a special incidence in prisons.

This current coronavirus pandemic has been difficult to manage in all countries and contexts. Prisons and other correctional facilities are, by their very nature, places of close physical proximity (the main frequent mechanisms of contagion and transmission ofCOVID-19), particularly sensitive to the impact of this pandemic (Bedford et al., 2020; Hoff et al., 2009; WHO, 2020b).

On March 11, 2020, after 3 months of intense epidemiological monitoring of COVID-19, the WHO officially declared the state of a global pandemic (Contini et al., 2020; WHO, 2020a). It is producing devastating effects around the world in terms of public health, economy, and social relations (Campbell & Doshi, 2020; Duarte et al., 2020; Ma et al., 2020). Its effects are spreading to all human activities and organizations, including prisons and other correctional systems as well.

The virulent expansion of this pandemic has forced urgent measures to be taken worldwide, sometimes very drastic and comprehensive (WHO, 2020c). They include legal measures of restriction of rights (in general, under the exceptional laws of alarm), confinement of the population in their homes, massive application of health tests, and other mandatory public health regulations (use of face masks, maintenance of social distance, closure of shops and leisure ...).

Analogous measures have also been logically applied in correctional systems, both in prisons and in the community, in order to limit and prevent the expansion and effects of the pandemic on their premises (CPCWG, 2020b; WHO, 2020a). Also, international organizations such as the Council for Penological Cooperation Working Group (CPCWG) of the Council of Europe, the European Organization of Prison and Correctional Services (European Prison Observatory, 2020; EuroPris, 2020a), the Confederation of European Probation (CPCWG, 2020a) or the Association Inter-American Public Defenders of Latin America (IACHR, 2020), have published guidelines and recommendations to adapt the operation of courts, corrections, and juvenile centers for preventing the incidence of COVID-19 on the health of inmates, the prison staff and their respective social environments (family, neighbors, etc.).

This paper primarily analyzes the impact of the COVID-19 pandemic in the correctional systems of Spain and Portugal, in the South of Europe, as well as the prevention measures adopted to prevent its spread. For a better understanding of the significance and consequences of the impact of COVID-19 and the measures applied in corrections, a general sociodemographic, criminal, and penitentiary view of these two countries is presented. Secondarily, although this was not the initial objective of the article, relevant information is also provided here on the evolution of crime in Spain and Portugal during the pandemic and the subsequent lockdown of citizens.

Before offering a current "still photo" (September 2020) of the situation of the pandemic issue in Spain and Portugal, a caveat must be made. Most of the sociodemographic, criminal, and prison data summarized here are quite accurate and valid. However, not all of them equally fulfill these properties for two reasons: firstly, due to the constant change of the COVID-19 epidemiological data; secondly, the absence of information on the medium and long-term consequences (in domains such as health, social, and economic) of this pandemic.

Being aware of these limitations, the sociodemographic data of the countries analyzed in this work, their epidemiological data from COVID-19, as well as their respective crime and prison rates, will be presented below. Lastly, the measures adopted in both Portuguese and Spanish penitentiary systems to confront this pandemic will be more precisely contextualized. Given that in Spain the region of Catalonia has a differentiated prison administration, some of the data presented below will also refer specifically to that Spanish region.

Sociodemographic factors and COVID-19 pandemic

Apart from their different sizes, Spain and Portugal are very similar countries in terms of their sociodemographic characteristics (https://datosmacro.expansion.com/paises/portugal; https://datosmacro.expansion.com/paises/espa%C3%B1a). In 2020, Spain had a population of 47,329,981 people with an average age of 43.4 years (19.49%, over 65) and a female rate of 50.98%. (Within this, the Spanish region of Catalonia has a population of 7,727,029 people, with an average age of 44.02 years –18.9% over 65 years– and a female population rate of 50.91%). Portugal has a population of 10,341,330 inhabitants, with an average age of 44.8 years (20.7% over 65) and a female population rate of 52.6%.

The first serious effects of COVID-19 on the Spanish population raised the government alarm in the first week of March 2020 (Millan, 2020). On March 13, the general confinement of the population in their homes and multiple mobility prohibitions were decreed (after approval of the state of alarm provided for in the Spanish Constitution): closure of schools and playgrounds, universities, almost absolute cessation of industrial and commercial activity (except essential services: health, police, and security, food supplies), closure of sports and leisure facilities, hotels, bars, and any public activity in closed and open places. This situation lasted 14 weeks, until June 21, 2020.

Portugal had the first confirmed case of COVID-19 on March 2. Since then, a set of measures were adopted to prepare both community and entities for the outbreak (European Union Agency for Fundamental Rights, 2020). The strict lockdown measures began on March 12 (Portuguese Council of Ministers of March 12, 2020; Sappal, 2020) and ended in early May. Despite the suspicions that, in Portugal, the number of reported cases would be probably underestimated (Duarte et al., 2020; Sánchez, 2020), according to the official data, unlike in Spain, the preventive effect of such measures seemed to be effective, producing a low rate of infections and deaths. During the pandemic, people have been mobilizing themselves to the social distance to prevent virus expansion. However, this protection may be difficult to be ensured for the incarcerated population. Typically, prisons are overcrowded (Aebi et al., 2016; UNODC, 2020) and maintaining the isolation of inmates seems not to be feasible. Over time, because of the massive use of imprisonment not only for violent and dangerous offenders but also for misdemeanors, a growth of the prison population started to be noticed (Coyle et al., 2016). For example, J. M. Byrne et al. (2015) carried out a macro-analysis of incarceration in different regions of the world, highlighting that the global number and incarceration/population rates continued to increase in most countries, despite the fact that in many crime decreased. Indeed, despite the expansion of alternative sanctions in the community, prisons' overcrowding remained a challenge with a significant impact on the conditions provided to the inmates.

To face the spread of the infection and its consequences for the population, both Spain and Portugal have followed the social and health guidelines recommended by the WHO and the health experts of each country (WHO Director-General's Special Envoys on COVID-19 Preparedness and Response, 2020). In both countries, different outbreaks of

COVID-19 have occurred since the end of the confinement. However, in neither of the two countries the epidemic alarm situations and the severity of the disease are up to now as severe as in the first wave of the pandemic. In Spain, until September2020, the cases of contagion were more of 677,000 confirmed by PCR analysis, with a population rate of detected infection of about 1.42%, and more than 30,663 deaths (a rate of 0.06% of the general population) (Zafra et al., 2020). In the Catalonia region, which represents the 16.41% of the Spanish population, more than 102,000 people were infected (a population rate of about 1.32%) and more than 5,725 died (a rate of 0.07%). In the case of Portugal, data from 28th July indicated that the number of those infected was 69,663 and of deaths 1,925, representing a population rate of 0.67% and 0.02%, respectively (Directorate-General of Health, 2020).

Prison population in Spain and Portugal

Essential information, to contextualize the preventive measures about COVID-19 adopted in the prison systems of Spain and Portugal, concerns the incarceration rates of these countries. Unlike what happened 5 years ago, both prison systems have experienced during the last years, a gradual decrease in the number of prisoners (Aebi et al., 2019; Cid, 2020). Accordingly, the analysis carried out here on the prison impact of the COVID-19 pandemic must be framed in a context of structural decline in prison figures.

In the European countries, in 2018, the average incarceration rate was 112.5 prisoners per 100,000 inhabitants, ranging from 51 prisoners in Finland to 235 in Lithuania (Aebi & Tiago, 2018). At the beginning of 2020, Spain had a total number of 58,374 prisoners, which implies a prison rate of 123 prisoners per hundred thousand inhabitants (Catalonia has a rate of 110 prisoners), while Portugal has a prison population of 11,053 inmates, corresponding to a rate of 102 (World Prison Brief, 2020).

Globally, Spain, with a rate of 45.6 crimes per 1000 inhabitants, and Portugal, with a rate of 38.2 crimes per 1000 inhabitants, have low crime rates (MI, 2020a; Redondo & Frerich, 2014; Redondo & Garrido, 2013). Despite this, their prison sentences tend to be longer than those established in most European countries (Cid, 2008, 2020). This tendency could explain why Spain and Portugal have, despite their low criminal rates, incarceration figures above the European average.

Epidemiological and public health studies (Bedford et al., 2020; Di Lorenzo & Di Trolio, 2020; Hu et al., 2020) indicate that the prominent risk factors for increased virulence of COVID-19 infection are being elderly, being male, smoking, suffering from asthma, obesity, diabetes, chronic hypertension, obstructive pulmonary disease, immunosuppression, chronic kidney disorders and having a low level of social development. This last risk factor is a global measure of social disadvantage and structural inequality. It includes poor housing conditions, insufficient hygiene, poor nutrition, drug addiction, smoking problems, and difficulties in accessing health, education, and other personal resources (Hoff et al., 2009; WHO, 2020b).

The prison population is composed mainly of men, from disadvantaged social groups, lower cultural and educational levels (Moreira & Martins, 2019), and, in many cases, from ethnic, religious, or political minorities. Their health is generally weaker than that of their reference population (Penal Reform International, 2020; UNODC, 2020), with a higher risk of getting infections and developing serious illnesses such as tuberculosis, AIDS, hepatitis, or mental disorders (Fazel & Baillargeon, 2011; Flanigan et al., 2009; Liebrenz et al., 2020; Stoliker & Galli, 2019). Hence, a simple glance at the aforementioned risk factors and, in parallel, the characteristics of many incarcerated people, allows to easily verify that the prison population may be especially vulnerable to the impact of COVID-19, and particularly to the effects of the type 2 coronavirus causing severe acute respiratory syndrome (SARS-CoV-2) (Bedford et al., 2020; Sanchez et al., 2020). Apart from their special personal vulnerability, prison inmates live in close proximity during their routines, which increases the risk of the coronavirus dissemination (Gonçalves et al., 2019; WHO, 2020b).

Studies focused on other previous pandemics have emphasized the high prevalence of the communicable and infectious disease among correctional populations, particularly prisoners, and the lack of preparedness of correctional services to address this problem and ensure effective care for inmates and other sentenced people (Hoff et al., 2009; Liebrenz et al., 2020). Considering the danger of COVID-19 contagion for those who have a higher risk of illness, protecting the health and wellbeing of the correctional population seems to be a priority to prevent a serious outbreak in both sentenced subjects and prison staff. As noted by Duarte et al. (2020), it is important to make efforts to fight the virus' dissemination based on the lessons learned by other emergencies, such as H5N1 avian influenza, SARS, H1N1 Pandemic and MERS-CoV. Moreover, experiences and lessons from earlier pandemics should be considered not only to enhance the responses to address the risks for physical but also for mental health (Afonso, 2020).

Method

To collect information for this study, a series of questions were asked to experts and managers of the prison systems of Spain (including the national and the Catalan prison administration) and Portugal. These questions were developed around five main axes: 1) main sociodemographic and correctional characteristics; 2) health impact of the COVID-19 pandemic in the society and in corrections (infections, sick, deceased); 3) measures of lockdown and others within prisons and community corrections (interrupted activities: visits, education, work, treatment...); 4) sanitary (protection, hygiene...) and preventive measures adopted (such as the possible release of prisoners and the use of community measures); 5) lessons that can be derived from this experience for the prison system and future prospects.

The questions raised for the purpose of this work were answered both by sending written reports and verbally. The authors of this work (academic and professional experts in corrections) reviewed, summarized, and consensually ordered the data and information presented here.

Results

Correctional measures against COVID-19

Studies developed in the context of pandemic influenza have already underlined the need to develop infection control plans that address the reallocation of the space and regrouping of prisoners (Maruschak et al., 2009). However, other measures should be pondered, particularly to solve the problem of prison overcrowding (UNODC, 2020). Indeed, overpopulation results in a higher risk for any situation of transmittable diseases (Penal Reform International, 2020). It might be recommendable to release those who do not represent a real danger for the society, and who do not have committed violent or sexual crimes

(UNODC, 2020). In addition, alternatives such as community orders could be a priority, especially for those who are at high-risk risk (such as elderly, prisoners with chronic diseases, and pregnant women) (Penal Reform International, 2020; UNODC, 2020).

Consistent with these and other similar considerations, various measures have been taken to combat the COVID-19 pandemic, both in the countries analyzed here (Spain and Portugal) and in the European countries as a whole. We will begin by describing briefly the European panorama and later, more extensively, what happened in Spain and Portugal.

Europe

When they became aware of the spread of the COVID-19 pandemic in Europe, the European correctional systems established various measures of confinement (consistent with those adopted by the general health institutions). EuroPris has so far published on its website three reports on the situation of the COVID-19 pandemic and the measures adopted in the prisons of the EU countries. The second report corresponds to April 22, 2020. It includes the following main information (European Prison Observatory, 2020; EuroPris, 2020a; https://www.europis.org/covid-19-prevention-measures-in-european-prisons/):

- Of the 27 member states of the EU, 21 documented by April cases of *infections and quarantines* among inmates and staff, while 6 countries had not detected infections. In line with the greater impact of the pandemic in their respective societies, the countries with the highest prevalence of infections were Spain (with 46 prisoners and 238 staff infected) and Italy (with 37 infected prisoners and 163 staff members).
- In all countries, all *physical visits* related to probation, mediation, and religious services were interrupted (except the interviews, with the necessary sanitary control, with the legal counsel services, the consular officers, and the religious counselors).
- A particularly negative impact of this situation has derived, from the suspension of *family visits*, for the children of the inmates (women and men). To alleviate these harmful effects, various countries have created support groups for children and packs that imprisoned mothers could send to their children and Family Video Visits.
- Most states interrupted the educational, sports, group, and professional training *activities* usually carried out in prisons. Although some, if they had the possibility of specialized staff and space, held one-on-one activities, distance learning, or certain workshops. Some workshops have been aimed for the production of protective clothing and masks for health services.
- Generally, the correctional facilities allowed inmates to *shower* daily and laundry services have remained active.
- Kitchen services have been kept running during de pandemic, but *meals* were usually held in the cells.
- Providing prisoners with comprehensive and clear *information* has been critical to an adequate understanding and acceptance of the restrictive and lockdown measures applied. In some cases, telephone information lines were activated for prisoners and their families.
- Different *compensatory measures* have been used for the negative effects of the situation: more time for phone calls (including defraying the cost of the calls in some cases),

videoconferences, free television, extra food, and financial compensation (to counteract the suspension of paid workshops).

- Most countries have maintained the use of *shared cells* (except for infected prisoners).
- Most facilities have medicalized *quarantine units* to serve those incarcerated with symptoms of infection. In general, medical personnel and access to ambulances and hospitals have been considered sufficient. Infection tests are usually carried out by prison health services or the general health system on prisoners or prison staff who have symptoms of infection.
- Regarding *personal protection materials*, most countries prescribe the use of masks only for inmates who are infected or at higher risk of infection (when transferred, those who carry out tasks of greater contact with others). However, it is generally expected that the prison staff in direct contact with the inmates will wear protective clothing and mask.
- In coordination with the police and the prosecution office, efforts have been made to *avoid new prison incomes* (e.g., those sentenced to short sentences or pre-trial prisoners) except for violent crimes. Alternatively, house arrest, electronic monitoring, and fines have been used. Potential new admissions have been medically monitored and quarantined. In some cases, as a result of these measures, a significant reduction in the prison population has been observed.
- Different countries have *released in advance* prisoners who have been sentenced to short sentences or had certain nonviolent crimes. Aebi and Tiago (2020) have analyzed in the European countries their respective percentages of reduction of the prison population (as of April 15, 2020, during COVID-19′ confinement) in relation to the previously existing population as of January 1 2020. Various European countries have experienced significant reductions in their respective prison populations: Spain (7.7%-4,505 prisoners less; according our data), Italy (9.4%), Ireland (12.1%), Norway (13.3%), France (14.4%), Portugal (11.7%-1,289 prisoners less; according to our own data), and the Spanish region of Catalonia (17%).
- With regard to *prison staff*, in many countries, general preventive measures have been initially adopted: staying at home for staff members with COVID symptoms, chronic diseases, people over 60 and pregnant women. Secondly, a series of specific measures for work in prisons have been applied: creation of small stable work groups, to always work together; spacing between guards; suspension of training courses; temporary suspension of work permits; psychological help.
- Following the same report, most countries were focused by April on the day-to-day life of the pandemic and its prevention; they had not yet begun to make forecasts for possible outbreaks of the infection. Some countries had already started to prepare for the "after lockdown" and a gradual restoration of prison activities and family visits. It was considered that, as a general principle, all these actions should be closely linked to the measures adopted for citizens in the outside.

Spain

For the management of the health crisis situation caused by COVID-19 in Spanish prisons, the following main measures and restrictions were established (DGEPRS, 2020a, 2020b):

(1) The suspension of all external communications and of all leave exits, except for reasons of force or extreme necessity. Inmates classified in the third degree (open regime) or in a flexible regime could only leave in the case of having to carry out essential activities such as purchasing food, going to health centers, traveling to workplaces, care of dependent people, etc. (as provided in article 7 of the Decree 463/2020, of March 14, by which the Spanish government declared a state of alarm).
(2) Prohibition of access to prisons of any person (volunteers, collaborating entities, etc.) who are not part of the prison staff, unless their work inside was considered essential.
(3) Suspension of teaching activity and production workshops of external companies.
(4) Suspension of inmates' transfers, except for health of judicial reasons.
(5) Authorization for the inmates to stay voluntarily in their cells.
(6) Establishment of turns in the dining rooms for daily meals, as well as for the inmates' stay in common areas (leisure rooms, playgrounds…), in order to promote social distancing.
(7) Carrying out informative talks to the inmates about the current health crisis and the measures adopted for its prevention in the prison facilities.
(8) Free telephone calls for those inmates without resources and installation of free software for videoconferences. For this, more than 200 mobile phones were sent to the prisons to facilitate inmates to make phone and video calls with their families.
(9) Manufacture of masks in the workshops of some prisons.
(10) Permanent distribution of sanitary material supplied by the Spanish Ministry of Health.
(11) Use of military doctors in correctional facilities where necessary. Disinfection of prison facilities by the Spanish Army's Military Emergency Unit.
(12) Suspension of the possibility of voluntary presentation in prisons from freedom, to serve a sentence, except in justified exceptional circumstances.
(13) Possibility of applying random telephone controls (while a telematic control device is installed) to individuals in an open or flexible regime authorized to remain at home.

Various specific measures were also adopted for the management of alternative measures as community service and treatment programs (Fiscal de Sala Delegado de Vigilancia Penitenciaria, 2020). In total, 2,273 educational workshops and 8,884 face-to-face treatment programs were halted with the proper judicial authorization. These programs have been developed as far as possible through telephone or telematic follow-up of the prison staff or of the expert in charge of each activity.

Information campaigns have been carried out with imprisoned subjects about the health crisis unleashed by COVID-19 and about the necessary measures for its prevention. These information campaigns about the pandemic have been especially intense with certain vulnerable groups, such as prisoners with intellectual or developmental disabilities, who have been provided with a document in the form of "Easy Reading." Also, foreign inmates have been provided with information in their own language.

Regarding prison staff, since the beginning of the pandemic, indications, and criteria were established regarding working hours, flexible hours, teleworking, special work shifts for management teams, and videoconference meetings. These measures have reduced the physical presence in prisons of prison staff to the minimum number essential in each functional area: offices, interior of the centers, treatment, workshops, training activities, etc.

For the coordination of all these actions, a work team was created, made up of those responsible for all the areas of management and prevention (health, human resources, treatment, security, transfers, material resources, inspection, institutional relations, prison work, and job training). Its actions were managed through telematic communication channels, permanently coordinating with the penitentiary centers.

The Catalan prison administration

In Catalonia the management of the COVID-19 crisis has gone through three key periods (SMPRAV, 2020b):

(A) Period of confinement (March 13-May 10), when the most intense protection measures were taken in the prison services.
(B) Transition period (May 11-July 19), during which began the recovering of the interrupted prison activities.
(C) Resumption, from July 20, which purpose is recovering the full functioning of the penitentiary system, while maintaining some protection and prevention measures until the pandemic is fully controlled.

Special attention will be paid here to the measures and circumstances of the first period of lockdown (SMPRAV, 2020a), which have been the following:

(1) External barrier measures adopted to prevent the infection from entering prisons:

- Quarantine of 14 days for admissions to prisons.
- Suspension of face-to-face communications between inmates and families.
- Limitation of transfers to cases strictly necessary for security or prison management reasons.
- Suspension of outings and ordinary permits. Extraordinary permits were limited to exceptional cases and with quarantine on return.
- Suspension of the access to the prisons of the collaborating, voluntary and cult entities, except for necessary attention, with the due protection, to the foreign population (cultural mediators), to severe drug addictions cases, or people with intellectual or developmental disabilities.
- Attention by lawyers was channeled through videoconferencing (with the difficulty that bar associations were closed due to community lockdown).
- Avoid contact between inmates of different modules.
- The maximum capacity of group activities was reduced, and protection measures were tightened.
- Prison schools closed at the beginning of the confinement. The contact between the teaching staff and the students (for doing some educational tasks) has been maintained in part through videoconference. The lack of technological and structural means in prisons have not allowed to maintain this activity sufficiently.

(2) Protection of vulnerable people

At the beginning of the crisis, the health services screened imprisoned people who, due to their age or health vulnerability, had a higher risk if they became infected. From this, 70 inmates were identified, and the following measures were applied depending on their health, social, and legal situation:

(1) Referral to their home (what the law allows in certain cases) or to an external resource where they could be cared for,
(2) Destination to another prison with follow-up by the sanitary services.
(3) Release measures and reduction of the concentration of people in prisons

A relevant initiative in this regard has been to send some subjects, in legal conditions for it, to their own home or to community resources. The two legal figures used for this have been: an increase (from 1.649 cases – 27% of classified prison population – to 1.916 cases – 30% of prison population–) of the classifications in the third degree of treatment, or open regime; a substantial increase in the application of community measures (from 302 inmates to 1.694, un increase of 461%), which allow subjects to remain in their homes with some controls. This measure has probably had, firstly, a preventive effect of contagion, as there has been a 12% reduction in the concentration of inmates in ordinary prison units. With this, the region of Catalonia has experienced the largest decrease in the prison population that has occurred in Europe, as previously seen. Furthermore, the extension of the open regime and community measures has not led to an increase in breaches of sentence, but contrary to its decrease (10 breaches of sentence during confinement in front of 18 breaches in the same time interval of 2019). This could indicate that community supervision measures have worked well and that a more open model of prison management is feasible. Although the global increase in social control resulting from the confinement of the population could also have contributed to preventing the breach of sentences.

(5) Maintaining contact with the outside

An increased number of phone and video calls were used in the Catalan prisons in order to maintain the contact of the inmates with their families and other close people. Also, different measures have been taken to keep the prison population and their families informed (by management teams, prison staff, infographics…), both on the individuals' situation and of the measures taken during the lockdown.

(6) Attention to vulnerable subjects

The impact of the health crisis on prisons critically affects inmates with more vulnerability factors, in relation to which the following measures have been taken: a) financial support for inmates without economical resources; b) a plan for action to prevent substance abuse and possible overdoses, including informative actions, awareness sessions with the population at risk, and greater coordination between the different prison teams for the detection and care of cases with a higher risk. Fortunately, the incidence of overdose has not increased during confinement and during the transition compared to 2019.

(7) Decrease in the prison population

At the same time, during the health crisis, the population of prisons has been reduced, largely as a result of the decline in the activity of the courts and, probably also, by a decrease in the criminal activity during the lockdown. This would have resulted in a 53% reduction in the number of prison admissions (359 people in the period between March 16 and May 10, 2020; compared to 830 during the same period of 2019).

Portugal

The Portuguese government, through its Minister of Justice and the General Directorate of Prisons and Social Reinsertion (DGRSP) approved and released the Contingency Plan for COVID-19 as early as February 17 (then referred as containment phase). The structural lines of the Contingency Plan included, in a synoptic way, the following procedures:

(1) Creation of two rearwards infirmaries, one at the Porto Prison and the other at the São João de Deus Prison Hospital in Caxias, for the internment of infected prisoners; and the availability of the security pavilions in two other central prisons. Moreover, eight tents were installed in several other prisons but there was no need to resort to any of these structures.
(2) Since March 9, visits to prisoners were suspended and only resumed, on June 15, in 14 prisons, and on June 24, they already took place in 42 prisons. Visits to the remaining six prisons resumed until the end of June.
(3) Recommendations to prevent the entry of washed clothes or other goods from the outside were also implemented. Since there were security procedures to be followed, a delay between 24 and 72 hours should be considered between its reception and delivery to the inmates.
(4) Facilitating contact with family and friends, allowing for three daily telephone calls lasting 5 min each.
(5) Definition, for each geographical region, of which prison establishments would allow the entrance of new inmates to remain in prophylactic isolation, with due clinical monitoring, for a period of 14 days.
(6) Suspension of transfers of prisoners between facilities, unless security reasons so determine. Work activities with external entities and leisure activities were also suspended. Regarding school classes and professional training, a distance learning procedure was implemented, following the same procedure used in the outside. Moreover, short-term leaves within warden's duties were suspended and there was the possibility of deferring jurisdictional leaves, granted by the Penal Execution Court, over time. Short-term leaves and judicial leaves for prisoners were gradually resumed after the state of emergency was lifted, with returning prisoners following prophylactic isolation and clinical monitoring for a period of 14 days.
(7) Determination for prisons to reassign and to differentiate the schedules of the inmates' daily routines to try to separate, as much as possible, prisoners considered most vulnerable (aged more than 60, with immunosuppression or chronic disease, namely respiratory, hypertension, and diabetes).
(8) Definition of the protocol of procedures to be followed in the case of infection (following the guidelines of public health services).

(9) Distribution, by all prison clinical services, of a "Protective Kit" for all individuals. Besides, a plan was prepared with the daily needs estimated by each facility, based on the differentiation of each prison. Up till now, a lot of personnel protective equipment have been distributed throughout all the facilities.
(10) A significant part of the civilian workers was put on teleworking and/or in shift work with rotation, following the procedures and recommendations of the public health services, to prevent social and interpersonal contact.
(11) For prison officers, DGRSP declared the Status of Permanent Promptness, in compliance with the declaration of State of Emergency adopted in the country that ceased in accordance with the gradual regularization of activities.
(12) On April 10, Law No. 9/2020 was published stating the "Exceptional regime for easing the execution of sentences and freedom measures in the context of the COVID-19 disease pandemic." This law grants a partial pardon of prison sentences for convicts whose sentences were no longer than 2 years and a pardon for those whose sentences were longer than the aforementioned, if the time remaining time would not exceed 2 years. It was also granted a special regime of pardon for prisoners with 65 years old or more, carrying physical or mental diseases, or with a degree of autonomy incompatible with life in prison in the context of the pandemic. From these two measures were excluded prisoners serving sentences for domestic violence, sexual crimes, or homicides among other violent crimes.

This Law also granted an extraordinary administrative leave for a period of 45 days for prisoners under an open regime who have already successfully enjoyed a judicial leave or to those under common regime who have successfully enjoyed two jurisdictional leaves. Additionally, for those who have successfully handled these leaves, the Court of Execution of Sentences may anticipate the release on parole, for a maximum period of 6 months.

Incidence of the COVID-19 in corrections

A summary table of the main data on the impact of COVID-19 pandemic in the correctional system of Spain and Portugal is presented in Table 1.

Spain

In the prison facilities dependent on the central Spanish prison administration, the impact of the COVID-19 pandemic has been much less than that produced in the social community (DGEPRS, 2020d): total infections have been four times less, hospitalizations seven times less, and deaths 10 times less. Specifically, in a population of 49,998 inmates, 3 have died, and in a group of 24,000 prison staff, 5 staff have died. In the context of Catalonia prison administration, 91 inmates had been infected of which, as of July 12, there were 9 active cases. Among the staff, 167 prison staff were infected of which 19 were still active on July 19. During the month of June, the Department of Health of Catalonia carried out a screening through PCR tests on the entire prison population. This screening has resulted in 0.62% of the ordinary population presenting a positive result in the detection test.

Initially, there was concern about possible violent incidents in prisons, derived from restrictions associated with confinement (this had been the case, for example, in Italy).

Table 1. Main data on the impact of Covid-19 pandemic and the applied measures in the correctional systems of Spain and Portugal (March-October, 2020).

	Central Spanish prison administration		Catalan prison administration		TOTAL SPAIN		PORTUGAL	
	Lockdown period (March 15-June 20)	Return to "new normal" /June 21-October)	Lockdown period (March 15-June 20)	Return to "new normal" /June 21-October)	Lockdown period (March 15-June 20)	Return to "new normal" /June 21-Octover)	Lockdown period (March 12-May 2)	Return to "new normal" /May 3-October)
COUNTRY DATA								
Country population (2020)			7,727,029 (16% of Spanish population)		**47,329,981 (average of 43.4 years; 19.56 over 65)**		**10,341,330 (average of 44.8; 20.7% over 65)**	
Country infection cases (September 22, 2020)			102,000		**671,000**		**69,663**	
PCR positive: % of analyzed population			1.32%		**1.42%**		**0.67%**	
Country deaths (% of population) (September 22, 2020)			5,725 (0.07%)		**30,663 (0.065%)**		**1,925 (0.02%)**	
CORRECTIONAL POPULATION								
Prison population, January 2020 (rate/100,000 inhabitants)	998 (127)		8,376 (109)		**58,374 (123)**		**11,053 (102)**	
Reduction of prison population	6.9% (3,462 prisoners less)		12% (1,043 prisoners less)		**7.7% (4,505 prisoners less)**		**11.7% (1,289 prisoners less)**	
CORRECTIONAL IMPACT OF THE PANDEMIC								
Infected prisoners (accumulated)	46	+71 new cases	91	+72 new cases (PCR tests to all new admissions: 0.62% positive)	**137**	**+143 = 280**	**5**	**+25 = 30 (700 tests on prisoners)**
Dead prisoners	2	+1	0	0	**3**		**0**	
Infected prison staff (of analyzed cases)	238	+176	167	+197	**405**	**+373 = 778**	**17**	**+30 = 47 (3.300 tests on prison staff)**
Dead prison staff	5/24,000 global prison staff		0		**5**		**0**	

However, fortunately, this concern was soon diluted, as there was a low number of incidents and a low incidence on the safety of the centers.

Connected to this, a relevant effect that must be highlighted is the absence in prisons of deaths from drug overdoses during lockdown (compared to what happened in the same period of 2019, in which six inmates died from overdoses between March 1 and 25 of April). The confinement situation, by causing a forced abstinence from drugs (when its main routes of introduction disappear: visits, convicts who return from a permit. . .), could in theory have stimulated stress and violence in drug addicts' prisoners. But this has not been the case. Paradoxically, even some drug addicts, forced by the situation to non-consumption, had asked to enter into de-addiction programs through the use of methadone. In Catalonia, despite the stress caused by the health crisis and the measures taken in prisons, the conflicts have not increased significantly. During the confinement period, there was a slightly higher rate of incidents/1,000 inmates (135 compared to a rate of 104 for the same period of 2019). Afterward, the rate has been steadily decreasing: 110 for the transition period and 102 during the "new normal" period (until September 9).

Another striking fact during the pandemic and lockdown is the significant decrease in the prison population (2020c, 2020d, 2020e). In the Spanish prisons administrated by the General Secretariat of Penitentiary Institutions (apart from Catalonia) has been a reduction of 3,462 inmates (between 14 March and June 18). To find a similar reduction in the number of prisoners we must refer to a date as far away as 2002. This net reduction in the prison population results from the difference experienced in this period between the number of prisons admissions (which was 3,847) and the number of discharges (7,273). The lower number of prison admissions was probably related to two connected phenomena during the pandemic: a significant reduction in crime, as will be detailed later; less activity of the courts of justice, as a consequence of confinement.

However, this decrease of prison population cannot be attributed to a significant number of measures of release due to the pandemic. The release measures adopted (community programs, electronic monitoring. . .) have not formally decreased the *quantum* of the prison population. These measures made it possible for some inmates to serve the final periods of his sentence in more flexible life regimes, out of prison. Specifically, while as of March 13 there were 2,684 convicts serving sentences in an extra-prison regime (telematic means, face-to-face controls, extra-prison monitoring. . .) as of June 18, that figure was 5,670 (an increase greater than 200%).

Finally, the irruption of the disease COVID-19 and the measures adopted for its prevention have had a very negative impact, in all countries, on multiple rights and freedoms of citizens (European Union Agency for Fundamental Rights, 2020). These negative effects have probably been worse in prisons, due to their already restrictive nature of rights. These restrictions have drastically limited some of the legitimate rights and interests of those incarcerated (European Prison Observatory, 2020; EuroPris, 2020a; Solar & Lacal, 2020): cancellation of exit permits, communications and visits, education and training, labor, therapeutic, sports, cultural, religious activities, etc.

To avoid that these limitations of rights (as a result of the pandemic) could become *de facto* a suspension of such rights, at the Spanish prisons a series of alternatives have been adopted (DGEPRS, 2020a, 2020b):

-Concerning the inmates' right to communications, as mentioned, telephone calls have been maintained with family and friends, increasing their frequency, and adding the possibility of making video calls. Videoconferencing technology has also been promoted between prisons and in relation to judicial authorities, the prosecutor's office, lawyers, the ombudsman, consulates, and embassies.

-Regarding the right to exit permits, extraordinary permits have been maintained (for serious reasons) with health prevention measures. Ordinary permit applications have continued to be studied and authorized by the Treatment Boards of the Penitentiary Centers, for their eventual enjoyment after lockdown.

-Regarding the right to prison treatment, face-to-face treatment sessions have continued, with due sanitary measures, by prison technical staff who have continued to carry out their activity in person.

In Catalonia, the pandemic has had a negative impact on the jobs of inmates in the productive workshops developed in prisons (Centre d'Iniciatives per la Reinserció, 2020): 47% of the collaborating companies have ceased their activity in prisons definitively or temporarily (as of 31 May); part of the employment activity contracted with the public sector has also been affected, except for the production carried out by the healthcare system; as a result, there has been a 35% reduction in jobs in industrial workshops; the employment of interns has also been reduced as a result of the health and social crisis.

Portugal

According to the Portuguese Code of Enforcement of Prison Sentences, imprisonment should be applied to protect the society and to enhance the reintegration of inmates by preparing them for the return to the community (Gonçalves et al., 2019). Indeed, the intent to punish criminals should not imply their loss of the right to health care (Hoff et al., 2009; Liebrenz et al., 2020). The sanctions foresee not only offenders' punishment but also their treatment and control (Gonçalves, 2007). Despite this, often, the lack of conditions during the sentences – which is also a result of the prisons' overcrowding – makes difficult the achievement of such purposes.

By June 24, there were three positive asymptomatic cases (enterprise employees providing Services to DGRSP) for COVID-19, contaminated in society. In addition to these three active cases, from the beginning of the pandemic until June 24, were detected another 17 cases that were all recovered. Of these, seven were prison officers, one a medical doctor, two nurses, one a health assistant, and another an administrative assistant. Among detainees, five prisoners tested positive, all coming from community, except one who caught the disease in a unit hospital that had a COVID-19 focus at the time where he had a consultation there.

Since the first positive cases in the DGRSP, reported by the end of March, 700 tests had been carried out by July on prisoners, for screening suspects and contacts of suspects. Starting on May 4, and following a protocol signed between DGRSP and health services, screening tests for prison workers were made available, having already carried out about 3,300 tests on workers and employees assigned to all 49 Portuguese prisons. Until July, there were only four positive cases to COVID-19 (one remained asymptomatic and already recovered while the other three, equally asymptomatic, remain active). This systematic screening currently proceeds in all Portuguese prisons.

Concerning the preventive measures to avoid contagion in prisons, 1,289 prisoners were released under the pardon (article 2 of Law 9/2020), and 701 orders for authorization of Extraordinary Administrative Leave (article 4 of Law 9/2020) were sent to prisons. Besides, 14 acts of grace were conceded. All these release measures provided the creation of separated spaces in prisons, allowing for greater social distance both in canteens and in the playgrounds.

A great part of the 45 days leaves have already ended. The guidelines are the renewal of the license, in accordance with the provisions of the law, meaning that successful leaves might imply further authorizations. So far, 10 prisoners have not requested the renewal of these leaves while 12 others did not get the renewal due to unfavorable reports provided by monitoring staff. Additionally, there were 44 revocations for noncompliance with the defined containment rules and three voluntary returns to prison. In this universe of 701 licenses, 84 individuals reach the mid-term of their sentences in the meanwhile and were granted parole, as 12 others who benefit from the pardon. Finally, and until the time of writing this text, among the 1289 released under Pardon, there were 10 returns to prison following the commission of new crimes.

Lockdown and crime

The analysis of criminality was not the primary objective of this work. However, as the authors delved into the preparation of this paper, a significant relationship was detected between population confinement and crime. Hence, given the relevance of this phenomenon, it has been decided to incorporate this analysis here mainly for the case of Spain. The analyzed data come from official sources (police and judicial) and correspond to the period 2017–2020 (See Table 2).

The first observation that must be made is that Spain and Portugal generally have a low crime rate within the framework of European countries (Aebi & Tiago, 2020; Cid, 2020; EuroPris, 2020a; Redondo & Garrido, 2013). These low rates of crime are exemplified below from three types of offenses (corresponding to 2017): crimes against property, homicide, and cars' theft. The comparison unit will be the arrests per 100,000 inhabitants. The crime rates against property in Spain and Portugal were, respectively, 144 and 115 (the European country with the highest rate was Belgium with 167). As for homicide, the highest rate in Europe was that of Latvia, with a value of 5.6 homicides per year for every 100,000 inhabitants. In contrast, Spain and Portugal present identical rates of 0.7 homicides per year per 100,000 inhabitants, which are among the lowest in Europe and in the world. Regarding vehicle theft crimes, the highest rate in the EU was 328 in Luxembourg, contrasting this with that of Spain, which was 69, and that of Portugal, 109.

Given these structural crime figures, what has happened to the crime during these months of lockdown and application of extraordinary measures of control? From the outset, it would be expected that the important changes produced in the social dynamics, regarding the interruption of industrial production, trade, the radical decrease in travel and tourist exchanges, would have produced a global decrease in the rates of criminality (Duwe & Clark, 2017; Felson, 2006, 2008, 2014; Redondo, 2015; Stickle & Felson, 2020). The data of the Spanish Police does indeed reflect a generalized narrowing of some crimes during COVID-19 confinement. For example, street crimes have abruptly decreased, up to 80%, including all crimes associated with leisure and tourism activities. This is probably due to the closure of entertainment venues and the almost absolute absence of tourists. Likewise, the dramatic decline in people using public transportation (metro, bus, trains) has also been associated with a significant reduction in crime in these contexts. Offenses related to driving have also deeply diminished during lockdown (up to 80%), in association with the radical drop in road traffic.

Table 2. Lockdown and variations in crime in Spain.

Crimes that have decreased	
Global reported crimes	73.8% (greater reduction in more urban areas: 80.3% in Catalonia; 84.1% in Madrid)
Global reported property crimes	From 56,460 (same period of 2019) to 10,628 (during lockdown)
Global street crimes	80%
Thefts	90.18%
Vehicle theft crimes	69%
Driving offences	80%
Frauds and scam crimes	86.6%
Illegal occupation of buildings	79.7%
Direct hate crimes	73.1%
Partner murders	Reduction from 4-5 monthly murders to a total of 5 murders over three months
Juvenile delinquency	Drastic reduction, according to the Spanish Juvenile Prosecutor's Office
Police arrests (two first weeks of lockdown)	77.94
Crimes that have not decreased, but rather modified their topography	
Drug trafficking	Use of couriers or taxi drivers as drug dealers
Crimes that have increased	
Cyber-crimes associated with domestic violence	Increase in phone calls to police and family support services
Probably frauds by internet, cyber-bulling, grooming sexting, "malware", hate crimes online, hoaxes and "fake news"	Increased "cyber" space
Detainees for resistance and disobedience (generally to police requirements to comply with sanitary restrictions)	519% increase

In contrast, other crimes have not exactly decreased, but they have varied in topography to adapt to the social circumstances of the pandemic. For example, drug trafficking has taken advantage during the confinement of new distribution mechanisms (couriers, taxi drivers...); thefts have focused on pharmacies and supermarkets (which were open as essential services).

Opposite, the crimes that take place in the "cyber" space have exploded during the lockdown. Cyber-crimes associated with domestic violence have in general increased, if telephone calls to aid services and police interventions in family contexts are taken into account. However, some sexual and gender cyber-crimes have decreased. In particular couple murders in Spain have dropped sharply, from an average of 4–5 monthly murders to a total of five couple murders during the 3 months of confinement. Nevertheless, as for economic and other cyber-crimes, it is early to know the criminogenic effects of the pandemic in family and sex crimes, since many of them can be discovered with significant temporal latency.

Criminal phenomena such as scams or frauds, "pishing," cyber-bullying, grooming, sexting, "malware," hate crimes online, hoaxes, and "fake news" have been triggered for structural reasons. The "cyber" space has become the new reality of the main social exchange: such a high volume of cyber-interactions -even if only for epidemiological reasons- the increase in these crimes is probably been favored (Miró, 2011; Ngo & Paternoster, 2011; Redondo, 2008, 2015).

The Spanish National Police published on May 1, 2020, a report that compares, firstly, the rates of reported crime between 2019 and 2020, for two defined intervals: from March 1 to 13 and from March 14 to 31 (for 2020, before sanitary confinement and during confinement). Data show an increase in crime in 2020 of 8% in the first period (without confinement) and a decrease of 73.8% in the second (with confinement), in contrast to the same periods of 2019. The police of Catalonia also informs that during the lockdown the reported rate of crimes decreased by 80.3% in relation to the same period of 2019. Contrarily, once the confinement ended, a clear increase of crime has been observed, although not up to the same criminal level that existed in 2019, only half of that previous level (Mossos d'Esquadra, 2020).

These data show that in Spain the crime rate has changed in the context of the COVID-19 crisis in a very sensitive way (following a dose-effect pattern): where the epidemic has been more serious, the offenses have decreased more. For example, in the region and city of Madrid, where the epidemic has been especially critical, in the first months of confinement crime reached a reduction of 84.1%, significantly greater than the average reduction in Spain of 73.8% (MI, 2020a, 2020b; Policía Nacional, 2020).

As expected, the largest decreases during lockdown have occurred in property crimes. An analysis of 2 months (March–April 2020) shows that 10,628 property offenses were reported to the police, in front of 56,460 informed in the same period of 2019. Crimes of scam decreased by 86.6% and those of illegal occupation of buildings by 79.7%. Thefts (which are the most frequent property crime) decreased by 90.2%, from 23,200 known cases in the second half of March 2019 to 2,278 in the same period of 2020. The depletion in other less frequent crimes, such as hate crimes, was 73.1%.

The reduction in the number of reported crimes has also been reflected in a decrease in police arrests: there would have been only 12,047 arrests during the first two weeks of confinement compared to 54,634 during the same period of 2019 (77.9% less). In contrast, the detainees for resistance and disobedience to authority (generally, disobedience to police requirements to comply with the restrictions derived from the state of alarm) increased during confinement by 519.1% (reaching 6,700 arrests).

What has happened to juvenile delinquency (vandalism, youth gangs, etc.) during the lockdown resulting from the COVID-19 pandemic? Although there are still no detailed reports in this regard, there are indications that many juvenile offenses have decreased. The prosecutor in charge of the Juvenile Prosecutor's Office in Spain has stated that "since the State of Alarm was declared in Spain due to the coronavirus pandemic, the rate of crimes of minors has decreased dramatically." And similarly to what happened in the adult crime, there was also a "certain rise, during the first fortnight of the confinement, of intra-family violence committed by minors, especially against their brothers or parents"; as well as a decrease in this violence in the first two weeks of lack of confinement (Declarations from the prosecutor to a TV news network, 4/26/2020).

De-escalation planning and resumption of normalcy

As above-mentioned, many countries are in the de-escalation stages of the previous sanitary confinement, and back to "new normality." However, there is great uncertainty about the future evolution of the pandemic, and about the possible measures that must be adopted, including the possibility of new infections and new lockdowns. Corrections logically do not escape this uncertainty about the future. In both Spanish and Portuguese prisons and community corrections, transition processes toward unconfinement begun with the aim of recovering the main programs and activities related with prisoners' lives (*i.e.*, communications, exit permits, an increase of open regime, return of volunteers, collaborating entities, education, treatment programs, face-to-face attention of the social services, visits at home, etc.).

However, this return of correctional institutions to "normality" continues to be subject to various eventualities and shocks, depending on the evolution of the pandemic in each country. So that, let us summarize the evolution of the pandemic in recent months and the measures applied in the correctional systems of Spain and Portugal as well as globally in Europe.

Spain

As commented, on June 20, the period of "new normality" began in Spain. As of the end of June, all the prison activities that had been suspended during the declaration of the state of alarm were gradually restored (DGEPRS, 2020f, 2020g). As expected, with the restoration of the inmates' contact with the outside world (exit permits, visits...) some infections began to appear in various prisons, particularly in the Spanish regions and cities with the highest incidence of outbreaks (including Madrid, the Basque Country, and other). Overall, the accumulated number of infected prisoners since the end of the state of alarm until the beginning of September was 71, out of a prison population of 47,703 inmates (a total of contagious since March to September of 117 prisoners, a figure still four times less than that observed in the general population). As a consequence of these new infections, family and intimate visits were temporarily suspended in the prisons of the risk regions (DGEPRS, 2020h).

Nevertheless, a positive fact in this context is that the Spanish prison authorities have decided to maintain, with the proper prevention measures, the resumption of school activities from the month of September (DGEPRS, 2020i). Contrarily, an especially negative fact is that, since the reestablishment of family visits, there has been a significant increase of deaths in prison due to drug overdoses. This points to the plausible hypothesis that a large part of the drug would enter the prison through these visits.

Regarding the open regime (DGEPRS, 2020j), as of March 13 (before the pandemic), there were 2,684 inmates serving their sentences in an extra-prison life regime (through the use of telematic means, face-to-face controls, monitoring by community institutions, etc.). As of June 18 (at the end of the critical stage of the pandemic) that figure was 5,670 individuals, that is, almost 3,000 more. As of August 5, in the unconfined phase, the number of subjects in the extra-penitentiary regime had decreased to 5,176.

In Catalonia, between June and July, the routines of contact of the prisoners with the outside, also interrupted during confinement, were progressively recovered. The number of cases of infection remained quite stable in relation to the beginning of the transition phase: on May 10 there were 10 active cases and 61 accumulated in Catalan prisons and on July 20 there were 9 active cases and 102 accumulated. However, in anticipation of the existing risks, it was agreed to once again suspend face-to-face family communications and leaves of those inmates residing in geographic areas with outbreaks of the infection. PCR tests were also carried out on new admissions to prison, with the corresponding period of preventive quarantine until the result of the test was known (SMPRAV, 2020c).

As of September 9, there were 16 active cases in Covid-19 in the prisons of Catalonia and 72 new infected cases. Among the personnel, 24 positive active, and 197 new infected (Internal data of the Department of Justice). Nonetheless, the interrupted activities were partially recovered (exit permits; face-to-face visits, with limitations in the number of visitors and the duration: SMPRAV, 2020d).

Since the beginning of the crisis in Catalan prisons, two main actions, as referred, were carried out, aimed at reducing the concentration of inmates in ordinary prison units: 1) increasing the open prison population; 2) refer as many prisoners as possible, with proper controls, to remain in their own homes or inappropriate community resources.

These measures had had a great impact in everyday operation of open prisons. Before confinement, 65% of the inmates of such open centers (801 people) occupied residential places: they could be away during the day and on weekends (work, family life. . .), but had to return at night. The remaining prisoners in the open regime (35% of them) were authorized to remain continuously in their homes or in the assigned community resources. However, with the Covid-19 pandemic, the high concentration of people in these open units, but which daily contact the outside world, posed a high risk of infection and spreading the virus among all residents. For this reason, it was established that the majority could remain in their homes, without the obligation to return to the center at night. This drastically reduced the occupation of residential places in open regime, to a minimum of only, as of May 13, of 40 people (3.44% of the total of the places theoretically available in the open regime). This made it necessary to quickly modify the supervision procedures for these prisoners authorized to reside in the community. Face-to-face contacts and community visits by the staff of open prisons were reduced to a minimum, with supervision carried out through telephone calls, video calls, and geolocation, in addition to the regular use of electronic controls.

However, with the gradual return to the "new normal", a part of the previous residential occupation of the open prisons has been recovered: 22.6% (232 people) as of July 22 and 29.7% (312 people) at September 9. Even so, it is considered a priority to maintain a low residential occupancy of the open regime, and to maximize the protection measures against contagion in these facilities.

A final relevant issue here is to what degree the impact of the pandemic in the correctional context has been able to affect the private sector that provides services and technology to the correctional system. There is a growing international trend toward the privatization of the correctional systems, regarding the management of both institutional and community corrections (J. M. Byrne et al., 2019; J. M. Byrne et al., 2015). It is true that in most European countries, including Spain and Portugal, the majority of correctional services are currently developed by the public sector of the government (generally, ministries of Justice, Interior, Health, Education). But so is it, as J. Byrne et al. (2019) have documented, that in various countries, including Spain, some services related to food, health care, maintenance of facilities, rehabilitation, and video surveillance have been privatized. For example, in Catalonia, part of the rehabilitation and reintegration programs (drug addiction, community reintegration, care for the disabled, residential units in the community, etc.) are contracted with private entities (NGOs). During the health crisis and confinement, out of 55 contracts in program developed by external entities (with a budget of five million euros), 5 contracts had to be interrupted. Nevertheless, this has not led to an economic decrease for the providers, but they have been compensated for the time they have not been able to provide their services in prisons.

Portugal

From March 1 to September 7, there were 57 cases of Covid-19 in the Portuguese prison system. These 57 cases, mostly asymptomatic, concern 30 workers (15 from Prison Administration staff and 15 from private companies that provide/sell services to DGRSP), 25 prisoners, and 2 juveniles from educational centers. At the present date (September 7, 2020), there are 12 active cases of Covid-19, all of them related to prisoners previously in freedom. These cases were detected during the quarantine to which are subjected newcomers or furlough prisoners from society. Five cases were persons handed over by police after arrest and court confirmation. The other seven were returning prisoners after benefiting from Extraordinary Exit License (art. 4 of Law 9/2020 of April 10), jurisdictional exit license, and short-term exit license. The remaining 45 cases – 15 of DGRSP workers, 15 of workers from private companies providing services, 13 of prisoners, and 2 juveniles in educational centers refer to people who have already recovered from the illness (available on https://dgrsp.justica.gov.pt/Estatísticas-e-indicadores).

Concerning the adopted measures, between January and August this year, the operative activity of the Portuguese correctional system experienced a sharp drop, except for the penalties and measures inspected by electronic surveillance. This decrease was of 20.33% failures in technical assistance to judicial decision-making (reports and hearings; Estatística Mensal das Penas e Medidas com Vigilância Eletrónica, August 2020) and 12.49% in penalties and measures being implemented in the community (Assessoria Técnica à Tomada de Decisão Judicial Execução de Penas e Medidas na Comunidade Áreas Penal e Tutelar Educativa, August 2020). In the opposite sense, only the penalties and measures inspected by electronic surveillance increased by 9.03%. In addition, in the juvenile area, technical assistance for judicial decision-making (reports and hearings; Estatística Mensal Centros Educativos, August 2020) decreased by 23.01%, the measures being implemented in the community fell by 16.89% and the number of young people confined to juvenile facilities decreased by 18% (see https://dgrsp.justica.gov.pt/Estatísticas-e-indicadores).

Although is too early to draw definitive conclusions regarding these declines, it is possible that these breaks result from the combination of a decrease in the work of the courts (suspension of hearings and trials) and the confinement rules accorded for people in general. This aspect reduced the exposure of potential victims and therefore affected the rates of low-intensity criminal activity that tends to be the main cause for imprisonment.

The issue related to the impact of Covid-19 pandemic in the private sector providing services to the correctional system does not strictly apply to Portugal, since no private sector supply areas of activity that remain under the jurisdiction of the General Directorate of Reinsertion and Prison Services. Accordingly, electronic surveillance, community measures, and juvenile justice depend entirely on organic units of this General Directorate and are under state responsibility. When it comes to service providers, we refer to providing meals and cleaning central services or security services, in the case of educational centers for juveniles. At a state level, there were no dismissals, maintaining the tenders for hiring new workers that were planned, as it is the case of the tender for the admission of new prison guards.

Europe

The most recent report from EuroPris corresponds to July 24, 2020. Its most important insights in relation to the evolution of the pandemic in European correctional systems are the following (EuroPris, 2020b):

-In most countries, the strong restrictions at the start of the pandemic have been relaxed. However, in general, *correctional systems continue to experience great pressure* to lessen the impact of Covid-19. There is concern that the prolongation of this situation could diminish the motivation of the staff and increase the dissatisfaction of the inmates.

-The most severe impact of the pandemic in prisons is the *restriction of family visits* (number of visits and visitors, duration of visits...), which largely continues today. A good palliative mechanism has been videoconferences, which have allowed prisoners to have more frequent and extensive contacts with their families; and even the possibility, in some countries, of being able to read bedtime stories to their children. However, it is appreciated that videoconferences should be a complementary instrument, but not a substitute for in-person visits.

-There is great variability between countries on the greater or lesser obligation to use masks within correctional facilities: from the obligation to always use them to their occasional use for certain contacts or activities.

-In many countries, tests are carried out (similar to the community) to those who present symptoms (either prisoners or staff members) and to all those people with whom they have had contact. In some systems, random tests are also performed on the inmates and the prison staff.

-In most countries, medical care for prisoners is face-to-face, although many correctional systems have generated complementary remote health consultation services.

-As a health protection mechanism, many countries try to reduce the prison occupancy rate through measures such as the following: early release, suspension, or postponement of the application of sentences, increased community measures, increased prisons' capacity, or use of single-person cells.

-Among the measures adopted that have shown greater effectiveness in managing the pandemic in prisons are: the combination of restriction of visits, exits from and admissions to prison; the application of compensatory measures with the prisoners (video colling, distant education); clear and continuous communication on the measures adopted and their justification; the provision of sanitary protection equipment to the prison staff and their access to Covid-19 testing.

Discussion

The global health crisis due to COVID-19 is causing a serious stress in all societies, who have suddenly seen threatened the health of their citizens, their economies and, more globally, their way of life. The impact of this pandemic on the correctional systems has also been acute, including both the inmates (and their families) and the prison staff (Ashby, 2020). To fight this crisis in prisons and other correctional facilities, extraordinary restrictive measures had to be adopted, for preventing the epidemic itself and for minimizing the negative effects of the applied restrictions. The results obtained can probably offer us some important lessons in order to improve and strengthen the prison system when the crisis is over.

Fortunately, the infections by Covid-19 have been few by now in the prison systems of Spain and Portugal, probably due to the prompt adoption of the diverse preventive measures referred in this paper (lockdown, suspension of visits and exit permits, interruption of education and work programs...); the commendable "professionalism and dedication" of prison staff and managers; the excellent response of the inmates (aware of the seriousness of the situation); the availability of appropriate infrastructures that allowed the inmates to be in acceptable conditions of comfort and well-being.

Among the critical measures adopted has been the almost absolute suspension of the external visits of inmates with their family and friends. Adaptation to life in prison is usually very difficult for inmates, particularly due to the lack of frequent contact with their relatives. For example, a study of Gonçalves and Gonçalves (2012) in Portugal showed that a reduced number of prison visits was associated with a higher level of aggressiveness and a lower level of adaptation to prison live. If the isolation is in principle desirable to protect the virus' dissemination, this deprivation may increment at the same time the prisoners' psychological vulnerability (Afonso, 2020) for experiencing some mental and emotional disorders as higher levels of anxiety and stress (Liebrenz et al., 2020).

To deal with such problems, during the crisis, a relevant strategy has been to maximize the information given to inmates and their families (as well to the prison staff) to involve them in the responsibility of preventing contagion within prisons. As a favorable consequence, their understanding and collaborative responses have contributed to a better management of this critical situation. In particular, the established "family telephone service" with the prisoners' families have proven to be a very successful initiative to improve the quality of the support offered to inmates and their close contexts, to which they will later return. In this framework, actions have also been taken (in collaboration with health services, social organizations, and families) to prevent drug use within prisons and the risk of drug overdose. For those measures, the use of the new devices and advances in communication technology has been greatly accepted for all the users. The lesson learned is that these communication mechanisms, extremely useful for the daily dynamics of prisons, should be consolidated as a stable complementary prison service for prisoners and their families, beyond this crisis.

During the lockdown, something has happened that has profound implications for the prison system, and more broadly, for the entire penal system. Throughout the most severe stage of the pandemic, the prison systems of Spain and Portugal have applied more open-ended and community-based measures to thousands of prisoners. These measures, which decrease the concentration of inmates in prisons by 9%, probably contributed to the prevention of massive infections within prisons. But, beyond this, these open-ended and community measures could have favored the processes of social reintegration of the released prisoners (without a significant increase in new crimes being observed). From now on it would be necessary to assess precisely to what extent this provisional discharge may have truly favored a greater social adjustment of individuals. If such analysis reveals that discharged offenders were able to start a new non-criminal life, new policies regarding community sentences for other offenders could be considered.

With the return to "normality," although the population in open regime remains in a significantly higher proportion than before, the global rate of inmates residing outside the prison has decreased. Some prosecution and penitentiary surveillance courts are revoking part of the previous applications of this measure, understanding that its use was exceptional for the health crisis but not necessary or convenient in a "normal" situation.

The authors of this article want to express their opinion contrary to these restrictive considerations. In the advanced societies of the 21st century, it is certainly anachronistic to continue to attribute to prison sentences primarily punitive purposes, instead of those of rehabilitation and social reintegration, particularly for nonviolent offenders (Atkin-Plunk, 2020; Moss et al., 2018). For that, the measures of approaching ex-offenders to their family and social context have proven to be a critical factor (Cullen, 2007; Duwe & Clark, 2017; Martín et al., 2019; Redondo, 2017). Going even further, J. M. Byrne et al. (2015) concluded, based on their international macro-analysis of incarceration, that in order to significantly improve the current negative prison reality (disproportionate rates of prisoners, overcrowding, recidivism…) it would not be enough to improve the quantity and quality of rehabilitation prison programs: "[It] will not fundamentally change the life course of prisoners, resulting in continued high return-to-prison rates for these offenders. (…) For the United States [and this could also apply to most of the countries of the world] … we will need to rethink our approach to crime and punishment (…) we call for the development of corrections and sentencing policies – and the hiring of corrections personnel – based on the new goal of corrections: individual and community rehabilitation" (p. 421). In other words, in the opinion of these authors, correctional systems are in need of more than just improvement: they need, as they have literally pointed out in the title of their paper, a "Global Rehabilitation Revolution."

Although the analysis of crime was not an initial objective of this work, the authors have considered it important to incorporate it here. In particular, the analysis made of the evolution of crime in Spain has shown a spectacular reduction in crimes during confinement (73.8%), in comparison to the same period of 2019 and the periods before and after the confinement. Some criminological theories and multiple empirical studies have endorsed the importance that social exchanges, and the criminal opportunities generated by them, have as precipitators of crime (Felson, 2008; Redondo, 2015; Stickle & Felson, 2020). Probably, the abrupt reduction in social exchanges (as a result of lockdown) has produced a decrease in the opportunities for "common" crimes on the street; while the return to social and urban relations (at the end of strict lockdown) has been linked to a further increase in street crime (Lum et al., 2020).

Opposite, during lockdown there have been an increase in cybercrimes, which some experts have estimated around 70–80% (Mossos d'Esquadra, 2020). Just as criminal opportunities for street crime would have diminished, confinement might have favored increased opportunities for certain family crimes and cybercrime (by spending more time at home and making greater use of communication technologies and social networks). Within this framework, there could have been also an increase of certain personal and social criminogenic risk factors, such as the perception of a greater anonymity and impunity, increased economic or emotional needs, or group influence and pressure; and, in parallel, a decrease in some protective factors as social control (physical absence of teachers, more unsupervised leisure time…). This combination of increased risk factors and decreased protective factors could have contributed to the increase, for example, of family offenses and cybercrimes.

As lockdown has been linked to a sharp decline in street crime (up to 70.3% in the first 15 days of confinement), the return to normality (the so-called "new normality," without strict confinement) has been associated – as if it were a "natural experiment" – with an intensive increase in crime, especially street crime, such as theft, robbery, drug trafficking, road crime, etc. Other crimes that have experienced ups and downs, in a reactive manner to confinement/lack of confinement, are cyber-crimes, family violence, crimes at work and the economic context, hate crimes and terrorism.

All these observations clearly endorse the decisive role played by social exchanges, and the opportunities created by them, in the generation of crimes (Stickle & Felson, 2020). Certainly, not in an absolute and exclusive way, but in conjunction with the risk factors and criminal motivation of the individuals themselves (Bobbio et al., 2018; Farrington et al., 2012; Redondo, 2015; Reyns et al., 2014; Ward & Fortune, 2016). These results on the impact of this pandemic on crime, which were not initially the object of this analysis, has, however, relevant implications for basic criminological investigation. The time ranges, prevalence, variability, and idiosyncrasy of the evolution of each type of crime should be analyzed with greater precision hereinafter.

In conclusion, the prison systems of Spain and Portugal have quickly put in place multiple measures, as showed, to prevent Covid-19 infection within prisons, which have so far been quite effective. Nevertheless, the risk posed by the pandemic in the social environment and in prisons remains active. Therefore, prisons must still maintain the most effective prevention measures applied, like the ones discussed in this paper.

Disclosure statement

No potential conflict of interest was reported by the author(s).

References

Aebi, M. F., Berger-Kolopp, L., Burkhardt, C., & Tiago, M. M. (2019). *Prisons in Europe 2005-2015 – Volume 2: Sourcebook of prison statistics*. Council of Europe.

Aebi, M. F., & Tiago, M. M. (2018). *SPACE I - 2018 – Council of Europe Annual Penal Statistics: Prison populations*. Council of Europe.

Aebi, M. F., & Tiago, M. M. (2020). *Prisons and prisoners in Europe in pandemic times: An evaluation of the short-term impact of the COVID-19 on prison populations*. Council of Europe. http://wp.unil.ch/space/files/2020/06/Prisons-and-the-COVID-19_200617_FINAL.pdf

Aebi, M. F., Tiago, M. M., & Burkhardt, C. (2016). *Council of Europe Annual Penal Statistics SPACE I: Prison populations. Survey 2015*. Council of Europe.

Afonso, P. (2020). The impact of the COVID-19 pandemic on mental health. *Acta Medica Portuguesa*, *33*(5), 351–358. https://doi.org/10.20344/amp.13877

Ashby, M. P. J. (2020). Initial evidence on the relationship between the coronavirus pandemic and crime in the United States. *Crime Science*, *9*, 6. https://doi.org/10.1186/s40163-020-00117-6

Assessoria Técnica à Tomada de Decisão Judicial Execução de Penas e Medidas na Comunidade Áreas Penal e Tutelar Educativa [Judicial Court Decisions for Adults and Juveniles on Penal and Community Sentences Statistics]. (2020, August). CCCRE/DGRSP.

Atkin-Plunk, C. A. (2020). Should all violent offenders be treated equally? Perceptions of punishment and rehabilitation for violent offenders with varying attributes. *Victims & Offenders*, *15*(2), 218–242. https://doi.org/10.1080/15564886.2019.1711277

Bedford, J., Enria, D., Giesecke, J., Heymann, D. L., Ihekweazu, C., Kobinger, G., Ungchusak, K., Oh, M.-D., Sall, A. A., Schuchat, A., Ungchusak, K., Wieler, L. H., & Lane, H. C. (2020). COVID-19: Towards controlling of a pandemic. *The Lancet*, *395*(10229), 1015–1018. https://doi.org/10.1016/S0140-6736(20)30673-5

Bobbio, A., Arbach, K., & Vazsonyi, A. T. (2018). Self-control and deviance: A test of the general theory of crime in Argentina. *Victims & Offenders, 14*(1), 119–142. https://doi.org/10.1080/15564886.2018.1552222

Byrne, J., Kras, K. R., & Marmolejo, L. M. (2019). International perspectives on the privatización of corrections. *Criminology & Public Policy, 18*(2), 477–503. https://doi.org/10.1111/1745-9133.12440

Byrne, J. M., Pattavina, A., & Taxman, F. F. (2015). International trends in prison upsizing and downsizing: In search of evidence of a global rehabilitation revolution. *Victims & Offenders, 10*(4), 420–451. https://doi.org/10.1080/15564886.2015.1078186

Campbell, K. M., & Doshi, R. (2020). The coronavirus could reshape global order. *Foreign Affairs*, 18.

Centre d'Iniciatives per la Reinserció. (2020). *Informe sobre l'afectació de la COVID-19 a l'activitat laboral als centres penitenciaris* [Report on COVID-19 at work in prisons]. Unpublished internal report. Departament de Justícia.

Cid, J. (2008). El incremento de la población reclusa en España entre 1996-2006: Diagnóstico y remedios [The increase of prison population in Spain between 1996-2006]. *Revista Española de Investigación Criminológica (REIC) Art. 2, Núm 6*, 1–30.

Cid, J. (2020). El futuro de la prisión en España [The future of imprisonment in Spain]. *Revista Española de Investigación Criminológica (REIC), Art. 1, Núm., 18*, 1–32.

Contini, C., Di Nuzzo, M., Barp, N., Bonazza, A., De Giorgio, R., Tognon, M., & Rubino, S. (2020). The novel zoonotic COVID-19 pandemic: An expected global health concern. *The Journal of Infection in Developing Countries, 14*(3), 254–264. https://doi.org/10.3855/jidc.12671

Coyle, A., Fair, H., Jacobson, J., & Walmsley, R. (2016). *Imprisonment worldwide: The current situation and an alternative future.* Policy Press.

CPCWG. (2020a, April). *COVID-19 related statement by the members of the Council for Penology Cooperation Working Group.* PC-CP (2020) 5. Council of Europe.

CPCWG. (2020b). *Statement of principles relating to the treatment of persons deprived of their liberty in the context of the coronavirus disease (COVID-19) pandemic.* CE print. CPT/Inf(2020)13. Council of Europe.

Cullen, F. T. (2007). Make rehabilitation corrections' guiding paradigm. *Criminology & Public Policy, 6*(4), 717–728. https://doi.org/10.1111/j.1745-9133.2007.00469.x

DGEPRS. (2020a). *Actuaciones de contención del virus en los establecimientos penitenciarios* [Actions to contain the virus in prison facilities]. Unpublished internal report. Dirección General de Ejecución Penal y Reinserción Social, Secretaría General de Instituciones Penitenciarias Ministerio del Interior.

DGEPRS. (2020b). *Nuevas actuaciones en los centros penitenciarios para la gestion de la situación de crisis sanitaria ocasionada por el Covid-19.* Unpublished internal report. Secretaría General de Instituciones Penitenciarias, Ministerio del Interior.

DGEPRS. (2020c). *Informe sobre la evolución de los internos clasificados en regimen abierto y regimen de vida extra-penitenciario* [Report on the evolution of prisoners classified in open and extra-prison life regimes]. Unpublished internal report. Dirección General de Ejecución Penal y Reinserción Social, Secretaría General de Instituciones Penitenciarias Ministerio del Interior.

DGEPRS. (2020d). *Informe sobre los movimientos de altas y bajas que efectan a la ocupación de los centros penitenciarios* [Report on the movements of discharges and discharges that affect the occupation of penitentiary centers]. Unpublished internal report. Dirección General de Ejecución Penal y Reinserción Social, Secretaría General de Instituciones Penitenciarias Ministerio del Interior.

DGEPRS. (2020e). *Informe sobre los penados clasificados en cada grado de tratamiento penitenciario* [Report on the convicts classified in each grade of prison treatment]. Unpublished internal report. Dirección General de Ejecución Penal y Reinserción Social, Secretaría General de Instituciones Penitenciarias Ministerio del Interior.

DGEPRS. (2020f). *Medidas Nueva Normalidad (COVID-19* [New normal measures (COVID-19)]. Dirección General de Ejecución Penal y Reinserción Social, Secretaría General de Instituciones Penitenciarias Ministerio del Interior.

DGEPRS. (2020g). *Aclaración Nueva Normalidad (COVID-19)* [Clarifications New Normal (COVID-19)]. Unpublished internal report. Dirección General de Ejecución Penal y Reinserción Social, Secretaría General de Instituciones Penitenciarias Ministerio del Interior.

DGEPRS. (2020h). *Medidas actuación (COVID-19).* [Action measures (COVID-19)]. Unpublished internal report. Dirección General de Ejecución Penal y Reinserción Social, Secretaría General de Instituciones Penitenciarias Ministerio del Interior.

DGEPRS (2020i). *Actividades educativas 20/21* [Educational activities 20/21]. Unpublished internal report. Dirección General de Ejecución Penal y Reinserción Social, Secretaría General de Instituciones Penitenciarias Ministerio del Interior.

DGEPRS. (2020j). *Informe sobre penados clasificados 27/ 08/2020* [Report on the convicts classified 27/08/2020]. Unpublished internal report. Dirección General de Ejecución Penal y Reinserción Social, Secretaría General de Instituciones Penitenciarias Ministerio del Interior.

Di Lorenzo, G., & Di Trolio, R. (2020). Coronavirus disease (COVID-19) in Italy: Analysis of risk factors and proposed remedial measures. *Frontiers in Medicine*, *7*, 140. https://doi.org/10.3389/fmed.2020.00140

Directorate-General of Health. (2020). *Situation report of Portugal.* Ministry of Health. https://covid19.min-saude.pt/ponto-de-situacao-atual-em-portugal/

Duarte, R., Furtado, I., Sousa, L., & Carvalho, C. (2020). The 2019 novel coronavirus (2019-nCoV): Novel virus, old challenges. *Acta Medica Portuguesa*, *33*(3), 155–157. https://doi.org/10.20344/amp.13547

Duwe, G., & Clark, V. (2017). The rehabilitative ideal versus the criminogenic reality: The consequences of warehousing prisoners. *Corrections*, *2*(1), 41–69. https://doi.org/10.1080/23774657.2016.1240596

Estatística Mensal Centros Educativos [Educational Centers Statistical Indicators]. (2020, August). CCCRE/DGRSP.

Estatística Mensal das Penas e Medidas com Vigilância Eletrónica [Electronic surveillance Statistics]. (2020, August). CCCRE/DGRSP.

European Prison Observatory. (2020). *COVID-19: What is happening in European Prisons?* (Update #3). European Prison Observatory. http://www.prisonobservatory.org/upload/17042020European_prisons_during_covid19%233.pdf

European Union Agency for Fundamental Rights. (2020). *Coronavirus COVID-19 outbreak in the EU Fundamental Rights Implications.* European Union Agency for Fundamental Rights. https://fra.europa.eu/sites/default/files/fra_uploads/portugal-report-covid-19-april-2020_en.pdf

EuroPris. (2020a, March 30). *Overview of European prison services' responses to the COVID-19 crisis.* EuroPris. https://www.europris.org/covid-19-prevention-measures-in-european-prisons/

EuroPris. (2020b, July 24). *Overview of European prison services' responses to the COVID-19 crisis* (3rd ed.). EuroPris. https://www.europris.org/covid-19-prevention-measures-in-european-prisons/

Farrington, D. P., Loeber, R., & Ttofi, M. M. (2012). Risk and protective factors for offending. In B. Welsh & D. P. Farrington (Eds.), *The Oxford handbook of crime prevention* (pp. 46–69). Oxford University Press.

Fazel, S., & Baillargeon, J. (2011). The health of prisoners. *The Lancet*, *377*(9769), 956–965. https://doi.org/10.1016/s0140-6736(10)61053-7

Felson, M. (2006). *Crime and nature.* Sage.

Felson, M. (2008). Routine activity approach. In R. Wortley & L. Mazerolle (Eds.), *Environmental criminology and crime analysis* (pp. 1–18). Willam Publishing.

Felson, M. (2014). *Lectio: El estudio científico del delito* [Lectio: The Scientific Study of Crime]. Ceremonial of the academic act of investiture as Doctor Honoris Causa of Professor Marcus Felson at the Miguel Hernández University. Universidad Miguel Hernández.

Fiscal de Sala Delegado de Vigilancia Penitenciaria. (2020, Abril). *Nota de Servicio 2/2020: Efectos de la paralización de los programas de trabajos en beneficio de la comunidad por razones de emergencia sanitaria* [Service Note 2/2020: Effects of the stoppage of community service programs for reasons of health emergency]. Fiscalía General del Estado.

Flanigan, T. P, Zaller, N., Taylor, L., Beckwith, C., Kuester, L., Rich, J., & Carpenter, C. C. J. (2009). HIV and infectious disease care in jails and prisons: Breaking down the walls with the help of academic medicine. *Transactions of the American Clinical and Climatological Association, 120*, 73–83.

Gonçalves, L., & Gonçalves, R. A. (2012). Agressividade, estilo de vida criminal e adaptação à prisão [Aggressiveness, criminal lifestyle and adaptation to prison]. *Psicologia USP, 23*(3), 559–584. https://doi.org/10.1590/S0103-65642012005000013

Gonçalves, R. A. (2007). Promover a mudança em personalidades anti-sociais e psicopatas: Punir, tratar e controlar [Promoting change in antisocial personalities and psychopaths: Punishing, treating and controlling]. *Análise Psicológica, 25*(4), 571–583. https://doi.org/10.14417/ap.466

Gonçalves, R. A., Valente, D., Andrade, J., & Castro-Rodrigues, A. (2019). How inmates and prison officers perceive prison: An exploratory study. In G. Mowll (Ed.), *A closer look at prisons and prison inmates* (pp. 1–36). Nova Science Publishers.

Hoff, G., Fedosejeva, R., & Mihailescy, L. (2009). Prison preparedness for pandemic flu and the ethical issues. *Public Health, 123*(6), 422–425. https://doi.org/10.1016/j.puhe.2009.04.003

Hu, L., Zhang, W., Jin, R., Liang, L., Xu, B., & Hu, Z. (2020). Risk factors associated with clinical outcomes in 323 COVID-19 hospitalized patients in Wuhan, China. *Clinical Infectious Diseases, 52* (7), 498–505. https://doi.org/10.1093/cid/ciaa539

IACHR. (2020). *IACHR calls on states to protect and preserve the work of human rights defenders during the COVID-19 pandemic.* Inter-American Commission on Human Rights. https://www.oas.org/en/iachr/

Liebrenz, M., Bhugra, D., Buadze, A., & Schleifer, R. (2020). Caring for persons in detention suffering with mental illness during the COVID-19 outbreak. *Forensic Science International: Mind and Law, 1*, Article 100013. https://doi.org/10.1016/j.fsiml.2020.100013

Lum, C., Maupin, C., & Stoltz, M. (2020). *The impact of COVID-19 on law enforcement agencies (wave 1).* International Association of Chiefs of police. https://www.theiacp.org/sites/default/files/IACP-GMUsurvey.Pdf

Ma, C., Rogers, J. H., & Zhou, S. (2020). *Global economic and financial effects of 21st century pandemics and epidemics.* SSRN.

Martín, A. M., Padrón, F., & Redondo, S. (2019). Early narratives of desistance from crime in different prison regimes. *The European Journal of Psychology Applied to Legal Context, 11*(2), 71–79. https://doi.org/10.5093/ejpalc2019a2

Maruschak, L., Sabol, W., Potter, R., Reid, L., & Cramer, E. (2009). Pandemic influenza and jail facilities and populations. *American Journal of Public Health, 99*(2), S339–S344. https://doi.org/10.2105%2FAJPH.2009.175174

MI. (2020a). *Balance de criminalidad de 2019* [Crime in Spain in 2019].

MI. (2020b). *Balance de criminalidad. Primer trimestre del año 2020* [Crime balance. First quarter of the year 2020].

Millan, P. (2020, June 18). Coronavirus España: Cifras, contagiados y última hora de la nueva normalidad, en directo [Coronavirus Spain: Figures, infected and last minute of the new normal, live]. *La Vanguardia* (Newspaper).

Miró, F. (2011). La oportunidad criminal en el ciberespacio. Aplicación y desarrollo de la teoría de las actividades cotidianas para la prevención del cibercrimen [The criminal opportunity in cyberspace. Application and development of the routine activities theory for the prevention of cybercrime]. *Revista Electrónica de Ciencia Penal y Criminología*, 13–07, 1–55. http://criminet.ugr.es/recpc

Moreira, J., & Martins, M. (2019). Estatísticas [Statistics]. *Sombras e Luzes, 2*, 181–230. https://dgrsp.justica.gov.pt/Revista-Sombras-e-Luzes

Moss, S. A., Lee, E., Berman, A., & Rung, D. (2018). When do people value rehabilitation and restorative justice over the punishment of offenders? *Victims & Offenders, 14*(1), 32–51. https://doi.org/10.1080/15564886.2018.1539688

Mossos d'Esquadra. (2020). *Informe sobre la delinqüència en Catalunya* [Report on Crime in Catalonia]. Departament d'Interior.

Ngo, F. T., & Paternoster, R. (2011). Cybercrime victimization: An examination of individual and situational level factors. *International Journal of Cyber Criminology, 5*(1), 773–793.

Penal Reform International. (2020). *Coronavirus: Healthcare and human rights of people in prison.* Briefing note. Penal Reform International. https://www.penalreform.org/resource/coronavirus-healthcare-and-human-rights-of-people-in/

Policía Nacional. (2020). *Informe sobre la delincuencia en España* [Report on crime in Spain]. Ministerio del Interior.

Portuguese Council of Ministers of March 12. (2020). *Medidas extraordinárias de resposta à epidemia do novo coronavirus* [Extraordinary measures to respond to the new coronavirus epidemic]. Goverment of Portugal. https://www.portugal.gov.pt/pt/gc22/governo/comunicado-de-conselho-de-ministros?i=330

Redondo, S. (2008). *Individuos, sociedades y oportunidades en la explicación y prevención del delito: Modelo del Triple Riesgo Delictivo (TRD)* [Individuals, societies and opportunities in the explanation and prevention of crime: Model of Triple Risk Factors for Crime (TRD)]. *Revista Española de Investigación Criminológica, Artículo 7, N. 6.* www.criminologia.net

Redondo, S. (2015). *El origen de los delitos: Introducción al estudio y explicación de la criminalidad* [The origin of crimes: Introduction to the study and explanation of crime]. Ed. Tirant lo Blanch.

Redondo, S. (2017). *Evaluación y tratamiento de delincuentes* [Assesment and treatment of offenders]. Ed. Pirámide.

Redondo, S., & Frerich, N. (2014). Crime and justice reinvestment in Europe: Possibilities and challenges. *Victims & Offenders, 9*(1), 13–49. https://doi.org/10.1080/15564886.2013.864525

Redondo, S., & Garrido, V. (2013). *Principios de Criminología (4ª ed.)* [Principles of criminology]. Tirant lo Blanch.

Reyns, B. W., Henson, B., & Fisher, B. S. (2014). Digital deviance: Low self-control and opportunity as explanations of sexting among college students. *Sociological Spectrum: Mid-South Sociological Association, 34*(3), 273–292. https://doi.org/10.1080/02732173.2014.895642

Sanchez, A., Simas, L., Diuana, V., & Larouze, B. (2020). COVID-19 in prisons: An impossible challenge for public health. *Cadernos de Saúde Pública, 36*(5), 1–5. https://doi.org/10.1590/0102-311x00083520

Sánchez, F. (2020, July 10). Portugal entra en la lista negra por el azote del virus [Portugal enters the blacklist due to the scourge of the virus]. *El País* (Newspaper).

Sappal, P. (2020, April 23). Portugal starts mass testing for Covid-19 to help lift lockdown restrictions quicker & attract tourists back. *Euroweekly.*

SMPRAV. (2020a). *Pla d'acció per a la transició del confinament pel COVID-19 als centres penitenciaris* [Action plan for the transition from COVID-19 confinement at the prison context]. Unpublished internal report. Secretaria de Mesures Penals, Reinserció i Atenció a la Víctima, Departament de Justícia.

SMPRAV. (2020b). *Protocol d'actuació als centres penitenciaris de Catalunya per a la gestió de la situació de crisi sanitària ocasionada pel COVID-19* [Protocol of action in the prison centers of Catalonia for the management of the situation of sanitary crisis caused by the COVID-19]. Unpublished internal report. Secretaria de Mesures Penals, Reinserció i Atenció a la Víctima, Departament de Justícia.

SMPRAV. (2020c). *Adaptació de la fase de represa als centres peniteciaris* [Adaptation of the resumption phase to prisons]. Unpublished internal report. Secretaria de Mesures Penals, Reinserció i Atenció a la Víctima, Departament de Justícia.

SMPRAV. (2020d). *Adaptació de la fase de represa als centres peniteciaris. Mesures provisionals per la represa progressiva de les comunicacions especials a partir del 21 de setembre* [Adaptation of the resumption phase to prisons. Provisional measures for the gradual resumption of special communications from 21 September]. Unpublished internal report. Secretaria de Mesures Penals, Reinserció i Atenció a la Víctima, Departament de Justícia.

Solar, P., & Lacal, P. (2020). Europa ante el Covid-19. Referencias específicas al Derecho penitenciario. *Revista Aranzadi Unión Europea, N. 7.*

Stickle, B., & Felson, M. (2020). Crime rates in a pandemic: The largest criminological experiment in history. *American Journal of Criminal Justice, 45*(4), 525–536. https://doi.org/10.1007/s12103-020-09546-0

Stoliker, B. E., & Galli, P. M. (2019). An examination of mental health and psychiatric care among older prisoners in the United States. *Victims & Offenders*, *14*(4), 480–509. https://doi.org/10.1080/15564886.2019.1608883

UNODC. (2020). *COVID-19 preparedness and responses in prison*. UNODC. https://www.unodc.org/documents/justice-and-prison-reform/UNODC_Position_paper_COVID-19_in_prisons.pdf

Wade, L. (2020, May). From Black Death to fatal flu, past pandemics show why people on the margins suffer most. *Science*, *368*(6492), 700–703. https://doi.org/10.1126/science.abc7832

Ward, T., & Fortune, C. A. (2016). The role of dynamic risk factors in the explanation of offending. *Aggression and Violent Behavior*, *29*(July–August), 79–88. https://doi.org/10.1016/j.avb.2016.06.007

WHO. (2020a). *Preparedness, prevention and control of COVID-19 in prisons and other places in detention*. (Interim guidance). WHO. http://www.euro.who.int/__data/assets/pdf_file/0019/434026/Preparedness-prevention-and-control-of-COVID-19-in-prisons.pdf?ua=1

WHO. (2020b). *WHO announces COVID-19 outbreak a pandemic*. WHO. https://www.euro.who.int/en/health-topics/health-emergencies/coronavirus-covid-19/news/news/2020/3/who-announces-covid-19-outbreak-a-pandemic

WHO. (2020c). *2019 novel coronavirus (2019-nCoV): Strategy preparedeness and response plane*. https://www.who.int/publications/i/item/strategic-preparedness-and-response-plan-for-the-new-coronavirus

WHO Director-General's Special Envoys on COVID-19 Preparedness and Response. (2020). WHO. https://www.who.int/emergencies/diseases/novel-coronavirus-2019/who-director-general-s-special-envoys-on-covid-19-preparedness-and-response

World Prison Brief. (2020). *World prison brief data: Portugal*. World Prison Brief. https://www.prisonstudies.org/country/portugal

Zafra, M., Blanco, P., & Sevillano, L. (2020July17). Casos confirmados de coronavirus en España y en el mundo [Confirmed cases of coronavirus in Spain and in the world]. *El País* (Newspaper).

Telematic Control and Semi-Freedom as a Response to the Pandemic: The Spanish Penitentiary System Experience

Esther Montero Perez de Tudela

ABSTRACT

In response to the pandemic that started in early 2020, prison systems around the world have adopted various strategies to prevent the spread of Covid-19 (coronavirus disease 2019). In Spain, the main strategy used by the State Penitentiary Administration against the pandemic has focused on the use of the "third degree" of prison or "semi-freedom" with telematic control (or electronic monitoring, as it is better known in the rest of the world). While in closed prisons the main measures to manage the pandemic have been focused on avoiding contact with outside, in open prisons inmates who could have introduced the virus into prison facilities due to their semi-freedom have been released and sent "home," in order to prevent the spread of the virus. The author analyzes the data provided by the Spanish prison statistics during the pandemic, illustrating the evolution of the numbers of convicts classified in "open regime" and under electronic monitoring. At the same time, the author highlights some of the ethical and public security implications that might be posed by the quasi-massive release supported by the expansion in the use of open regime with telematic control, and some recommendations thereon are proposed.

Introduction

As in other countries, in Spain the coronavirus disease 2019 (Covid-19) crisis has had an important impact on the penitentiary system. Leaving aside the measures adopted within the penal system's prisons to face the pandemic (suspension of prison leave, suspension of communication and visits, etc.), the most important effect of Covid-19 on the penitentiary system has been the reduction of the prison population, not only in absolute numbers, but also in the number of inmates serving their sentence inside the prison walls. This article will cover mainly the administration of Spain—the State Administration. The autonomous region of Catalonia enjoys extensive autonomy in the field of sentence execution, and therefore can deviate from state policy and practice in this respect. This article does not cover Catalonia.

According to the most recent data provided by the statistic of the Council of Europe (called Space I), from mid-March to mid-April, "the spread of the pandemic had a direct effect on imprisonment: the vast majority of prison administrations showed decreasing or stable prison population rates" (Aebi & Tiago, 2020, p. 1). According to this data, Spain is considered as one of the countries showing a stable evolution during the first month of the confinement.[1] Aebi and Tiago (2020) argued that there are three reasonable explanations that can explain the decrease (or stability) of the prison population in Europe: a drop in crime, a reduction of judicial activity in the penal system, and the release of inmates. Concerning the first explanation, and according to the situational-based criminological theories (Clarke & Felson, 1993; Wikström, 2014; Wikström & Treiber, 2016; Wortley & Tilley, 2014), it makes sense to think that the confinement or lockdown has had an impact on the criminal activities, reducing opportunities to commit a crime. On the one hand, the restrictions on leaving one's home and the closures of businesses affect crime rates, at least as far as traditional crimes are concerned. On the other hand, judges, prosecutors, and judiciary staff have been confined as the general population, and consequently fewer people has been involved in a penal process during this period, and fewer therefore sent to prison. Concerning the third explanation, the release of inmates, one should exercise some degree of caution. There are various types of "release" from prison around the world (e.g., conditional release, open regime or semi-freedom, home detention, liberty under telematic control [or electronic monitoring, as it is better known in the rest of the world], etc.; Van Kalmthout & Durnescu, 2008, see also Dünkel et al., 2018; Padfield et al., 2010), and some of these mechanisms do not reduce the total prison population number. A person placed in open regime or under telematic control continues serving the prison sentence initially imposed. In Spain, prison population data includes, in addition to the persons on pretrial detention or remand (i.e., persons being in prison awaiting trial), all sentenced persons serving their prison sentences, even if they are doing it outside prison walls. Therefore, convicts placed in open regime and under telematic control are still counted as part of the prison population.

In Spain, custodial sentence implementation is quite flexible. The judge establishes the formal sentence (the length of the sentence). Still, the manner in which it is implemented depends on several factors, mainly relating to the behavior of the convict. Thus, the sentenced person can progress to the open regime or third penitentiary degree (the semi-liberty regime, which will be explained subsequently) from the very beginning of the sentence, with a few exceptions.[2] Spain's open regime has several different modalities, each offering different levels of freedom. One involves electronic monitoring or telematic control (as it is called in Spanish legislation), resembling conditional release in other jurisdictions: the convict has a normal life, is living at home, and, among other possible measures, has to communicate regularly (call, visit, or meet) with the prison officer in charge of their case.

Covid-19 confinement was ordered on March 14[3] in Spain, and although during the first month the confinement did not have a significant impact on the prison population, one can observe a decline in the following months. In addition to this decline, an increase in the use of the open regime in its "remote control" modality has taken place, decreasing de facto the Spanish prison population. In order to better understand the evolution of the prison population in Spain and the most important effects of Covid-19, this article will be divided in four sections. The first section will be focused on a brief introduction of the Spanish penitentiary system, to provide the reader with a global overview of its functioning and with information that can be useful to understand the data presented subsequently. The second section will be focused on the evolution of Spanish prisons during the last months. The Spanish strategy against the pandemic will be covered in the third section. Finally, the fourth section will be dedicated to discussing some of the eventual ethical issues related to the expansion in the use of electronic monitoring, and some possible recommendations to monitor or supervise the eventual impacts of the Spanish penitentiary strategy in the face of the Covid-19 pandemic.

The Spanish penitentiary system in brief: The use of open regime and telematic control

The Spanish Penitentiary Administration is responsible for the execution of almost all sanctions and measures imposed by the Spanish penal justice system. Leaving aside the execution of some penal measures (mainly disqualifications)[4] that are under the supervision of the State Security Forces, custodial penalties and the community sanctions and measures are the domain of the Penitentiary system. Thus, the Spanish Penitentiary Administration involves the prison and probation systems in Spain (Montero Pérez de Tudela & García, 2016).

The Spanish penitentiary system is not in a strict sense a "progressive system." Aiming to achieve the full re-education and social reintegration of sentenced persons, the Spanish system is based on the "scientific individualization principle" (Aranda Ocaña, 2013; Cid & Andreu, 2017; Montero Pérez de Tudela, 2019, p. 230; Pastor & Torres, 2017, p. 127). This principle implies that an individual treatment program (oriented to the rehabilitation of the offender) is developed for each convict. In addition, the Spanish Penitentiary system is divided in three "degrees" or regimes (each degree corresponds to a regime). In the context of custodial sentences, depending on the content of the treatment program and the profile of the offender, the individual will be classified in one of the three penitentiary treatment degrees (Cid Moliné, 2002; Montero Pérez de Tudela & García, 2016, p. 4; Nistal Burón, 2016). The first degree is dedicated to the most dangerous offenders and is focused on security and restricted movement. Inmates classified in first degree are placed in the closed regime. The second degree constitutes the ordinary regime, and is open to the vast majority of prisoners. This last regime is characterized by more freedom of movement within the prison and the availability of many activities. The ordinary regime is applied to inmates classified in second degree, but also to those awaiting trial (in pretrial detention) or not yet classified. The third degree, or open regime, comprises a semi-free mode of life (see Cid Moliné, 2005). There are different modalities of third degree (see Figure 1), some of which fall within the concept of "probation," as understood in the rest of Europe and United States (i.e., a set of measures and sanctions—alternatives to imprisonment—involving the supervision of the offender in the community; Abadinsky, 2009; Labrecque, 2017; Taxman, 2012; Van Kalmthout & Durnescu, 2008).

Broadly, in order to classify a convict into one of the three penitentiary degrees, an assessment of the behavior and evolution of the sentenced person is made by a technical team, taking into account factors such as their personality, the seriousness of the offense, their criminal history, family and social circumstances, etc. In the Spanish penitentiary system, each convict has a technical team responsible for their case, composed of jurists (prison lawyers), psychologists, educators, and social workers. This team plans and monitors the execution of sentences, develops an individual treatment program for each convict,

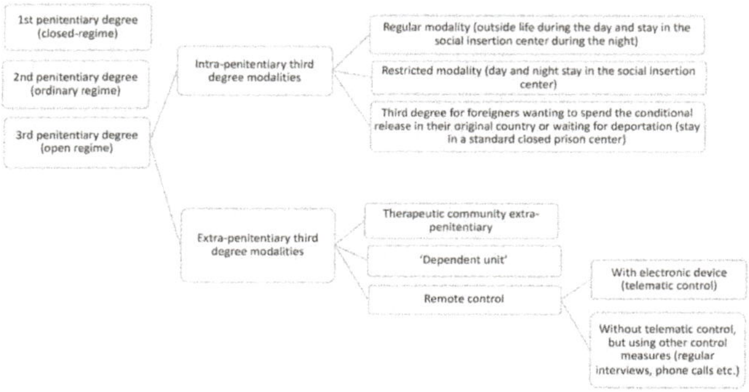

Figure 1. Spanish penitentiary modalities of third degree.

and presents its proposals to the prison's decision-making body (in both open or closed prisons), known as the treatment board. In all the prison facilities the treatment board revises the classification and the treatment program of each convict every six months.

A convict can be classified directly and initially to third degree—without having to transition through the lower grades—as long as the individual meets the necessary conditions. Briefly, to be classified to third degree (open regime) the convict has to meet the requirements both of being ready and of making good use of the semi-liberty.[5] Those classified in third degree are sent to the social insertion centers, a kind of "open prison" for people placed in the open regime. These establishments are usually placed near cities in order to allow their residents or those allocated to them to have a "normalized life." Inmates classified in the third degree, including those under electronic monitoring, those conditionally released, those sentenced to an alternative penalty or measure, and those whose sentence has been suspended under certain kinds of conditions that require follow-up, are assigned to a Social Insertion Center (Montero Pérez de Tudela & García, 2016, p. 5), always depending on the Spanish Penitentiary Administration.

In this context, two major groups of third-degree modalities can be discerned: extra-penitentiary and intrapenitentiary. It is the first group that has been promoted during the pandemic.

Depending on the aim pursued by the classification in open regime (e.g., to achieve the semi-liberty, to receive drug treatment, to take care of children or another relative, to undergo supervision with electronic monitoring, etc.), and depending on the personal conditions, the convict will either stay in Social Insertion Centers, or will enjoy an extra-penitentiary third-degree regime. Thus, normally, those inmates placed in open regime live in Social Insertion Centers, can go out during the day (e.g., to work, to find a job, to visit the doctor, etc.) and spend the night in the center. But there are other situations in which they can stay at another location—one which differs from a prison facility (Martí-Barrachina, 2019, p. 215):

-To provide care for relatives and children, because of illness, or for employment which requires particular time conditions, the convict can be placed under telematic control, known worldwide as electronic monitoring, and can live at home. In these cases, electronic control can be replaced for another type of appropriate remote-control measure (regular visits to the prison officer responsible for the case, phone calls, etc.)

-When a convict had (or still has) important drug problems, instead of being sent to a Social Insertion Center, the individual can be placed—directly from prison—in a therapeutic community extrapenitentiary (i.e., external to the prison facilities).

-In addition, a convict can also stay—although this is not a common scenario—in a "dependent unit." These units are residential facilities outside the prisons, managed through the collaboration of public or private entities, to facilitate the achievement of specific objectives of penitentiary treatment of inmates classified in third grade (e.g., to accommodate mothers with babies when the parent is serving a sentence but the child is too old to live inside the prison).[6]

These three modalities, which have in common that the sentenced person does not reside within the Social Insertion Center, together constitute the group of extrapenitentiary third-degree modality.

It can be also noted here that foreigners may have access to the third degree when they want to spend their conditional release in their country of origin, or when they are going to be deported, but these cases have not increased (rather the opposite) during the pandemic. In the same line, together with this modality, there is another category of third degree that has decreased drastically during the pandemic: restricted modality of third degree (Cid & Ibàñez, 2019), which involves the obligation for the convict to remain in the Social Insertion Center the whole day (with a few exceptions).[7] As will be argued subsequently, the cases classified in third degree in these last two modalities have decreased during the pandemic in favor of extrapenitentiary modalities, mainly in favor of open regime under telematic control.

Focusing on telematic control, it should be noted that the Spanish penitentiary system has several varieties of means available to control inmates from a distance. Specifically, a bracelet or anklet linked to a telephone detector and the personal locator via GPS are the most used measures for inmates classified in third degree and for prison leaves.[8] When electronic monitoring is used for those classified in third degree, convicts enjoy a regime of life practically akin to freedom. As understood throughout the rest of the world and explained by Nellis (2015), the long established and widely-used "term 'semi-liberty' captures quite well the kind of control that electronic monitoring imposes" (p. 16). Certainly, in Spain, although the open prison regime or third degree might be regarded as a semi-parole system (Cid & Ibàñez, 2019), and when used with electronic monitoring or other kind of remote control (and therefore without the obligation of being in a prison facility), it constitutes a regime of life in practical terms similar, if not equal, to the conditional release or parole regime (as known in United States). Of course, these electronic monitoring systems can provide restrictions on movement that may be considered appropriate, depending on each case, to support social integration and public safety (Secretaría General de Instituciones Penitenciarias, 2014, p. 24). Nevertheless, the same disposition allowing the use of telematic control also allows the use of "other measures" to monitor the convict remotely. The Spanish Prison Rules, dating from 1996, states that "in general, the minimum time of stay at the Center (social insertion center) will be eight hours a day, having to spend the night in the Establishment, except when, on a voluntary basis, the convict accepts the control of his presence outside the Center by means of adequate telematic devices, provided by the Penitentiary Administration, or other sufficient control mechanisms, in which case the convict will only have to stay in the Establishment during the time established in his (or her) treatment program to carry out treatment activities, interviews and face-to-face controls" (art. 86.4). Note that the remote control regulated in this modality of third degree can be implemented through electronic devices or not, requiring only "sufficient" control measures (e.g., regular interviews). This is an important point because this possibility allows to apply this remote control modality of open regime even when electronic devices are not available, which has been also used eventually to face the pandemic situation in the penitentiary facilities in a few cases, as will subsequently be seen.

In the Spanish State General Administration,[9] when telematic control is applied during the execution of the custody sentence—as an extrapenitentiary modality of third degree—is directly managed by the Penitentiary Administration. The electronic devices are provided by a private enterprise (Attenti Group)[10]; however the management of telematic control falls within the Penitentiary Administration's central services, in practice under the competence of the Telematic Control Area.[11] The central management of the available electronic devices and the centralized control of the users under telematic control is implemented by the Electronic Surveillance Operational Center (sp. COVE), located in the Social Insertion Center of Victoria Kent (in Madrid). In relation to the facility-based services, to monitor those users under telematic control in each province, social insertion centers generally have a telematic control unit, responsible for the supervision of convicts placed under electronic monitoring.

Evolution of the prison population before and during the pandemic

The Spanish penitentiary population has been decreasing during the last decade, being somewhat stable during the last three years (Secretaría General de Instituciones Penitenciarias, 2019, p. 21).

As illustrated previously in Figure 2, from mid-2016, the evolution of the Spanish prison population has had almost no variation.

Nevertheless, during the period of Covid-19 confinement the decrease of the prison population has been more pronounced. Focusing on the pandemic period, from the beginning of March to the end of June 2020, can be observed a decrease of, approximately, 3,000 persons in the Spanish prison population (Figure 3).

The State of Alert was decreed in Spain on March 14, 2020, establishing the period Covid-19 confinement one day later. The de-escalation started on May 4, with the State of

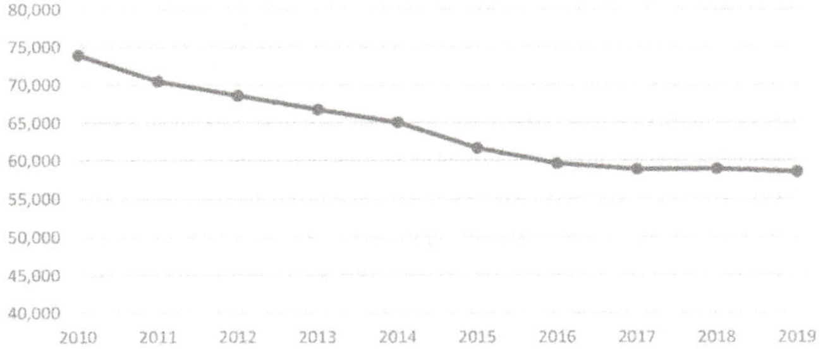

Figure 2. Evolution of the Spanish prison population from 2010 (data at December 31 each year). Source: based on the data provided by General Secretariat of Penitentiary Institutions.

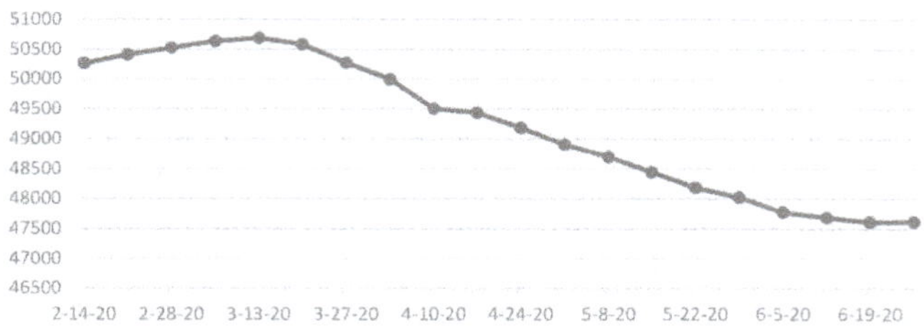

Figure 3. Evolution of the Spanish prison population during the State of Alert. Source: based on the data provided by General Secretariat of Penitentiary Institutions.

Alert ending completely on June 21, 2020. The evolution of the Spanish penitentiary population thus shows a clear decreasing trend during the whole State of Alert.

If these figures are compared with those from last year, the variation results in an important decrease. At the end of June 2019[12] the prison population was 59,398, compared with the same date in 2020,[13] at which it was approximately 47,600 (a variation of −19.83%). Focusing on the pandemic period, in March 2020,[14] at the beginning of State of Alert, the prison population in Spain was 50,635, so the resulting percentage variation was finally, approximately, −6%.

That means that Spain, in relation to the impact of Covid-19 on the penitentiary systems in the European context, the prison population can be considered as "decreasing," rather than "stable." In fact, in June 2020 the Spanish prison population figures dropped to an all-time low.

There is one main cause of this decrease in absolute figures: a fall in admissions to prison during this period. People from outside the penitentiary system, especially those who are not familiar with the accounting treatment of the prison data, may conclude that the diminution of the prison population in Spain is due to the expansion in the use of the open regime. It is a fact that (as will be seen in the next section) thousands of inmates have been sent "home" in third degree under remote control, but as explained in the first section of this article, all these convicts placed in third degree (even in an extrapenitentiary modality) are included in the total prison population figures in Spain.

According to the data provided by the General Secretariat of Penitentiary Institution, between March 14 and June 18, 2020, there were 3,847 new admissions into prison facilities, compared with 7,273 releases from penitentiary centers. Certainly, before the Covid-19 confinement, approximately 2,000 new persons per month were placed in the penitentiary institutions regularly. In April 2020, this figure was 806,[15] which was also the figure for May.

Differentiation should therefore be made between two distinctive aspects. The promotion of the open regime and the expansion in the use of the telematic or remote control is the strategy adopted by the Spanish Prison Administration to face the pandemic, in order to stop the spread of the Covid-19 virus. This involves an active role by the administration. But the main cause explaining the reduction of the prison population in absolute figures is the sharp reduction of the prison admissions since March 2020, principally due to the slow-down of judicial activity in the penal system (and the eventually diminution of the traditional criminality), as natural consequence of the confinement.

The Spanish strategy against the pandemic: Open regime and telematic control as a remedy to prevent the spread of Covid-19

As explained previously, in order to avoid the spread of the Covid-19 virus, the Spanish prison administration has opted for relocating inmates outside prison establishments. By doing so, the administration avoided direct contact between convicts and prison officers, as well as between convicts themselves. The decision has been to downsize the number of prisoners held in the Social Insertion Centers dedicated to the open regime (and semi-liberty modalities), and to place as many prisoners as possible under telematic control.

While in closed prisons (for inmates in second and first degree or those not classified)[16] the main measures have been focused on avoiding contact with outside (cutting communication and visits, suspending prison leave etc.), in open prisons (for those placed in third degree with daily contact with outside) the strategy has been focused on the promotion of the extrapenitentiary modalities of third degree, mainly the release of convicts under telematic control.

As explained previously, in the context of the Spanish State General Administration, the management of the telematic control falls within the competence of the Prison Administration (public administration), but the electronic devices are provided by a private enterprises. On average, approximately 6,000 electronic devices are available to be installed to users of the Spanish prison system.

According to the data described previously, once the State of Alert Decree was issued (on March 14), the increase in the use of the extrapenitentiary modalities of third degree did not stop until the first week of May, at which point the de-escalation started, having reached record highs (see Figure 4).

Looking closely, it can be observed that most third-degree cases during the pandemic were under the modality of telematic control. Certainly, about 200–250 cases on average (per month) were placed in an external therapeutic community (for drug addicts) or a "dependent unit" (as explained previously). Almost 96% of the 5,915 convicts classified in extrapenitentiary modalities of third degree at the beginning of May 2020 were under "remote control." Most of these inmates were carrying an electronic device (Figure 5).

On the other hand, the number of prisoners placed in various open regime modalities, which oblige convicts to remain permanently within the social insertion center or other prison facility have decreased during the pandemic period. In practice, two modalities are included in this category: third degree for foreigners awaiting expulsion or deportation, and

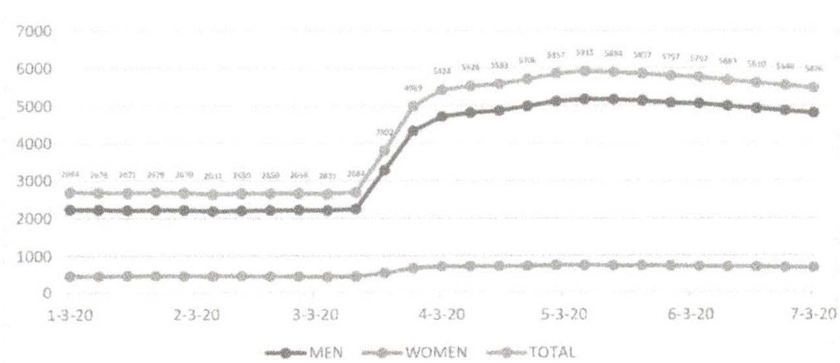

Figure 4. Evolution of the extrapenitentiary modalities of third degree during the pandemic. Source: based on the data provided by General Secretariat of Penitentiary Institutions.

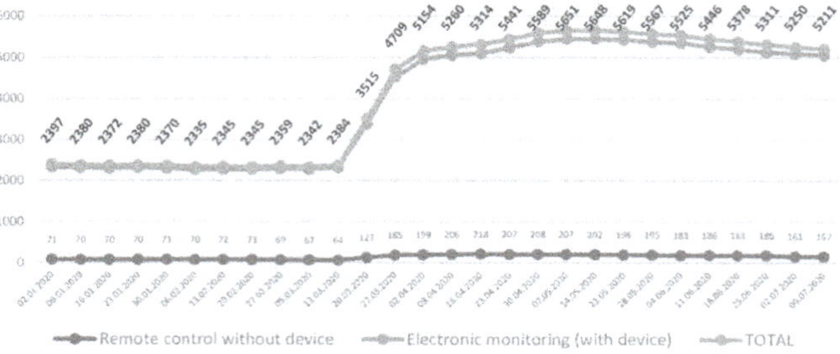

Figure 5. Evolution of the remote-control modality of third degree during the pandemic. Source: based on the data provided by General Secretariat of Penitentiary Institutions.

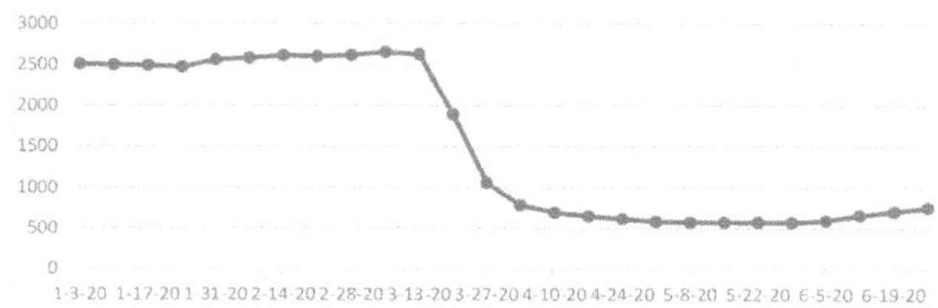

Figure 6. Evolution of the restricted modalities of third degree during the pandemic. Source: based on the data provided by General Secretariat of Penitentiary Institutions.

third degree restricted modality (explained in the first section of this article). These restricted modalities of third degree have decreased during the pandemic period (Figure 6).

The evolution of the total number of people placed in closed and ordinary regimes also follows a similar decreasing trend during the period of the pandemic. Looking at the number of convicts placed in ordinary and closed regimes, and also taking into account people sentenced who are placed in an intrapenitentiary modality of third degree and therefore have the obligation of staying in a social insertion center (physically occupying a cell), it can be observed how the number of persons actually placed "behind bars" has reduced (Figure 7).

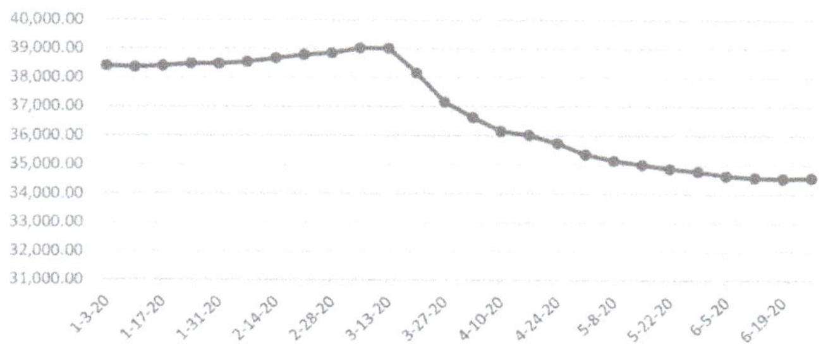

Figure 7. Evolution of the number of inmates in ordinary and closed regime, and in an intrapenitentiary modality of open regime. Source: based on the data provided by General Secretariat of Penitentiary Institutions.

So, the real number of prisoners physically serving their sentence in prison has gone down during the pandemic period. This promotion of the extrapenitentiary modalities of open regime or third degree, together with the reduction of the number of admissions in the Spanish prisons (more than 1,000 cases less per months) has made the prison population in Spain more manageable in real terms.

Evidently, in a situation of alert, the treatment perspective behind the promotion of the open regime and semi-liberty modalities of third degree has been sacrificed in the favor of a sanitary one. To face the pandemic, the Spanish Penitentiary Institution has encouraged and promoted measures allowing the enforcement of the sentence outside the penitentiary establishments, by promoting the expansion in the use of alternative measures to imprisonment. The reason behind this decision was clear: to avoid the interaction of convicts who were enjoying regular contact with society. Therefore, more than 3,000 convicts have been placed in third degree under telematic control during the pandemic period.

Leaving aside the debate about the readiness of de facto released people to enjoy freedom, one can observe that the strategy implemented by the Spanish prison administration has been quite effective. The impact of the pandemic in the penitentiary centers of the General Secretariat of Penitentiary Institutions (eg excluding the Catalonia penitentiary centers),[17] has been four times less significant in prisons—in terms of the number of infections—than in the rest of Spanish society. The mortality rate and the hospitalization rate have been 10 times less and 7 times less in prisons than outside, respectively. Only two inmates have died due to Covid-19 (out of more than 50,000 prisoners held in penitentiary facilities in March 2020). In relation to the officers, this figure rises to four deceased staff out of about 24.000 penitentiary professionals working in the prison system. For the reasons described previously and observing outcomes it can be concluded that the Spanish strategy to stop the spread of Covid-19 virus was effective.

Discussion and recommendations. Complex and ethical issues

Starting from the idea that the decisions taken by the Penitentiary Administration during the pandemic have proved to be appropriate and effective, it cannot be forgotten that more than 3,000 persons, who were not under telematic control at the beginning of the pandemic, have been "sent home" during the confinement. This quasi-massive release can raise some ethical questions (see Bülow, 2014). One can ask: Were all this people ready to be reincorporated into society?

As seen previously, an individual assessment of each convict is made when the penitentiary classification or revision of the classification is implemented, and several factors (e.g., personality, criminal history, family and social circumstances, treatment progress, etc.) are assessed. Thus, it can be argued that if all the people—later placed under telematic control—that had not been classified in an extrapenitentiary modality of open regime before the confinement, it is because they did not meet the conditions. Therefore, it can be argued that all the resolutions relating to the modality of third degree under electronic monitoring have been taken mainly because of the pandemic. This fact may be reprehensible from a treatment point of view.

Certainly, if the State of Alert had not been decreed, the majority of the people placed under electronic monitoring during March and April 2020 would have remained in a prison facility (mainly in a social insertion center), so it can be claimed that all these administrative resolutions have been "instrumental" and not justified on the behavioral evolution and the treatment progress of these convicts. This fact can pose some questions about the public safety, and some research should be implemented during the next months to follow and monitor the recidivism rates. When a convict is released too late and is not included in a transitional program (dealing with criminogenic needs and improving the convict's social bonds) the risk of recidivism is higher (Dünkel et al., 2010; Petersilia, 2003). Early release followed by constructive supervision is one of the factors that can reduce reoffending (Capdevila, 2015; Luque et al., 2004). But applying early release when the person is not yet ready, the treatment program is not completed or the social conditions are still not adequate, can have arguably a detrimental effect on recidivism. Because more than 3,000 cases placed under electronic monitoring were assessed with great haste and based on health-related criteria, it would be recommended that they are revised once the pandemic over.

In addition, even if today there is no doubt about how cost- and socially effective the use of electronic monitoring is (Bagaric et al., 2018; Padgett et al., 2006; Whitfield, 1997; Yeh, 2015), and that new electronic monitoring technologies open up new monitoring and surveillance possibilities (Graham & McIvor, 2017), authors have warned of the risk that excessive focus on control might omit the treatment perspective (Nellis, 2015).[18] As suggested in the recommendations of the Council of Europe (2014, p. 4), electronic monitoring "should be combined with other professional interventions and supportive measures aimed at the social reintegration of offenders." Certainly, electronic monitoring is not rehabilitative itself, and needs to be accompanied by a treatment program (Nellis, 2015, p. 16). There is an international evidence-based consensus on the need to use electronic monitoring in tandem with supervision and support, in order to maximize the opportunities of rehabilitation and desistance for the offender (Belur et al., 2017; Graham & McIvor, 2015; Nellis et al., 2013). "Without complementary supervision and support, the impact of Electronic Monitoring may be limited to its duration, with only modest short-term benefits when monitoring ends" (Graham & McIvor, 2017, p. 10). The manner in which the classifications in third-degree with telematic control has been produced during the pandemic (with urgency and conditional on health requirements), might give the impression that the rehabilitative perspective is presumably missing in these decisions, or is at least partially absent. Thus, when possible, a reassessment of the cases under telematic control from a rehabilitative perspective could be recommended, in order to properly develop treatment interventions.

In line with this rehabilitative perspective, the question of using remote surveillance to replace human contact has recently been reported by other authors (McNeill, 2017; Nellis, 2015, 2014; see also Pattavina & Corbett, 2019), but in the present case, the expansion in the use of electronic monitoring has been promoted precisely to avoid human contact during the pandemic period, in order to prevent the spread of Covid-19. Thus, no criticisms can be made in this respect regarding confinement time. It can only be hoped that once the pandemic has finished, the use of electronic monitoring focused on control and supervision—unrelated to the human contact—is not here to stay. As explained by Nellis (2015), "the potential of Electronic Monitoring to make a positive difference to penal practice in Europe is clear, but equally its misuse could impose dangers for traditional, but still desirable, forms of probation supervision" (p. 54).

In this respect, and precisely contrary to the first question posed at the beginning of this section, the segment could be concluded wondering if all those convicts placed under telematic control really needed to wear an electronic device. Certainly, one of the risks highlighted by authors is the excessive use of this new technologies just because they are accessible and available. Electronic monitoring can be very intrusive, and to track a person continuously may be unnecessary, invasive, and disproportionate in many cases, even potentially infringing human rights (Black & Smith, 2003; Fitzalan Howard, 2020, p. 18; Nellis, 2019, 1991). Electronic monitoring is not proportionate (or disproportionate) in itself, but rather depends on the circumstances of the convict. In practice, the type of technology used and the duration of the supervision should be proportionate to the seriousness of the offense and the level of risk presented by the offender (Nellis, 2015; 18 et seq; Graham & McIvor, 2015, p. 96). Thus, some questions about compliance with the proportionality principle can be raised in the context of the expansion in the use of the electronic monitoring during the Covid-19 pandemic. It may be that if all those convicts placed under electronic monitoring semi-freedom were to have been granted an extrapenitentiary modality of third-degree following the "standard procedure" (without acceleration and without the influence of priorities other than rehabilitation goals), they may have been placed in a modality of remote control without the obligation to wear an electronic device (e.g., just subject to regular monitoring visits or regular phone calls).

Thus, in line with the previous recommendations, this perspective should also be considered when a revision of the cases placed under telematic control during—and because of—the Covid-19 confinement takes place.

Conclusions

In conclusion, the strategy of Spanish Penitentiary Administration against the spread of Covid-19 was based on the reduction of the number of prisoners which are effectively serving time behind bars. Although they are still included in the total number of prisoners, more than 3,000 of them were serving their prison sentence outside penitentiary establishments—on telematic control. The decrease of the number of prisoners was also supported by the reduction of new admissions, due to the limited activity of judiciary during the State of Alert.

As both the number of those infected with Covid-19 and the number of related deaths among prisoners and staff were quite low compared with the general population, one can argue that the Spanish strategy against the spread of Covid-19 was effective. Of course, this impressive outcome had as additional contributory factors all the internal measures that ensured less contact between inmates, between inmates and staff, fewer interactions between inmates and the outside world, and so on.

On the one hand, from a criminological point of view, several more months must pass before any assessment of the potential impact of all these releases -even under telematic control- on the crime rate and public safety. It is still too early to evaluate whether or not the Spanish strategy of dealing with the pandemic as it affected the penitentiary system has had any effect in terms of recidivism (understood as the commission of a new crime). Future criminological research will reveal whether or not there has been collateral damage related to the expansion in the use of semi-liberty modalities of the prison regime, specifically the expansion of electronic monitoring, during the Covid-19 pandemic. Shall we find an increase in the crime rate the next months? Shall we find a diminution due to the benefits related to the use of alternative to detention measures? It may be that no repercussions will be revealed.

On the other hand, the assessment and revision of electronic monitoring cases applied during the upcoming months will show how many cases actually required, or did not require, being under technological supervision.

In any event, one positive effect of this Covid-19 pandemic can be pointed out: the Spanish prison population has reached an historical low. And this is without counting the "de facto" reduction of the Spanish penitentiary population through the increase of sentenced persons undergoing electronic monitoring. However, this decrease in the prison population should be assessed in dialog with the transformations that take place in the community supervision field. More research should be conducted in studying to what extent this decrease fuels the so-called mass-supervision phenomenon.

Nevertheless, in absolute figures, the reduction of the Spanish prison population may be considered as moderate, and the strategy based on the use of the extramodalities of third degree under electronic monitoring as adequate, pending the results of the future researches and the next swings of the pandemic, as the sanitary alert is still in force according to the World Health Organization.

Notes

1. The countries that showed a variation between −4 and +4% in relation to the prison population during the pandemic have been considered as "stable" prison administration.
2. Mainly one: in case of serious offenses, when the length of the sentence is longer than five years the judge can order that the classification in third degree (i.e., the placement of the convict in open regime) does not take place until half of the sentence has been served inside.
3. State of Alarm accorded by Royal Decree 463/2020, published on the Official State Gazette, Madrid, Spain, on March 14, 2020.
4. The control of some noncustodial sentences, such as the "prohibition to reside in a particular place or come to it" are the responsibility of the State Security Forces, as is the implementation of one of the deprivation of freedom penalties known as "permanent location." This penalty was introduced into the Spanish Penal Code in 2003 and corresponds to what is usually known as "home detention," one of the most used alternatives to incarceration.
5. Normally, to evaluate the capacity of the sentenced person to live in the open regime, the conditions taken into account are the length of the sentence, the time served in prison (although there is no specified minimum period of time), the sentenced person's penitentiary evolution and behavior, their level of participation in activities, their involvement in treatment programs, their use of leave (in cases where the person enjoyed any periods of leave from prison), etc. The assessment is individualized and flexible. As explained, only in cases of serious offenses for which the sentence is longer than five years of prison, will the convict have to complete at least the half of the sentence before being classified as third degree.
6. Spanish penitentiary law also provides mothers with the right to keep their children with them in prison until the children reach the age of three (see Cerezo, 2016).
7. Normally this modality of "restricted open regime" with less time outside of the prison, is applied because of the risk of recidivism or the lack of outside work. These prisoners are allocated in semi-open facilities but cannot go out ordinarily.
8. Also, some alcohol intake analyzers with a face viewer (even personal identification voice detectors) are available, but are residually used; according to the data provided by the General

Secretariat of Penitentiary Institutions in 2019 there are registered approximately 10 cases of the use of alcohol intake analyzers with a face viewer.

9. Which does not include Catalonia. The autonomous region of Catalonia enjoys implementing powers on prison management. Catalonia is the only Spanish autonomous region that has assumed penitentiary competences. Relating to prisons and probation services, the rest of the autonomous regions are under the competence of the State General Administration, whose data and information are explained in this article.
10. Information available on: https://www.attentigroup.com/intl/.
11. Which belongs to the General Deputy Direction of Open Regime and Alternative Sanction and Measures, of the General Secretariat of Penitentiary Institutions. Information available on: https://www.institucionpenitenciaria.es/es/web/home/el-medio-abierto/control-telematico.
12. Data provided at June 30, 2019.
13. Data provided at June 26, 2020.
14. Data provided at March 6, 2020.
15. Data provided directly by the General Secretariat of Penitentiary Institutions.
16. An inmate can be without classification because the individual is waiting to be classified, that is, to be evaluated by the technical team, or because the individual is in pretrial detention (awaiting trial).
17. As explained previously, the autonomous region of Catalonia enjoys prison management implementation powers. While the basic legislation (the Spanish prison rules) is common for the whole country, implementation powers have been delegated to Catalonia. Therefore this region can deviate from state policy and practice, and has its own penitentiary instructions.
18. I should note that some authors warned that there is a real possibility that without proper controls in place, the expansion of alternative sanctions using electronic monitoring could even increase prison populations because of technical violations that can provoke the return to prison of users under electronic supervision (see Byrne, 2016).

Disclosure statement

No potential conflict of interest was reported by the author(s).

ORCID

Esther Montero Perez de Tudela http://orcid.org/0000-0001-9068-2284

References

Abadinsky, H. (2009). *Probation and parole: Theory and practice* (10th ed.). Pearson Prentice Hall.

Aebi, M., & Tiago, M. M. (2020). *Prisons and prisoners in Europe in pandemic times: An evaluation of the short-term impact of the COVID-19 on prison populations*. Special SPACE I report. Council of Europe statistics. Retrieved July 19, 2020, from http://wp.unil.ch/space/files/2020/06/Prisons-and-the-COVID-19_200617_FINAL.pdf

Aranda Ocaña, M. (2013). *Prison conditions in Spain*. Antigone Edizioni. Retrieved July 19, 2020, from http://www.ub.edu/ospdh/sites/default/files/documents/PrisonconditionsinSpain.pdf

Bagaric, M., Hunter, D., & Wolf, G. (2018). Technological incarceration and the end of the prison crisis. *Journal of Criminal Law and Criminology*, *108*(1), 73–135. Retrieved July 19, 2020, from https://scholarlycommons.law.northwestern.edu/jclc/vol108/iss1/2

Belur, J., Thornton, A., Tompson, L., Manning, M., Sidebottom, A., & Bowers, K. (2017). *A systematic review of the effectiveness of electronic monitoring of offenders*. College of Policing.

Black, M., & Smith, R. G. (2003). Electronic monitoring in the criminal justice system. *Trends and Issues in Crime and Criminal Justice*, *254*, 1–6. Retrieved July 19, 2020, from https://apo.org.au/sites/default/files/resource-files/2003-07/apo-nid7949.pdf

Bülow, W. (2014). Electronic monitoring of offenders: An ethical review. *Science and Engineering Ethics*, *20*(2), 505–518. https://doi.org/10.1007/s11948-013-9462-3

Byrne, J. (2016). Smart sentencing revisited: Assessing the policy/practice implications of research on electronic monitoring and other intermediate sanctions (chapter 18). In T. G. Blomberg, J. M. Brancale, K. Beaver, & W. Bales (Eds.), *Advancing criminology and criminal justice policy* (pp. 249–264). Routledge.

Capdevila, M., (Coord.) (2015). *Tasa de reincidencia penitenciaria 2014* (*Reincarceration Rate 2014*). Centro de Estudios Jurídicos y Formación Especializada. Retrieved July 19, 2019, from http://cejfe.gencat.cat/web/.content/home/recerca/cataleg/crono/2015/taxa_reincidencia_2014/tasa_reincidencia_2014_cast.pdf

Cerezo, A. I. (2016). Women in prison in Spain: The implementation of bangkok rules to the Spanish prison legislation. *European Journal on Criminal Policy and Research*, *23*(2), 133–151. https://doi.org/10.1007/s10610-016-9323-0

Cid, J., & Andreu, A. (2017). European prison policy and Spanish prison practice: Confluences and gaps. In T. Daems & L. Robert (Eds.), *Europe in prisons* (pp. 255–289). Macmillan.

Cid, J., & Ibàñez, A. (2019). Prisoner resettlement in Spain—Good practices for early-released prisoners and prisoners lost in transition that fully serve their sentence. In F. Dünkel, I. Pruin, A. Storgaard, & J. Weber (Eds.), *Prisoner resettlement in Europe*. Routledge Frontiers of Criminal Justice.

Cid Moliné, J. (2002). El sistema penitenciario en España. *Jueces para la democracia*, *45*, 15–27. Retrieved July 7, 2020 http://www.juecesdemocracia.es/revista/jpd_num_45.pdf

Cid Moliné, J. (2005). The penitentiary system in Spain: The use of imprisonment, living conditions and rehabilitation. *Punishment & Society*, *7*(2), 147–166. https://doi.org/10.1177/1462474505050439

Clarke, R. V., & Felson, M. (1993). Introduction: Criminology, routine activity, and rational choice. In R. V. Clarke & M. Felson (Eds.), *Routine activity and rational choice. Advances in criminological theory* (Vol. 5; pp. 1–14). Transaction Publishers.

Council of Europe. (2014) *Recommendation CM/Rec(2014)4 of the committee of Ministers to member States on electronic monitoring*. Adopted by the Committee of Ministers on 19 February 2014. Council of Europe. Retrieved June 19, 2020, from https://pjp-eu.coe.int/documents/41781569/42171329/CMRec+%282014%29+4+on+electronic+monitoring.pdf/c9756d5b-be0e-4c72-b085-745c9199bef4

Dünkel, F., Pruin, I., Storgaard, A., & Weber, J. (Eds). (2018). *Prisoner resettlement in Europe (Routledge frontiers of criminal justice)*. Routledge. https://doi.10.4324/9781315194592

Dünkel, F., van Zyl Smit, D., & Padfield, N. (2010). Concluding thoughts. In N. Padfield, D. van Zyl Smit, & F. Dünkel (Eds.), *Release from prison. European policy and practice* (pp. 395–444). Willan.

Fitzalan Howard, F. (2020). The experience of electronic monitoring and the implications for effective use. *The Howard Journal of Crime and Justice*, *59*(1), 17–43. https://doi.org/10.1111/hojo.12351

Graham, H., & McIvor, G. (2015). *Scottish and international review of the uses of electronic monitoring*. Scottish Centre for Crime and Justice Research (SCCJR). Retrieved July 17, 2020, from https://www.sccjr.ac.uk/wp-content/uploads/2015/08/Scottish-and-International-Review-of-the-Uses-of-Electronic-Monitoring-Graham-and-McIvor-2015.pdf

Graham, H., & McIvor, G. (2017). *Electronic monitoring in the criminal justice system. Institute for research and innovation in social services. Insights, 40*. IRISS. Retrieved July 19, 2020, from https://dspace.stir.ac.uk/bitstream/1893/26188/1/insights-40_0.pdf

Labrecque, R. (2017). Probation in the United States: A historical and modern perspective. In O. Hayden Griffin & V. Woodward (Eds..), *Handbook of corrections in the United States*. Routledge. Retrieved July 19, 2020, from https://pdxscholar.library.pdx.edu/cgi/viewcontent.cgi?article=1029&context=ccj_fac

Luque, E., Ferrer, M., & Capdevila, M. (2004). *La reincidencia penitenciaria en Cataluña (Reincarceration in Catalonia)*. Centro de Estudios Jurídicos y Formación Especializada. Retrieved July 19, 2020, from http://cejfe.gencat.cat/web/.content/home/recerca/cataleg/crono/2004/reincidenciaPenitenciaria_CA.pdf

Martí-Barrachina, M. (2019). Prisoners in the community: The open prison model in Catalonia. *Nordisk Tidsskrift for Kriminalvidenskab, 2019*(2), 211–231. Retrieved July 19, 2020, from https://www.researchgate.net/publication/336281552_Prisoners_in_the_community_the_open_prison_model_in_Catalonia/citations#fullTextFileContent

McNeill, F. (2017). Post-script: Guide, guard and glue—Electronic monitoring and penal supervision. *European Journal of Probation*, *9*(1), 103–107. https://doi.org/10.1177/2066220317700544

Montero Pérez de Tudela, E. (2019). La reeducación y la reinserción social en prisión: El tratamiento en el medio penitenciario español. *Revista de estudios socioeducativos (RESED)*, *7*, 227–249. https://doi.org/10.25267/Rev_estud_socioeducativos.2019.i7.16

Montero Pérez de Tudela, E., & García, ca. 2016. Probation in Spain. In A. M. Van Kalmthout & I. Durnescu (Eds.), *Probation in Europe (updated)* (pp. 1–62). Confederation of European Probation. Retrieved July 9, 2019, from https://www.cep-probation.org/wp-content/uploads/2018/10/probation-in-europeChapter-Spain-final.pdf

Nellis, M. (1991). The electronic monitoring of offenders in England and wales: Recent developments and future prospects. *The British Journal of Criminology*, *31*(2), 165–185. https://doi.org/10.1093/oxfordjournals.bjc.a048096

Nellis, M. (2014). Upgrading electronic monitoring, downgrading probation: Reconfiguring 'offender management' in England and Wales. *European Journal of Probation*, *6*(2), 169–191. https://doi.org/10.1177/2066220314540572

Nellis, M. (2015). *Standards and ethics in electronic monitoring*. Council of Europe. Retrieved June 29, 2019, from https://rm.coe.int/handbook-standards-ethics-in-electronic-monitoring-eng/16806ab9b0

Nellis, M. (2019). Clean and dirty electronic monitoring. Justice Trends Magazine, 3. Retrieved July 19, 2020, from https://justice-trends.press/shaping-lives-the-use-of-electronic-monitoring/

Nellis, M., Beyens, K., & Kampinski, D. (2013). Introduction: Making sense of electronic monitoring. In B. K. Nellis & D. Kampinski (Eds.), *Electronically monitored punishment: International and critical perspectives* (pp. 1–18). Routledge.

Nistal Burón, J. (2016). El sistema penitenciario español "de un vistazo." Editorial Criminología y Justicia.

Padfield, N., Zyl Smit, D., & Dünkel, F., Eds. (2010). *Release from prison: European policy and practice*. Willan.

Padgett, K. G., Bales, W. D., & Blomberg, T. G. (2006). Under surveillance: An empirical test of the effectiveness and consequences of electronic monitoring. *Criminology & Public Policy*, *5*(1), 61–91. https://doi.org/10.1111/j.1745-9133.2006.00102.x

Pastor, E., & Torres, M. (2017). El sistema penitenciario y las personas privadas de libertad en España desde una perspectiva internacional. *Política Criminal, 12, 23*(5), 124–150. Retrieved July 19, 2020, from http://www.politicacriminal.cl/Vol_12/n_23/Vol12N23A5.pdf

Pattavina, A., & Corbett, R. P. (2019). How smartphone technology can link the theoretical, policy, and practical contexts of community supervision reform: Voices from the field. *Victims & Offenders*, *14*(7), 777–792. https://doi.org/10.1080/15564886.2019.1659894

Petersilia, J. (2003). *When prisoners come home. Parole and prisoner reentry*. Oxford University Press.

Secretaría General de Instituciones Penitenciarias. (2014). *The Spanish prison system*. Ministerio del Interior - Secretaría General Técnica. Retrieved July 19, 2020, from https://www.institucionpenitenciaria.es/documents/20126/72836/SIS._PENITENCIARIO_2014_ING_acc_2.pdf/1c51adf8-d3e7-cab8-4bea-eabdf18adf7e

Secretaría General de Instituciones Penitenciarias. (2019). *Informe general de 2018*. Ministerio del Interior. Retrieved July 19, 2020, from https://www.institucionpenitenciaria.es/documents/20126/72836/Informe_General_2018_acc.pdf

Taxman, F. S. (2012). Probation, intermediate sanctions, and community-based corrections. In J. Petersilia & K. R. Reitz (Eds.), *The Oxford handbook of sentencing and corrections* (pp. 363–385). Oxford University Press.

Van Kalmthout, A. M., & Durnescu, I. (Eds.). (2008). *Probation in Europe*. Wolf Legal Publishers (WLP).

Whitfield, D. (1997). *Tackling the tag: The electronic monitoring of offenders*. Waterside Press.

Wikström, P.-O. H. (2014). Why crime happens: A situational action theory. In G. Manzo (Ed.), *Analytical sociology: Actions and networks* (pp. 74–94). Wiley.

Wikström, P.-O. H., & Treiber, K. (2016). Situational theory: The importance of interactions and action mechanisms in the explanation of crime. In A. R. Piquero (Ed.), *The handbook of criminological theory* (pp. 415–444). John Wiley.

Wortley, R., & Tilley, N. (2014). Theories for situational and environmental crime prevention. In G. Bruinsma & D. Weisburd (Eds.), *Encyclopedia of criminology and criminal justice*. Springer. https://link.springer.com/referencework/10.1007/978-1-4614-5690-2

Yeh, S. S. (2015). The electronic monitoring paradigm: A proposal for transforming criminal justice in the USA. *Laws*, *4*(1), 60–81. https://doi.org/10.3390/laws4010060

Sweden's Response to the COVID-19 Outbreak

Maria Lindström, Emma Ahlstrand, and Jenny Kärrholm

ABSTRACT

The Swedish Prison and Probation Service (SPPS) formed a national crisis management team on March 12, 2020, in response to the global Covid-19 pandemic. The team, consisting of experts from multiple departments within the SPPS, coordinated efforts within the government agency to support the jails, prisons, probation offices, and national transportation service in managing the pandemic while upholding operational security and the safety of staff and inmates. The SPPS handled the Covid-19 outbreak by taking measures to minimize the risk of contagion spread, consistent with the recommendations of the Public Health Agency in Sweden. These recommendations differ from those introduced in many other countries. For example, Sweden chose to avoid a general lockdown. The SPPS's measures to minimize contagion spread included: canceling all visitation at-and furlough from-jails and prisons, placing inmates with suspected and confirmed Covid-19 infections in isolation, creating digital solutions to minimize travel and in-person meetings, as well as providing protective gear to manage infected inmates and inmates within a risk group. To date, the SPPS has had 143 confirmed inmate cases of Covid-19 and no deaths due to the virus.

Sweden and the Covid-19 pandemic

With the spread of Covid-19 in Sweden, all government agencies prepared for major changes in day-to-day operations. The Public Health Agency in Sweden maintains authority over recommendations and restrictions placed on citizens during a pandemic and chose an approach to minimizing contagion spread that differs from most other countries. Instead of enforcing strict general lockdowns or quarantines, the Public Health Agency in Sweden provided all Swedish citizens with recommendations to control and minimize the contagion, such as proper hand washing procedures, social distancing, working from home if possible, walking or bicycling to work instead of using public transportation, and avoiding crowds. Beyond these recommendations, the Public Health Agency in Sweden put forth measures to facilitate public compliance, including canceling sporting events and restricting shows and other gatherings to a maximum of 50 people. Currently, the Public Health Agency in Sweden reports 84,985 (8,415 per 1,000,000 inhabitants) confirmed cases of Covid-19 of which 2,574 have been treated at an intensive care unit and 5,835 (577 per 1,000,000) have died (Public Health Agency in Sweden, 2020). Figure 1 specifies the contagion spread in Sweden throughout 2020.

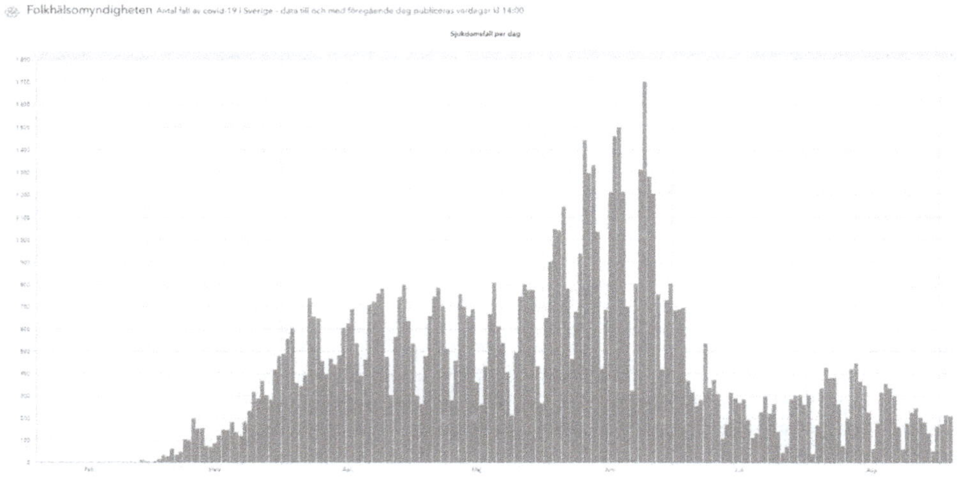

Figure 1. Number of confirmed Covid-19 cases in Sweden – The Public Health Agency In Sweden.

The national crisis management team

The Swedish Prison and Probation Service (SPPS) is the Swedish government agency responsible for all correctional operations in the country, specifically jails, prisons, probation offices, and transportations within the SPPS and on assignment for other government agencies. The SPPS national crisis management team for Covid-19 formed on March 12, 2020 in response to the WHO classifying Covid-19 as a pandemic, as well as the start of contagion spread in Sweden. The SPPS appointed the head of the Security Department as the chairperson of the team and recruited experts from the security intelligence, HR, logistics, security, inmate placement, and legal departments. The national crisis management team met every day to evaluate potential and required measures for the SPPS. The team organized into five main operational tracks to allow the representatives to focus on their specific areas of expertise; the five operational tracks included security, staff, contagion spread, communications and legal. The team swiftly moved into action while the Director General decided on canceling all visitation at, and furlough from, jails and prisons while providing the inmates with no-charge phone calls as compensation.

In the months that followed, the national crisis management team made multiple decisions and specified instructions on how to enforce those decisions to control the pandemic to the best of the SPPS's ability, while complying with the recommendations of the Public Health Agency in Sweden. Table 1 outlines the most prominent actions taken by the national crisis management team.

The security operational track

Representatives of the security operational track in the national crisis management team focus on the general security and safety of all SPPS units across the nation. These representatives maintain communications with units that have flare ups due to Covid-19 outbreaks or reactions within the inmate population in response to decisions made by the SPPS. The first major reactions came immediately following the decision to cancel all visitation and furlough on

Table 1. Timeline for the SPPS national crisis management team.

March 12	The SPPS national crisis management team formed
	Visitation and furlough canceled
March 13	No-charge phone calls for all inmates
	Specific Covid-19-site on the staff-only internal website
	Shorter staff training programs canceled
	All non-essential in-service trips canceled
March 14	Only "absolutely necessary" transports of inmates with confirmed or suspected Covid-19 will be carried out
March 16	Probation offices switch to digital meetings
	Legal track added
March 17	All close-contact staff training canceled
March 23	The national correctional officer training program paused, students return to work at their respective units
March 24	Distribution of protective gear to all units
March 27	Working from home, if possible, recommended for staff at the SPPS headquarters
	Decision to test inmates with symptoms of Covid-19, as soon as such tests are available
	Headquarter staff inventory for potential reallocation of resources at jails, prisons, probation offices and national transportation service
March 30	First confirmed inmate case of Covid-19
April 1	First outbreak at a SPPS unit, five confirmed cases of Covid-19 and high rate of sick leave within the staff at the unit
April 15	Skype available for treatment programs at probation offices
April 27	Skype-calls on tablets available for video calls to inmates' children
April 29	Instructions regarding handling of inmates with confirmed or suspected Covid-19 as well as inmates within certain risk groups published to the staff website
May 7	Staff magazine with Covid-19 focus published
May 9	800 reusable protective visors, produced in prison workshops, distributed to units
June 4	Compiled "terminology and instructions" document published to the staff-only Covid-19 page
June 5	Training materials regarding Covid-19 for summer staff distributed
June 23	Decision to commence the national correctional officer training program during the fall
June 25	Decision to gradually return to "regular" probation office services starting July 1, with regular practices in place by September 1
	Decision to gradually return to regular visitation and furlough from prison starting July 1, with regular practices in place, at the lowest security class prisons, by September 1
July 13	New directives for protective gear, must be CE-marked upholding the European Union security demands
July 21	CE-marked protective gear distributed to units

March 12. Two of the low security prison populations engaged in minor mass actions; at one of the prisons, the inmates activated the fire alarm and refused the nightly lock-down. At the other prison, some inmates attempted to create a barricade, but when the special tactics force entered the wards all inmates followed instructions and returned to their respective cells.[1] The SPPS transported the instigators to higher security facilities. That night, three inmates escaped from the prison. However, it is important to highlight that the lowest security class in Sweden requires minimal supervision, with no use of cameras or fences. The inmates simply removed their ankle monitors and ran away. Two of the three escapees have been caught and placed at higher security facilities (TT, 2020). As escaping from a prison is not considered a crime in Sweden, the escapees' sentences were simply paused until they were caught. With support from representatives of the security operational track, local crisis management teams managed to resolve the situations with no injuries or further incidents. Other prisons had some minor reactions with inmates refusing to attend their mandated prison jobs. The local units managed to deescalate these situations and return to normal practice quickly. The refusal to work continued peacefully at one unit until March 19. The motive behind the refusal to work could also have been the changes in rules regarding commissary fund transfers from family and relatives, as the SPPS discontinued transfers to inmate commissary accounts only a few weeks before the cancelation of visitation and furlough.[2] The decision to stop commissary fund transfers and the Covid-19 outbreak were unrelated, but the unfortunate timing most likely influenced the inmates' emotional reactions.

The decision to allow inmates no-charge phone calls was a strategic move to compensate the inmates for the loss of visitation and furlough as well as a way to maintain the treatment plans of many inmates who need prosocial contacts as a part of their rehabilitation. The positive reactions that followed from the inmate population allowed the representatives of the security operational track time to focus on creating risk analyses in preparation for future decisions, possible new outbreaks of Covid-19, and other potential situations that may arise throughout the pandemic. They also coordinated with representatives from the contagion spread track to create practical solutions for managing suspected and confirmed infected inmates. One of these practical solutions was to create a template that was sent out to all SPPS regional offices requesting information about the number of inmates with Covid-19, suspected and confirmed, and the number of inmates within a risk group.[3] Each of the six regions utilized the template to compile reports provided by their local units and sent it back to the national crisis management team. This action provided the national crisis management team with daily structured information for the contagion spread, staff, and security operational tracks.

The national crisis management team continually reviews the decision regarding the no-charge phone call policy each month. By the first update of the decision, the SPPS decided to keep providing no-charge phone calls within Sweden but to charge all international calls at half the normal rate. The SPPS made this decision based on a major increase in the cost of international phone calls. Because inmates may not leave Sweden while on furlough and visits from family and friends from other countries are rare, the reduced charge for international calls serve as a form of compensation for the restrictions in place during the pandemic.

A common problem during the spring of 2020 has been new inmates feeling threatened, as the inmates in their wards feared the new inmates would be infected with Covid-19 and spread it within the population. The SPPS has the option of placing inmates in isolation for a variety of reasons, one of which is to minimize the risk of spreading a disease (Chapter 6, section 7, Act on Imprisonment (Sveriges Riksdag, 2010)). This regulation allowed the security operational track to create routines to use isolation as a form of quarantine for new inmates, as well as inmates with suspected or confirmed Covid-19. Because someone can be asymptomatic for Covid-19, representatives from the security, legal, and contagion spread operational tracks created instructions to place new inmates in isolation until the jail/prison health care professionals could ensure that they would not introduce the virus into the ward.

The security operational track supports all SPPS units in specific cases of inmates acting out due to the virus; however, the security situation has remained stable throughout the pandemic. The SPPS accredit this maintained security mainly to the staff's ability to follow new instructions and maintain good communication with the inmates, but also to the quick decisions made by the national crisis management team. Many units have had weekly information meetings with inmates; a strategy to keep the inmates aware of the situation in society but also to inform them of the different measures taken by SPPS to keep them safe. The SPPS remains cautiously optimistic regarding future security threats and reactions from the inmate population since the SPPS has proved able to handle the rare and uncertain situation of a global pandemic.

The staff operational track

The representatives of the staff operational track of the national crisis management team solely focus on the SPPS staff. They observe trends in staff sick leave, maintain communications with the unions, and provide support in all staff-related issues connected to Covid-19, while safeguarding the staff's protection during the pandemic. At each meeting of the national crisis management team, the representatives of the staff operational track report the sick leave on a national basis, divided into four main groups: jails/prisons, the national transportation service, probation offices, and headquarters. Sick leave spiked quickly at the beginning of the pandemic and became the highest recorded sick leave within the SPPS.[4] However, the rate started to decline in April and, currently, the SPPS sick leave is at an all-time low. The reasons for the low sick leave rate have not been investigated yet; however, it may be attributed to a large portion of the staff working from home and the opportunity of working from home on days they would not typically attend work due to minor symptoms. In addition, the government enforced new legislation to remove the qualifying period of one day required for receiving sick pay in order to encourage people with symptoms to stay home. The SPPS also quickly enforced these rules and ensured staff felt comfortable to work only if they were completely healthy. These actions may also have had a big impact on sick leave and minimizing contagion spread in the workplace.

One of the first actions of the national crisis management team was to cancel all shorter staff training programs. Most of the staff in these short programs needed to travel by train and other forms of public transportation to and from the programs, which the Public Health Agency identified as hot spots for the spread of Covid-19. By March 23, all training programs and physical practices, including the national correctional officer training program, were paused or canceled. This decision proved to be one of the most successful actions of the national crisis management team. The reason for the decision was threefold; first, minimizing the risk of contagion spread between staff at the training facilities; second, minimizing travel by public transportation to and from the training facilities, and; third, providing the SPPS units with more staff to cover for the projected increase in sick leave while minimizing the need to bring temporary workers into the units. Temporary workers often work in multiple units and would therefore increase the risk of contagion spread, and more effective use of regular staff reduced the number of different people passing through each unit. Along with the cancelation and pausing of training programs, the SPPS canceled all non-essential work trips consistent with the recommendations from the Public Health Agency to minimize travel by public transportation – the SPPS's preferred form of work-related transportation.

As the pandemic spread in Sweden, the representatives of the staff operational track proactively searched for solutions to a possible shortage of correctional officers at the units due to sick leave as the number of overtime hours at the units began to rise. One of the measures taken was to do an inventory at the SPPS headquarters to identify staff who previously had worked at jails, prisons or probation offices, or for the national transport service. The plan was to reallocate resources to units that may have a large volume of sick leave cases due to the pandemic. The units of SPPS cannot run without staff and as an important public function of Swedish society, the work cannot be paused or stopped. However, largely due to the return of students from the national correctional officer training programs, the SPPS, thus far, has not needed to reallocate any headquarter staff.

During the early stages of the pandemic, representatives of the staff operational track worked closely with the units and kept monitoring recommendations from the Public Health Agency in Sweden to develop strategies to protect staff within the identified risk groups for Covid-19. A few of the staff were excused from work and asked to stay home with pay since the SPPS did not have the necessary information and instructions to protect them from the virus. This safeguard was a manageable measure for the SPPS as the units were over-staffed due to the return of correctional officers from the national correctional officer training program. The units also received extra staff from the national transportation service because of a decrease in transportations conducted. All units completed a voluntary inventory of staff who may be within a risk group and these individuals were not to interact with inmates with suspected or confirmed Covid-19. In May, the national crisis management team decided that all staff who had worked with inmates with confirmed cases of Covid-19, without the necessary protective gear, were to stay at home with pay for 14 days. The goal of this decision was to protect staff and inmates from potential asymptomatic Covid-19 carriers.

As sick leave began to reduce, the staffing situation within the SPPS stabilized and, as previously mentioned, the staff sick leave has been at an all-time low. Currently, the representatives of the staff operational track focus on the restart of the national correctional officer training program and solutions to protect students by minimizing the risk of contagion spread, while providing them with the necessary tools to be confident and competent correctional officers.

The contagion spread operational track

The representatives of the contagion spread operational track focus on the risks of contagion spread, handling of suspected or confirmed cases of Covid-19, organizing protective gear for staff, and providing support to experts creating creative solutions for the new "normal operations" for the SPPS throughout the life span of the pandemic. One of the first actions of the contagion spread operational track was to identify all inmates within any of the known risk groups to know the actual number of inmates who might need extra protection from Covid-19.[5] The national crisis management team realized early on that the SPPS needed strategies to obtain the necessary protective gear to protect both staff and inmates since no such inventory was readily accessible within the government agency. As such, the representatives of the contagion spread operational track made a request to the Swedish Armed Forces to borrow protective masks; the Swedish Armed Forces provided the SPPS with some borrowed masks to use until the SPPS could obtain protective gear from manufacturers. At this time, prison workshops across the nation began to produce temporary protective gear and the SPPS used the communications operational track to inform all staff and inmates about hand washing procedures and the importance of general hygiene and social distancing.

The Covid-19 outbreak required mitigation strategies both inside prisons and in the community corrections system. An important step in minimizing risk of contagion spread in community corrections was to discontinue most in-person meetings at probation offices. All operational tracks coordinated with departments at the SPPS headquarters to introduce a digital form of probation office services. The probation officers were able to conduct meetings and treatment programs over FaceTime and Skype. Probation offices nationwide identified a few of their clients as having a high-risk of recidivism and need for control; these clients required in-person meetings to ensure personal and public safety. At this time, the SPPS does not have records of an aggregated total of these individuals as the identification and decision process was delegated to each individual probation office. The probation officers conducted the in-person meetings in accordance with the recommendations of the

Public Health Authority in Sweden. Thus, the SPPS could minimize the risk of contagion spread while continuing the necessary rehabilitation activities and upholding safety for individuals on probation.

On March 30, a medium security prison reported the first confirmed inmate case of Covid-19. While supporting the units with confirmed and suspected infection, the contagion spread operational track focused on creating clear and correct instructions to minimize contagion spread of Covid-19 within the SPPS. The instructions covered, for example, safe placement strategies for inmates with suspected or confirmed Covid-19 and inmates within risk groups, use and disinfection of protective gear, and transportation of inmates during the pandemic.

The SPPS confirmed the first cluster of infected inmates at a medium security prison on April 1. Five inmates tested positive for Covid-19 and the prison acted immediately, following the instructions issued by the SPPS national crisis management team. The infected inmates were isolated and staff used proper precautionary actions when in contact with the inmates. This first cluster case allowed the contagion spread operational track to learn and develop better strategies for future outbreaks. One of the measures taken was to conduct webinars with heads of all SPPS units to provide information and lessons learned from the first major outbreak. The head of the unit with the cluster of infected inmates led the webinars. He provided his colleagues all over Sweden with first-hand information regarding Covid-19 procedures, questions and reactions from inmates and staff, and lessons he and his staff learned from the experience. By the end of the webinars, the unit heads shared their appreciation for the information and that they felt better prepared for future outbreaks and clusters of infected inmates.

To date, the SPPS has had 143 Covid-19 cases among the inmates. The testing procedures for each unit differ since the Swedish health care system of each county has different conditions and opportunities for testing. The SPPS only receives data about inmates at jails and prisons; clients reporting to the probation offices handle their own health care, and the SPPS does not have access to their potential test results. Most of the cases can be connected to local outbreaks at a few isolated units and there have been no deaths. Most of the 143 inmates have recovered, with only a handful requiring health care at a hospital. Those who are yet to recover are handled according to the instructions and routines provided by the national crisis management team. The SPPS expects more cases of Covid-19 with the intake of new inmates and contagion through asymptomatic staff. However, all units prepare for the contagion spread with instructions in place for the safe management of Covid-19, making new confirmed cases a part of day-to-day operations. Currently, the representatives of the contagion spread operational track are working closely with the jail/prison and probation office departments at the SPPS headquarters. The goal is to provide them with enough information and competence to handle all Covid-19 related questions and issues starting in September 2020. The primary focus is to provide support to all units in preparation for visitation, regular furlough, and normal probation services while managing social distancing and using creative solutions in situations where social distancing is not possible. One of these solutions is to use Plexiglass to separate individuals during meetings at the probation offices or during visitation at jails and in prisons.

The communications operational track

Throughout the pandemic, the communications operational track has provided information regarding the SPPS's work with Covid-19 to the SPPS staff and inmates as well as the media. The communications operational track acted fast after the formation of the national crisis management team and created a dedicated Covid-19 page on the internal staff website by March 13. Representatives of the communications operational track maintain the website and publish all decisions, instructions, videos, and news related to Covid-19 for all staff to see. The site also has a Frequently Asked Questions page to streamline the information staff most commonly ask for. In addition, the staff magazine May edition focused on the Covid-19 pandemic (Swedish Prison and Probation Service, 2020).

The communications operational track created informational posters that featured proper hand washing techniques, information about the importance of social distancing, and general Covid-19 information. The SPPS encouraged all units to post the posters in both staff and inmate areas. As the national crisis management team made decisions, the communications operational track created and used channels of communication with units to provide all inmates and staff with updated information in the most efficient way possible. By June 1, the communications operational track provided inmates with general Covid-19 information in the four most commonly spoken languages in Swedish jails and prisons (English, Arabic, Spanish, and Russian). In preparation for summer temporary workers, the communications track coordinated with all other operational tracks to create educational packets to expedite the learning process regarding Covid-19 for all new correctional officers.

There has been a steady public and media interest for the SPPS's operations and actions during the Covid-19 pandemic. Many of the articles posted by media outlets have been in response to the cancelation of visitation and furlough. Family members and friends of inmates have spoken out in media about what they consider inhumane treatment since they are restricted from visitation. For example, a local newspaper in the southern region of Sweden published an article about a six-year-old boy named Vincent who had not met his father for four months because of the cancellation of visitation. The article describes the negative emotional impact on children when denied access to a parent and comments on the SPPS's decision to maintain the prohibition of visits for so long (Wester et al., 2020). At the end of April 2020, before the article was published, the SPPS provided all units with tablets set up for video calls via Skype. These tablets may only be used for video calls to the inmates' children; the inmates may use the no-charge phone calls for communication with their adult family members and friends. Many media outlets requested information regarding specific units where Covid-19 has spread. Along with the legal operational track, the communications operational track referred to the protection of information related to inmates' health care. However, due to the Swedish public access principle, media representatives made freedom of information requests to obtain decisions relating to the isolation of inmates. These decisions are public information according to Chapter 6, section 7 in the Act on Imprisonment (isolation in order to prevent risk to another inmate) and media representatives could therefore identify the units with Covid-19 spread.

The legal operational track

The national crisis management team identified the need for a separate track to manage the many legal issues that surfaced and would arise during the pandemic and therefore added the legal operational track on March 16. Most of the decisions made by the national crisis management team could have legal ramifications and the representatives of the legal operational track ensured that the SPPS would follow all laws and regulations in the management of the pandemic. While correctional departments in some countries decided to release some of their inmates due to the pandemic, Sweden did not and the SPPS handled the situation with all inmates serving their sentences as ordered by the courts.

The cancelation of all furloughs and visitations initiated many questions and appeals from inmates, since inmates maintained their right to apply for furlough. The SPPS denied all requests because of the Covid-19 pandemic. The legal department and the representatives of the legal operational track assisted the units in how to formulate furlough decisions during this time, while handling the appeals from inmates. Following the changes of some of the national recommendations from the Public Health Agency in Sweden, and as the understanding of the virus grew, the SPPS could grant a few furlough requests; however, all furloughs require staff monitoring to ensure the inmate follows the social distancing recommendations.

In April, a parliamentary ombudsman investigated the SPPS actions in response to the Covid-19 outbreak. The investigation was completed and delivered to the SPPS by June 30 (Katarina Påhlsson, 2020). The parliamentary ombudsman criticized the SPPS's preparedness for the pandemic, questioned the large restrictions placed on inmates through the cancelation of visitation and furlough, and regarded the information to the inmates as poor. The parliamentary ombudsman requested a quick return to "regular" visitation and furlough operations, with measures to minimize contagion spread. Before the parliamentary ombudsman finished their report, the SPPS decided on June 25 to return to normal operations starting July 1, with "new regular procedures" in place for the low security prisons by September 1, and a team working to create solutions for medium and maximum security jails and prisons. The parliamentary ombudsman also criticized the SPPS for the common practice of using one-person cells for two inmates as they pointed to the impossibility to practice social distancing and minimizing contagion spread. Currently, and over the past year, the SPPS has placed two inmates in one-person cells due to overcrowding. Within the SPPS, standard practice is to provide each inmate with their own cell, however, because the inmate population in relation to the capacity is continuously reaching well over 90% and even over 100% at times since 2019, two inmates per cell has become a strategy to handle the large inmate population. On October 2, 2019, the SPPS identified overcrowding as a "special event" requiring the formation of a national crisis management team with operations focused on solutions to prepare for larger inmate populations (The Swedish Prison and Probation Service, 2019). The overcrowding issue still stands (currently 97% of capacity filled and rising (World Prison Brief, 2020)) and the national crisis management team for overcrowding is still active. The SPPS is building more facilities but the progress cannot keep pace with the continuing large intake of inmates. Importantly, the SPPS has never, and never will, allow an inmate with suspected or confirmed infection to share a cell with another inmate. The head of the national crisis management team, along with the communications operational track, issued a statement to clarify this standpoint.

Other functions within the national crisis management team

Beyond the head of the national crisis management team and the operational tracks, the team has a few other representatives. The national transportation service representative provides information about transportations both within the SPPS and transportations conducted for other government agencies; due to the reduction of inmate transportations during the pandemic, the national transportation service provided jails and prisons with extra staff and transported protective gear to units within the SPPS. The security intelligence representative allows the national crisis management team to keep track of security threats and general security within the SPPS. The IT department representative provides information about technical solutions needed to successfully take the SPPS through the pandemic; these solutions included increasing capacity for video meetings and the inmate telephone system (as phone calls increased when the SPPS offered no-charge calls). Representatives from the logistics department provide the national crisis management team with solutions regarding equipment distribution and procurement. Lastly, a representative from the security department handles administrative organization, notes, all-around assistance for the head of the national crisis management team, e-mail administration, and local, national, and international news monitoring to ensure that the national crisis management team stays up-to-date with Covid-19-related information.

Current operations and preparations for the future

The workload of the national crisis management team is reducing and will cease in September 2020. The representatives assist the jail/prison and probation office departments in overtaking Covid-19-related questions and issues in their day-to-day operations. The current focus is to create the best possible conditions for visitation and furlough. The SPPS prepares for the pandemic to continue and possibly worsen; regardless, the SPPS has strategies in place to handle the Covid-19 pandemic.

Closing remarks

In summary, the SPPS has taken a structured approach to managing the Covid-19 pandemic through the initiation of a national crisis management team, with important lessons learned. The investigation by the parliamentary ombudsman shed some light on what the SPPS as a government agency needs to improve on in the future, and the Covid-19 process has provided the SPPS with an opportunity to learn and prepare for future pandemics. Even though the SPPS's handling of the pandemic was not perfect, the government agency can take some pride in that to date, the SPPS has not had any deaths due to Covid-19 and maintains a low contagion count. The pandemic is not yet over, and systematic evaluation is needed to draw conclusions regarding the quality and efficiency of SPPS's crisis management. With that said, perceived facilitating factors of the SPPS's management of the Covid-19 pandemic include: the rapid formation of the national crisis management team; competent and compliant staff who managed to minimize the contagion spread even before they had access to proper protective gear; the swift decision to cancel all furlough and visitation; the cancelation of the national correctional officer training program to provide additional staff for the units; and lastly, continuous communication with our units, staff, and inmates. The SPPS met many challenges, mostly due to the lack of knowledge about the virus and the lag in updated national recommendations from the Public Health Agency in Sweden. In addition, the shortage of protective gear globally required creative solutions, such as producing temporary protective gear in the prison workshops. The SPPS prepared for more and worse reactions from the inmate population, but the negative reactions were few. The SPPS attributes these beneficial outcomes to the hard work of correctional officers and other staff as they managed to keep the inmate population calm and informed during these trying times.

It is too early to foresee the potential long-term impact of the SPPS Covid-19 strategies, especially since the pandemic is still active. However, the experience of handling Covid-19 has given the SPPS insight into future needs of correctional practices. The SPPS will need to consider the necessary infrastructure when building new units, such as options to isolate and place inmates in quarantine quickly and efficiently, ability to utilize video services for meetings, probation meetings, and maintaining relationships between inmates and their children, as well as readily available protective gear in preparation for future outbreaks of Covid-19 or other viruses. The SPPS has focused on managing the pandemic and keeping up with the national recommendations from the Public Health Agency in Sweden throughout the spring and summer of 2020. A systematic evaluation of the SPPS's actions is necessary to draw conclusions and evaluate the long-term impact of both the pandemic and the SPPS's actions in response to it.

Notes

1. Observation by coauthor EA present at the unit during the mass action.
2. On February 24, 2020, the SPPS decided to discontinue transfers to inmate commissary accounts to eliminate the possibility to laundered money though the government agency. (Ny hantering av intagnas medel, 2020).
3. The Public Health Authority in Sweden classified risk groups for Covid-19 as individuals of high age, anyone who has received an organ transplant, has cancer, neurological disorders, obesity, chronical breathing disorders, heart disease, or liver disease. (The Public Health Agency in Sweden, 2020). The average rate of SPPS inmates within the risk group from March 2020 to August 2020 has been 4.7%.
4. The average recorded rate of sick leave from March 9, 2020 to August 24, 2020 was 12.7% (jails/prisons: 13.1%, National transportation service: 16.8%, Probation offices: 12.0%, Headquarters: 8.8%). The average sick leave between March 9, 2020 to August 24, 2020 has been 5.4%. On August 24, 2020, the sick leave average was 3.4%.
5. The average rate of SPPS inmates within the risk group from March 2020 to August 2020 has been 4.7%.

Disclosure statement

No potential conflict of interest was reported by the author(s).

References

Katarina Påhlsson. (2020, June 30). *Initiativ angående Kriminalvårdens åtgärder med anledning av covid-19 och konsekvenserna för intagna*. Riksdagens Ombudsmän.

Public Health Agency in Sweden. (2020, September 4). *folkhalsomyndigheten.se*. https://www.folkhalsomyndigheten.se/globalassets/statistik-uppfoljning/smittsamma-sjukdomar/veckorapporter-covid-19/2020/covid-19-veckorapport-vecka-35-final.pdf

The Public Health Agency in Sweden. (2020, July 10). *folkhalsomyndigheten.se*. Folkhälsomyndigheten. https://www.folkhalsomyndigheten.se/smittskydd-beredskap/utbrott/aktuella-utbrott/covid-19/skydda-dig-och-andra/rad-och-information-till-riskgrupper/

Sveriges Riksdag. (2010, June 10). *riksdagen.se*. https://www.riksdagen.se/sv/dokument-lagar/dokument/svensk-forfattningssamling/fangelselag-2010610_sfs-2010-610

The Swedish Prison and Probation Service. (2019, October 2). *Beslut i stort för hantering av den höga beläggningen i Kriminalvårdens anstalter och häkten.*

Swedish Prison and Probation Service. (2020, May). *OMKRIM.*

Ny hantering av intagnas medel. (2020, February 24). *Norrköping.* The Swedish Prison and Probation Service.

TT. (2020, March 23). *Två av tre förrymda fångar hittade.* SVT.

Wester, T., Erlandsson, M., & Svensson, S.-E. (2020, July 21). *Besöksförbud gör att Vincent, 6, inte får träffa sin häktade pappa.* Helsingborgs Dagblad.

World Prison Brief. (2020, September 9). Institute for Crime & Justice Policy Research. https://www.prisonstudies.org/country/sweden

Responses Taken to Mitigate COVID-19 in Prisons in England and Wales

Pauline K. Brennan

ABSTRACT

The purpose of this paper is to discuss and evaluate how prison administrators in England and Wales responded to the coronavirus disease (COVID-19). The first case of COVID-19 was confirmed in the United Kingdom (UK) in late January 2020. In the days that followed, the number of positive cases grew exponentially; by the end of March thousands of new cases were detected daily and several hundred people had died of COVID-19. In response to the pandemic crisis, Prime Minster Boris Johnson mandated a national lockdown on March 23 and prison administrators were told to immediately begin implementing Exceptional Regime Management Plans. These Plans included (1) strategies to minimize the risk of transmission of the virus within prisons, (2) measures to reduce the potential for the virus to enter prisons, and (3) methods to manage prison populations in order to contain the virus. Overall, 6 months into the coronavirus crisis, the adopted measures appear to have helped curtail the spread of the virus within prisons, but at a great cost to the inmates and their families.

Introduction

The first confirmed case of COVID-19 in the United Kingdom (UK) was on January 29, 2020 (Kay, 2020, p. 2). By the beginning of March, there were 36 confirmed cases and health experts warned widespread transmission of the virus was "highly likely" (BBC News, March 2, 2020). Fourteen days later, more than 1,000 people in the UK had tested positive for the virus and 21 had died of COVID-19 (Van Wagtendonk, 2020). About a week later, on March 23, the number of positive cases had increased to 6,650 and 335 had died, which lead Prime Minster Boris Johnson to order a police-enforced lockdown across the country (Rawlinson, 2020). Citizens were told to stay home, but were given permission to leave for essential items, exercise alone outdoors, and go to work if necessary (Stewart et al., 2020).

Experts feared what could happen in prisons. The first case of COVID-19 in an English prison was reported on March 18, 2020 (Jarvis, 2020). Soon after (on March 21), epidemiologists warned that more than 800 inmates could die if appropriate measures were not taken by prison administrators (Townsend et al., 2020). The COVID-19 pandemic hit England and Wales in the midst of a period of mass incarceration, overcrowding, underfunding, and growing concerns over substandard conditions within prisons. Overall, prisons provide hotbeds for outbreaks of infectious diseases such as COVID-19; cramped environments, in particular, make mitigation strategies (such as social distancing and hygienic protocols) challenging for both inmates and staff to follow.

In this paper, I discuss and evaluate how prison administrators in England and Wales[1] responded to the pandemic, with focus placed on the following three questions: (1) What were the conditions within prisons before COVID-19?; (2) How did prison administrators manage the pandemic inside prisons? and (3) What were the immediate effects of the responses taken? To address these questions, I relied on multiple sources of information, including available databases, reports from NGOs, governments, and international organizations, newspaper articles, and other publically available documents. Combined, these documents provided information on the types of responses taken in prisons in England and Wales to mitigate transmission of COVID-19 and their effects. My review and analysis of the measures employed is preliminary and should be cautiously taken, as the pandemic is ongoing and a viable vaccine has not yet been identified.

Pre-COVID realities in prisons in England and Wales

COVID-19 hit prisons in England and Wales in the midst of decades-long challenges to the correctional system: crowded conditions, budget cuts, staff shortages, poor infrastructure, and inmate unrest. The system, in other words, was "struggling to cope" before the pandemic (Corker, 2020, p. 27). The myriad of pre-COVID struggles added to the difficulty administrators faced in trying to mitigate the spread of the coronavirus within their institutions.

Overcrowding

England and Wales incarcerate more people and at a higher rate than other western European nations (Abei & Tiago, 2020). As of August 28, 2020, there were 79,443 prisoners housed within 118 facilities across England and Wales (World Prison Brief, 2020). About 14% were pretrial detainees (World Prison Brief, 2020). In addition, English and Welsh prisons were operating above their rated capacities during the pandemic (World Prison Brief, 2020), which meant they were overcrowded.

Prisons in England and Wales have been overcrowded for years. As a solution, the Government planned to "build 10,000 new prison beds by 2020, but due to financial pressures only delivered 206" (Davies et al., 2020, p. 60). In the months before the coronavirus pandemic began, 60% of prisons in England and Wales were overcrowded (Davies et al., 2020), and at least 10 were operating at over 140% of their rated capacity (Howard League for Penal Reform, 2020). In overcrowded facilities prisoners share cells designed for fewer people. Within these crammed spaces, incarcerated individuals sleep, eat, and go to the toilet. Before COVID-19, members of the House of Commons' Health and Social Care Committee provided the following description of one of the prisons they visited:

> We were shown a three-bed cell, consisting of a bunk bed on the left-hand side and another bed up against the opposite wall. The gap between the two beds appeared to be about a metre wide. Room to move around the cell was limited; if all three men were standing there was not enough space for them to pass each other without touching. To the right-hand side of the entrance there was a sink, a plastic bin and a tiny mirror, about the size of a small paperback book. There was a toilet in the right-hand corner of the room. The toilet had a small door or screen with

> a small gap below and above. However, not all cells have a screen or door. The main door to the room was not barred, but the wall on the other side had a fairly large window, providing some natural light in the cell. There were two cupboards either side of the window, both broken. (House of Commons' Health and Social Care Committee, 2018, para. 35)

Independent inspectors have made similar observations, and have pointed out that some of the cells at Her Majesty's Prison (HMP) Pentonville and HMP Nottingham violated international standards because they were too small (Corker, 2020, p. 29). Prior to the pandemic, most inmates regularly left their cells to shower, attend educational classes, work, and freely interact with others in housing wings and exercise yards. But, after lockdown measures were employed on March 24, 2020, inmates spent very little time out of their cells.

Budget cuts, staffing shortages, underinvestment in infrastructure

As noted, budget cuts have affected available prison space. Indeed, prison spending was 10% lower in 2018/19 than in 2009/10 (Davies et al., 2020, p. 54). Due to spending cuts, there are 11% fewer prison officers today than a decade ago, and the ratio of prisoners to staff is among the highest in the European Union (Davies et al., 2020, p. 55; see also Atkins et al., 2019). In addition, prison officers "are now on average substantially less experienced than they were 10 years ago" (Davies et al., 2020, p. 57, see also Atkins et al., 2019). In June 2019, prison inspectors acknowledged that staffing shortages across prisons in England and Wales resulted in difficulties to "deliver acceptable and consistent regimes" and prisons were struggling to assure safe environments due to a "high proportion of inexperienced young staff" (Independent Monitoring Boards, 2019, p. 4).

Budget cuts have also meant that prisons have been in a chronic state of disrepair. A recent report from the National Audit Office revealed that numerous prisons had leaking roofs, pest control problems, failed heating and plumbing systems, outdated electrical wiring, and broken cell windows (Comptroller and Auditor General, 2020). A quarter of the prisons in England and Wales were built before 1900 (Corker, 2020, p. 27), and the vast majority of all the prisons there entered the pandemic with "severe maintenance backlogs" that would cost £916 million to address (Comptroller and Auditor General, 2020, p. 7). Moreover, in 2019, 41% of the prisons were deemed to require "major repair or replacement in the next three years" and 2% were at risk of "imminent breakdown" (Comptroller and Auditor General, 2020, p. 7). Longstanding maintenance issues compromised the health and safety of both inmates and prison staff before the pandemic hit and presented considerable challenges when all prisons were locked down.

In addition, telephone and video-conferencing capabilities were limited across prisons in England and Wales before COVID-19. While an estimated 60% of prisons there have in-cell telephones that allow outgoing calls at certain times of the day (Davies et al., 2020), inmates in many prisons must share phones located within communal areas in their housing blocks; some of these phones may be broken (Clarke, May 5, 2020). As for video-conferencing, the government planned to introduce such technology into 22 prisons several years ago, in order to reduce the cost and time involved in having staff transport prisoners to court. But, by November 2019 the equipment had been installed in only 7 prisons, due to budget cuts to the program in 2016 (Comptroller and Auditor General, 2020, p. 31).

Inmate unrest

Staffing shortages and unfavorable living conditions contributed to inmate unrest before the coronavirus crisis. Since 2012, notable increases in the extent of violence and self-harm among inmates have been reported (Davies et al., 2020). The number of self-harm incidents reached a "record high" in 2019, and were "up 14% from the figure for the previous 12 months" (House of Commons' Justice Committee, July 27, 2020, para. 17). Overall, even during the pre-COVID period, the prison environment was not ideal.

Pandemic plans

Given that violence is a reality within prisons, all the prisons in England and Wales had lockdown procedures in place before COVID-19. They also had pandemic plans in place, because "prisons regularly experience regular outbreaks of flu, norovirus and other conditions among prisoners, [which means that management plans must] include precise details of how to deploy staff to cope with staff shortages and infections among inmates" (Davies et al., 2020, p. 49).

On March 12, 2020, the Minister of State issued a statement about how prepared prisons were to deal with the pandemic. Within that statement, she indicated

> Prisons have existing, well-developed policies and procedures in place to manage outbreaks of infectious diseases. This means prisons are well prepared to take immediate action whenever cases or suspected cases are identified, including isolating individuals where necessary. (Frazer, March 12, 2020, para. 3)

She added that informational posters promoting basic hygiene had been placed in all prisons and that prisoners had access to handwashing facilities "not just in cells but other shared areas such as education blocks and kitchens" (Frazer, March 12, 2020, para. 4). Also, the Minister of State indicated that staff and visitors were able to wash their hands, and there were adequate supplies of soap and cleaning materials. Her statement further stipulated that prisons would operate normal regimes for as long as possible, which meant that visits to prisoners would continue as long as friends and family members did not have coronavirus symptoms (Frazer, March 12, 2020). But, existing plans could not sufficiently address how prisons would operate once the coronavirus crisis actually hit prisons.

COVID-19 in prisons in England and Wales

The first case of the coronavirus within a prison in England was reported at HMP Manchester on March 18, 2020 (Jarvis, 2020), which was about 2 months after the first case was reported in the community (Kay, 2020). By March 30, 65 prisoners across 23 prisons and 14 prison staff across 8 prisons had tested positive for the virus (Corker, 2020, p. 14). By April 15, the number of confirmed cases more than doubled, and the virus was known to be in more than half of all prisons in England and Wales (Howard League for Penal Reform, April 17, 2020, para. 4). About a month later, by May 12, 404 inmates were infected with the coronavirus, and 21 inmates and 7 staff had died (Beard, 2020, p. 2). These figures serve to demonstrate how quickly the virus spread amongst prisoners and staff.

Epidemiologists from the University College London predicted that viral infection could lead to 800 deaths among prison inmates if sufficient protocols were not enacted (Townsend et al., 2020). On March 23, the day Prime Minster Boris Johnson imposed a lockdown of the country, prisons went into "command mode" (Her Majesty's Prison and Probation Service – HMPPS, April 3, 2020). The next day, prison administrators moved to "an exceptional model of delivery," which meant that prisons were locked down; prisoners were allowed very little time outside their cells, visits were suspended, non-essential employment ceased, and educational programming was severely reduced (House of Commons' Justice Committee, July 27, 2020, p. 2). On March 27, 2020, administrators were tasked with implementing Exceptional Regime Management Plans (Davies et al., 2020, pp. 49, 51). These Plans included (1) strategies to minimize the risk of transmission of the virus within prisons, (2) measures to reduce the potential for the virus to enter prisons, and (3) methods to manage prison populations in order to contain the virus. In the sections below, I discuss each of these strategies and provide an assessment of their immediate effects and the issues raised.

Strategies used to minimize the risk of transmission within prisons: effects and issues

The primary strategies used to reduce the risk of transmission within prisons included the distribution of personal protective equipment (PPE) to staff, routine testing of prison officers, isolated confinement of inmates for social distancing purposes, and added handwashing facilities. Limited PPE was provided to staff on March 24, prompting the Justice Secretary to make an urgent request for more supplies (Davies et al., 2020). By mid-May, prison staff were well-equipped with PPE (Davies et al., 2020).

The testing of prison staff was prioritized on April 27th and those who tested positive were instructed to quarantine (Beard, 2020). At that time, the Justice Secretary hoped routine testing would be extended to prisoners (Beard, 2020). However, as of September 28, 2020, prisoners have not yet been routinely tested. Limited testing capability makes it difficult for prison administrators to estimate the true magnitude of the pandemic outbreak within their facilities.

Beyond distribution of PPE and testing, stringent social distancing protocols were implemented across prisons in England in Wales on March 24 when prisons went into complete lockdown. In oral testimony to the House of Commons' Justice Committee, the head of the Prison and Probation Service noted the following:

> From today [24 March], [the inmates] will spend more time in their cells, but we will be making sure that people come out for meals, to make phone calls to family or other people that they need to phone, and to have their health attended to and to take showers. We will also be making arrangements for people to exercise in the open air with proper social distancing. (House of Commons' Justice Committee, March 24, 2020)

By July 27, the prisons had been in lockdown for 15 weeks and prisoners had spent most of their time in their cells (House of Commons' Justice Committee, July 27, 2020, p. 2; see also Beard, 2020). Furthermore, inspections of prisons by government officials revealed:

> The vast majority were locked up for nearly the whole day with usually no more than half an hour out of their cells. We found some examples of even greater restrictions. In one prison, a small number of symptomatic prisoners had been isolated in their cells without any opportunity to come out for a shower or exercise for up to 14 days. (Clarke, April 28, 2020, p. 7)

Moreover, independent inspectors reported that the amount of allotted time outside of cells varied considerably across prisons, with some only allowing "as little as 30 minutes a day out of a cell, or exercise only every other day" (Owers, 2020, p. 2).

Concerns were also raised about the level of sanitation within prisons. Although the Minister of State acknowledged on March 12 that basic hygiene was necessary to combat the virus and that handwashing facilities were made available to inmates and staff, questioning of witnesses by members of the House of Commons' Justice Committee on March 24 indicated that "buckets of warm or hot water and liquid soap ha[d] been placed outside prisons at the gates – one in particular – and staff [were] told to wash their hands in a bucket on their way into work" (House of Commons' Justice Committee, March 24, 2020). When asked to comment, the Head of the Prison and Probation Service stated:

> I have not heard that, and I would be very shocked if it [were] true. If it is true, however, it would be good to know that example because we would want to put a stop to that. We have been providing hand sanitation for staff coming into prisons and facilities for both staff and prisoners to have adequate access to handwashing facilities and soap, but I certainly would not be expecting people to use a bucket outside a prison gate. (House of Commons' Justice Committee, March 24, 2020, Response to Question 48)

And, on April 28th, the Chief Inspector of Prisons issued a report detailing the conditions within local prisons. In his account of a facility where inmates did not have sinks or toilets in their cells, he wrote:

> The result was that prisoners, faced with long waits to use the communal facilities, resorted to using buckets in their cells. ... prisoners faced waits of up to two hours during the night. In addition, communal toilets and showers were not cleaned often or thoroughly enough. The situation at Coldingley was likely to improve with the imminent addition of 48 temporary single cells within a week or two, but the difficulties faced by prisoners living in cells without sanitation raised the question of whether these cells should be currently occupied. The situation was exacerbated by the fact that prisoners had to eat their meals in these same cells, and that by the time of this visit hand sanitiser had not been provided. (Clarke, April 28, 2020, p. 7)

In response to these concerns, the Ministry of Justice and Her Majesty's Prison and Probation Service (hereafter, HMPPS) stated that "the unique nature of the prison environment will not always allow for [hand-washing] to be practical, and prison levels plans must identify where exceptions will be made, justify why the exception is proportionate and the additional mitigations that will be put in place to manage this" (Ministry of Justice and HMPPS, June 2, 2020, p. 3).

By the end of April, officials from Public Health England cautiously announced that the outbreak of the coronavirus appeared to have been contained within prisons (O'Moore, 2020) and the Justice Secretary said that the numbers of prison cases and deaths were lower than "originally predicted" (Beard, 2020, p. 1). Despite the optimism from the Government, Crook and Dawson (2020) warned the extreme measures taken within prisons to prevent transmission would take a toll on inmates. In their joint letter to the Justice Secretary, on behalf of the Howard League for Penal Reform and the Prison Reform Trust, they warned of the heightened risk of self-harm and suicide among prisoners who were "effectively in solitary confinement" and who were living in horrific conditions for prolonged periods of time (Crook & Dawson, 2020). Similar concerns had been raised by the INQUEST charity on March 23, when the prisons began to go into lockdown; the charity cautioned that levels of anxiety and uncertainty would increase during periods of prolonged isolation (INQUEST, 2020, p. 6). Sadly, at the end of May, Grierson (2020) reported there had been 16 self-inflicted deaths in prisons in England and Wales after lockdown restrictions were imposed, and five of the deaths occurred over a six-day period. A few days later, the Chairwoman of the Independent Monitoring Boards provided an update to the House of Commons' Justice Select Committee on findings from recent inspections (Owers, 2020). Within that update she noted that while prisons overall remain "stable and reasonably calm, [...] a number of prisons are now starting to report an increase in self-harm and self-inflicted deaths, and there are also some spikes in violence" (Owers, 2020, pp. 1, 2). By late July, members of the House of Commons' Justice Committee indicated:

> we share concerns about the potential long-term impact current restrictions will have on the health and wellbeing of prisoners themselves. We are unclear what additional support is being provided to those struggling with their mental health. Before the Covid-19 pandemic, prisons already faced alarmingly increased levels of self-harm and the current situation in prisons may serve to make that situation worse. (House of Commons' Justice Committee, July 27, 2020, para. 22)

A month later, Davies et al. (2020) argued that current conditions were not sustainable, and that prison administrators may be "left with a difficult choice between stricter lockdown with greater risk of violence and self-harm, or easing restrictions but risking increased infections" (p. 61).

Measures taken to reduce the potential for the virus to enter prisons: effects and issues

In accordance with the Exceptional Regime Management Plans, which necessitated the lockdown of prisons, prison administrators took immediate action to minimize the potential for the virus to be introduced into their facilities by restricting contact between incarcerated people and the outside world. Administrators moved to immediately "temporarily" eliminate in-person visits and suspended educational programs and non-essential work. By comparison, before the first case of COVID-19 was confirmed in a prison, prisoners regularly moved between cell blocks to work, go to the gym, engage in educational programming, meet with counselors, visit with their families, and so on. Prisoner movement into and between prisons was also common for a variety of other reasons. For example, charged individuals who were remanded into custody from court often left prisons for required in-person court hearings and returned later. In addition, prisoners could be moved to higher or lower security prisons, if warranted, or from one prison to the next to manage prison capacity. And, those nearing their automatic release dates could be moved to facilities with reintegration supports (Kay, 2020).

All inter-prison transfers (IPT) ended on March 31, 2020, and a directive from Her Majesty's Prison and Probation Service stated the policy would remain in effect for the duration of the COVID-19 crisis (HMPPS, March 2020). The policy was imposed to help "reduce opportunities for transmission of COVID-19 between prisons, prevent the introduction of infection into prisons where there is no outbreak and reduce the chance of new prisoners becoming infected" (HMPPS, March 2020, p. 2). Only under exceptional circumstances, such as the need to move an inmate for unusual legal reasons, security necessity (e.g., transfer of a high escape risk to a more secure facility), emergency contingency (e.g., during a fire or after a natural disaster), mental health treatment outside the prison (followed by subsequent return), and/or immigration removal would inmates be allowed to move into and out of prisons (HMPPS, March 2020). Notably, transfer from one prison to another was not permitted for the purpose of helping prison governors alleviate crowding in prisons that were operating over capacity (House of Commons' Justice Committee, April 7, 2020).

Movement from prisons to courts (and vice versa) effectively stopped on March 23, when all jury trials in England and Wales were suspended; no new trials were allowed to begin and ongoing trials paused pending the implementation of safety measures (Giodarno, 2020). This policy had immediate effects for remanded defendants facing serious charges. For defendants charged with less serious offenses, where imprisonment is an unlikely outcome, court hearings were allowed to continue remotely by video and by phone (Giodarno, 2020). But, the more serious pretrial defendants waited in prison. By early May, case backlogs were mounting and outcry was increasing. For example, a barrister from Wales expressed his alarm over the stalled legal process:

> We're nearly up to 300,000 people just waiting to find out what's going on with the cases they are involved in, this is the equivalent to a city the size of Swansea. That's quite a frightening prospect. (BBC News, May 3, 2020)

By September 6, 2020, there were more than 500,000 cases awaiting court hearings in England and Wales, and the British Parliament had introduced a statute that would allow people to be held in prison for 8 months while awaiting their adjudication (Somerville, 2020). Therefore, the policy to halt jury trials has had serious legal consequences for pretrial detainees. There have also been legal consequences for prisoners serving time for convictions. Specifically, in-person parole hearings were suspended on March 23 (Corker, 2020, p. 31), which effectively resulted in the denial for consideration of early release for some prisoners.

Other cautionary measures taken have likely added to levels of frustration among both pretrial and sentenced prisoners. Since lockdown began on March 24, prisoners have been given few, if any, opportunities to work or learn because many staff members and volunteers were deemed non-essential and, consequently, were prohibited from entering prisons. In regard to schooling, the

> [e]ducation provision in the prison setting [has been] minimal, consisting primarily of in-cell work packs. Many education departments have closed, and education providers have withdrawn from prisons. Peter Clarke, Chief Inspector of Prisons, in all of his recent reports on short scrutiny visits has found that education provision across the prisons inspected was variable, and that face-to-face education had been largely suspended in most prisons. (House of Commons' Justice Committee, July 27, 2020, para. 12)

In the few instances where educational programming continued, delivery left much to be desired. For example, at one prison for women – HMP Bronzefield – restricted face-to-face education was provided at cell doors (Clarke, May 19, 2020) and at one institution for younger offenders – HMP Parc – limited face-to-face education with social distancing took place (Clarke, April 19, 2020).

Prisoners were also prevented from having in-person visits with their families and friends beginning on March 24 (Ministry of Justice, March 24, 2020). To supplement the loss of in-person visits, the Government

> announced that 55 prisons were to receive 900 secure phone handsets to help maintain family contact during the COVID-19 outbreak and the Prison Service was also exploring the use of video calls at six pilot sites, to allow prisoners to be called by their families in a secure environment with strict safeguards. (Corker, 2020, p. 31; see also Ministry of Justice, March 24, 2020)

In addition, as was the case during the pre-COVID-19 period, friends and family members could contact prisoners through the "Prison Voicemail Service, the email a prisoner service, and by writing letters" (Beard, 2020, p. 3). And, in mid-May, the Government announced prisoners would be given extra phone credit (Beard, 2020) and secure video-calling technology would be introduced in 10 prisons, with more to follow (Ministry of Justice & HMPPS, May 15, 2020). By the end of May, video calls were available in 26 prisons (Prison Reform Trust & Prison Policy Network, 2020).

As of September 28, 2020, many prisoners have gone without visitation for months, although prison visits were allowed to resume with Government approval in July, 2020 when the Ministry of Justice reduced the national alert level (Inside Time Newspaper, 2020). The prisons approved for reopening were required to make "major changes" to their operations, which resulted in more restrictive visitation (e.g., shorter sessions, face coverings, separation screens between prisoners and visitors) (Inside Time Newspaper, 2020). But, "some families found the new rules so distressing, especially for children unable to hug a jailed parent," that they have decided to refrain from visiting inmates (Inside Time Newspaper, 2020, para. 7). And, some of the prisons that reopened have recently shut down due to surging cases of COVID-19 in their surrounding communities (Inside Time Newspaper, 2020). "From the evidence, this extensive period of separation, which initially induced feelings of frustration, is now causing extreme distress and desperation" (Prison Reform Trust & Prison Policy Network, 2020, p. 7). Moreover, outcry has been raised over the inadequacy of the compensatory measures taken to address the lack of in-person visitation. According to critics, what the Government did

> amounted to in-cell telephones in fewer than half the prisons; 900 mobile phones distributed across the remainder; and video calls, initially at six prisons, rising to 26 by the end of May. . . . the inadequacy of compensation is obvious. With up to 40,000 prisoners given very little time out of cell, the demand for 900 mobile phones spread over 55 prisons was certain to overwhelm the supply. The additional phone time these provided could never offset the profound impact of cutting off family contact. (The Prison Reform Trust & The Prison Policy Network, 2020, p. 6)

In addition, prisons have been using antiquated technology that is struggling to catch up. A report released in February, 2020 by the National Audit Office highlighted just how far behind the prisons were in updating communications equipment. In the month before prisons went into lockdown, the Government's

> Reconfiguration Project [was] more than two years behind schedule and not expected to be completed before February 2023. As at November 2019, Her Majesty's Prison and Probation Service had changed the function of two prisons with a combined operational capacity of 2,208 (6% of its 37,000 target). In addition, it installed video conference centres (VCCs) in seven of its

> 17 priority prisons but had originally identified 22 prisons that needed this technology. It scaled back plans when the programme board reduced the project's budget by 20% in 2016 (from £79 million to £59 million) to bring the overall programme costs within budget. (Comptroller and Auditor General, 2020, p. 31)

Years of underfunding, therefore, made it difficult to get communication options up and running once the pandemic hit.

On June 30, months into lockdown, the Government acknowledged that network and connectivity issues have been in problem in some prisons (Prison Reform Trust & Prison Policy Network, 2020, p. 14). Moreover, the rollout of the technology across prisons was slow and uneven, which resulted in added frustration for inmates and their families. As one person put it:

> I haven't seen my partner's face in over 12 weeks ... 11 weeks ago they said they were piloting video visits. 20 prisons have the service out of 117. Some that have received video visits also have in cell phones! How is that fair? We have no clear plan on exit strategy. The framework just like the phones, video visits is a lip service document to keep us quiet and give us false hope. (as reported by the Prison Advice and Care Trust to The Prison Reform Trust & The Prisoner Policy Network, 2020, p. 15)

Concerns were also raised about the amount of time prisoners were given to make calls, due to limited out-of-cell time. In particular,

> Where prisons do not have phones in cells, they largely rely instead on communal wing phones. This makes it 'difficult for prisoners to speak to family or friends at length given the brief" time they have out of their cells during the lockdown – time that might otherwise be used for showering, exercise or other activities. (Davies et al., 2020, p. 59)

Overall, prisoners and their families have been left feeling "forgotten and disregarded" by the Government, and their ill-feelings toward the prison service have been heightened by broken promises that have caused "anxiety, hopelessness, and anger" (The Prison Reform Trust & The Prisoner Policy Network, 2020, p. 16).

Methods employed to manage prison populations: effects and issues

On March 24, 2020, the Ministry of Justice and HMPPS announced measures that would help prison administrators and staff manage existing prison populations. These measures included the early release of some prisoners, the addition of temporary accommodations across prisons, and the implementation of a "cohorting" strategy (House of Commons' Justice Committee, July 27, 2020). Efforts were also made to increase prison officer availability through the introduction of "the COVID19 Special Payment Schemes" on March 23 (Davies et al., 2020, p. 56). Once activated, prison staff were able to earn up to "an additional £4,126 over a 12-week period, or £1,292 over four weeks, for working nine hours of weekly overtime" (Ridler, 2020, para. 3).

By the time the lockdown went into effect, 3,500 prison staff (10% in total) were out sick or in self-isolation (House of Commons' Justice Committee, March 24, 2020) and the Head of the Prison Governors Association "warned that a combination of prison overcrowding, prisoner lockdown and staff shortage ... meant that the system was facing unprecedented pressure" (Pegg & Allison, 2020, para. 4). But, overtime incentives and stringent regimes imposed on prisoners have allowed prisons to operate successfully, according to Davies et al. (2020, p. 56). Nonetheless, low staffing numbers will make it difficult for activities to resume while social distancing measures are in place and staff–prisoner relations will be tested once restrictions are eased (Davies et al., 2020, p. 57).

Other than attempts to assure sufficient prison staff coverage through overtime incentives, the Government announced that the prospect of temporary release was being given careful consideration (House of Commons' Justice Committee, July 27, 2020, p. 2). Such a possibility was welcomed and encouraged by the Prison Reform Trust and the Howard League for Penal Reform (Beard, 2020). On March 31, the Government issued a press release stating that, pending risk assessments, pregnant women in custody and prisoners in Mother and Baby Units would be allowed temporary release from prison (Ministry of Justice, HMPPS, & Buckland, March 31, 2020). On April 4, the opportunity for release was extended to other low-risk inmates who were within 2 months of their release dates (Ministry of Justice, April 4, 2020). However, the Ministry of Justice also acknowledged that many prisoners would not be eligible. Specifically,

> No high-risk offenders, including those convicted of violent or sexual offences, anyone of national security concern or a danger to children, will be considered for release, nor any prisoners who have not served at least half their custodial term. Additionally, no offender convicted of COVID-19 related offences, including coughing at emergency workers or stealing personal protective equipment, will be eligible. No prisoner would be released if they have symptoms of coronavirus or without housing and health support being in place. (Ministry of Justice, April 4, 2020, paras. 4, 5)

Even with these exclusions, Government officials estimated that up to 4,000 prisoners would qualify for temporary release (Beard, 2020). The Prison Governors' Association (PGA, 2020), however, disagreed. Instead, its members believed that no more than 2,000 prisoners would be able to meet the Government's strict criteria for release, and urged officials to reconsider stipulated requirements (PGA, 2020). The PGA (2020) also said that 15,000 inmates – well over the Government's projected figure – would need to be released in order to free up enough prison space to protect inmates and staff.

By mid-April, when only 18 male and female prisoners had been allowed release, it became apparent that few prisoners would benefit from the temporary release policy (Howard League for Penal Reform, April 17, 2020). This became all the clearer on April 18 when the policy was put on hold, after errors were discovered in the release of six prisoners (BBC News, April 18, 2020). On April 24, the Ministry of Justice revamped eligibility criteria and provided clearer guidance for the process by which prisoners could be released (Beard, 2020, p. 5). But, on May 10 the Government announced the temporary release policy was no longer necessary "as the coronavirus outbreak has eased pressure on the prison system with fewer cases going to the courts" (BBC News, May 10, 2020, para. 2). When all was said and done, only 55 prisoners had left prisons on temporary release, including 21 pregnant women (Beard, 2020, p. 6).

On April 7, the head of HMPPS testified before members of the House of Commons that the temporary release of prisoners was not the only strategy that had been considered to manage the prison population (House of Commons' Justice Committee, April 7, 2020). She went on to say that there are different ways to protect inmates and that temporary prison accommodations would be installed across prisons (House of Commons' Justice Committee, April 7, 2020). On April 9, a press release from the Government indicated "work to expand the prison estate by installing the first 500 temporary single-occupancy cells [had begun]" (Ministry of Justice & HMPPS, April 9, 2020, para. 1). By April 29 temporary cells had been installed at three prisons and efforts were underway to further expand single-cell capacity by reopening two former prisons – Medway Secure Training Center and HMP Rochester (Ministry of Justice and HMPPS, April 29, 2020). More substantial progress had been made by the end of May, when the Minister of State reported to the House of Commons that nearly 600 temporary cells had been delivered to 17 prisons, 48 were already in use, and the remainder were expected to be occupied in the coming weeks pending final inspections (Frazer, May 22, 2020). She added that there were plans to install a total of 2,000 temporary cells, exceeding previous goals (Frazer, May 22, 2020).

While the Government argued that the installment of temporary accommodations was necessary to allow for single-cell occupancy to reduce the potential for the coronavirus to spread, critics argued the Government used the pandemic as a vehicle to expand prison capacity and feared the so-called "temporary accommodations" would remain long after the crisis was over (Garside, 2020; Kay, 2020). Critics also pointed out that the added "accommodations" amounted to nothing more than adopted shipping containers, which did not qualify for suitable housing (Kay, 2020). By the end of July, members of the House of Commons' Justice Committee requested information from the Minister of State in regard to how the Government planned to "re-deploy these cells in the long-term" (House of Commons' Justice Committee, July 27, 2020). In addition, because the planned installation of 2,000 temporary cells had not yet occurred, the Justice Committee asked for a more definitive timeline (House of Commons' Justice Committee, July 27, 2020).

Faced with overcrowded facilities where single-cell occupancy was not a given, prison administrators announced on March 24 that efforts were being made to "cohort" prisoners, an idea adopted from a policy used to manage an outbreak of influenza within prisons in 2010 (Kay, 2020, p. 7). At the end of March, HMPSS implored prison governors to take "proactive local steps to reduce the risk of COVID-19 spreading through their establishments by re-engineering the way prisoner locations are determined" (HMPPS, March 2020, p. 3). In so doing, HMPPS published a guidance document specifying how areas or units within the prison could be used to protect specific groups within the prison population and/or delay the spread of the virus (HMPPS, March 2020). Identified areas of separation were referred to as "cohort units" and the process by which inmates would be grouped together was called "cohorting" (HMPPS, March 2020, p. 3). In short, three distinct types of cohort units were noted: (1) a 7-day Protective Isolation Unit for prisoners with symptoms of the virus who could not be isolated in their cells, (2) a 14-day Isolation Unit (also referred to as a Reverse Cohort Unit) for asymptomatic prisoners who may have been exposed to the virus and those new to the prison, and (3) a Shielding Unit for high-risk individuals who could die if infected (HMPPS, March 2020; PGA, 2020). In essence, the cohorting strategy aimed to assure that new prisoners were not mixed with the existing population and that the risk of infection among vulnerable individuals would be minimized.

In early April the Justice Secretary reported that efforts were underway within prisons to create different cohorts of prisoners (House of Commons' Justice Committee, April 7, 2020). But, the Prisoner Governors' Associated voiced "significant concerns in the ability to achieve this [objective] if prisons are full and cells remain doubled," and added it would be necessary to reduce the prison population by 15,000 inmates in order to assure the safety of inmates and staff (PGA, 2020, para. 4). By April 21, about a month after prisons were locked down, only 25% of prisons were able to fully implement the Government's "cohorting" policy (O'Moore, 2020, p. 4). Several months later, by the end of July, 98% of all prisons had "cohorting" in place (House of Commons' Justice Committee, July 27, 2020).

While the strategy of separation seemed logical, infectious disease experts and others were skeptical about whether the effort would make a difference in mitigating the spread of COVID-19 (Kay, 2020; O'Moore, 2020). The incubation period for the coronavirus varies from individual to individual, and it may take between two and 14 days for symptoms to appear. Moreover, some people who are contagious may fail to display symptoms (Kay, 2020). In the absence of testing, it would be difficult (if not impossible) for prison officers to determine exactly who should be isolated for 7 or 14 days. Also, the types of symptoms for COVID-infected people can vary widely, which would make it difficult to determine, without testing, whether someone has COVID-19 or some other illness. "As such, utilizing cohorting measures solely on the basis of prisoners presenting with symptoms is insufficient" (Kay, 2020, p. 8). Nonetheless, in late April, the Government issued a press release stating that the collective actions taken across prisons, including "isolating those with symptoms and quarantining new arrivals" have "successfully limit[ed] the transmission of the virus" (Ministry of Justice & HMPPS, April 29, 2020, para. 2).

Discussion and concluding comments

Prisons provide hotbeds for outbreaks of infectious diseases such as COVID-19 because social distancing and handwashing protocols are not easily implemented in cramped environments where sanitation is questionable. In the pre-COVID period, prisons in England and Wales were overcrowded (Howard League of Penal Reform, 2020) and suffered from "severe maintenance backlogs" (Comptroller & Auditor General, 2020). Consequently, well before the coronavirus, prisoners shared single-occupancy cells that were in a state of disrepair with others. Years of funding cuts, moreover, limited the Government's ability to expand prison capacity, hire necessary staff, and update antiquated communications technology across prisons. In addition, due to staffing shortages and unfavorable living conditions, incidents of inmate self-harm and violence were on the rise. Overall, less than ideal prison conditions in England and Wales in the pre-COVID period made it challenging for prison administrators to respond once the pandemic hit.

On March 23, prisons went into "command mode" (HMPPS, April 3, 2020) and were locked down as prison administrators moved to "an exceptional model of delivery" (House of Commons' Justice Committee, July 27, 2020, p. 2). On March 27, 2020, administrators began implementing Exceptional Regime Management Plans (Davies et al., 2020, pp. 49, 51) that included (1) strategies to mitigate the risk of transmission of the virus within prisons, (2) measures to reduce the potential for the virus to enter prisons, and (3) methods to manage prison populations in order to contain the virus.

With regard to steps taken to reduce viral transmission within prisons, PPE was successfully distributed to prison staff, prison officers were routinely tested, handwashing facilities were added, and inmates were locked in their cells. Testing of staff was prioritized on April 27, but (as of September 28) prisoners have not yet been routinely tested, which makes it difficult for Government officials to estimate the true magnitude of ongoing pandemic. Concerns have also been raised about the level of sanitation within prisons, as testimony before the House of Commons' Justice Committee and inspector reports have indicated inadequate access to soap and water for both inmates and staff (House of Commons' Justice Committee, March 24, 2020; Clarke, April 28, 2020). Moreover, prisoners in some facilities are living in dirty cells where they eat their meals next to the buckets they use for toilets (Clarke, April 28, 2020). These realities are made even worse when one considers that by July 27 prisons had been in lockdown for 15 weeks and the vast majority of inmates spent 23 hours a day in their cells (Clarke, April 28, 2020).

The prisoners have been given few, if any, opportunities to work, learn, or visit with their families or friends. As of September 28, 2020, many prisoners have gone without visitation for months, and the compensatory measures taken to address the lack of in-person visitation has left much to be desired as prisons with antiquated technology are struggling to provide inmates with modern phone and video-calling equipment (The Prison Reform Trust & The Prison Policy Network, 2020). Combined, these realities have caused "extreme distress and desperation" for both inmates and their families and have left them feeling "forgotten and disregarded" (Prison Reform Trust & Prison Policy Network, 2020, pp. 7, 16). Crook and Dawson (2020), on behalf of the Howard League for Penal Reform and the Prison Reform Trust, warned that extreme periods of isolated confinement would put inmates at a heightened risk of self-harm and suicide. Unfortunately, by the end of May, a couple of months after stringent lockdown measures were imposed, 16 inmates in England and Wales had killed themselves (Grierson, 2020). By the end of July, members of the House of Commons' Justice Committee wondered what mental health supports had been provided to inmates, while voicing their concerns over the potential long-term impact of prolonged isolation (House of Commons' Justice Committee, July 27, 2020).

Concerns have also been raised about the growing backlog in court cases and the related serious legal consequences for pretrial detainees. All jury trials in England and Wales were effectively stopped on March 23 because social distancing protocols could not be realistically put in place within courtrooms. Therefore, many defendants charged with serious offenses have spent their time awaiting court hearings while detained in prison for months. This state of pretrial legal limbo may be allowed to continue for some time. And, some sentenced prisoners have had to put their hope of early release on hold due to the suspension of in-person parole hearings. For both categories of inmates, one could reasonably argue that justice has not been forthcoming.

Opportunities for temporary release, however, were briefly considered for certain categories of low-risk prisoners who were within months of their release dates. But, when all was said and done, only 55 inmates were granted temporary release before the Government declared the policy no longer necessary (BBC News, May 10, 2020; Beard, 2020), which was probably because other measures taken – including added temporary cells and "cohorting" of inmates – helped prison administrators to manage existing prison populations. By mid-May, the Government announced plans to install 2,000 temporary cells in prisons across England and Wales in order to add single-cell capacity where needed (Frazer, May 22, 2020). But, by the end of July, members of the House of Commons' Justice Committee questioned the timeline for final installation and wondered what the plans were to "re-deploy these cells in the long-term" (House of Commons' Justice Committee, July 27, 2020). Related to this, critics argued the Government used the pandemic as a mechanism to expand prison capacity with "accommodations" that amounted to nothing more than adopted shipping containers ill-suited for housing (Garside, 2020; Kay, 2020). These critics fear the so-called temporary cells will remain long after the crisis is over.

As for the "cohoring" strategy, in early May, efforts were underway to separate prisoners into distinct cohort units based on whether they had symptoms of the virus, had possibly been exposed to the virus or were new to prison, or were at a high risk of death if infected. While implementation of the strategy was not immediate, 98% of all prisons in England and Wales had "cohorting" in place by late July (House of Commons' Justice Committee, July 27, 2020). Critics questioned whether the strategy would prove useful without the routine testing of inmates, but Government officials believed it would successfully limit the transmission of the virus within the prison population (Ministry of Justice & HMPPS, April 29, 2020).

Did the strategies taken by the Government reduce the spread of COVID-19 within prisons? The most recent available figures indicate that 16 prison officers and 23 inmates died of COVID-19 since the pandemic began (Ministry of Justice, August 20, 2020), which is well below the number predicted by epidemiologists in early 2020. Since the start of the pandemic, a total of 560 prisoners across 87 facilities were confirmed to have the coronavirus (Ministry of Justice, September 11, 2020). Recent figures indicate that infections continue, but the pace of transmission seems to have slowed among inmates and staff. In fact, there have only been 20 newly confirmed cases among inmates from July to September 2020 (Ministry of Justice, September 11, 2020). The relatively low number of cases may lead some to believe that the virus has, for the most part, been successfully managed across prisons in England and Wales.

Some may say that sufficient numbers of prisoners were released to allow for effective social distancing within facilities. There were 4,058 fewer prisoners in facilities across England and Wales at the end of July than when lockdown measures were first implemented in March (House of Commons' Justice Committee, July 27, 2020). However, the temporary release scheme put in place by the Government had little effect on these numbers because only 55 prisoners were granted the opportunity for temporary release before the policy was abandoned. Instead, "reduced court activity, meaning fewer new prisoners, and the scheduled release of prisoners at the end of their sentences has driven the reduction in the overall prison population" (House of Commons' Justice Committee, July 27, 2020, p. 2). In other words, when court activity resumes, prison populations will increase once again, which will make it more difficult for prison officers to "separate and cohort prisoners in the way that is presently being done" (House of Commons' Justice Committee, July 27, 2020, p. 2).

Others may point out that the addition of temporary accommodations has made a difference. But, by the end of July, it was not clear exactly how many of the so-called temporary cells were actually occupied by inmates or whether the added capacity would remain once the pandemic ended (House of Commons' Justice Committee, July 27, 2020). Arguably, the stringent restrictions that went along with the lockdown of all prisons on March 24 probably had the greatest impact on containing the coronavirus, but these restrictions have come at a great price for inmates and their families. As months went by in 2020, the number of inmate suicides, self-harm incidents, and acts of violence increased. Moreover, justice has been denied to many because of case stagnation and inability to meet face-to-face with parole boards. Moreover, the families of inmates have suffered collateral damage due to the difficultly that COVID-19 has presented for visitation and other forms of contact. Overall, the pandemic aggravated many problems that existed for years in prisons in England and Wales and exposed the poor living conditions of those profoundly isolated behind prison walls.

Many hoped the worst days were over when restrictions slowly began to ease in late summer 2020. Unfortunately, daily rates of infection began to again rise sharply in mid-September, which suggested the UK entered the second wave of COVID-19 (BBC News, September 18, 2020). After having eased restrictions in the community over the summer, Prime Minister Boris Johnson peddled back on September 22, 2020 when he indicated that "working from home when possible, a 10 p.m. closing time for pubs and restaurants and increased fines for breaking laws on gatherings and mask use" could be in effect for the next 6 months (Smith-Schoenwalder, 2020, para. 2). As of September 28, 2020, a full return to lockdown had not occurred. However, the Prime Minister left the option on the table. A full lockdown during the second wave of COVID-19 may be even more difficult for inmates and prison officers to bear, because frustrations will certainly grow when signs of a return to normal seem too distant. Prison administrators, therefore, may be "left with a difficult choice between stricter lockdown with greater risk of violence and self-harm, or easing restrictions but risking increased infections" (Davies et al., 2020, p. 61).

Note

1. Prisons in England and Wales are administered at the national level by Her Majesty's Prison and Probation Service (HMPPS); one entity provides oversight of prisons in both countries. As such, Government mandates apply to prisons in both England and Wales and data for both countries are aggregated in documents, press releases, and websites.

Disclosure statement

No potential conflict of interest was reported by the author(s).

References

Abei, M. F., & Tiago, M. M. (2020). *Prisons and prisoners in Europe in pandemic times: An evaluation of the short-term impact of the COVID-19 on prison populations*. University of Lausanne: UNIL. http://wp.unil.ch/space/files/2020/06/Prisons-and-the-COVID-19_200617_FINAL.pdf

Atkins, G., Davies, N., Wilkinson, F., Pope, T., Guerin, B., & Tetlow, G. (2019). *Performance tracker 2019: A data-driven analysis of the performance of public services*. Institute for Government and the Chartered Institute for Public Finance and Accountancy. https://www.instituteforgovernment.org.uk/sites/default/files/publications/performance-tracker-2019_0.pdf

BBC News. (2020, April 18). *Coronavirus: Early prison release scheme suspended after errors*. https://www.bbc.com/news/uk-52334848

BBC News. (2020, March 2). *Coronavirus: Widespread transmission in UK 'highly likely'*. https://www.bbc.com/news/uk-51700604

BBC News. (2020, May 10). *Plans for prisoner early release shelved by government*. https://www.bbc.com/news/uk-politics-52607618

BBC News. (2020, May 3). *Coronavirus: Courts must resume to deal with 'backlog of cases'*. https://www.bbc.com/news/uk-wales-52523074

BBC News. (2020, September 18). *Covid: UK seeing second wave, says Boris Johnson*. https://www.bbc.com/news/uk-54212654

Beard, J. (2020, May 18). *Coronavirus (prisons): England and Wales* (Briefing Paper, Number 8892). House of Commons. https://commonslibrary.parliament.uk/research-briefings/cbp-8892/

Ministry of Justice, Her Majesty's Prison and Probation Service, & Buckland, R. (2020, March 31). *Pregnant Prisoners to be temporarily released from custody* (press release). https://www.gov.uk/government/news/pregnant-prisoners-to-be-temporarily-released-from-custody

Clarke, P. (2020, May 5). *Report on short scrutiny visits to Category C training prisons.* Her Majesty's Inspectorate of Prisons. https://www.justiceinspectorates.gov.uk/hmiprisons/wp-content/uploads/sites/4/2020/05/Cat-C-training-prisons-web-SSV-2020.pdf

Clarke, P. (2020, April 28). *Report on short scrutiny visits to Local Prisons.* Her Majesty's Inspectorate of Prisons. https://www.justiceinspectorates.gov.uk/hmiprisons/wp-content/uploads/sites/4/2020/05/Locals-SSV-web-2020.pdf

Clarke, P. (2020, May 19). *Report on short scrutiny visits to Prisons holding women.* Her Majesty's Inspectorate of Prisons. https://www.justiceinspectorates.gov.uk/hmiprisons/wp-content/uploads/sites/4/2020/06/Womens-prisons-SSV-2020.pdf

Clarke, P. (2020, April 19). *Report on short scrutiny visits to young offender institutions holding children.* Her Majesty's Inspectorate of Prisons. https://www.justiceinspectorates.gov.uk/hmiprisons/wp-content/uploads/sites/4/2020/05/YOIs-SSV-Web-2020-1.pdf

Comptroller and Auditor General. (2020). *Improving the prison estate (Session 2019-20, HC 41).* National Audit Office. https://www.nao.org.uk/wp-content/uploads/2020/02/Improving-the-prison-estate.pdf

Corker, R. (2020). *Expert report: Covid-19 and prisons in England and Wales.* Howard League for Penal Reform and the Prison Reform Trust. http://prisonreformtrust.org.uk/portals/0/documents/COKER_Report_HL_PRT.pdf

Crook, F., & Dawson, P. (2020). *Covid19: The need for immediate release of prisoners.* Prison Reform Trust and the Howard League for Penal Reform. http://prisonreformtrust.org.uk/portals/0/documents/letters/Covid-19%20open%20letter%20to%20SoS%20020420.pdf

Davies, N., Atkins, G., Guerin, B., & Sodhi, S. (2020, August). *How fit were public services for coronavirus?* Institute for Government and the Chartered Institute for Public Finance and Accountancy (CIPFA). https://www.instituteforgovernment.org.uk/sites/default/files/publications/how-fit-public-services-coronavirus.pdf

Frazer, L. (2020, March 12). *Coronavirus (COVID-19) prison preparedness: Lucy Frazer statement.* Ministry of Justice and Her Majesty's Prison and Probation Service. https://www.gov.uk/government/news/coronavirus-covid-19-prison-preparedness-lucy-frazer-statement

Frazer, L. (2020, May 22). *Deployment of temporary accommodations across the prison estate as part of COVID-19 mitigation plan* (Letter to the House of Commons' Justice Committee Chair). Ministry of Justice. https://committees.parliament.uk/publications/1339/documents/12153/default/

Garside, R. (2020). *Prisons need to emerge from the lockdown* (commentary). Centre for Crime and Justice Studies. https://www.crimeandjustice.org.uk/resources/prisons-need-emerge-lockdown

Giodarno, C. (2020, March 23). Coronavirus: All jury trials suspended in England and Wales. *The Independent.* https://www.independent.co.uk/news/uk/crime/coronavirus-trials-suspended-cancelled-jury-england-wales-a9417436.html

Grierson, J. (2020, May 28). Alarm over five suicides in six days in prisons in England and Wales: Campaigners fear restrictive regime to contain coronavirus is taking toll on inmates. *The Guardian.* https://www.theguardian.com/society/2020/may/28/alarm-over-five-suicides-in-six-days-at-prisons-in-england-and-wales

Her Majesty's Prison and Probation Service—HMPPS. (2020, March). *Cohorting guidance for prisons during the COVID-19 period.* https://howardleague.org/wp-content/uploads/2020/05/6.-HMPPS-Cohorting-guidance-31-March-2020-upd.-15-April-2020.pdf

Her Majesty's Prison and Probation Service—HMPPS. (2020, April 3). *COVID-19 operational guidance —Exceptional regime & service delivery* (Version 3.0). https://howardleague.org/wp-content/uploads/2020/05/1.-Exceptional-regime-and-service-delivery-27.03.20_Redacted.pdf

House of Commons' Health and Social Care Committee. (2018). *Annex 1: Visit to Greenwich cluster.* https://publications.parliament.uk/pa/cm201719/cmselect/cmhealth/963/96302.htm

House of Commons' Justice Committee. (2020, July 27). *Coronavirus (Covid-19): The impact on prisons.* https://publications.parliament.uk/pa/cm5801/cmselect/cmjust/299/29902.htm

House of Commons' Justice Committee. (2020, March 24). *Oral evidence: The work of the Lord Chancellor, HC 225.* https://committees.parliament.uk/oralevidence/248/html

House of Commons' Justice Committee. (2020, April 7). *Summarized note of the meeting with the Lord Chancellor from April 7: All questions asked and answered.* https://publications.parliament.uk/pa/cm5801/cmselect/cmjust/correspondence/200407-Justice-Committee-meeting-Robert-Buckland-note1.pdf

Howard League for Penal Reform. (2020). *Howard League prison watch.* https://howardleague.org/prisons-information/

Howard League for Penal Reform. (2020, April 17). *Judicial review: Howard League and Prison Reform Trust issue government with letter before action over its response to coronavirus in prisons.* https://howardleague.org/news/judicial-review-howard-league-and-prison-reform-trust-issue-government-with-letter-before-action-over-its-response-to-coronavirus-in-prisons/

Independent Monitoring Boards. (2019). *National Annual Report 2018-19.* https://s3-eu-west-2.amazonaws.com/imb-prod-storage-1ocod6bqky0vo/uploads/2019/06/IMB-NATIONAL-ANNUAL-REPORT-PUBL-5-JUNE-2019.pdf

INQUEST. (2020). *INQUEST briefing on COVID-19: Protecting people in places of custody and detention.* https://committees.parliament.uk/publications/611/documents/2587/default/

Inside Time Newspaper. (2020, September 20). *Leicester is the only prison still closed for social visits.* https://insidetime.org/three-prisons-still-closed-for-social-visits/

Jarvis, J. (2020, March 18). First UK prisoner with coronavirus confirmed at HMP Manchester. *Evening Standard.* https://www.standard.co.uk/news/health/uk-prison-coronavirus-case-confirmed-hmp-manchester-a4390981.html

Kay, C. (2020, May 21). COVID-19 in custody: Responding to pandemics in prisons in England and Wales. *British Journal of Community Justice.* Published online. https://www.mmuperu.co.uk/assets/uploads/bjcj_files/BJCJ_Kay_2020.pdf

Ministry of Justice. (2020, August 20). *HM Prison and Probation Service COVID-19 experimental statistics for staff.* https://assets.publishing.service.gov.uk/government/uploads/system/uploads/attachment_data/file/910307/hmpps-covid-19-staff-stats-jun-2020.pdf

Ministry of Justice. (2020, September 11). *HM Prison and Probation Service COVID-19 official statistics.* https://assets.publishing.service.gov.uk/government/uploads/system/uploads/attachment_data/file/919130/HMPPS_COVID19_AUG20_Pub_Doc.pdf

Ministry of Justice. (2020, April 4). *Measures announced to protect NHS from coronavirus risk in prisons* (press release). https://www.gov.uk/government/news/measures-announced-to-protect-nhs-from-coronavirus-risk-in-prisons

Ministry of Justice. (2020, March 24). *Prison visits cancelled* (press release). https://www.gov.uk/government/news/prison-visits-cancelled

Ministry of Justice & Her Majesty's Prison and Probation Serivce—HMPPS. (2020, May 15). *Secure video calls to help prisoners maintain family ties: Family video calls will be introduced at prisons and young offender institutions across England and Wales.* https://www.gov.uk/government/news/secure-video-calls-to-help-prisoners-maintain-family-ties

Ministry of Justice & Her Majesty's Prison and Probation Service—HMPPS. (2020, June 2). *Covid-19: National framework for prison regimes and services.* https://www.gov.uk/government/publications/covid-19-national-framework-for-prison-regimes-and-services

Ministry of Justice & Her Majesty's Prison and Probation Service—HMPPS. (2020, April 29). *Further expansion of prison estate to protect NHS* (press release). https://www.gov.uk/government/news/further-expansion-of-prison-estate-to-protect-nhs

Ministry of Justice & Her Majesty's Prison and Probation Service—HMPPS. (2020, April 9). *Prison estate expanded to protect NHS from coronavirus risk* (press release). https://www.gov.uk/government/news/prison-estate-expanded-to-protect-nhs-from-coronavirus-risk

O'Moore, E. (2020). Briefing paper: Interim assessment of impact of various population management strategies in prisons in response to COVID-19 pandemic in England. Her Majesty's Prison and Probation Service. https://assets.publishing.service.gov.uk/government/uploads/system/uploads/attachment_data/file/882622/covid-19-population-management-strategy-prisons.pdf

Owers, A. (2020). *Letter to the Judicial Select Committee, update on the Independent Monitoring Board findings*. National Monitoring Boards. https://committees.parliament.uk/publications/1416/documents/12925/default/

Pegg, D., & Allison, E. (2020, March 25). Release inmates or face jail pandemic, say prison governors. *The Guardian*. https://www.theguardian.com/society/2020/mar/25/release-prisoners-or-face-jail-pandemic-says-chief

Prison Governors Association (PGA). (2020). *Prison Governors' Association (PGA) evidence to Justice Committee on COVID-19*. https://prison-governors-association.org.uk/prison-governors-association-pga-evidence-to-justice-committee-on-covid-19/

Prison Reform Trust & Prisoner Policy Network. (2020). *How prisons are responding to Covid-19: Briefing #1, Families and communications* (a component of the Covid-19 Action Prisons Project: Tracking Innovation, Valuing Experience—CAPPTIVE). http://www.prisonreformtrust.org.uk/Portals/0/Documents/CAPPTIVE_families_webfinal.pdf

Rawlinson, K. (2020, March 23). UK coronavirus: Boris Johnson announces strict lockdown across country – As it happened, closing summary. *The Guardian*. https://www.theguardian.com/politics/live/2020/mar/23/uk-coronavirus-live-news-latest-boris-johnson-minister-condemns-people-ignoring-two-metre-distance-rule-in-parks-as-very-selfish

Ridler, F. (2020, May 7). Prison officers will get £4,100 extra for doing nine hours a week more during Covid-19 crisis while nurses get nothing. *Daily Mail (online version)*. https://www.dailymail.co.uk/news/article-8295855/Prison-officers-4-100-extra-doing-nine-hours-week-Covid-19-crisis.html

Smith-Schoenwalder, C. (2020, September 22). England's coronavirus restrictions could last into '21 as Europe struggles with second wave. *U.S. News and World Report*. https://www.usnews.com/news/world-report/articles/2020-09-22/coronavirus-restrictions-in-england-could-last-into-2021-as-europe-struggles-with-second-wave

Somerville, E. (2020, September 6). People can now be held in prison for eight months while awaiting trial as Government extends time limit. *iNews*. https://inews.co.uk/news/court-cases-backlog-coronavirus-uk-lockdown-crime-nightingale-633814

Stewart, H., Mason, R., & Dodd, V. (2020, March 23). Boris Johnson orders lockdown to be enforced by the police. *The Guardian*. https://www.theguardian.com/world/2020/mar/23/boris-johnson-orders-uk-lockdown-to-be-enforced-by-police

Townsend, M., Savage, M., & Doward, J. (2020, March 21). Prisons 'could see 800 deaths' from coronavirus without protective measures. *The Guardian*. https://www.theguardian.com/uk-news/2020/mar/21/prisons-could-see-800-deaths-from-coronavirus-without-protective-measures

Van Wagtendonk, A. (2020, March 15). The UK backs away from "herd immunity" coronavirus proposal amid blowback. *Vox*. https://www.vox.com/world/2020/3/15/21180414/coronavirus-uk-herd-immunity-vallance-johnson

World Prison Brief. (2020). *World Prison Brief data for the United Kingdom: England and Wales*. https://www.prisonstudies.org/country/united-kingdom-england-wales

North America Regional Overview and Reports from USA and Canada

An Examination of COVID-19 Outbreaks in Prisons and Jails in North America, Central America, and the Caribbean

Sabrina S. Rapisarda, James M. Byrne, and Lina Marmolejo

ABSTRACT
This article documents the extent of COVID-19 outbreaks in the North American, Central American, and Caribbean regions, and then compares the country-specific COVID-19 mitigation strategies implemented in the largest prison systems in these regions. We offer a preliminary assessment of the short-term impact of the COVID-19 prison mitigation strategies used in these regions, within both correctional and community settings. At this time, it appears that the governments with greater success controlling COVID-19 outbreaks in these regions are the governments adopting early prison and jail population reduction strategies.

Introduction and overview

In the following review, we highlight data on the nature and extent of COVID-19 outbreaks in the largest prison systems in the above three regions,[1] and then describe the types of mitigation strategies used to respond to these outbreaks. According to World Prison Brief (2020), 5 of the 50 largest prison systems in the world are located in the regions of North America, Central America, and the Caribbean, including the United States (ranked 1st), Mexico (ranked 11th), Cuba (ranked 34th), Canada (ranked 44th), and El Salvador (ranked 47th). Our review identifies within-region differences in both the extent of the problem and how the governments in these countries responded – and continue to respond – to this ongoing crisis.

Within-region variations in COVID-19 outbreaks and the mitigation strategies used

Table 1 highlights the extent of COVID-19 outbreaks in the five largest prison systems in this (combined) region, while Table 2 provides an overview of the various front-end, in-prison, and back-end mitigation strategies used to address these outbreaks. There is variation reported in the extent of COVID-19 outbreaks in the region's five largest prison systems, and in the use of mitigation strategies, that are important to consider. Given the evidence these governments offer on the short-term impact of initial mitigation strategies, it is apparent that some strategies have been more effective than others. Not surprisingly, governments that moved quickly to reduce the size of their prison and jail populations

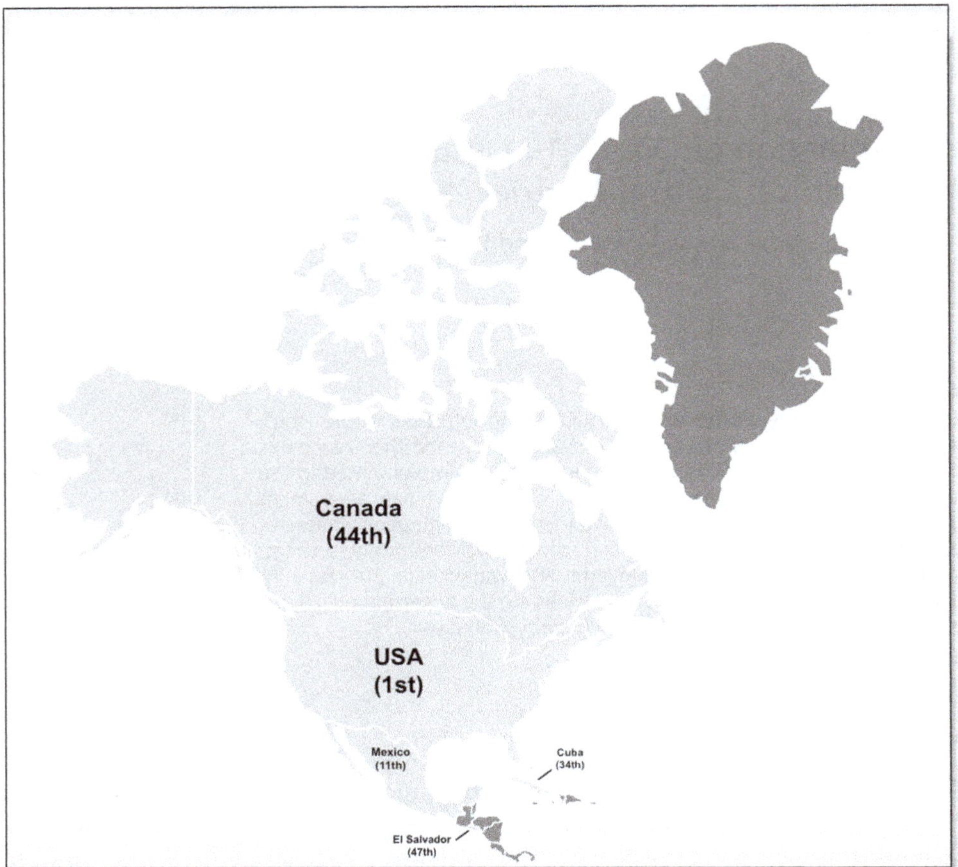

Figure 1. North & Central America and the Caribbean's largest prison systems. The labeled countries in Figure 1 are among the top 50 largest prison systems globally and represent the 5 largest prison systems in the North American, Central American, & Caribbean regions. Among the 50 largest prison systems, the USA is ranked 1st, Mexico is ranked 11th, Cuba is ranked 34th, Canada is ranked 44th, and El Salvador is ranked 47th (World Prison Brief, 2020).

report the most positive results through the end of August 2020. We provide additional context on the likely reasons for these differences in reporting rates and mitigations strategies by providing the following country-specific profiles.[2]

COVID-19 outbreaks in prisons and jails in the United States

We begin our regional overview by describing COVID-19 outbreaks in the region's largest prison system, the United States. The United States leads the world in the total number of individuals it incarcerates, at approximately 2.3 million individuals behind bars on any given day.[3] The U.S. has just under 2.1 million inmates within its federal and state prison systems, with an incarceration rate of approximately 639 inmates per 100,000 individuals (see Table 1). The U. S. also has a large jail system. In 2018, the Bureau of Justice Statistics reported that slightly under 740,000 of U.S. inmates were confined in jail settings; on an annual basis,

Table 1. North America, Central America, & the Caribbean's largest prison systems in the world's top 50 by prison population & COVID-19 prevalence.

Rank	Global Region	Country	Prison Population	Date of Most Recent Reporting	COVID-19 Case Count in Prison^
1	North America	USA[1,2]	2,094,000	2018	132,677*
11	North America	Mexico[1,3]	198,384	April 2019	3,200**
34	Caribbean	Cuba[1,4]	57,337	May 2012	–[8]
44	North America	Canada[1,5]	39,579	March 2018	360***
47	Central America	El Salvador[1,6]	36,693	August 2020	–[9]

Data were extracted from the World Prison Brief database[1], the U.S. Bureau of Justice Statistics[2], Animal Politico[3], El Diario Oficial Gfranma[4], Statistics Canada[5], & National Prison Administration[6]

^ Refers to the cumulative COVID-19 case count total in respective prison systems.

* Based on data provided by the Marshall Project on September 22, 2020.

** Based on data provided by ASILEGAL between April and mid-September, 2020.

[8]Cuba has not released official data pertaining to the number of inmates and prison staff afflicted by COVID-19, in terms of case or death prevalence. By late July, Cuba's National Institute of Epidemiology Director announced that Cuban prisons had 0 COVID-19 cases. One mitigation strategy used by Cuba includes early release, according to the Miami Herald.

*** Canadian prison-level data (updated on September 29, 2020) extracted from Correctional Service Canada.

[9]El Salvador has not released official data pertaining to the number of inmates and prison staff afflicted by COVID-19, in terms of case or death prevalence, to date. Various news articles provide context and the extent of suspected local outbreaks (e.g., see National Post).

nearly 11 million individuals were admitted to jail and averaged an estimated stay of 25 days (Zeng, 2020). Given the sheer magnitude of the U.S.'s incarcerated population, the documented poor quality of the prison and jail heath care system, and the percentage of individuals in prisons and jails with pre-existing conditions that place them at higher risk for infection, it comes as no surprise that cases of COVID-19 have mushroomed through prisons and jails alike (Byrne, et al., this volume; Heard, 2019; Nowonty & Piquero, 2020).

After having first instituted mass testing in prison systems among states such as Michigan, Ohio, Tennessee, and Texas in late April, cases initially peaked due to increased rates of testing but appeared to have flattened by June. However, cases within prisons peaked by mid-August, with at least 102,494[4] inmates in federal and state prisons cumulatively testing positive for COVID-19, a 7% increase from the week before (The Marshall Project, 2020). While 77,026 inmates have recovered as of mid-August, at least 889 confirmed deaths have been reported.[5] The recent growth in cases can be largely attributed to inmates testing positive in Florida, California, and the Federal Bureau of Prisons, in addition to outbreaks in Arkansas, Hawaii and Oklahoma (The Marshall Project, 2020). The emerging implication is that COVID-19 has been circulating among asymptomatic inmates and staff in greater amounts than previously known.

We examined the relationship between the prevalence of cases within states overall and the prisons that reside within those states, and found that the prison systems in states with the highest cumulative rates of COVID-19 were located in states with the highest reported community rates. For example, Florida currently has the second largest number of COVID-19 cases in the U.S. (N = 582,407; Centers for Disease Control and Prevention [CDC], 2020), while also reporting the second largest number of cases nationwide among its prison population (N = 15,170; The Marshall Project, 2020).[6] The rate of COVID-19 cases in Florida's prison system (1,718 per 10,000 inmates) is 536% higher than that of Florida's rate overall. California has the largest number of reported COVID-19 cases nationally (N = 644,751; CDC, 2020) and the third largest prevalence of cases in the U.S. among its prisons (N = 9,650; The Marshall Project, 2020).[3] A rate of 879 positive cases per 10,000

Table 2. A comparison of mitigation strategies used in North and Central American and Caribbean prisons.

Country (Rank)	Front-End	Within	Back-End
USA (1st)[a]	Suspension of visitation and prison transfers; New intakes for federal prisons only if offender being held for federal government in a state or local facility; Preventative screening for prison staff	Federal system-wide and state-level lockdowns; Widespread testing; Disbursement of masks, dispersal of hand sanitizer and other PPE among staff and inmates; Increased sanitation; Isolation of confirmed or suspected inmates; Remote legal counsel; Use of "field-ready" tents to maximize social distancing; "Stay at home" policy for prison staff manifesting COVID-like symptoms, coming in contact with individuals (including inmates) that have, or are suspected of having, COVID-19	Appx. 4.29% (N = 7,000) inmates in the federal system released to home confinement; Inmates in states such as CA, AL, CO, and MA have implemented early release (for inmates with low-level offenses or who are high-risk in terms of health)
Mexico (11th)[b]	Suspension of transfers; Reducing or eliminating visits; Suspended work-related activities that occurred outside of custody	Implemented policies for early detection, isolation, identification of severity, and evacuation of the seriously ill; Testing of inmates and staff; Restricted movement of people and staff inside the 525 state-level prisons, as well as suspended work and/or educational activities; Use of videoconferencing to reduce inmate trips to court	Amnesty for first-time, low level inmates, and/or inmates whose crimes were driven by poverty
Cuba (34th)[c]	Prohibiting workers or visitors with feverish symptoms or without masks to enter the premises; Limiting the total number of visitors	Providing hand disinfectants at points of access to units; Requiring inmates and staff to wear masks; Placing newly incarcerated individuals in isolation for 15 days; Conducting daily investigations twice per day to identify inmates with symptoms; Disseminating preventative medicines to boost inmates' immune systems; Providing specialized attention to vulnerable groups, such as those that are HIV positive and women who are pregnant	Appx. 11.47% (N = 6,579) inmates from within Cuba's prison system were released into the community
Canada (44th)[d]	Provisional suspension of arrests and court proceedings for minor offenses; Extended parole; Preparation of protocols for the transfer and hospitalization of inmates with severe cases of COVID-19; Screening inmates for COVID-19 before taking them in to custody	Isolation of persons who are, or are suspected of being, COVID-positive; Enhanced hygiene measures and of PPE; Increased training for staff to perform their roles while COVID-19 is a threat; Suspended inter-regional transfers	Release from prison of persons with the lowest risk of recidivism, of older inmates, and of persons with either mental or general health problems; Identification of infected and recovered staff who may have acquired greater immunity and could therefore be assigned to duties related to the hygiene and care of COVID-positive inmates
El Salvador (47th)[e]	Family visitation and transfer rates to other facilities have decreased	Extensive use of lockdowns; Restriction of programming and activities; Early in the pandemic, the Salvadorian government renewed the focus on "sanitary protocols to prevent Coronavirus in the prison population"	None

[a]See USA-based articles (e.g., Hummer, Novinsky et al., and Nowonty & Piquero) in this volume for more detail regarding the USA's mitigation strategies to combat COVID-19 within federal and state prisons; [b]See Agoff et al. and Marmolejo et al. (this volume) for more detail on Mexico's response to COVID-19 in its prison system; [c]See Gamez Torres (2020), Index Mundi (2020), and Prensa Latina (2020) for more details regarding Cuba's response to COVID-19 in its prison system; [d]See Murdoch (this volume) and Lemieux et al. (this volume) for more detail regarding Canada's mitigation strategies in response to COVID-19; [e]See Pitts & Inkpen (this volume), for more information on El Salvador, Guatemala, and Honduras' response to COVID-19 in its prison systems.

inmates equates to 449% higher than California's prevalence of COVID-19 overall. Texas is ranked first domestically for the number of COVID-19 cases in its prison system (N = 18,756; The Marshall Project, 2020), while placed third overall for cases nationwide (N = 562,559; CDC).[3] At a rate of 1,475 positive cases per 10,000 among Texan inmates, that is equal to a 677% higher rate than the state's prevalence of cases overall.

It is no coincidence that the states with the greatest prevalence of COVID-19 cases within their communities are the same states with prison systems struggling to contain the virus. By decreasing the risk of the virus's spread in prisons and jails, the risk of spread in communities also decreases. Increased spread of the virus in prisons and jails conversely increases the risk of spread in communities. Despite how "isolated" prisons and jails are thought to be, they are – in reality – heavily enmeshed, and play an important role, in the public health response to COVID-19.

According to The Marshall Project, 2020, the actual number of prison staff members currently working and being tested in U.S. prisons is largely unknown. The release of partial data regarding prison staff is likely due to the lack of systematic testing currently taking place, where documented cases include voluntary reporting of diagnoses in the course of calling out sick. As of August 20, 2020, there have been at least 22,544 positive COVID-19 cases and only 72 publicly reported deaths among prison staff nationwide (The Marshall Project, 2020). However, the sole method by which infections can infiltrate prisons and return to the community is via prison workers or other visitors entering and leaving prisons (e.g., lawyers, clergy workers, etc.). While it is important to better monitor the health statuses of prison staff through systematic and frequent testing, the solutions to combatting and preventing the further spread of the virus cannot strictly be limited to better monitoring and restricting who enters and leaves prisons, because infections have already entered and transmitted throughout many prisons across the U.S. The cases that already exist within prison populations, especially those that are asymptomatic, must also be contained. To do so, prison population sizes must be vastly reduced to allow for effective social distancing and quarantining of infected inmates.

Earlier in the pandemic, even in the case of jail settings, staff appeared to be the source of COVID-19 outbreaks, despite that individuals are newly admitted and released at much higher rates than prisons (Ollove, 2020). High turnover rates aid in increasing the opportunities for transmission of the virus. According to a report released in April by ACLU Analytics in tandem with Washington State University, University of Pennsylvania, and University of Tennessee, it was estimated that jails could potentially contribute anywhere from 99,000 to 188,000 individuals to the U.S. death toll, depending on how effective the safety precautions were/are exercised (e.g., social distancing, wearing personal protective equipment, etc.; American Civil Liberties Union, 2020). In order to reduce spreading of the virus, jails have released inmates, law enforcement agencies have been making less arrests, and courts have ordered administrative releases (Prison Policy Initiative, 2020b). States like California have implemented statewide reductions in the cost of bail for most misdemeanor and low-level felony offenses to 0 USD. Consequently, counties such as Los Angeles and Sacramento have experienced 30% decreases in their jail populations. Other counties such as San Diego and San Mateo released hundreds of individuals held in jail pre-trial. Many states have also opted to release inmates early that were soon-to-be released and/or medically vulnerable (Prison Policy Initiative, 2020b).

COVID-19 outbreaks in prisons and jails in Mexico

In comparison to the U.S., the next largest prison system in North America, Mexico, currently houses 198,384 inmates among 300 jails/penitentiaries (World Prison Brief, 2020). Between April and mid-September, according to ASILEGAL (2020), over 3,200 inmates have tested positive for COVID-19 and at least 316 deaths were reported among Mexican prisons. The prisons experiencing the brunt of COVID-19's impact can be found within Mexico City, Puebla, Baja California, and Veracruz (Bonello, 2020).

Despite that Mexico has a much smaller prison population and prevalence of nationwide COVID-19 cases relative to the U.S., prisons within Mexico are notorious for overcrowding, being poorly resourced and unsanitary, lacking transparency, and corruption (Bonello, 2020). According to the Instituto Nacional de Estadística y Geografía (Encuesta Nacional de Población Privada de la Libertad (ENPOL) 2016: Principales resultados, 2017), 46% of inmates throughout Mexico's prisons share a cell with at least 5 other inmates and 13% with more than 15 inmates. These conditions are likely contributing to the transmission of COVID-19 among inmates and, consequently, back into the community through staff and/or visitors. Overcrowding is not conducive to proper isolation strategies and social distancing practices, both of which aid in combatting the spread of the virus. Positive cases and deaths due to COVID-19 among inmates are likely underreported, given Mexico's history of lacking transparency, in addition to a lack of existing testing and information/data collection systems, which can be mainly attributed to Mexico's extremely underfunded prison systems (Agoff et al., this volume; Marmolejo, et al., this volume).

In response to the virus, the president and Mexican Congress passed a prisoner amnesty law in April, which was aimed at releasing nonviolent, low-level inmates as a containment measure, including those who have been convicted of robbery, small-scale drug possession, receiving abortions, and being coerced to work with criminal gangs (Felbab-Brown, 2020). The Mexican Congress approximated that 2,600 inmates would be eligible for release under this law (Felbab-Brown, 2020); however, not a single inmate has been released as of this review (Marmolejo, et al., this volume).

COVID-19 outbreaks in prisons and jails in Cuba

Cuba has the third largest prison system in the North/Central America & Caribbean regions (N = 57,337) and a much smaller total land mass size and population relative to countries like Canada, the U.S., and Mexico. However, they have a serious COVID-19 outbreak problem. As of August 21, 2020, 3,565 COVID-19 cases and 88 COVID-19 related deaths country-wide have been reported since the outbreak of the pandemic (Index Mundi, 2020). It appears that Cuba's prison system's response to the virus has been largely successful. At the end of July, the National Institute of Epidemiology revealed that there had been zero positive COVID-19 cases reported within Cuba's prison system.[7]

Cuba's success in abating COVID-19 within its prisons may be attributable to the government sending home 6,579 inmates – one the largest Cuban releases of inmates in decades – as part of a comprehensive prevention and control plan (Gamez Torres, 2020). By the end of April, other rigorous, preventative measures had been implemented including providing hand disinfectants at points of access to units, requiring inmates and staff to wear masks, prohibiting workers or visitors with feverish symptoms or without masks to enter the premises, placing newly incarcerated individuals in isolation for 15 days in order to detect potentially infected inmates and contain the spread, limiting the total number of visitors, conducting daily investigations twice per day to identify inmates with symptoms, disseminating preventative medicines to boost inmates' immune systems, and providing specialized attention to vulnerable groups such as those that are HIV positive and women who are pregnant (Prensa Latina, 2020).

COVID-19 outbreaks in prisons and jails in Canada

Despite that the U.S. and Canada have similar land mass sizes, the U.S. has approximately 8.64 times as many citizens as Canada.[8] Canada has a relatively small population in comparison to total land mass size. Moreover, Canada has less than 40,000 inmates incarcerated in its prisons, which is 53.6 times smaller than the U.S.'s prison population, despite sharing nearly the same total land mass size (World Prison Brief, 2020). Nevertheless, Canada houses the 44th largest prison system in the world (World Prison Brief, 2020). Collectively, according to the Canadian government, as of August 20, 2020, Canada has reported at least 123,873 positive COVID-19 cases and over 9000 deaths (Government of Canada, 2020). Despite the prevalence of positive COVID-19 cases and deaths among Canadian communities, by August 18, 2020, Canadian federal institutions have managed and contained the virus to a total of 360 positive cases (Correctional Service Canada [CSC], 2020).[9]

The low prevalence of positive tests in Canadian prisons may be attributed to the low number of tests being administered among inmates (i.e., according to CSC, as of mid-August, a total of 1534 tests had been administered relative to the near 40,000 inmates residing in Canadian prisons). Another explanation is that the proactive decision was made to release roughly 6,000 low-risk inmates in Canadian institutions, including provincial jails, between February and April (Statistics Canada, 2020, August 12). The average Canadian jail size decreased by 25% compared to a 1% decrease in prisons during the same time frame (Statistics Canada, 2020, August 12). To maintain the decrease in rates of incarcerated individuals, Canada also extended parole and implemented alternatives to those awaiting trial or sentencing (Cousins, 2020). As previously stated, due to the higher turnover rates within jails, which likely maximize opportunity for transmission, the Canadian government's decision to target jails early on in the pandemic may have contributed to better containing the virus. In managing the remaining correctional population behind bars, institutions reportedly provided inmates with increased access to hygiene and cleaning supplies, began screening inmates for COVID-19 before taking them in to custody, suspended inter-regional transfers, and allowed for video visitation sessions with loved ones (Cousins, 2020).

COVID-19 outbreaks in prisons and jails in El Salvador

Not unlike other Central America countries, El Salvador's prison system is wrought with overcrowding (i.e., built for a capacity of 18,000 inmates, yet houses over 36,000), poor quality of food and air, inconsistent access to clean water, and broadly, for its inhumane treatment of inmates (Cady Hallett, 2020; Human Rights Watch, 2020). For example, well before the pandemic ensued (i.e., 2016), at a local level, visitors/observers were already unable to enter Salvadorian prisons, thus entirely cutting off inmates from seeing and interacting with loved ones in-person. Even with continued "no contact" with the outside world, inmates are not capable of abiding by recommended safety guidelines such as social distancing and wearing masks. Stated simply, Salvadorian prisons are not equipped to combat the virus once it infiltrates. By late April, a total of 1,400 inmates and prison staff had tested positive for COVID-19 throughout El Salvador (Wion, 2020). Moreover, two separate outbreaks with 25 and 11 positive cases were reported among two prisons at the end of May (Reuters staff, 2020).

It has been reported that controversy unfolded in El Salvador due to the president's declaration of a strictly enforced, national, mandatory quarantine, which resulted in the arrest and detainment of thousands of citizens for violating quarantine restrictions, in addition to infringing on their individual rights (Cady Hallett, 2020; Human Rights Watch, 2020). These actions on behalf of the government call to question the president's intention in implementing strict lockdowns in prisons and within the community at large. In other words, is strictly enforcing lockdowns in the community via detainment counter-active to slowing the spread of the virus by failing to reduce (and thus increasing) the number of incarcerated individuals in its correctional system? Despite the pre-existing vulnerabilities within Salvadorian prisons as well as the punitive approach to addressing COVID-19 in the community, the Salvadorian prison system has implemented strategies that mainly focus on containing the virus, such as extensive lockdowns (therefore restricting the transfer of inmates to other facilities), restrictions on programming and other activities within prisons, and specific sanitary protocols (see Pitts & Inkpen, this volume).

Concluding comments

There are lessons to be learned from comparing how the governments of countries with large prison populations in these geographic regions have documented the extent of COVID-19 outbreaks in their prisons and jails, as well as how they have responded during the first several months of the pandemic. Two recommendations come immediately to mind: (1) governments need to be transparent about testing protocols, testing levels, and testing results; and (2) the most effective mitigation strategy currently used by the governments in these regions appears to be early prison and jail population reduction strategies.

Notes

1. We have combined these three geographic regions for the purpose of this review, but we recognize that the countries profiled here are from three distinct regions that need to be examined separately. See the country-specific profiles included in the special issue for more detail about the importance of regional culture and context.
2. For more detail, see the country-specific reviews included in this volume covering each of the five countries we profile here.
3. Jail population sizes fluctuate frequently. See Sawyer and Wagner (2020) and Prison Policy Initiative (2020a) for more details.
4. This total reflects the cumulative number of inmates that have tested positive for COVID-19 within U.S. prisons as of August 20, 2020. The total reflected in Table 1, has since been updated, thus reflecting a much larger cumulative total.

5. The inmate totals for deaths and those who have recovered is based on data provided on August 20, 2020 (The Marshall Project, 2020).
6. Data provided by the CDC on statewide COVID-19 case rates in Florida, California, and Texas were updated on August 21, 2020. Data provided by the Marshall Project on prison systems' COVID-19 case prevalence for corresponding states were updated on August 20, 2020.
7. The citizens of Cuba can be jailed for not wearing masks, but we do not have data on how often this occurs (Gamez Torres, 2020). Moreover, since the end of July, positive cases may have emerged; however, official statistics have not been released, to our knowledge.
8. Canada consists of 3.855 million square miles (Statistics Canada, 2020, January 17) with approximately 37.97 million inhabitants (Statistics Canada, 2020, June 18) while the U.S. consists of around 3.797 million square miles with approximately 328.2 million residents (U. S. Census Bureau, 2020a, 2020b).
9. The total reflected in Table 1 has since been updated, thus reflecting a larger cumulative total.

Disclosure statement

No potential conflict of interest was reported by the author(s).

ORCID

Lina Marmolejo http://orcid.org/0000-0002-2841-2627

References

A state-by-state look at Coronavirus in prisons. (2020, April 14). The Marshall Project. https://www.themarshallproject.org/2020/05/01/a-state-by-state-look-at-coronavirus-in-prisons

ASILEGAL. (2020). *Cifras a nivel nacional al 17 de septiembre de 2020*. Asistencia Legal por los Derechos Humanos. https://asilegal.org.mx/mapa-penitenciario-covid-19/

Bonello, D. (2020, August 18). *COVID may be killing hundreds of prisoners in Mexico*. Vice. https://www.vice.com/en_us/article/7kpq9g/covid-may-be-killing-hundreds-of-prisoners-in-mexico

Cady Hallett, M. (2020, March 29). *Mass arrests and overcrowded prisons in El Salvador spark fear of coronavirus crisis*. The Conversation. https://theconversation.com/mass-arrests-and-overcrowded-prisons-in-el-salvador-spark-fear-of-coronavirus-crisis-137673

Canada's population estimates, first quarter 2020. (2020, June 18). *Statistics Canada*. https://www150.statcan.gc.ca/n1/daily-quotidien/200618/dq200618b-eng.htm?HPA=1&indid=4098-1&indgeo=0

Centers for Disease Control and Prevention. (2020, April 19). *United States COVID-19 cases and deaths by state: Reported to the CDC since January 21, 2020*. CDC COVID Data Tracker. https://www.cdc.gov/covid-data-tracker/#cases

Changes in federal, provincial and territorial custodial populations during the COVID-19 pandemic, April 2019 to April 2020. (2020, August 12). Statistics Canada. https://www150.statcan.gc.ca/n1/daily-quotidien/200812/dq200812a-eng.htm?CMP=mstatcan

Coronavirus cases – Cuba. (2020, August 21). Index Mundi. https://www.indexmundi.com/coronavirus/country/cu

Coronavirus disease (COVID-19): Outbreak update. (2020, August 20). Government of Canada. https://www.canada.ca/en/public-health/services/diseases/2019-novel-coronavirus-infection.html

Cousins, B. (2020, August 12). *Provincial jails released thousands of inmates amid calls to slow the spread of COVID-19*. CVT News. https://www.ctvnews.ca/canada/provincial-jails-released-thousands-of-inmates-amid-calls-to-slow-the-spread-of-covid-19-1.5061829?cache=piqndqvkh%3FautoPlay%3Dtrue%3FclipId%3D89926

COVID-19 model finds nearly 100,000 more deaths than current estimates, due to failures to reduce jails. (2020). American Civil Liberties Union. https://www.aclu.org/sites/default/files/field_document/aclu_covid19-jail-report_2020-8_1.pdf

Encuesta Nacional de Población Privada de la Libertad (ENPOL) 2016: Principales resultados. (2017). Instituto Nacional de Estadística y Geografía. https://www.inegi.org.mx/contenidos/programas/enpol/2016/doc/2016_enpol_presentacion_ejecutiva.pdf

Felbab-Brown, V. (2020, May 22). *Mexico's prisons, COVID-19, and the amnesty law.* Brookings. https://www.brookings.edu/blog/order-from-chaos/2020/05/26/mexicos-prisons-covid-19-and-the-amnesty-law/

Gamez Torres, N. (2020, May 1). *Cuba releases thousands of prison inmates amid coronavirus fears.* Miami Herald. https://www.miamiherald.com/news/nation-world/world/americas/cuba/article242435511.html

Geography. (2020, January 17). Statistics Canada. https://www150.statcan.gc.ca/n1/pub/11-402-x/2011000/chap/geo/geo-eng.htm#archived

Heard, C. (2019). *Towards a health-informed approach to penal reform? Evidence from ten countries.* Birkbeck Institutional Research Online. https://eprints.bbk.ac.uk/id/eprint/27743

Human Rights Watch (2020, April 29). *El Salvador: Inhumane prison lockdown treatment.* https://www.hrw.org/news/2020/04/29/el-salvador-inhumane-prison-lockdown-treatment

Inmate COVID-19 testing in federal correctional institutions August 18, 2020. (2020). Correctional Service Canada. https://www.csc-scc.gc.ca/001/006/001006-1014-en.shtml

Inmates in El Salvador suffer as Latin American prisons breed COVID-19. (2020, April 28). Wion News. https://www.wionews.com/world/inmates-in-el-salvador-suffer-as-latin-american-prisons-breed-covid-19-295382

New report, Arrest, Release, Repeat, *reveals how many people go to jail each year and how many times they go.* (2020a, August 26). Prison Policy Initiative. https://www.prisonpolicy.org/blog/2019/08/26/arrests-report/

Nowonty, K. M., & Piquero, A. R. (2020). The global impact of the pandemic on institutional and community corrections: Assessing short-term crisis management and long-term change strategies. *Victims & Offenders* (this volume). https://doi.org/10.1080/15564886.2020.1813229

Ollove, M. (2020, July 1). *How COVID-19 in jails and prisons threatens nearby communities.* Pew Research Institute. https://www.pewtrusts.org/en/research-and-analysis/blogs/stateline/2020/07/01/how-covid-19-in-jails-and-prisons-threatens-nearby-communities

Prensa Latina. (2020, April 23). *Cuban prisons without Covid-19 cases.* Agencia de Noticias Latinoamericana. https://www.plenglish.com/index.php?o=rn&id=54921&SEO=cuban-prisons-without-covid-19-cases

Responses to the COVID-19 pandemic. (2020b, August 18). Prison Policy Initiative. https://www.prisonpolicy.org/virus/virusresponse.html

Reuters staff. (2020, May 25). *Thirty-six inmates test positive for coronavirus in Salvadoran prisons.* Reuters. https://www.reuters.com/article/us-health-coronavirus-elsalvador/thirty-six-inmates-test-positive-for-coronavirus-in-salvadoran-prisons-idUSKBN23208O

Sawyer, W., & Wagner, P. (2020). *Mass incarceration: The whole pie 2020.* Prison Policy Initiative. https://www.prisonpolicy.org/reports/pie2020.html

State area measurements and internal point coordinates. (2020a). United States Census Bureau. https://www.census.gov/geographies/reference-files/2010/geo/state-area.html

U.S. and world population clock. (2020b, August 21). United States Census Bureau. https://www.census.gov/popclock/

World Prison Brief. (2020, August). *World prison brief data.* Institute for Crime & Justice Policy Research (ICPR). https://www.prisonstudies.org/world-prison-brief-data

Zeng, Z. (2020). *Jail inmates in 2018.* U.S. Department of Justice, Bureau of Justice Statistics. https://www.bjs.gov/content/pub/pdf/ji17.pdf

Institutional Responses to the COVID-19 Pandemic in American Prisons

Meghan A. Novisky, Chelsey S. Narvey, and Daniel C. Semenza

ABSTRACT

The COVID-19 pandemic infiltrated the United States in early 2020, with correctional facilities becoming hot spots for the novel coronavirus shortly thereafter. Using data gathered from Departments of Corrections' official websites, we provide a summary of state and federal prison system responses to COVID-19 as of June 2020. We highlight strengths and deficiencies in system responses as well as pertinent variations across jurisdictions. We conclude with a call for scholars and grant funders to prioritize incarceration-based data collection efforts on COVID-19 so the short and long-term consequences of the pandemic, and systemic responses to it, can be more fully assessed.

Introduction

The novel coronavirus (COVID-19) pandemic was first documented in the U.S. in early 2020 and spread quickly throughout the country thereafter. As of September 8, 2020, the United States is responsible for 23% of the world's confirmed cases of COVID-19 (n = 6,318,978) and 21% of the world's COVID-19 deaths (n = 189,456), despite making up only about 4.25% of the global population (Johns Hopkins University, 2020). As with the rest of the world, the pandemic has placed major strains on the United States and has presented substantive challenges to a number of different social institutions, including nursing homes, schools, and churches. Correctional facilities serve as particularly salient examples of vulnerable spaces in the U.S., incarcerating nearly 1.5 million people in prisons (Bronson & Carson, 2019), and processing over 10 million annual jail admissions annually (Zeng, 2020).

The sheer volume of people incarcerated throughout the U.S., coupled with common environmental features of correctional facilities, including overcrowding, reduced sanitation, insufficient access to healthcare, poor ventilation, and inabilities to socially distance, have posed unique challenges and risks for incarcerated persons and staff during the pandemic (Nowotny et al., 2020). People incarcerated in jails and prisons also tend to have worse health than the general population (Binswanger et al., 2009; Wilper et al., 2009), meaning that these spaces disproportionately house health-compromised individuals at baseline. It is therefore not surprising that at the time of this writing, the 15 largest hotspots or "clusters" of COVID-19 cases in the U.S. were all identified as correctional facilities (New York Times, 2020).

Given these circumstances, correctional system responses to the pandemic in the U.S. warrant closer attention. In this paper, we contribute to the literature by providing an overview of institutional responses to COVID-19 in prisons across the United States using data gathered from Department of Corrections' official websites in June 2020. We focus our analysis on the strengths and deficiencies of system responses as well as pertinent variations that occurred across jurisdictions. We conclude with a discussion of the results of our analysis and offer recommendations for improving correctional responses to the COVID-19 pandemic moving forward.

Background

In response to the COVID-19 pandemic, governments across the globe have enacted stay-at-home and social distancing orders to mitigate the spread of the virus. These orders mandate that individuals stay home and refrain from interacting with large groups of people to the extent possible, or limit interactions to small groups as needed. Where interaction is unavoidable, the Centers for Disease Control and Prevention (CDC) suggests that people maintain a distance of at least 6 feet from one another, wear personal protective equipment (PPE) such as facemasks, and practice rigorous hand-washing hygiene (Centers for Disease Control and Prevention [CDCa], 2020). Despite these recommended strategies, many prisons and jails have struggled to adhere to basic public health guidelines, largely as a result of inherent limitations within the structure and function of correctional facilities.

Prisons and jails are high-risk settings for the spread of COVID-19 due to a higher background prevalence of other infectious diseases, limited access to healthcare services relative to community settings, and a greatly reduced capacity for practicing social distancing measures in most facilities (Akiyama et al., 2020; Hawks et al., 2020; Kinner et al., 2020). Many institutions are overcrowded in the U.S., further driving residents and correctional officers into close quarters and rendering outbreak prevention more difficult because of greater population density in many prisons and jails (Hawks et al., 2020). Since correctional settings represent particularly high-risk locations for COVID-19 outbreaks, researchers and medical professionals have concluded that many jails and prisons are likely to experience COVID-19 outbreaks and that targeted preventive efforts for correctional facilities must be included in any nationwide outbreak mitigation strategies (Kinner et al., 2020; Marcum, 2020; Montoya-Barthelemy et al., 2020; Wurcel et al., 2020). Specifically, public health and medical professionals have recommended a series of preventive efforts to reduce the risk of COVID-19 outbreaks in correctional facilities that include increased provision of cleaning and sanitizing supplies, rapidly improving testing and isolation capacity, granting early release for medically high-risk and low-level offending segments of incarcerated populations, and consulting with experts in gerontology to prepare for the unique challenges posed by COVID-19 to older incarcerated adults (Malloy et al., 2020; Okano & Blower, 2020; Prost et al., 2020; Wurcel et al., 2020).

It appears that correctional authorities in many states have taken action against the spread of COVID-19, often in response to state-mandated guidelines. Research shows that places like Los Angeles county, for instance, have adopted preventive measures such as the early release of people convicted of low-level offenses or admitting fewer people into jails (Okano & Blower, 2020). A number of states, including Alabama, Colorado, Massachusetts, Michigan, Ohio, Pennsylvania, and Texas have also reduced their jail or prison populations by releasing people considered to be at low-risk of criminal behavior, as well as those considered to be high risk as far as health status (Prison Policy Initiative, 2020). Despite these efforts, it remains unclear how various states and facilities are incorporating local and federal guidance into actionable policies within facilities to prevent and mitigate the spread of the virus.

Furthermore, scholars are concerned that mitigation efforts to reduce the spread of COVID-19, such as visitation suspensions and isolation strategies, are likely to have unintended consequences, including poorer mental health among prisoner populations (Hewson et al., 2020; Kothari et al., 2020). For instance, incarcerated persons may face increased risks for self-harm and depression due to diminished social contact. Reduced abilities to see loved ones face to face or communicate with them verbally in the midst of a pandemic may raise anxieties and fears about risks for infection, both personally and out of concern for loved ones. Risks for infractions may also increase given that incarcerated individuals who maintain visits are less likely to commit misconduct (Cochran, 2012; Reidy & Sorensen, 2020). Abrupt changes in prison operations, including mask mandates, physical distancing requirements, and reductions in movement, may also increase the potential for misconduct reports given the rapid introduction of new rules that require substantial changes in behavior. Demand for contraband items, including cell phones to connect with family and drugs to cope with likely increases in stress, may escalate. Accumulation of such infractions could then have detrimental impacts on institutional privileges, custody status, and judicial release decisions.

To date, what is known about COVID-19 in correctional facilities across states has largely been culled by data collection efforts from groups like the COVID Prison Project (2020) and the Marshall Project (2020), based on information supplied by cooperating Departments of Corrections. As of September 8th, 2020, the COVID-19 Prison Project reports that 119,858 prisoners and 23,695 correctional staff have tested positive for COVID-19. Of those that have contracted the virus, 974 prisoners and 67 staff have died as a result of complications related to COVID-19, bringing the total correctional death toll in the United States thus far to 1,041.

The national case rate of COVID-19 in prisons and jails is estimated to be about 3,251 per 100,000 prisoners, or roughly 5.5 times that of the general U.S. population (Saloner et al., 2020). However, case rates vary considerably across jurisdictions, ranging from .23 (Hawaii) to 321.39 (Arkansas) per 1,000 prisoners as reported by the COVID Prison Project (2020). Adjusted for age and sex distribution, the death rate in prisons is about 39 deaths per 100,000 prisoners, or roughly 3 times higher than the U.S. in general. To illustrate, the number of prisoner deaths range from zero in states like Hawaii, North Dakota, Rhode Island, South Dakota, and Utah to upwards of more than 140 deaths in Texas alone (a rate of about 11 deaths per 10,000) (Marshall Project, 2020). Although updated year-over-year mortality data will be needed to make a firm determination, it is probable that the disproportionate death rate in prisons has contributed to an increase in the all-cause mortality rate in prisons in 2020 compared to 2016 (303 per 100,000 prisoners), the most recent year for which prison and jail mortality data are available (Carson & Cowhig, 2020). Significant heterogeneity in basic testing and mortality statistics related to COVID-19 among correctional facilities suggests that a better understanding is needed regarding the actual policies put into practice and what is most effective at reducing outbreaks across locales (Malloy et al., 2020).

In addition, largely missing from the research on COVID-19 in correctional facilities are the perspectives of residents confined in prisons and jails. However, Pyrooz et al. (2020) offer an initial qualitative assessment of the challenges of COVID-19 in correctional facilities, based on interviews with a sample of 31 men incarcerated in a maximum security prison in Oregon. The findings demonstrate that prisoners perceive their risk of contracting COVID-19 "not as a matter of if, but rather as a matter of when," the virus will spread throughout the prison system (Pyrooz et al., 2020, p. 8). Incarcerated individuals are particularly concerned about community spread in correctional facilities via correctional officers who come in and out of the facilities. Yet the respondents in Oregon were not particularly concerned about contracting the virus themselves, in part due to restrictive housing policies that were perceived as advantageous within the context of the pandemic. While many of the respondents in this study felt that Oregon correctional facilities were taking virus mitigation efforts seriously, they also did not trust that an outbreak could be contained once let loose among incarcerated persons. This study provides preliminary insight into the perceptions of risk and treatment availability among incarcerated individuals living in one particular correctional setting, however a greater comparative approach to understanding COVID-19 responses across states is needed to more fully assess the efficacy of actions being taken.

Current study

In this paper, we present a comparative approach to understand patterned jurisdictional variations in correctional system responses to COVID-19. This is valuable because although prisons and jails are high risk sites for the spread of infectious disease generally (Massoglia, 2008; Nowotny et al., 2020), the severity of the public health threats posed by COVID-19 spread in correctional facilities is likely to fluctuate across states and even individual institutions. Variations may reflect factors including correctional population size and efforts to implement mitigation efforts, for example. In many ways, the fragmented response of the country's state and federal correctional systems is symbolic of the broader approach to the pandemic throughout the United States as a whole. Thus, our analysis can help to highlight the unique challenges that face an often divided and polarized country that has struggled to confront the singular threat of COVID-19.

Understanding differences in correctional responses is important. Beyond the substantial medical risks of COVID-19 infection in correctional facilities (Reinhart & Chen, 2020), experiences during incarceration can predict access to medical care and perceptions of the correctional health care system (Novisky, 2018). Health conditions are also related to the likelihood of successful reentry (Link et al., 2019; Semenza & Link, 2019). Differences in responses can influence the mental health toll of being incarcerated during a pandemic. This is the case not only because the availability of mental health services in the context of COVID-19 may fluctuate (Liebrenz et al., 2020), but also because the humaneness of confinement during this time is directly dependent upon the measures taken by prisons and jails to protect their confined populations. In short, understanding patterned differences in correctional responses to the pandemic across jurisdictions is likely to assist with assessing the longer-term consequences of the pandemic tied to physical and mental health, recidivism, and potential 8th amendment litigation efforts.

Methods

To assess correctional system responses to COVID-19 in the U.S., we relied on a manual web-based data scraping methodology. We first made a list of all 50 state Department of Correction (DOC) websites plus the Federal Bureau of Prisons (BOP)[1] website (total n of websites = 51). These government websites became the sources for this project. As a team, we created a database in advance of data collection to establish consistency regarding what data needed to be pulled from each website to address our research question. Upon implementation, our database was designed to track the following for each of the 51 correctional jurisdictions: correctional population size; first confirmed COVID-19 case; total tests, cases, hospitalizations, recoveries, and deaths reported among prisoners; total tests, cases, hospitalizations, recoveries, and deaths reported among staff; visitation policy changes; provision of PPE; mitigation efforts; and other important notes about COVID-19 response efforts (e.g., whether there were frequent updates on the reporting website or if these data were easy to find). Thus, we ultimately collected a combination of quantitative and qualitative data to inform our final results.

It is important to note that assessing correctional responses to COVID-19 during the pandemic involves somewhat of a moving target. Information on the number of positive cases and tests change daily, for example.[2] Thus, our goal was to analyze system responses based on the information available across jurisdictions *at that designated point in time*. To accomplish this, we split the labor of scraping data from the 51 sources equally across the research team and did all of our data gathering on the same day. On June 16, 2020, we filled in the data from our respective jurisdictions simultaneously and communicated as a research team while we did so. This helped us to begin establishing similarities and departures in responses across jurisdictions early on. This protocol also allowed us to be responsive in incorporating additional columns in our database during data collection as needed. It became apparent early on, for example, that we should collect information on the extent to which prisoners were being asked to manufacture PPE, as this information emerged multiple times during data collection efforts. We therefore ended up adding a column on prisoner manufacturing of PPE to our database during data collection.

As we entered the data from each website, we also saved copies of supporting documents (e.g., posted response plans, FAQ to family) and screenshots (e.g., announcements about visitation cessation, memos detailing first confirmed COVID-19 cases). We later conducted a content analysis of these documents, adding additional details to our database from them as appropriate. Once all of the quantitative and qualitative data were collected, we analyzed all state and federal systems for commonalities across a number of metrics and categories to identify similarities and differences. The results presented in the next section reflect these efforts and ultimately highlight the patterned strengths and deficiencies in institutional responses to the pandemic within prisons that emerged during data analysis.

Results

Strengths

(I) *Access*

All 51 correctional jurisdiction websites provided some type of online access point for COVID-19 updates. With few exceptions, this access point was readily identifiable and accessible from each website's homepage. Thus, as a whole, correctional jurisdictions were responsive in adding web-based access points so the public could locate COVID-19 information relevant to each correctional jurisdiction. Although the depth of information provided varied across jurisdictions, these web links tended to include information about testing data (e.g., number tested, number of positive cases), COVID-19 related announcements (i.e., changes in visitation policies), information about the precautions being taken, and news releases. While 94% of correctional websites (n = 48) posted a direct COVID-19 link housed within the correctional system's official website, in some cases links to COVID-19 information directed users to the state's Department of Health website (e.g., North Carolina, West Virginia) or social media website (e.g., Rhode Island).

(II) *Testing*

Eighty-two percent of correctional agencies (n = 42) also made efforts to post information about the first confirmed cases to enter their jurisdictions (see Table 1). Of the jurisdictions providing this information, 64% (n = 27) reported their first cases in March, with the first infection reported in Washington on March 12th, 2020. Thirteen more states reported their first cases in April, with Utah and Montana reporting their first cases as late as May and June, respectively. Notably, more than half of the first cases reported across the 42 jurisdictions (n = 23) were infections of staff members.

(III) *Visitation*

All 51 correctional jurisdictions suspended prisoner visitation to reduce the volume of traffic coming in and out of prisons at any given time, with the vast majority implementing these changes in mid-March. To help offset visitation freezes, 72% of states (n = 37) provided incarcerated men and women some combination of free phone calls, video visits, e-mails, and stamps. Among states providing these supplementary communication opportunities, the number of communications and the length of communications varied substantially.

Provision of phone calls ranged from one free five minute call per week (Iowa) to ten free fifteen minute calls per week (Utah). Availability of video visits ranged from one free video visit per week (North Dakota) to three free video visits per week (Kansas). As for e-mails, incarcerated individuals were given anywhere from to one (Missouri) to eight (Ohio) free e-mails weekly. Four jurisdictions (Michigan, New Jersey, New York, and Virginia) highlighted their efforts to provide free stamps to enhance communication opportunities in lieu of in person visits. While visitations were halted across the U.S., 18% of jurisdictions (n = 9) did specify that these suspensions did not apply to prisoner meetings with attorneys.

Table 1. First reported COVID-19 cases.

	March (n = 27)			April (n = 13)	
	First Infection	Person Infected		First Infection	Person Infected
Washington	3–12	Staff	North Carolina	4–1	Prisoner
Georgia	3–18	Staff	Oregon	4–2	Prisoner
New York	3–18	Prisoner	Arkansas	4–3	Staff
Wisconsin	3–18	Staff	New Hampshire	4–3	Staff
Alabama	3–19	Staff	Tennessee	4–3	Prisoner
FBOP	3–19	Prisoner	Nebraska	4–4	Staff
Maine	3–21	Staff	Delaware	4–6	Prisoner
California	3–22	Prisoner	Arizona	4–7	Prisoner
Florida	3–22	Staff	Iowa	4–10	Staff
Michigan	3–22	Prisoner	Wyoming	4–10	Staff
Connecticut	3–23	Staff	Mississippi	4–13	Prisoner
Missouri	3–23	Prisoner	Indiana	4–14	Staff
South Dakota	3–23	Prisoner	Alaska	4–26	Prisoner
Texas	3–23	Staff			
Vermont	3–23	Staff	May (n = 1)		
Illinois	3–24	Staff			
Colorado	3–26	Staff	Utah	5–29	Prisoner
Louisiana	3–26	Staff			
Nevada	3–26	Staff	June (n = 1)		
South Carolina	3–27	Staff			
Ohio	3–29	Staff	Montana	6–9	Prisoner
Pennsylvania	3–29	Prisoner			
Rhode Island	3–29	Staff			
Maryland	3–30	Prisoner + Staff			
Minnessota	3–30	Prisoner			
Kansas	3–31	Staff			
Virginia	3–31	Prisoner			

First infection data were not reported for the following states: HI, ID, KY, MA, NJ, NM, ND, OK, WV.

(IV) *Other Mitigation Efforts*

Other preventive responses to the pandemic to protect incarcerated people and correctional officers appear to vary widely from state to state. While sanitization efforts throughout facilities have increased across correctional jurisdictions, sanitation responses ranged from vague descriptions such as "deep cleaning," to more detailed efforts, including spraying bleach-based disinfectant on surfaces, providing greater accessibility of cleaning supplies to correctional workers and prisoners, spraying the hands of incarcerated individuals with disinfectant, increasing the frequency with which surfaces are cleaned, and placing hand sanitizer dispensers in common areas. Seven jurisdictions (Alabama, Alaska, BOP, Maine, New Mexico, Missouri, Utah) described efforts to post preventive signage and pamphlets regarding hand washing and social distancing measures to reduce the risk of spreading the virus. Others went as far as to host educational townhalls (Pennsylvania) and "sanitation broadcasts" (BOP). Nearly one-third of jurisdictions (n = 15) also noted providing increased access to soap for prisoners at no cost to help encourage frequent hand washing and further assist with sanitation efforts.

Many correctional systems also indicate implementation of preventive screening for correctional officers and staff in some capacity. Forty-one percent of jurisdictions (n = 21) posted materials detailing their policies for mandatory temperature readings and verbal symptom screenings for all staff. Some departments specify that screening is also required for all new prisoners and those being released, although this does not appear to apply to departments where transfers have been halted or new prisoners are not being accepted. However, regular screening does not generally appear to apply to those prisoners that are already in residence for the majority of the state correctional systems. Thus, screening is largely used to test for symptomatic positive COVID-19 cases among those most frequently moving in and out of the individual facilities. Finally, a number of departments outline a quarantine policy for new prisoners, transfers, and any residents displaying symptoms of the virus. These isolation practices were not outlined for many departments, however, and most state responses appear to focus largely on broader preventive efforts to reduce viral spread.

Deficiencies

(I) *Testing*

COVID-19 data posted across jurisdictions were not comprehensive and often lacked transparency. One of the driving factors regarding poor data transparency was an obvious lack of testing. In general, mass testing of the incarcerated population was not occurring at the time of our data collection. Thirty-five percent of jurisdictions (n = 18) did not include any information on the number of prisoners they had tested for COVID-19 at all, making their testing efforts impossible to assess (see Table 2). Of the jurisdictions that did provide this information (n = 33), the number of tests ranged from 31 (New Hampshire) to 107,684 COVID-19 tests (Texas). Collectively, many states (n = 14) had tested less than 5 percent of their prisoner population for COVID-19, with few exceptions testing more than 50% of the incarcerated population (Michigan, Minnesota, Rhode Island, Tennessee, Texas, Vermont, West Virginia).

Testing of staff, which is just as important to understanding the scope of infection rates in correctional facilities, was generally described on jurisdiction websites as the individual responsibility of employees (Texas was one exception). More specifically, the number of confirmed COVID-19 cases reported on jurisdiction websites among staff were based on employees' self-reported disclosures. This means that if staff did not take initiatives to get tested for COVID-19, if they did not call off work because of COVID-19 symptoms, or if they did not share testing information or symptoms with their employers, those data would not be reported under the COVID-19 staff data. As shown in Table 3, only 19% of jurisdictions (n = 10) provided data on the number of COVID-19 tests administered among staff. Of the jurisdictions that did provide this information, the number of tests ranged from 17 (Montana) to 31,547 COVID-19 tests (Texas).

Tables 2 and Tables 3 further outline the availability of COVID-19 testing data at the time of our data collection regarding prisoners and staff, respectively. The most common COVID-19 data offered about prisoners was the number of confirmed positive prisoner cases. As indicated in Table 2, all jurisdictions made this information available, although three jurisdictions (Hawaii, Idaho, Wyoming) reported no positive cases to report at the time of data collection. The majority of jurisdictions (n = 30) also posted data on the number of deaths of incarcerated people due to COVID-19, although 17 jurisdictions reported no deaths at the time of data collection and four jurisdictions (South Carolina, Washington, West Virginia, and Wisconsin) included no data on prisoner mortality at all. While 64% of jurisdictions (n = 33) provided data on the number of prisoners who had recovered from COVID-19, nearly one-third of jurisdictions (n = 15) included no data on

Table 2. Availability of COVID-19 prisoner data.

	# of Tests	# of Positive Cases	# Hospitalized	# of Deaths	# Recovered
Alabama	✓	✓	–	✓	✓
Alaska	✓	✓	–	*	✓
Arizona	✓	✓	–	✓	✓
Arkansas	✓	✓	–	✓	✓
California	✓	✓	–	✓	✓
Colorado	✓	✓	–	✓	✓
Connecticut	–	✓	–	✓	✓
Delaware	–	✓	–	✓	✓
FBOP	✓	✓	–	✓	✓
Florida	✓	✓	–	✓	–
Georgia	–	✓	–	✓	✓
Hawaii	✓	*	*	*	*
Idaho	✓	*	*	*	*
Illinois	✓	✓	–	✓	✓
Indiana	✓	✓	–	✓	✓
Iowa	✓	✓	–	*	✓
Kansas	–	✓	–	✓	✓
Kentucky	–	✓	–	✓	✓
Louisiana	–	✓	–	✓	✓
Maine	✓	✓	–	*	–
Maryland	✓	✓	–	✓	✓
Massachusetts	–	✓	–	✓	–
Michigan	✓	✓	–	✓	✓
Minnesota	✓	✓	✓	*	✓
Mississippi	✓	✓	–	✓	–
Missouri	✓	✓	–	✓	✓
Montana	–	✓	–	*	–
Nebraska	–	✓	–	*	–
Nevada	–	✓	–	*	–
New Hampshire	✓	✓	–	*	–
New Jersey	–	✓	–	✓	–
New Mexico	–	✓	–	✓	–
New York	–	✓	–	✓	✓
North Carolina	–	✓	–	✓	–
North Dakota	–	✓	–	*	–
Ohio	✓	✓	–	✓	✓
Oklahoma	✓	✓	–	*	✓
Oregon	✓	✓	–	✓	✓
Pennsylvania	✓	✓	–	✓	✓
Rhode Island	✓	✓	–	*	✓
South Carolina	–	✓	–	–	✓
South Dakota	✓	✓	–	*	✓
Tennessee	✓	✓	–	✓	✓
Texas	✓	✓	–	✓	✓
Utah	✓	✓	–	*	*
Vermont	✓	✓	*	*	✓
Virginia	–	✓	✓	✓	–
Washington	✓	✓	–	–	–
West Virginia	✓	✓	–	–	✓
Wisconsin	✓	✓	–	–	✓
Wyoming	–	*	–	*	–

✓ = Data Available; – = Data Unavailable; * = 0 Cases Reported.

prisoner recoveries at all. The largest gap in information involved hospitalization data, as only two jurisdictions (Minnesota, Virginia) reported data on the number of incarcerated individuals hospitalized as a result of COVID-19.

As with incarcerated persons, the most frequent COVID-19 data offered about correctional staff was the number of positive cases among staff. As can be seen in Table 3, with the

Table 3. Availability of COVID-19 staff data.

	# of Tests	# of Positive Cases	# Hospitalized	# of Deaths	# Recovered
Alabama	–	✓	–	*	✓
Alaska	–	✓	–	*	✓
Arizona	–	✓	–	✓	✓
Arkansas	✓	✓	–	✓	✓
California	–	✓	–	✓	✓
Colorado	–	✓	–	*	✓
Connecticut	–	✓	–	*	✓
Delaware	–	✓	–	*	✓
FBOP	–	✓	–	✓	✓
Florida	–	✓	–	*	–
Georgia	–	✓	–	✓	✓
Hawaii	–	–	*	*	–
Idaho	–	*	*	*	*
Illinois	–	✓	–	*	✓
Indiana	✓	✓	–	✓	✓
Iowa	–	✓	–	*	✓
Kansas	–	✓	–	✓	✓
Kentucky	–	✓	–	*	✓
Louisiana	–	✓	–	✓	✓
Maine	–	✓	–	*	–
Maryland	✓	✓	–	✓	–
Massachusetts	–	✓	–	*	–
Michigan	–	✓	–	✓	–
Minnesota	–	✓	–	*	✓
Mississippi	✓	✓	–	*	–
Missouri	–	✓	–	*	✓
Montana	✓	✓	–	*	–
Nebraska	–	✓	–	*	–
Nevada	–	✓	–	*	–
New Hampshire	–	✓	–	–	–
New Jersey	–	✓	–	–	–
New Mexico	–	✓	–	*	–
New York	–	✓	–	✓	–
North Carolina	–	✓	–	✓	–
North Dakota	–	✓	–	*	–
Ohio	–	✓	–	✓	✓
Oklahoma	–	✓	–	*	–
Oregon	–	✓	–	*	✓
Pennsylvania	✓	✓	–	✓	✓
Rhode Island	✓	✓	–	*	✓
South Carolina	–	✓	–	–	✓
South Dakota	✓	✓	–	*	✓
Tennessee	–	✓	–	–	✓
Texas	✓	✓	–	✓	✓
Utah	–	✓	–	–	–
Vermont	–	✓	–	*	✓
Virginia	–	✓	–	–	–
Washington	–	✓	–	–	–
West Virginia	✓	✓	–	–	✓
Wisconsin	–	✓	–	–	✓
Wyoming	–	✓	*	*	✓

✓ = Data Available; – = Data Unavailable; * = 0 Cases Reported.

exception of Hawaii, all jurisdictions made this information available (however, one jurisdiction, Idaho, reported no positive cases among staff at the time of data collection). Most jurisdictions (n = 30) also provided data on the number of staff who had recovered from COVID-19. As with the prisoner data, hospitalization data on staff were especially lacking. In fact, the only available COVID-19 staff hospitalization data came from three jurisdictions that reported no hospitalizations had taken place among staff at the time of data collection (Hawaii, Idaho, Wyoming). As for mortality data, 29% of jurisdictions (n = 15) provided data on the number of correctional staff who had died of COVID-19 at the time of data collection, while 53% (n = 27) reported no correctional staff deaths and 17% (n = 9) provided no data on staff mortality at all.

(II) *Personal Protective Equipment*

Regarding PPE, we found that while 55% of jurisdictions (n = 28) did provide some type of equipment for incarcerated persons and correctional staff by mid-April, distribution of these supplies, as well as guidelines for their use, varied considerably across jurisdictions. For example, in Michigan, all prisoners and staff were provided with three masks per person and were expected to wear masks at all times. Yet, in other jurisdictions, masks for incarcerated individuals were actually banned for wear due to security reasons (e.g., Nevada), were only provided to a portion of the prisoner population (e.g., Delaware), were provided, but not required for wear (e.g., Oregon, Pennsylvania, South Carolina), or were set aside for staff first (e.g., Florida, South Dakota). The Federal Bureau of Prisons' policy stated that staff were required to wear masks when working in certain areas (e.g., quarantine or isolation units), but could "opt not to wear masks when walking on the compound." In Hawaii, masks were only required for symptomatic prisoners and staff. Other jurisdictions were more difficult to assess, such as West Virginia, which stated that those in quarantine should wear face masks "only if there is a sufficient supply," Florida, which stated masks were "provided as needed," and Tennessee, which stated masks were "being distributed as they are being produced."

(III) *Other Mitigation Efforts*

As for other mitigation efforts, we recognize that hand sanitizer is generally not available to incarcerated persons due to its high alcohol content and its classification as contraband in many prisons and jails. Our analysis determined that these parameters largely remained, even in the face of a pandemic. Specifically, we found only 10 jurisdictions that stated hand sanitizer was freely available in the prisons: Alaska, California, Delaware, Indiana, Massachusetts, New York, South Carolina, Tennessee, Vermont, and Wisconsin. In some cases, bans on hand sanitizer were temporarily lifted to make it available, but restrictions remained. For example, correctional officers were permitted to distribute hand sanitizer to prisoners in limited quantities in Ohio and South Dakota, and exceptions for hand sanitizer were permitted "for medical workers with approval of the superintendent" in West Virginia. Explanations were provided in some cases for continued bans on hand sanitizer, including that hand sanitizer can result in "potential alcohol misuse" (e.g., Colorado).

Discussion

In summary, most prison jurisdiction systems across the United States have provided information on their public websites regarding the measures being taken to prevent the spread of COVID-19 across their facilities. The majority of the systems have engaged in certain preventive measures to reduce the risk of virus spread by educating prisoners on hand washing and social distancing measures, increasing sanitization efforts, providing staff and prisoners with some cleaning supplies, and regularly screening correctional officers and staff members. Yet, as with many issues in the American criminal justice system, responses have not been uniform and often vary substantially from one jurisdictional system to the next. This is most apparent when considering the deficiencies in response to the COVID-19 pandemic within correctional facilities. Thus, the overall correctional response to the pandemic has largely mirrored the broader response from the United States government as a whole, relying on individual states and fragmented systems to implement their own policies rather than working to protect citizens through coherent and unified guidance.

We offer three main recommendations to correctional departments for strengthening the efficacy of their responses to COVID-19. First, mass testing in all facilities is needed (see also Marcum, 2020). More than a third of jurisdictions (n = 18) did not provide any information on the number of prisoners tested for COVID-19 and 80% of jurisdictions (n = 41) did not provide any information on the number of staff tested for COVID-19. Hospitalization data was rarely reported for either prisoners or staff. These gaps in information severely limit correctional jurisdictions from documenting the full scope of the problem that prisons are grappling with, thereby hindering the deployment of crucial resources and response efforts. Central to mass testing should be a requirement for correctional facilities to test all of their staff at no cost to the staff themselves, increasing the likelihood that asymptomatic cases of COVID-19 will be detected. Even if greater testing is occurring than is being reported online, greater transparency regarding the results of this testing to the public and the families of those in correctional facilities is needed.

Second, correctional jurisdictions must work to ensure adequate provision of PPE and availability of tools for proper hand hygiene, including hand sanitizers. The public health harms related to deficiencies in the provision of PPE and hand sanitizer in some U.S. jurisdictions are substantial. Facial coverings are a critical preventive tool in reducing risk for COVID-19 infection, as they can reduce the spray of respiratory droplets when worn properly (Konda et al., 2020). According to the CDCb (2020), masks are especially necessary for prevention in close quarters where social distancing measures range from difficult to impossible to implement. Such circumstances undoubtedly include prisons. Yet, multiple jurisdictions either did not provide unrestricted access to facial coverings or did not require staff or prisoners (or both) to use them – even months into the pandemic. The importance of hand hygiene in combatting the spread of COVID-19 is also vital (Kratzel et al., 2020). This is especially true when people lack unrestricted access to sinks for hand washing, which is the case in many prisons where incarcerated persons share bathrooms with dormitories of dozens, if not hundreds, of other adults. If hand sanitizer must remain a restricted from of contraband for those in prisons, then facilities should look to find ways of distributing the sanitizer in select amounts via correctional officers on a regular basis.

Notably, these barriers to prevention were in place for incarcerated persons while 21 jurisdictions posted details – and in some cases promotional videos – on their websites detailing incarcerated persons' efforts to mass produce COVID-19 equipment (e.g., masks, hospital gowns, sanitizer, soap, disinfectant, face shields). We note an important regional difference here in that mass production efforts of COVID-19 supplies by prisoners were most often described by southern jurisdictions (Florida, Georgia, Kentucky, Louisiana, North Carolina, Oklahoma, South Carolina, Tennessee, Texas, Virginia). In Virginia and

Texas, incarcerated people were making 15,000 masks per day and 20,000 masks per day at the time of our analysis, respectively. Incarcerated individuals in North Carolina were responsible for producing 957,200 bars of soap, 281,376 bottles of disinfectant spray, 15,260 gallons of antibacterial liquid soap, and 7,952 gallon jugs of hand sanitizer.

As further illustration, individuals incarcerated in Tennessee were producing 1,000–5,000 masks daily at the time of our analysis, despite the fact that not all prisoners in Tennessee had access to masks. The Florida Department of Corrections released a memo on April 11th stating that prisoners would begin producing masks, which would first "be issued to correctional officers, probation officers, and staff in high risk geographic areas of the state" and "then to institutions which have large at-risk inmate populations." We argue that these parameters, which establish a culture of denying access to basic preventive health measures during a pandemic, while simultaneously exploiting as laborers the very individuals denied that access, is especially cruel. If those in correctional facilities are going to be producing PPE, it seems only humane that they should be provided full access to PPE themselves.

Finally, we underscore the need for those living in prisons and jails to have continued access to a means of connecting with family and friends when visitation rights have been suspended. Feelings of isolation, degraded mental health, and increased risk for violence and misconduct may all result from a lack of social contact and reduced support from family members and friends among prisoners, especially amidst the uncertainty and chaos of the global pandemic (Biggam & Power, 1997; Jiang et al., 2005). Although our analysis shows that many states have, in fact, increased opportunities for phone or video calls available to prisoners during the suspension of visitation privileges, there remains stringent time restrictions or fees associated with these methods of communication. As long as visitation rights remain suspended, we recommend that facilities consider offering more digital options (especially video conferencing via tablets) with fewer restrictions that are not cost-prohibitive. Doing so can assist with maintaining well-being and social support for incarcerated individuals and their families.

As for future research directions, we call for research that explores how being incarcerated during the COVID-19 pandemic has impacted individuals' physical and mental health. Pandemic-related criminological research thus far has focused primarily on changes in crime rates due to COVID-19 (see Mohler et al., 2020; Payne & Morgan, 2020; Payne et al., 2020; Piquero et al., 2020), but the detrimental effects of the virus are more far-reaching than that. Beyond risks for COVID-19 infection, which are substantial, the stress of being incarcerated is likely to be elevated in the context of a pandemic given not only fears of infection, but the many policy changes that directly influence quality of life for incarcerated persons. For example, the increase in social isolation following cuts to familial visitation in an atmosphere that already lacks social contact might have especially detrimental effects, both in the short and long term. Reductions in institutional movement and lockdowns are likely to have resulted in decreased access to exercise, movement, and mobility, an especially important consideration for older incarcerated adults (Prost et al., 2020). Moreover, research indicates the physical and psychological harms of solitary confinement are severe and include sensory hypersensitivity and loss of identify (Reiter et al., 2020), post-traumatic stress disorder (Hagan et al., 2018), and chronic somatic diseases (Gamman, 1995; Haney, 2003). We encourage future scholars to explore how efforts to quarantine large numbers of incarcerated individuals during the pandemic may have increased exposure to solitary confinement-like living conditions for incarcerated persons, both in practice and in its effects.

Variations in correctional responses across institutions also warrant further study, especially with regard to whether or not more stringent policies mirroring evidence-based guidance and CDC guidelines significantly reduced the number of cases and collateral health consequences in those prisons and jails. One idea is to examine whether facilities that provided all staff and incarcerated persons with PPE *and* required wear of PPE had lower case rates or self-reported COVID-19 symptoms than facilities that did not. Moreover, a deeper understanding of why differences in correctional responses occurred in the first place would be beneficial. Considering the explicit recommendations made by the CDC, all correctional facilities should have adopted nearly identical responses to the pandemic in order to prevent outbreaks. Our results, however, demonstrate this did not occur.

Lastly, we encourage expansions in reentry and decarceration research. The pressing need to quickly reduce prison and jail population sizes across the country forced certain jurisdictions to release these persons early (see also Abraham et al., 2020). While we were unable to address these efforts in our study, moving forward this information can be highly beneficial to the study of reentry and risk assessment, as well as for sentencing reform (specifically sentencing reduction). If future research finds that those who were released early posed no increased threat of recidivism, this can serve as evidence in support of reductions in sentences and may hopefully contribute in some way to the problem of prison and jail overcrowding in general.

Like all research, ours must be considered with respect to its limitations. First, and related to our point above, there was a significant amount of missing information for certain metrics across facilities, especially in regard to testing and hospitalization data, as well as with respect to decisions on intakes, transfers, and early releases. These data were largely missing from DOC websites, yet hold significance for policy. For example, policies that permitted transfers of incarcerated individuals to continue across institutions – especially in large volume – likely exacerbated risks for spread of the virus by moving around potentially already-infected (perhaps asymptomatic) persons to new, uninfected locations. Alternatively, had correctional jurisdictions collectively pursued options for meaningful reductions in prison population sizes early on, overall risks for infection within institutions would have likely declined and options for incorporating CDC guidelines would have likely been more practical. Unfortunately, the current study gathered no data on the procedures or effects of these policies, mainly because such efforts were not highlighted in any kind of patterned manner by jurisdictions at the time of our data collection. It is clear that correctional departments must improve data collection and dissemination efforts to the public and these improved efforts can inform future research using more comprehensive data.

Secondly, our assessment necessarily only provides a snapshot of correctional system responses based on information available at one point in time. This means that our data cannot account for any changes made after the fact or policies that were potentially implemented but not communicated publicly through individual jurisdiction websites. Thus, our findings should be interpreted within that context. Yet, we were still able to gather a great deal of data across jurisdictions and our analysis does provide a comparative summary that can be used as a starting point for further analyses.

Another potential limitation is that all of the data here are provided by the correctional facilities themselves (rather than by incarcerated people, correctional officers, or other staff members). As such, the analysis reflects information provided in a public-facing context and may not necessarily reflect the reality of day-to-day life in certain prisons or the perspectives of those living and working in these facilities. This underscores the need for continued research that includes the perspectives of those embedded within facilities, as offered initially by Pyrooz et al. (2020). Lastly, despite the many adults incarcerated in U.S. jails, the current research did not include any information on jail-based responses to the COVID-19 pandemic. We encourage future scholars to conduct similar comparative analyses with jails to what we have offered here. However, such efforts will likely require substantial resources considering not only the number of jail jurisdictions throughout the U.S., but the more transient populations confined in jails relative to prisons.

Conclusion

The United States continues to disproportionately suffer the ravages of the COVID-19 pandemic, despite many instances of peer industrialized nations responding effectively to the virus in many parts of the world. Absent even remotely competent federal leadership, the correctional response to COVID-19 appears to reflect the broader response of the U.S. in many ways, often deferring to individual states and ad hoc policies for controlling outbreaks rather than following unified guidance across facilities and correctional systems. This shortcoming is particularly notable with respect to data collection and transparency regarding testing and hospitalization information for those in prisons, as well as in the provision of preventive supplies. Correctional facilities remain high-risk locales for outbreaks and it is imperative that policies moving forward protect those who are most vulnerable while ensuring equity in access to those protections.

Notes

1. While we include the Federal Bureau of Prisons (BOP) as one of fifty-one jurisdictions in our analysis, it was not our focus. The federal response is the focus of a separate article (Hummer, this issue).
2. To offer one further example, mortality data posted by the Ohio Department of Corrections changed midway through the pandemic from one indicator ("number of confirmed COVID-19 related inmate deaths") to two indicators ("number of probable COVID-19 related inmate deaths" and "number of confirmed COVID-19 related inmate deaths").

Disclosure statement

No potential conflict of interest was reported by the author(s).

Funding

This work was supported by the Scholars Strategy Network (SSN) of Northeast Ohio [Amplify & Apply Mini-Grant].

ORCID

Meghan A. Novisky http://orcid.org/0000-0003-4644-9148
Chelsey S. Narvey http://orcid.org/0000-0003-0672-6809
Daniel C. Semenza http://orcid.org/0000-0002-3843-9559

References

Abraham, L. A., Brown, T. C., & Thomas, S. A. (2020). How COVID-19's disruption of the U.S. correctional system provides an opportunity for decarceration. *American Journal of Criminal Justice*, *45*(4), 780–792. online first. https://doi.org/10.1007/s12103-020-09537-1

Akiyama, M. J., Spaulding, A. C., & Rich, J. D. (2020). Flattening the curve for incarcerated populations—Covid-19 in jails and prisons. *New England Journal of Medicine*, *382*(22), 2075–2077. https://doi.org/10.1056/NEJMp2005687

Biggam, F. H., & Power, K. G. (1997). Social support and psychological distress in a group of incarcerated young offenders. *International Journal of Offender Therapy and Comparative Criminology*, *41*(3), 213–230. https://doi.org/10.1177/0306624X97413002

Binswanger, I. A., Krueger, P. M., & Steiner, J. F. (2009). Prevalence of chronic medical conditions among jail and prison inmates in the USA compared with the general population. *Journal of Epidemiological Community Health*, *63*(11), 912–919. https://doi.org/10.1136/jech.2009.090662

Bronson, J., & Carson, E. A. (2019). *Prisoners in 2017*. U.S. Department of Justice, Bureau of Justice Statistics. Retrieved July 28, 2020, from https://www.bjs.gov/content/pub/pdf/p17.pdf

Carson, E. A., & Cowhig, M. P. (2020). *Mortality in state and federal prisons, 2001-2016-statistical tables* (NCJ # 251920). U.S. Department of Justice, Bureau of Justice Statistics. https://www.bjs.gov/content/pub/pdf/msfp0116st.pdf

Centers for Disease Control and Prevention (CDCa). (2020). *How to protect yourself and others*. U.S. Department of Health and Human Services. Retrieved August 2 2020, from https://www.cdc.gov/coronavirus/2019-ncov/prevent-getting-sick/prevention.html

Centers for Disease Control and Prevention (CDCb). (2020). *Considerations for wearing masks: Help spread the slow of COVID-19*. U.S. Department of Health and Human Services. Retrieved August 2 2020, from https://www.cdc.gov/coronavirus/2019-ncov/prevent-getting-sick/cloth-face-cover-guidance.html?CDC_AA_refVal=https%3A%2F%2Fwww.cdc.gov%2Fcoronavirus%2F2019-ncov%2Fprevent-getting-sick%2Fcloth-face-cover.html#recent-studies

Cochran, J. C. (2012). The ties that bind or the ties that break: Examining the relationship between visitation and prisoner misconduct. *Journal of Criminal Justice*, *40*(5), 433–440. https://doi.org/10.1016/j.jcrimjus.2012.06.001

COVID Prison Project. (2020). *National COVID-19 statistics*. Retrieved September 8, 2020, from https://covidprisonproject.com/data/data-v2/

Gamman, T. (1995). Hazardous health effect of isolation. A clinical study of 2 groups of persons in custody. *Journal of the Norwegian Medical Association*, *115*, 2243–2246. https://pubmed.ncbi.nlm.nih.gov/7652720/

Hagan, B. O., Wang, E. A., Aminawung, J. A., Albizu-Garcia, C. E., Zaller, N., Nyamu, S., Shavit, S., Deluca, J., & Fox, A. D., & Transitions Clinic Network. (2018). History of solitary confinement is associated with post-traumatic stress disorder symptoms among individuals recently released from prison. *Journal of Urban Health*, *95*(2), 141–148. https://doi.org/10.1007/s11524-017-0138-1

Haney, C. (2003). Mental health issues in long-term solitary and "supermax" confinement. *Crime & Delinquency*, *49*(1), 124–156. https://doi.org/10.1177/0011128702239239

Hawks, L., Woolhandler, S., & McCormick, D. (2020). COVID-19 in prisons and jails in the United States. *JAMA Internal Medicine*, *180*(8), 1041. online first. https://doi.org/10.1001/jamainternmed.2020.1856

Hewson, T., Shepherd, A., Hard, J., & Shaw, J. (2020). Effects of the COVID-19 pandemic on the mental health of prisoners. *The Lancet Psychiatry*, *7*(7), 568–570. https://doi.org/10.1016/S2215-0366(20)30241-8

Jiang, S., Fisher-Giorlando, M., & Mo, L. (2005). Social support and inmate rule violations: A multilevel analysis. *American Journal of Criminal Justice*, *30*(1), 71–86. https://doi.org/10.1007/BF02885882

Johns Hopkins University. (2020). *Coronavirus resource center, confirmed cases by country/region/sovereignty*. Center for Systems Science and Engineering. Retrieved September 8, 2020, from https://coronavirus.jhu.edu/map.html

Kinner, S. A., Young, J. T., Snow, K., Southalan, L., Lopez-Acuña, D., Ferreira-Borges, C., & O'Moore, É. (2020). Prisons and custodial settings are part of a comprehensive response to COVID-19. *The Lancet Public Health*, *5*(4), e188–e189. https://doi.org/10.1016/S2468-2667(20)30058-X

Konda, A., Prakash, A., Moss, G. A., Schmoldt, M., Grant, G. D., & Guha, S. (2020). Aerosol filtration efficiency of common fabrics used in respiratory cloth masks. *ACS Nano*, *14*(5), 6339–6347. https://doi.org/10.1021/acsnano.0c03252

Kothari, R., Forrester, A., Greenberg, N., Sarkissian, N., & Tracy, D. K. (2020). COVID-19 and prisons: Providing mental health care for people in prison, minimising moral injury and psychological distress in mental health staff. *Medicine, Science, & the Law*, *60*(3), 165–168. online first. https://doi.org/10.1177/0025802420929799

Kratzel, A., Todt, D., V'kovski, P., Steiner, S., Gultrom, M., Thao, T. T. N., Ebert, N., Holwerda, M., Steinmann, J., Niemeyer, D., Dijkman, R., Kampf, G., Drosten, C., Steinmann, E., Thiel, V., & Pfaender, S. (2020). Inactivation of severe acute respiratory syndrome coronavirus 2 by WHO-recommended hand rub formulations and alcohols. *Emerging Infectious Diseases*, *26*(7), 1592–1595. online first. https://doi.org/10.3201/eid2607.200915

Liebrenz, M., Bhugra, D., Buadze, A., & Schleifer, R. (2020). Caring for persons in detention suffering with mental illness during the Covid-19 outbreak. *Forensic Science International: Mind and Law*, *100013*, 1–2. https://doi.org/10.1016/j.fsiml.2020.100013

Link, N. W., Ward, J. T., & Stansfield, R. (2019). Consequences of mental and physical health for reentry and recidivism: Toward a health-based model of desistance. *Criminology*, *57*(3), 544–573. https://doi.org/10.1111/1745-9125.12213

Malloy, G. S., Puglisi, L., Brandeau, M. L., Harvey, T. D., & Wang, E. A. (2020). The effectiveness of interventions to reduce COVID-19 transmission in a large urban jail. *MedRxiv*, online first. https://doi.org/10.1101/2020.06.16.20133280

Marcum, C. D. (2020). American corrections system response to COVID-19: An examination of the procedures and policies used in Spring 2020. *American Journal of Criminal Justice*, *45*(4), 759–768. online first. https://www.ncbi.nlm.nih.gov/pmc/articles/PMC7275927/

The Marshall Project. (2020). *A state by state look at coronavirus in prisons*. Retrieved June 17, 2020, from https://www.themarshallproject.org/2020/05/01/a-state-by-state-look-at-coronavirus-in-prisons

Massoglia, M. (2008). Incarceration as exposure: The prison, infectious disease, and other stress-related illnesses. *Journal of Health and Social Behavior*, *49*(1), 56–71. https://doi.org/10.1177/002214650804900105

Mohler, G., Bertozzi, A. L., Carter, J., Short, M. B., Sledge, D., Tita, G. E., Uchida, C. D., & Brantingham, P. J. (2020). Impact of social distancing during COVID-19 pandemic on crime in Los Angeles and Indianapolis. *Journal of Criminal Justice*, *68*, 101692. online first. https://doi.org/10.1016/j.jcrimjus.2020.101692

Montoya-Barthelemy, A., Lee, C. D., Cundiff, D., & Smith, E. (2020). COVID-19 and the correctional environment: The American prison as a focal point for public health. *American Journal of Preventive Medicine*, *58*(6), 888–891. online first. https://doi.org/10.1016/j.amepre.2020.04.001

New York Times. (2020). *Coronavirus in the U.S.: Latest map and case count*. Retrieved September 8, 2020, from https://www.nytimes.com/interactive/2020/us/coronavirus-us-cases.html?action=

click&module=Top%20Stories&pgtype=Homepage&action=click&module=Spotlight&pgtype=Homepage#states

Novisky, M. (2018). Avoiding the runaround: The link between cultural health capital and health management among older prisoners. *Criminology*, *56*(4), 643–678. https://doi.org/10.1111/1745-9125.12188

Nowotny, K., Bailey, Z., Omori, M., & Brinkley-Rubenstein, L. (2020). COVID-19 exposes need for progressive criminal justice reform. *American Journal of Public Health*, *110*(7), e1–e2. https://doi.org/10.2105/AJPH.2020.305707

Okano, J. T., & Blower, S. (2020). Preventing major outbreaks of COVID-19 in jails. *The Lancet*, *395* (10236), 1542–1543. https://doi.org/10.1016/S0140-6736(20)31015-1

Payne, J. L., & Morgan, A. (2020). COVID-19 and violent crime: A comparison of recorded offence rates and dynamic forecasts (ARIMA) for March 2020 in Queensland, Australia. *SocArXiv*, online first. https://doi.org/10.31219/osf.io/g4kh7

Payne, J. L., Morgan, A., & Piquero, A. R. (2020). COVID-19 and social distancing measures in Queensland, Australia, are associated with short-term decreases in recorded violent crime. *Journal of Experimental Criminology*, online first. https://doi.org/10.1007/s11292-020-09441-y

Piquero, A. R., Riddell, J. R., Bishopp, S. A., Narvey, C., Reid, J. A., & Piquero, N. L. (2020). Staying home, staying safe? A short-term analysis of COVID-19 on Dallas domestic violence. *American Journal of Criminal Justice*, *45*(4), 601–635. online first. https://doi.org/10.1007/s12103-020-09531-7

Prison Policy Initiative. (2020). *Responses to the COVID-19 pandemic*. Retrieved June 17, 2020, from https://www.prisonpolicy.org/virus/virusresponse.html.

Prost, S. G., Novisky, M. A., Rorvig, L., Zaller, N., & Williams, B. (2020). Prisons and COVID-19: A desperate call for gerontological expertise in correctional healthcare. *Gerontologist*, online first, 1–5. https://doi.org/10.1093/geront/gnaa088

Pyrooz, D. C., Labrecque, R. M., Tostlebe, J. J., & Useem, B. (2020). Views on COVID-19 from inside prison: Perspectives of high-security prisoners. *Justice Evaluation Journal*, 1–13. online first. https://doi.org/10.1080/24751979.2020.1777578

Reidy, T., & Sorensen, J. (2020). Visitation and misconduct among maximum-security inmates. *The Prison Journal*, *100*(4), 447–467. https://doi.org/10.1177/0032885520939289

Reinhart, E., & Chen, D. (2020). Incarceration and its disseminations: COVID-19 pandemic lessons from Chicago's Cook County Jail. *Health Affairs*, *39*(8), 1–5. https://doi.org/10.1377/hlthaff.2020.00652

Reiter, K., Ventura, J., Lovell, D., Augustine, D., Barragan, M., Blair, T., Chesnut, K., Dashtgard, P., Gonzalez, G., Pifer, N., & Strong, J. (2020). Psychological distress in solitary confinement: Symptoms, severity, and prevalence in the United States, 2017–2018. *American Journal of Public Health*, *110*(S1), S56–S62. https://doi.org/10.2105/AJPH.2019.305375

Saloner, B., Parish, K., Ward, J. A., DiLaura, G., & Dolovich, S. (2020). COVID-19 cases and deaths in federal and state prisons. *JAMA*, *324*(6), 602–603. https://doi.org/10.1001/jama.2020.12528

Semenza, D. C., & Link, N. W. (2019). How does reentry get under the skin? Cumulative reintegration barriers and health in a sample of recently incarcerated men. *Social Science & Medicine*, *243*, 112618. https://doi.org/10.1016/j.socscimed.2019.112618

Wilper, A. P., Woolhandler, S., Boyd, J. W., Lasser, K. E., McCormick, D., Bor, D. H., & Himmelstein, D. U. (2009). The health and health care of U.S. prisoners: Results of a nationwide survey. *American Journal of Public Health*, *99*(4), 666–672. https://doi.org/10.2105/AJPH.2008.144279

Wurcel, A. G., Dauria, E., Zaller, N., Nijhawan, A., Beckwith, C., Nowotny, K., & Brinkley-Rubinstein, L. (2020). Spotlight on jails: COVID-19 mitigation policies needed now. *Clinical Infectious Diseases*, *71*(15), 891–892. https://doi.org/10.1093/cid/ciaa346

Zeng, Z. (2020). *Jail inmates in 2018*. U.S. Department of Justice, Bureau of Justice Statistics. Retrieved July 28, 2020, from https://www.bjs.gov/content/pub/pdf/ji18.pdf

OPEN ACCESS

United States Bureau of Prisons' Response to the COVID-19 Pandemic

Don Hummer

ABSTRACT

As the SARS-CoV-2 (COVID-19) spread across the United States in spring 2020, the Federal Bureau of Prisons (BOP) made the startling announcement that of its 2,700 initial screenings of inmates for the virus, 2,000 had tested positive – an astounding 70% positivity rate. It is obvious to assume that prisons and jails would be locations of outbreaks and rapid community spread given the close quarters, limited access to preventive methods, and movement of both inmates and staff in and out of facilities. Yet, the speed of early transmission through the federal prison system led to questions of whether the BOP was adequately prepared to handle a contagion such as COVID -19, and if the steps that have ultimately been taken (such as moving inmates from prison to community using existing release mechanisms, suspending visitation, and increased screening of both inmates and staff) are sufficient to minimize new infections throughout the system. This article describes and assesses the BOP's COVID-19 mitigation strategies, details treatment programming challenges during the pandemic, and offers suggestions for future infectious disease outbreak response.

The incarcerated population is uniquely affected by the dramatic effects SARS-CoV-2 (COVID-19) has had globally. By August 15, 2020, the United States had over 118,742 confirmed cases of COVID-19 in its correctional facilities and 27,153 confirmed staff cases (UCLA Law COVID-19 Behind Bars Data Project, 2020). Early in the pandemic it was assumed that prisons and jails would be locations of outbreaks and rapid community spread given the close quarters, limited access to preventive methods, sanitary issues, and movement of both inmates and staff in and out of facilities that have led to the transmission of other infectious diseases (Ndeffo-Mbah et al., 2018; Niveau, 2006; Saloner et al., 2020). Unlike a number of other diseases that have impacted correctional facilities (e.g., HIV, hepatitis, various sexually transmitted infections, foodborne illnesses), the novel coronavirus has no vaccine, very limited treatment protocols, and is highly contagious via airborne transmission. The close quarters of a prison enhance viral spread. Compounding the issue is that the U.S. inmate population overall has a higher rate of multimorbidity, and an earlier onset of these risk factors, than the general population (Kinner et al., 2020). A byproduct of decades of American mass incarceration is the aging of the correctional population, with the number of inmates over the age of 55 increased by 280% between 1999 and 2016, expanding from 7% of the total inmate population to 10% (Akiyama et al., 2020; McKillop & Boucher, 2018).

The Bureau of Prisons (BOP) is the largest correctional system in the United States, with over 163,000 inmates in custody (Blakinger & Hamilton, 2020). In April 2020, the BOP instituted its first system-wide lockdown in a quarter-century, in an attempt to arrest the spread of the virus in its facilities[1] (Unlock the Box, 2020). Two months later, the BOP confirmed cases of coronavirus infection at over half of its 122 prisons; however, there are indications that these official figures represent just a fraction of the true number of infections, and that infections are present in the majority of BOP facilities (Blakinger & Hamilton, 2020). The federal government's testing protocol for inmates has been criticized as being too slow to respond to the expanding crisis in the early months of the pandemic, and for not being comprehensive enough to ascertain the true number of infections among inmates and staff. Based on figures from the BOP in early August 2020, 37,625 inmates were tested, with 10,621 positive results, equating to a 28.2% positivity rate (Bureau of Prisons [BOP], 2020). By late July 2020, 100 federal inmates had died of coronavirus contracted while in custody (Hymes, 2020). The August positivity rate was well below the initial rate of nearly 70% (Balsamo, 2020), which was likely inflated due to initial tests being focused on inmates experiencing symptoms of the virus, and those who had come in contact with infected inmates. However, even a positivity rate of almost 30%, if extrapolated to the entire federal correctional population, indicates a rate of infection four to five times higher than the BOP is reporting as of this writing. To give the current positivity rate more perspective, the percentage of positive tests in South Korea in May 2020 was 3%, and the national average in the United States at that time was about 13.2% (Masters, 2020). A spike in the positivity rate in Florida's Miami-Dade county in early July 2020 to 26% was labeled "staggering" (Waldrop, 2020). Initial assessments of death rates show, aggregating state and federal correctional facilities, that prisons had death rates 5.5 times higher than the general population of the U.S. (Saloner et al., 2020).

The widespread outbreak in BOP facilities is creating a number of unique areas of concern. From a public health standpoint, infections among BOP inmates threaten to overwhelm the system's capacity to handle COVID-19 cases in house, and, including prison employees who contract the virus, health care systems in the rural communities in which many federal facilities are located may be overwhelmed as well (Kinner et al., 2020). Offender supervision is a potential issue as well, given that a primary strategy of the BOP in arresting the spread in coronavirus in facility is to transition many "suitable" inmates to home confinement. U.S. Attorney General William Barr directed the BOP to use the expanded powers granted to it by Congress in the Coronavirus, Aid, Relief and Economic Security (CARES) Act to expedite the release of inmates at elevated risk of contracting the disease and posing low risks to public safety (Cassels, 2020). Presently, over 7,000 inmates have transitioned from in-facility to home confinement. The rapid influx of inmates to non-custodial settings places a strain on U.S. Probation and Pretrial Services, who are tasked with community supervision of federal offenders (Pew Charitable Trusts, 2017). The pandemic has all but eliminated the transitional step of releasing inmates to residential community corrections (RCC) facilities in preparation for release. This crisis presents BOP with a unique opportunity to conduct a natural experiment on the need for RCCs. These roughly 170 private-for-profit and private nonprofit contracted facilities are reimbursed per offender rather than based on performance-based contracts, which many other states now use (e.g., Pennsylvania). One other aspect of current reentry practice that could be tested is the impact of performance contracting.

Measuring the extent of COVID-19 via testing and other measures, or lack of data and testing among staff and inmates

Despite the serious effects a highly contagious virus could have on incarcerated populations, most BOP facilities had few or no preparations in place to address COVID-19 when it began to spread across America in the spring of 2020 (Williams et al. (2020)). Further, correctional administrators feared inmate violence, staffing shortages, and public backlash if the numbers of infected inmates and staff members in their facilities were known (ABC Audio, 2020). Thus, testing protocols differed dramatically from state to state, or within states from facility to facility. Some states (Michigan, Texas, Ohio, and Tennessee) very early on initiated testing of their state prison populations and, as such, had positivity rates far higher than states that did not test (Firth, 2020; The Marshall Project, 2020). Outbreaks were reported in states where the virus spread rapidly during the summer of 2020, such as California and Arkansas (The Marshall Project, 2020). Early testing of correctional populations was hampered for many of the same reasons testing lagged in the general population: a shortage of tests and labs to process them, priority of testing for "frontline" individuals, and a focus on testing only symptomatic individuals. As became evident in short order, asymptomatic spread of COVID-19 was driving the proliferation of the virus, thus testing only those with symptoms missed a large segment of the infectious population (Firth, 2020). In prisons and jails, as were the cases in other settings where people came into close contact with one another (such as nursing homes), this led to the virus circulating for days, or even longer, before the first symptomatic patients presented.

Other than the aforementioned structural impediments to wholesale testing in correctional facilities, inmates could opt out of testing. There is evidence from other pandemics affecting American prisons that even mandatory testing falls short of full coverage of the institutional population. At the height of HIV/AIDs in the United States, the federal prison system and most state prison systems required inmates to be tested for HIV as part of the intake process; however, facilities had a difficult time enforcing this mandate (Andrus et al., 1989). For example, if a non-offender refused to be tested for HIV, they would not, for example, be permitted to donate blood or join the military. But what recourse does a correctional facility have for an inmate that refuses testing? In the case of COVID, if a facility's policy is quarantining COVID-positive inmates until they are no longer contagious, a refusal of testing could mean automatic quarantine. This has ramifications for the health of the inmate, outcomes, and possible liability for the facility if an otherwise healthy inmate is quarantined with known COVID-positive inmates and subsequently becomes ill. Despite these risks, facilities may have no other recourse to prevent the spread of the virus. Unlike other diseases common in correctional settings, there are no specific behaviors from which inmates can refrain (such as sexual activity or intravenous drug use) to prevent infection.

If COVID-19 progresses on a track similar to other diseases common in correctional settings (in addition to HIV/AIDS, viral hepatitis and tuberculosis occur at greater rates among the incarcerated population then the general public), high positivity rates can be assumed (see Tavoschi et al., 2018). However, this does not mean that the rampant spread of any infectious disease is imminent in correctional settings, or that nothing can be done to prevent outbreaks in facilities (Hammett, 2006).

The BOP response – website, media reports, government documents

The BOP communicated its response to the COVID-19 outbreak by establishing a dedicated page on its website. Protocols that are commonplace in society generally are also germane, if not somewhat more difficult to accomplish, in the correctional setting, such as mask wearing, social distancing, and isolation of those confirmed or suspected of being infected. Other strategies are unique to the prison context: suspending visitation, halting transfers between facilities, and remote consultations with legal counsel (Akiyama et al., 2020). Besides testing and home confinement information, the BOP webpage serves as a way to detail its efforts and debunk rumors/myths that have circulated in the media, in government circles, and among prison stakeholders such as staff, attorneys, and relatives of inmates. Examples of these myths include masks not being provided to all staff and inmates, and staff being forced to report for work even when they are exhibiting symptoms or have had close contact with an infected inmate or other person (BOP, 2020). It could be argued that the need to debunk rumors via the agency's webpage is a function of ineffective communication at the onset of the pandemic. Family members of inmates have reported a lack of information being provided about medical conditions of inmates, transfers within the system, and decisions on home confinement. This reluctance or inability to share information, both system-wide and from individual facilities, continued to be an issue into the summer of 2020, when local officials in communities where federal prisons were located reported that their requests for information were being ignored (Cheves & Musgrave, 2020).

Criticism of the Bureau's efforts to mitigate risk has come from a number of constituencies, with the most direct criticism came from inside. The union representing prison workers filed a complaint with the Occupational Safety and Health Administration (OSHA) shortly after the first inmates infected with COVID-19 were confirmed that cited "imminent dangers" within the system due to the lack of preparedness and implementation of mitigation strategies (Buble, 2020). Very early in the pandemic, before the BOP halted all inmate transfers in March 2020 (Segura, 2020), it has been asserted that the BOP moved what were believed to be COVID-19 negative inmates from facilities with outbreaks to facilities thought to not have coronavirus cases. This directive from Washington may have inadvertently spread COVID-19 to facilities – and by extension communities – that had few known or suspected cases (Buble, 2020). If, as mentioned earlier, a small number of "hot spot" facilities were driving overall numbers, then it is logical to infer that as the virus spreads in the community, these hot spot locations will likely change. Without an effective preparedness strategy, the BOP was forced to react to the disease with questionable effectiveness.

Wearing of masks

The BOP (2020) maintains that adequate numbers of masks and other personal protective equipment (PPE) such as gowns, gloves, face shields, and hand sanitizers have been provided to staff and inmates. This was done as soon as the Centers for Disease Control (CDC) guidance called for such measures when social distancing was not possible.[2] This statement, featured on the BOP's coronavirus response webpage, is at odds with reports that masks and other PPE were not available to either inmates or staff, including as part of the lawsuit brought against the BOP by the union representing employees (Balsamo, 2020; Buble, 2020). The nationwide shortage of PPE, particularly at the onset of the pandemic, meant that prisons and jails at the federal, state, and local levels were behind medical facilities, first responders, schools, and other institutions in priority (Barr, 2020). As a result, there were delays in getting PPE to BOP facilities, and when it did arrive, there were widespread concerns about its quality (Hamilton & Newhauser, 2020).

Inmate transfers

Movement of inmates throughout the system – for example, transferring inmates nearing their release dates to less secure facilities in preparation for release to residential community corrections or home confinement – ground to a halt early in the pandemic, sometimes so quickly that inmates in transit were caught in limbo between facilities in temporary housing (Segura, 2020). Keeping more of the inmate population in place during the initial rapid spread of the virus in spring 2020 was sound logic from a public health standpoint (Akiyama et al., 2020). If it were assumed that inmates were highly likely to have come in close contact with someone infected with COVID-19, then quarantining within facilities represents the best course of action in the short term.

Of course, not all movement of inmates (or staff, visitation, and others entering facilities) could be suspended throughout the system (e.g., Hawks et al., 2020). Though the BOP asserts that transfers were reduced by 95% between the outbreak of the pandemic and late April 2020, in May 2020, the Bureau transferred nearly 7,000 inmates within and into the system for a variety of reasons including for forensic studies, medical or mental health treatment, residential reentry, intake of federal offenders being housed in local jails, and inmates who had detainers by other jurisdictions (Balsamo & Sisak, 2020).

The BOP has established protocols and screening tools for specific constituent groupings that enter facilities, and a set of guidelines and contingencies for those individuals who may pose a risk of bringing infection into a facility (BOP, 2020). Even with these measures in place, BOP has met resistance from local elected officials and legal action to stop the transfer of inmates to facilities in communities with lower infection counts (Plum, 2020). In May 2020, the U.S. District Court for the Northern District of Ohio ordered the BOP, in detail, to "determine the appropriate means of transferring" elderly and medically vulnerable inmates out prisons with high numbers of coronavirus infections to other facilities within the system (Howe, 2020). A month later, the court was not satisfied with the BOP's response and instructed the agency to explain, within 7 days, why ineligible inmates could not be moved to another prison "where social distancing is possible (Howe, 2020)." In response, the BOP released a statement that emphasized the numbers of inmates who had recovered from COVID-19 and indicated how facilities were managing outbreaks through testing, use of "field-ready" tents to maximize social distancing, and providing protective gear where resources permit (Satija, 2020). Directives such as these from the courts are indicative of a system-wide inmate transfer plan that was inconsistent with safe and secure facility management and placed inmates and staff at risk.

Policies for staff who are ill

Protocols for staff to self-isolate and not report for work if they have come into contact with an infected inmate, family member, or other person, have been established within the BOP. But, there have been claims[3] that staff have felt compelled to come to work even if they have been exposed to a COVID-19 positive individual or were even exhibiting symptoms themselves (Buble, 2020). More problematic to prison workers has been the BOP's policy of outsourcing coronavirus testing to local institutions and community partnerships (Bur, 2020). There has been criticism of testing protocols generally in the United States since the pandemic began, beginning with faulty tests, insufficient numbers of testing kits, and an inability of many to access testing. Even as of this writing, in August 2020, delays in obtaining results of administered tests in many communities continue to be a vexing problem for communities trying to limit the spread of the virus in their jurisdictions. A prison employee, therefore, who is tested, is asymptomatic, and returns to work, but has to wait for a week or more for the results of their test could potentially contract and/or pass the virus to many others in a correctional setting, rendering the initial test useless, or worse yet, erroneous.

Being cautious with staff who have come in contact with an infected inmate, have COVID-19-like symptoms, or are at higher risk themselves of medical complications if they were to become infected, and not having them report to work, is fully in line with CDC guidelines. These employees are not part of the total institution, and leave facilities after each shift, potentially bringing with them into their households and communities coronavirus infection. Over 1400 BOP employees had been infected as of late August 2020, demonstrating the symbiotic relationship between prisons and the communities in which they are situated, and the difficulties inherent in preventing the spread of the disease during the course of the employee's everyday work (Bellware, 2020).

Impact of COVID-19 on implementation of the First Step Act

Before the global coronavirus pandemic began, almost exactly 1 year earlier, President Donald J. Trump signed the First Step Act into law in 2019. Lauded by some as the most significant federal criminal justice reform bill in years, the components of the First Step Act collectively sought to reduce the size of the federal prison population while maintaining public safety (Cohen, 2019; James, 2019). The act reauthorized the Second Chance Act of 2007 (James, 2019) and mandated that the Fair Sentencing Act of 2010 be applied retroactively to some federal offenses, resulting in lesser sentences for many criminal offenders (Ferrill, 2020). Lastly, the First Step Act promoted correctional reform via the establishment of a risk/needs assessment within BOP facilities (James, 2019). Specifically, the last component of the First Step Act:

> ...requires the Department of Justice (USDOJ) to develop a risk and needs assessment system to be used by BOP to assess the recidivism risk of all federal prisoners and to place prisoners in programs and productive activities to reduce this risk. Prisoners who successfully complete recidivism reduction programming and productive activities can earn additional time credits (i.e., "earned time credits") that will allow them to be placed in prerelease custody (i.e., home confinement or a Residential Reentry Center) earlier than they were previously allowed. The act prohibits prisoners convicted of any one of dozens of offenses identified in the chart above from earning additional time credits,though these prisoners can earn other benefits, such as additional visitation time, for successfully completing recidivism reduction programming." Defender Services Office Training Division, 2020)

By January of 2020, the USDOJ should have posted a full list of approved programs on www.bop.gov, and the BOP should have completed initial risk and needs assessments for each prisoner and begin to assign programming (James, 2019). What constitutes "effective programming and productive activity" was not at first delineated, though a subsequent report produced on behalf of the First Step Act Independent Review Committee provided an assessment of which programs demonstrated positive results after empirical testing, as well as programs that were deemed promising but for which not enough evidence had been accumulated to deem a particular strategy a "success" (Byrne, 2019).

Ostensibly, the complete formula for how program participation and completion would translate to earned time credits would be provided as well. While some elements of the First Step Act were implemented immediately after the bill was signed by President Trump, such as sentence reductions for newly sanctioned offenders and for certain offenders sanctioned under prior, disproportionate sentencing guidelines (e.g., powder vs. crack cocaine) (Grawert, 2020), the risk and needs assessment has proven to be more of a challenge – a challenge complicated by a global pandemic that struck just as the key January deadlines occurred. The USDOJ produced a detailed report in July 2019 that outlined the development of a risk and needs assessment system, as well as recommended steps for the implementation of such a system across BOP facilities (United States Department of Justice [USDOJ], 2019). Byrne's (2019) report on behalf of the First Step Act Independent Review Committee concludes that the programming the BOP has implemented in its facilities and labeled as "approved Evidence-based Recidivism Reduction (EBRR) Strategies and Productive Activities (PAs) [as] required by law" (USDOJ, 2020a, 2020b) has not been evaluated sufficiently to determine if they are effective. Specifically, the First Step Act Independent Review Committee Report states:

> Serious, formal evaluations of current BOP programming are too scarce to tell us much about the effectiveness of that programming. The Bureau's Directory of National Programs appears to suggest that only 3 of the 18 "national program models" have ever been directly evaluated, and only one of them during the past two decades. Based on the research evidence currently available, no reliable judgment can be made about the recidivism reduction effects of particular BOP programs now in operation. [T]he effects of current BOP programs are most accurately described as "unknown. (Byrne, 2019, p. 16)

It seems somewhat counterintuitive to be constructing a recidivism risk mitigation strategy with untested behavioral programming, yet the BOP is left few options given the wording of the First Step Act, and the roster of programs available that can be feasibly implemented in a majority of BOP facilities. USDOJ recommended programs that have become EBRR strategies and PAs were derived mostly from already implemented programs at the federal, state, and local correctional levels. There is also the question of whether inmates are appropriately matched with programming best suited to facilitate their desistence from crime upon release from supervision. As part of First Step Act implementation, the BOP has a comprehensive needs assessment system that is used to assign appropriate EBRR and PAs based on an inmate's criminogenic needs and other needs that are associated with an increased risk of recidivism, such as anger & hostility, dyslexia, and financial literacy (USDOJ, 2020b).

Keeping these issues in mind, the COVID-19 pandemic has had profound impacts on the implementation, and therefore inmate participation in, EBRR and PAs. From its own internal memo in August 2020, the BOP appears to indicate that some First Step Act programming was altered or suspended in the wake of COVID-19, impacting facilities (USDOJ, 2020a). The memo directs facilities to "resume programs" in both residential and nonresidential contexts, without restrictions based on group size (e.g., groups with more than ten participants) (USDOJ, 2020a). Facilities are encouraged to maintain social distance for program participants – for example, by offering meetings in outdoor or "unused" spaces – however, the caveat remains in place to make exceptions to any of the programming directives if the safety of staff and inmates cannot be assured (USDOJ, 2020a). Ambiguities, therefore, remain in determining the extent to which programming is even being offered at various BOP facilities, much less how inmate participation is being translated into hours awarded for completion of programs and, ultimately, the amount of time reduced from an inmate's sanction per the provisions of the First Step Act. It is unclear is whether the pandemic prevented the implementation of First Step Act components and the training of BOP employees on system procedures and protocols. The implementation timeline by the USDOJ is somewhat nebulous, though provisions in the act assert that BOP was to have completed initial assessments of *all* inmates (James, 2019). At this same point, staff training was to be completed, as was the establishment of EBRR and PAs at BOP facilities such that an annual audit by the USDOJ could be performed to monitor and ascertain how the components of the act had been operationalized throughout the BOP (USDOJ, 2020a).

It is unclear how the pandemic has affected the flow of funds for the implementation of First Step Act programming. It has yet to be determined how the COVID-19 pandemic has impacted specific parts of the federal budget. With trillions of dollars going toward sustaining small businesses and stimulus payments to citizens, it seems inevitable that monies earmarked for EBRR and PAs have/will be impacted. Finally, the status of those tens of thousands of inmates who had commenced programming, such as drug treatment and vocational training, prior to the COVID-19 outbreak remains unclear. While the BOP has established guidance for continuing programming while attempting to mitigate infections, the key question becomes whether sufficient resources will be available to sustain First Step Act implementation or if the Department of Justice will need to work with Congress to identify an alternate funding stream. Most importantly, the global pandemic hit 3 months *after* the FSA's risk reduction focused system was required to start. It may certainly be argued that the BOP missed an opportunity to have a defensible population reduction strategy in place *prior* to the start of the pandemic. This opportunity was not realized due to a lack of implementation of both the Prisoner Assessment Tool Targeting Estimated Risk and Need ("PATTERN") risk instrument, and the programming that is at the core of the BOP's risk-driven early release strategy (USDOJ, 2020d). Since these changes were mandated externally by the United States Congress, and not the result of an internal policy/practice/strategic initiative, it is certainly possible that resistance to organizational change was at least partially responsible for the delay. Even more likely, BOP line and mid-level managers were working in a turbulent environment, due to no less than three leadership changes between August 2019 and February 2020 (Phillips, 2020).

Recommendations

As the coronavirus pandemic continued through the summer of 2020 and hit hard the correctional populations of some U.S. states that had widespread COVID-19 infection in the overall population (such as California), the BOP continued to take measures to reduce the spread of the virus in its facilities. Because the trajectory of the pandemic nationally is yet to be determined, any strategies or recommendations are predicated on changing rates of infection, potential breakthroughs in treatment regimens, and, ultimately, whether a vaccine is developed relatively quickly, ending the pandemic. Until such a time comes about, all of the society will need to rely on social distancing, wearing of masks, self-isolation when ill, contact tracing of those infected or who were in contact with a known infected person, and other preventative measures. Prisons are not optimal settings for these practices to take place, but steps can be put into place to limit the spread of this highly contagious coronavirus, and help ensure the safety of those living and working in BOP facilities.

Better and ongoing testing of inmates and staff to prevent spread within the system and in communities where facilities are located

Widespread testing has been consistently shown, globally, to be a key first step in arresting the spread of COVID-19. Although the scope, institution, and effectiveness of testing have become politicized in the United States, what is clear is that without an accurate accounting of the extent of infection in a given setting, there is no way to effectively devise a strategy to isolate those infected and contain the spread. An ineffective testing strategy will either overinflate the extent of infections or underreport the true number of infections within a facility. For example, by testing those individuals who are already symptomatic and were exposed to the virus, testing is simply confirming an assumed outcome. This example was seen in some BOP facilities early in the pandemic when outbreaks were first reported in specific facilities, and then testing implemented afterward. The second likely outcome is the result of a lack of testing, which misses asymptomatic or pre-symptomatic carriers of the virus who go on to infect others, in an exponential fashion, when proper social distancing does not occur.

The screening tools for inmates, staff, and visitors/volunteers/contractors presently in use by the BOP (BOP, 2020) are helpful to a limited extent; however, to mitigate COVID-19 spread in closed institutions, a continual testing regimen would need to be in a place that tested a majority of those already in or entering facilities. Further, these tests would preferably be “rapid result” tests or at the very least allow for results to be returned in 2 days or less. Without widespread testing, and with people flowing into and out of facilities, it is impossible to obtain accurate reflections of the number of infections and how fast the virus is spreading throughout facilities in the BOP system.

Limiting/halting inmate transfers

The BOP maintains that it has limited inmate movement within the system as much as possible and that transfers between March 13, 2020, and April 23, 2020, were down 95% compared to the same time period in 2019 (BOP, 2020). While this was certainly the correct action to take, it is problematic that, during February and early March of 2020, internal BOP records showed that inmate transfers proceeded normally until the middle of March, in all likelihood spreading the virus through the BOP system (Blakinger & Hamilton, 2020). Movement within the system should only be occurring when absolutely necessary, and when it cannot be avoided, protocols must be in place to protect the safety of the transferring inmate and the inmate population of the facility into which that inmate is entering. These protocols include screening inmates prior to transfer, use of PPE by both inmates and correction staff transporting the inmate, screening at intake into the new facility, and a 14-day quarantine to ensure the inmate is asymptomatic before being placed into the general population (BOP, 2020). These measures must be employed for every necessary inmate transfer, and BOP must coordinate with non-USDOJ entities so they are made aware of the BOP's requirements for accepting inmates into federal facilities.

Alternatives to incarceration/detention to prevent infections

Correctional facilities were not designed for social distancing. Space is always at a premium in any jail or prison; thus, the easiest way to maintain social distance is for there to be fewer inmates in facilities. The USDOJ and BOP maintain that there was an "immediate" response at the beginning of the pandemic to review all inmates in the federal prison system for COVID-19 risk factors and to move suitable inmates to home confinement (BOP, 2020). Despite this action item being prominently featured on the BOP's coronavirus response webpage, data from the Marshall Project and the Associated Press indicate that by June 2020, the BOP's total inmate population had only been reduced by roughly 10%; roughly the same proportion as the states of Nevada, Mississippi, Utah, and Iowa (Sharma et al., 2020). The first months of the pandemic have shown the coronavirus spreads easily and rapidly in closed environments (indoors) where people are not socially distanced. Even using PPE, the risk of infection in a correctional facility is greater than elsewhere in society. One initial assessment determined the coronavirus infection rate to be three times higher in prisons than in the population at large (Unlock the Box, 2020).

It is clear that one tool for preventing COVID-19 infections in BOP facilities is to reduce the overall populations within them. The assessments that USDOJ called for early in the pandemic should be altered slightly, and determinations perhaps not made based on which inmates *could* be released, but rather on inmates that *should not*, thus hastening the rate at which BOP inmates are moved to home confinement. There will, of course, always be a subjective element to such assessments; however, if the key criteria become release from incarceration if an inmate is not deemed a significant risk to public safety, the process may lead to a faster reduction of total inmate populations.[4] There are reports that Prisoner Assessment Tool Targeting Estimated Risk and Need ("PATTERN") scores, the tool designed by BOP to measure recidivism risk of inmates, have been quietly revised by the USDOJ to make minimum scores required to qualify for home confinement more difficult to attain (Grawert, 2020). The implications of this unilateral modification are potentially grievous in the midst of a deadly pandemic.[5]

A final concern of not reducing inmate populations significantly enough during the pandemic is that facilities will fall back on the use of solitary confinement to either isolate COVID-positive inmates or protect non-infected inmates from potentially contracting the virus. There is evidence to suggest this practice had been occurring in BOP facilities – in early June of 2020, the BOP acknowledged that it had instituted a "total lockdown" in response to growing numbers of inmates contracting coronavirus, which in many cases includes cutting off telephone communications and video visits (Unlock the Box, 2020). These are measures typically instituted when there is violence, unrest, and/or contraband found in a facility. The deleterious effects of solitary confinement while incarcerated are well-documented (e.g., Haney, 2018; Smith, 2006; Wildeman & Andersen, 2020) – home confinement serves as a better alternative for the overall well-being of the inmate during the course of the pandemic, likely with minimal risks to public safety.[6] The process by which compassionate release occurs in the federal system under the First Step Act is rather convoluted, with the BOP acting as an intermediary between the inmate and the courts (who make a final determination on release). Whether an inmate's case proceeds, and the BOP requests it from the court, or rejects the petition, potentially initiating an appeals process, it is too much of a bureaucratic slog during a pandemic (Merkl, 2020). Inmate welfare would be better served if the USDOJ and BOP could work with the courts to streamline the process.

Conclusions

There are questions about how the Department of Justice (USDOJ) and the BOP managed their coronavirus response plan, and it is likely will be even more questions in the future. Some reports labeled the response as slow to be initiated, and, once up and running, was not flexible enough to respond to a dynamic viral outbreak in specific BOP facilities (Pavlo, 2020). Further, given the data collected thus far during the pandemic from correctional facilities nationwide, the strategies in place to mitigate spread are insufficient to control the spread, and more effective infection control is needed (Saloner et al., 2020).

For those inmates who do not win compassionate release under the provisions of the First Step Act, it is imperative that the reforms incorporated in the First Step Act be maintained so that inmates can continue working toward the reduction of their sentences through participation in EBRR and PAs, despite the challenges posed to federal prisons by the COVID-19 pandemic. The latest report (June 2020) released by the USDOJ on First Step Act implementation represents initiatives in place primarily during the calendar year 2019 (USDOJ, 2020c). It is almost certain there was interruption to programming – the USDOJ's (2020a) internal memorandum indicates as much when it indicates that programs are to "immediately resume" – as priority was placed on short-term assessments and PATTERN scores, while longer ranging goals of the First Step Act were understandably placed on the back burner. However, once the majority of inmates are assessed, attention should turn back to those components of the First Step Act that were established to make sentences fairer.

Notes

1. It has been reported that a small number (under 10) of the more than 120 federal prisons accounted for over 70% of all reported cases, but this information cannot be confirmed. There is no mention of "hot spot" federal prisons on the BOP website. Coronavirus cases spread across the country over summer 2020 from the east and west coasts, likely changing hot spot locations.
2. It is near impossible, of course, to follow the CDC mandate on social distancing in any correctional facility in the United States.
3. It must be emphasized that these are unsubstantiated, anecdotal perceptions of individual employees.
4. Conversely, it would be erroneous to say there is no public safety risk in compassionate release. There is both the public safety component and potential political fallout of releasing, as an example, a low-risk offender who commits another crime. It is not so much the probability as it

is the possibility in these cases, and who takes the blame if such an incident were to occur (see Byrne, 2019).

5. It must be noted that Grawert (2020) is basing his views on the assumption that the revised PATTERN was being used during this time period. If indeed it is being used to reduce inmate scores, this would require both program completion AND reassessment and rescoring of the risk instrument for FSA-eligible inmates. Because of staffing shortages due to COVID illnesses in facilities, assessment staff have been temporarily reassigned to correctional officer duties. Therefore, it is doubtful that there are personnel – and a system – available to even assess and reduce scores.
6. As the pandemic and its impacts continue, it is necessary to examine suicide rates and changes/ deterioration in mental health associated with in-prison mitigation strategies.

Disclosure statement

No potential conflict of interest was reported by the author(s).

ORCID

Don Hummer http://orcid.org/0000-0003-3026-0287

References

ABC Audio. (2020). Fearing outbreaks and riots, nation's prison and jail wardens scramble to respond to COVID-19 threat. https://www.wxhc.com/fearing-outbreaks-and-riots-nations-prison-and-jail-wardens-scramble-to-respond-to-covid-19-threat/

Akiyama, M. J., Spaulding, A. C., & Rich, J. D. (2020). Flattening the curve for incarcerated populations — Covid-19 in jails and prisons. *New England Journal of Medicine*, *382*(22), 2075–2077. https://doi.org/10.1056/NEJMp2005687

Andrus, J. K., Fleming, D. W., Knox, C., McAlister, R. O., Skeels, M. R., Conrad, R. E., Horan, J. M., & Foster, L. (1989). HIV testing in prisoners: Is mandatory testing mandatory? *American Journal of Public Health*, *79*(7), 840–842. https://doi.org/10.2105/AJPH.79.7.840

Balsamo, M. (2020). *Over 70% of tested inmates in federal prisons have COVID-19*. Associated Press. https://apnews.com/fb43e3ebc447355a4f71e3563dbdca4f

Balsamo, M., & Sisak, M. R. (2020). Federal prison system to begin moving nearly 7K inmates. *ABC 3340 News*. https://abc3340.com/news/nation-world/federal-prison-system-to-begin-moving-nearly-7k-inmates

Barr, L. (2020). Federal prisons facing shortages of resources amid coronavirus outbreak. *ABC News*. https://abcnews.go.com/Health/federal-prisons-facing-shortages-resources-amid-coronavirus-outbreak/story?id=69920966

Bellware, K. (2020). Prisoners and guards agree about federal coronavirus response: 'We do not feel safe'. *The Washington Post*. https://www.washingtonpost.com/nation/2020/08/24/prisoners-guards-agree-about-federal-coronavirus-response-we-do-not-feel-safe/

Blakinger, K., & Hamilton, K. (2020). "I begged them to let me die": How federal prisons became coronavirus death traps. *The Marshall Project/Vice News*. https://www.themarshallproject.org/2020/06/18/i-begged-them-to-let-me-die-how-federal-prisons-became-coronavirus-death-traps

Buble, C. (2020). *Federal prisons pose 'imminent danger' in spreading COVID-19, union says*. Government Executive. https://www.govexec.com/oversight/2020/04/federal-prisons-pose-imminent-danger-spreading-covid-19-union-says/164390/

Bur, J. (2020). BOP pushes staff COVID testing responsibility onto outside programs. *Federal Times*. https://www.federaltimes.com/management/2020/06/05/bop-pushes-staff-covid-testing-responsibility-onto-outside-programs/

Bureau of Prisons (BOP). (2020). *COVID-19, coronavirus resource page*. U.S. Department of Justice, Federal Bureau of Prisons. https://www.bop.gov/coronavirus/

Byrne, J. M. (2019). *The effectiveness of prison programming: A review of the research literature examining the impact of federal, state, and local inmate programming on post-release recidivism*. First Step Act Independent Review Committee. https://firststepact-irc.org/wp-content/uploads/2019/12/IRC-Effectiveness-of-Prison-Programming.pdf

Cassels, L. (2020). Inmates released to home confinement say too many remain in infected federal prisons. *Florida Phoenix*. https://www.floridaphoenix.com/2020/06/12/inmates-released-to-home-confinement-say-too-many-remain-in-infected-federal-prisons/

Cheves, J., & Musgrave, B. (2020). Ky. federal prison won't say if it released inmates to stop COVID-19 spread. *Corrections1*. https://www.corrections1.com/coronavirus-covid-19/articles/ky-federal-prison-wont-say-if-it-released-inmates-to-stop-covid-19-spread-Q8pmWlHbzbmejMuW/

Cohen, D. M. (2019). Justice, not jailbreak: The context and consequence of the First Step Act. *Victims & Offenders*, *14*(8), 1084–1098. https://doi.org/10.1080/15564886.2019.1671287

Defender Services Office Training Division. (2020). *Helpful Chart of First Step Act Earned Time Credits*. Administrative Office of the United States Courts. https://www.fd.org/news/helpful-chart-first-step-act-earned-time-credits

Ferrill, Q. H. (2020). Forgotten by the Fair Sentencing Act and the First Step Act: Federal Methamphetamine Sentencing Reform. https://ssrn.com/abstract=3623531

Firth, S. (2020). COVID-19 testing lags in prisons and jails. *MedPage Today*. https://www.medpagetoday.com/infectiousdisease/covid19/86391

Grawert, A. (2020). *What is the First Step Act — And what's happening with it?* Brennan Center for Justice. https://www.brennancenter.org/our-work/research-reports/what-first-step-act-and-whats-happening-it

Hamilton, K., & Newhauser, D. (2020). Federal prison staff say the government is 'getting hustled' with bogus coronavirus masks. *Vice News*. https://www.vice.com/en_us/article/884z4g/federal-prison-staff-say-the-government-is-getting-hustled-with-bogus-coronavirus-masks

Hammett, T. M. (2006). HIV/AIDS and other infectious diseases among correctional inmates: Transmission, burden, and an appropriate response. *American Journal of Public Health*, *96*(6), 974–978. https://doi.org/10.2105/AJPH.2005.066993

Haney, C. (2018). The psychological effects of solitary confinement: A systematic critique. *Crime and Justice*, *47*(1), 365–416. https://doi.org/10.1086/696041

Hawks, L., Woolhandler, S., & McCormick, D. (2020). COVID-19 in prisons and jails in the United States. *JAMA Internal Medicine*, *180*(8), 1041–1042. https://doi.org/10.1001/jamainternmed.2020.1856

Howe, A. (2020). Government asks court to block Ohio COVID-19 prisoner transfer. SCOTUSblog. https://www.scotusblog.com/2020/05/government-asks-court-to-block-ohio-covid-19-prisoner-transfer/

Hymes, C. (2020). Federal prisons reach grim milestone: 100 inmate deaths from coronavirus. *CBSNews*. https://www.cbsnews.com/news/coronavirus-100-federal-prison-inmates-covid-deaths/

James, N. (2019). *The First Step Act of 2018: An overview*. Congressional Research Service. https://fas.org/sgp/crs/misc/R45558.pdf

Kinner, S. A., Young, J. T., Snow, K., Southalan, L., Lopez-Acuna, D., Ferreira-Borges, C., & O'Moore, E. (2020). Prisons and custodial settings are part of a comprehensive response to COVID-19. *The Lancet*, *5*(4), E188–E189. https://doi.org/10.1016/S2468-2667(20)30058-X

The Marshall Project. (2020). *A state-by-state look at coronavirus in prisons*. https://www.themarshallproject.org/2020/05/01/a-state-by-state-look-at-coronavirus-in-prisons

Masters, K. (2020). What percent positivity can — And can't — Tell us about Virginia's COVID-19 epidemic. *Virginia Mercury*. https://www.virginiamercury.com/2020/05/14/what-percent-positivity-can-and-cant-tell-us-about-virginias-covid-19-epidemic/

McKillop, M., & Boucher, A. (2018). *Aging prison populations drive up costs*. Pew Charitable Trusts. https://www.pewtrusts.org/en/research-and-analysis/articles/2018/02/20/aging-prison-populations-drive-up-costs#:~:text=Estimates%20of%20the%20increased%20cost,cost%20differential%20may%20be%20wider

Merkl, T. A., (2020). *What's keeping thousands in prison during COVID-19*. Brennan Center for Justice. https://www.brennancenter.org/our-work/research-reports/whats-keeping-thousands-prison-during-covid-19

Ndeffo-Mbah, M. L., Vigliotti, V. S., Skrip, L. A., Dolan, K., & Galvani, A. P. (2018). Dynamic models of infectious disease transmission in prisons and the general population. *Epidemiologic Reviews, 40*(1), 40–57. https://doi.org/10.1093/epirev/mxx014

Niveau, G. (2006). Prevention of infectious disease transmission in correctional settings: A review. *Public Health, 120*(1), 33–41. https://doi.org/10.1016/j.puhe.2005.03.017

Pavlo, W. (2020). As Bureau of Prisons enters "Phase 9" of COVID-19 plan, BOP staff wonder if there is a real plan. *Forbes.com*. https://www.forbes.com/sites/walterpavlo/2020/08/07/as-bureau-of-prisons-enters-phase-9-of-covid-19-plan-bop-staff-wonder-if-there-is-a-real-plan/#5b35166326fc

Pew Charitable Trusts. (2017). *Number of offenders on federal supervised release hits all-time high*. https://www.pewtrusts.org/en/research-and-analysis/issue-briefs/2017/01/number-of-offenders-on-federal-supervised-release-hits-all-time-high

Phillips, M. (2020). AG Barr names new head of federal prison system after leadership shakeup following Epstein's death. *Fox News*. https://www.foxnews.com/us/ag-barr-names-new-head-of-federal-prison-system-after-leadership-shakeup-following-epsteins-death

Plum, K. (2020). Officials try to stop inmate transfers. *The Dominion Post*. https://www.dominionpost.com/2020/05/05/federal-and-state-elected-officials-seek-to-stop-or-change-the-way-the-u-s-bureau-of-prisons-bop-handles-inmate-transfers-to-quarantine-units/

Saloner, B., Parish, K., & Ward, J. A. (2020). COVID-19 cases and deaths in federal and state prisons. *JAMA, 324*(6), 602–603. https://doi.org/10.1001/jama.2020.12528

Satija, N. (2020). 'Come on, we're human beings': Judges question response to coronavirus pandemic in federal prisons. *The Washington Post*. https://www.washingtonpost.com/investigations/come-on-were-human-beings-judges-question-response-to-coronavirus-pandemic-in-federal-prisons/2020/05/12/925e5d32-912a-11ea-a9c0-73b93422d691_story.html

Segura, L. (2020). *The Coronavirus brought federal prison transfers to a halt. Now people are stuck in limbo*. The Intercept. https://theintercept.com/2020/07/19/coronavirus-prison-transfers-bop/

Sharma, D., Li, W., Lavoie, D., & Lauer, C. (2020). *Prison populations drop by 100,000 during pandemic*. The Marshall Project. https://www.themarshallproject.org/2020/07/16/prison-populations-drop-by-100-000-during-pandemic

Smith, P. S. (2006). The effects of solitary confinement on prison inmates: A brief history and review of the literature. *Crime and Justice, 34*(1), 441–528. https://doi.org/10.1086/500626

Tavoschi, L., Vroling, H., Madeddu, G., Babudieri, S., Monarca, R., Noordegraaf-Schouten, M. V., Beer, N., Gomes Dias, J., O'Moore, E., Hedrich, D., & Oordt-Speets, A. (2018). Active case finding for communicable diseases in prison settings: Increasing testing coverage and uptake among the prison population in the European Union/European Economic Area. *Epidemiologic Reviews, 40*(1), 105–120. https://doi.org/10.1093/epirev/mxy001

UCLA Law. (2020). COVID-19 behind bars project. https://law.ucla.edu/academics/centers/criminal-justice-program/ucla-covid-19-behind-bars-data-project

United States Department of Justice (USDOJ). (2019). *The First Step Act of 2018: Risk and needs assessment system*. United States Department of Justice, Office of the Attorney General.

United States Department of Justice (USDOJ). (2020a). *Internal memorandum, coronavirus (COVID-19) phase nine action plan*. United States Department of Justice, Federal Bureau of Prisons. https://prisonology.com/wp-content/uploads/2020/08/COVID-19-Phase-9-COVID-Action-Plan.pdf

United States Department of Justice (USDOJ). (2020b). *Evidence-based Recidivism Reduction (EBRR) Strategies and Productive Activities (PAs)*. United States Department of Justice, Federal Bureau of Prisons. https://www.bop.gov/inmates/fsa/docs/evidence_based_recidivism_reduction_programs.pdf

United States Department of Justice (USDOJ). (2020c). *First Step Act Implementation Fiscal Year 2020 90-day report*. United States Department of Justice. https://www.ncjrs.gov/pdffiles1/nij/254799.pdf

United States Department of Justice (USDOJ). (2020d). *The First Step Act of 2018: Risk and Needs Assessment System – UPDATE*. United States Department of Justice, Office of the Attorney General.

https://www.bop.gov/inmates/fsa/docs/the-first-step-act-of-2018-risk-and-needs-assessment-system-updated.pdf

Unlock the Box. (2020). *Solitary confinement is never the answer: A special report on the COVID-19 pandemic in prisons and jails, the use of solitary confinement, and best practices for saving the lives of incarcerated people and correctional staff.* unlocktheboxcampaign.org. https://static1.squarespace.com/static/5a9446a89d5abbfa67013da7/t/5ee7c4f1860e0d57d0ce8195/1592247570889/June2020Report.pdf

Waldrop, T. (2020). Coronavirus positivity rate: What the term means. *CNN.com*. https://www.cnn.com/2020/07/07/health/coronavirus-positivity-rate-explainer/index.html

Wildeman, C., & Andersen, L. H. (2020). Solitary confinement placement and post-release mortality risk among formerly incarcerated individuals: A population-based study. *Lancet Public Health, 5*(2), e107–e113. https://doi.org/10.1016/S2468-2667(19)30271-3

Williams, B., Ahalt, C., Cloud, D., Augustine, D., Rorvig, L., & Sears, D. (2020). Correctional facilities in the shadow of COVID-19: Unique challenges and proposed solutions. https://www.healthaffairs.org/do/10.1377/hblog20200324.784502/full/

Adaptations to COVID-19 in Community Corrections Agencies across the United States

Jill Viglione, Lucas M. Alward, Ashley Lockwood, and Sara Bryson

ABSTRACT

Currently, there are more than 4.3 million Americans are under some form of community supervision. Much of the experience of traditional community supervision relies on face-to-face interactions. Individuals on supervision often require treatment or services typically delivered in face-to-face settings. However, the COVID-19 pandemic has forced community corrections' agencies to quickly rethink how they do business, with limited existing research on how to adapt supervision protocols in the midst of a global pandemic. Using surveys of directors of community corrections' agencies across the United States, the goal of the current study was to examine how community corrections' agencies have adapted traditional supervision processes to address disease prevention and containment in addition to supporting client needs and community safety as a result of COVID-19. Changes implemented during the pandemic may have implications for the future landscape of community supervision. Understanding how and what agencies prioritize in a time of global crisis can provide a foundation for identifying sustainable changes as well as understanding future impacts on system and client-level outcomes.

Introduction

Currently, there are more than 4.3 million Americans under some form of community supervision (e.g., probation and parole), which represents the largest arm of the United States correctional system (Kaeble & Alpher, 2020). Individuals on community supervision typically have a host of requirements they must comply with, such as in-person office visits with their assigned supervision officer, occasional home visits by their officer, finding and maintaining employment, payment of fines, restitution, and fees, drug tests, and participation in treatment programs as appropriate (Petersilia, 1997). Much of the "experience" of traditional community supervision relies on face-to-face interactions between the supervision officer and individual on supervision (Andrews & Bonta, 2010). However, the global COVID-19 pandemic introduced significant challenges to these processes for the field of community supervision. With many states instituting "stay at home" orders in the first several months of the pandemic, community corrections' agencies were forced to rethink how they do business quickly, with limited existing research on how to change supervision protocols in the midst of a global pandemic.

There are little data currently synthesized on the prevalence of COVID-19 outbreaks amongst clients and community supervision staff. Reports have focused primarily on incarceration, with estimates indicating that roughly 95,000 individuals in U.S. prisons have tested positive for COVID-19 to date (The Marshall Project, 2020). In attempts to reduce transmission within correctional facilities, more than 100,000 individuals were released from state and federal prison between March and June 2020 (Sharma et al., 2020) with similar reductions occurring in local jails across the country (Prison Policy Initiative, 2020). While specific rates amongst community supervision agencies are not known at this time, many of these released individuals were placed on parole or probation, suggesting possible routes of community transmission (Prison Policy Initiative, 2020). Individuals of lower socioeconomic status and without access to health care are most vulnerable during the current pandemic (Ahmed et al., 2020), suggesting additional risk factors for community supervision populations. These populations are already medically vulnerable with increased risks of contracting infectious diseases due to the prevalence of preexisting medical risk factors (e.g., asthma, hepatitis, and sexually transmitted diseases) (Clark et al., 2013; Vaughn et al., 2012) as well as disproportionate levels of social and economic disadvantage (Vaughn et al., 2012), and behavioral risk factors (e.g., substance use) (Fearn et al., 2016). In addition, individuals on community supervision often require treatment or services typically delivered in face-to-face settings (e.g., mental health services, drug testing). The complex needs and increased risk factors for infectious disease present in community supervision populations, coupled with increased hardships as a result of the pandemic (e.g., increased unemployment, housing and food instability, lack of access to treatment and health care), have created significant challenges for correctional agencies and the populations they supervise.

Now, community supervision agencies must work to balance public safety, budgetary concerns, and public health and officers are now in charge of supporting at-risk populations while also considering their own job stability and health. As community corrections' agencies and officers are already asked to "do more with less" (Ginsburg-Kempany & Kaiser, 2017, p. 279), it is critical to understand how supervision agencies have adapted in response to COVID-19. Agencies have had to make quick, wide-scale policy decisions, which might have implications for the future landscape of community supervision. Understanding how and what agencies prioritize in a time of global crisis can provide a foundation for identifying sustainable changes as well as understanding future impacts on system and client-level outcomes.

Literature review

On March 11, 2020, the World Health Organization (WHO) declared a global pandemic following the rapid spread of COVID-19 (Campedelli et al., 2020). In an attempt to spearhead agency response to COVID-19, Exit: Executives Transforming Probation & Parole, a coalition consisting of current and former community supervision executives, and the Vera Institute of Justice (2020b) released statements with recommendations for community supervision agencies across the United States. To prevent the spread of COVID-19, these guidelines included immediate limitation of office visits for those on parole and probation, suspension, or limitation of technical violations throughout the pandemic, reduced intake to only those with an absolute need to be on probation and parole, reduced probation and parole terms, training for staff, and guidance for probationers and parolees. To contain the spread of COVID-19, Vera (2020b) recommended the use of Center for Disease Control (CDC) screening tools for all those on community supervision and sharing of educational information on COVID-19 with individuals on community supervision. Lastly, the Vera (2020b) guidelines provided guidance on responding to COVID-19, including creating medical care plans, training staff, and implementing policies to protect staff who become ill.

Taken together, these guidelines present huge transformations for the field of community supervision, including changes to methods of responding to noncompliance and integration of public health strategies completely new to the field. There is little in these guidelines that provide guidance for the many challenges that agencies may face in supervising their clients during the pandemic, such as the provision of mental health and substance use treatment and drug testing. Preliminary evidence suggests several challenges community corrections' agencies may have to grapple with for the foreseeable future. For example, since the start of the COVID-19 pandemic, poverty rates have increased (Sumner et al., 2020) and approximately three out of every 10 American's experienced a pay cut or were laid off as a direct result of COVID-19 (Igielnik, 2020), which will inevitably impact those on community supervision. Several correctional interventions and treatment services have been cancelled or temporarily replaced with telehealth initiatives (Schwartzapfel, 2020). However, little is known about how community corrections' agencies integrate telehealth services into treatment and whether individuals on supervision have reliable access to the technology (Schwartzapfel, 2020). Adapting to COVID-19 presents significant shifts in the daily operation and functioning of community supervision agencies. Community corrections' agencies will likely need to continue with altered supervision practices for the foreseeable future given there have been nearly 5.5 million confirmed cases and over 170,000 deaths in the United States as of August 2020 (Dong et al., 2020).

The current study

There is little existing research that examines how community supervision agencies adapt and respond to a global pandemic. The aim of the current study was to examine how community corrections' agencies have implemented changes to prevent, contain, and respond to COVID-19 while also serving the needs of the population they serve and maintaining public safety. This study examined the efforts community supervision agencies have taken to implement new policies and procedures designed to prevent, contain, and respond to the COVID-19 pandemic. Data from this study are designed to supply agencies with information regarding key barriers and strategies associated with the provision of community supervision services during a public health crisis.

Methods

Data collection

Data for this study are part of an ongoing, longitudinal, mixed-method study to examine how community supervision agencies are adapting to the COVID-19 pandemic. The current examination relied on self-reported survey data of community supervision agency administrators across the United States collected during June 2020. Data collection occurred in a series of stages.

First, a database was created that contained all existing counties and states in the United States. After every county in each state was identified, a list of county-level community supervision agencies was assembled along with a primary representative (e.g., director, chief probation officer, manager) for each corresponding organization. For every identified director, we collected all available contact information through publicly available directories and websites. For agencies with only phone numbers listed, the research team made phone calls to attain an e-mail address for an agency representative. The make-up of each state contact list varied depending on the structure of community corrections' system. For example, eight states were organized by regions and opted to have a regional director completes the survey for multiple counties while two states operated at the state-level and opted to have one representative from the state respond to the survey. In addition, the research team supplemented their community supervision contact database with access to an e-mail list-serve belonging to the Center for Advancing Correctional Excellence! (ACE!), which contains active subscribers of community supervision agency representatives from across the United States. This provided an avenue for the inclusion of additional supervision entities including juvenile and state agencies. Twelve states required approval from a centralized review board. At the time of data extraction, two states declined to participate in the research study and 10 had not yet approved participation.

Using a non-probability convenience sampling strategy, electronic surveys were distributed to all identified community supervision administrators using Qualtrics, a reliable and secure online survey service (Snow & Mann, 2013). Respondents were first sent an e-mail inviting them to participate in the study. The initial e-mail contained information detailing the purpose of the study, instructions to select only one representative within each supervision agency to complete the survey, guarantees about the voluntary nature of participation, and confirmed that all study methods were approved by the university's institutional review board. This e-mail also contained a link to the survey with an option for respondents to opt out of the study. To increase response rates, the administration of surveys followed an adapted Dillman (2000) method. After the initial e-mail invitation, respondents were sent reminder e-mails weekly for 3 weeks. The data examined in the current study represent completed surveys by the end of week four of data collection.

Sample

At the time of data extraction for the current study, a total of 1,295 community supervision administrators (chiefs, supervisors, directors) were invited to participate in the study. Of these individuals invited to complete the survey, 213 responded (16.4%). The response rates varied across states, ranging from 0% (n = 6) to 100% (n = 1). On average, the survey took approximately 35 minutes to complete. Agencies were represented from 37 states across the country.[1] Of the responding agencies, the majority reported they served rural areas (56.4%) and adults (90.6%). The majority of agencies were county probation agencies (60.1%) and supervised individuals on felony (83.6%) and misdemeanor (77.5%) supervision. Participating agencies employed on average 62 supervision officers supervising an average caseload of nearly 90 cases. Small agencies supervising between 20 and 499 individuals were the most prevalent in the sample (34.9%). At the time of data collection, all but two participating agencies were open and actively supervising individuals on community supervision (see Table 1).

Table 1. Sample characteristics (N = 213).

Variable	% (*n*)	*M* (*SD*)	Minimum	Maximum
Regions Served				
Rural	56.4% (119)			
Suburban	8.5% (18)			
Urban	9.5% (20)			
Rural/Suburban	6.2% (13)			
Rural/Urban	4.7% (10)			
Suburban/Urban	3.3% (7)			
Rural/Suburban/Urban	11.4% (24)			
Region of U.S.				
Northeast	13.1% (28)			
Midwest	32.9% (70)			
West	20.7% (45)			
South	33.3% (71)			
Populations Served				
Adults	90.6% (193)			
Youth	40.8% (87)			
Felony	83.6% (178)			
Misdemeanor	77.5% (165)			
Type of Supervision				
County Probation	60.1% (128)			
State Probation	39.9% (85)			
Federal Probation	1.4% (3)			
State Parole	26.8% (57)			
County Parole	10.3% (22)			
Caseload		89.8 (46.5)	10	300
Total Supervision Population		5169 (24,528)	20	250,000
20–499	34.5% (69)			
500–999	20.5% (41)			
1000–4999	33% (66)			
5000+	11% (22)			
Officers with Caseloads		62 (290)	1	3500
Office Status				
Open	99.1% (210)			
Closed	0.9% (2)			

Measures

The measures included in this study assessed whether and which type of prevention, containment, and response strategies were implemented in community supervision agencies across the United States.

Prevention strategies

Directors were asked to report whether officers were "meeting face-to-face with individuals on their caseload in the office," "in the field," "in another location," or if "no face-to-face meetings were occurring at that time" (1 = yes, 0 = no). If a respondent selected "another location," they were asked to specify which location(s) contact was occurring. We asked respondents to identify changes made to how face-to-face meetings are conducted compared to before COVID-19 (1 = yes, 0 = no), including whether officers "met in office, but somewhere other than their office," "outside an individual's home," and an open-ended space to provide other alternatives. We asked respondents to report who officers were meeting with face-to-face. Response options included "all who we normally would meet with," "high risk," "moderate risk," "low risk," and "individuals who needed a drug test," were "new to the agency," or other (1 = yes, 0 = no). Lastly, respondents were asked to report how frequently face-to-face meetings for specific types of caseloads (e.g., by risk level and special population status) were occurring compared to before COVID-19. This variable was measured on a 3-point Likert scale with response items including occurring less frequently, same frequency, and more frequently than before COVID-19.

Use of technology. The survey contained a dichotomous measure (1 = yes, 0 = no) asking directors to report which technologies officers were currently using to supervise individuals on their caseload. Items included "telephone calls," "texting," "e-mail," "postcards," "video conferencing," and "telehealth." Next, we asked directors to report whether the use of these technologies was occurring more or less frequently than before COVID-19. This scale was measured on a 4-point Likert scale, with response options ranging from not currently using, but we plan to use through using more frequently than before COVID-19.

Responses to behavior. The survey included two questions designed to measure the type of practices officers were currently implementing with their caseloads as well as violation practices. Both scales were measured on a 3-point Likert scale ranging from less frequently to more frequently than before COVID-19. First, we asked directors to report the frequency officers were implementing a variety of responses to individual behavior, such as "technical violations," "revocations," "drug testing," and "making referrals to mental health or substance use treatment." Next, we asked directors to report the frequency at which violations were issued for noncompliance behaviors, such as "failing a drug/alcohol test," "failure to attend a treatment program," "pay fines/fees," "find employment," and "committing a new crime."

Agency policies. Directors were asked to report whether collection of supervision fees was suspended, or if they were collecting fees and issuing violations for unpaid balances (1 = yes, 0 = no). Next, we asked directors to report whether any supervision terms were ended early (1 = yes, 0 = no). For those who responded yes, they were asked to provide information on the characteristics of individuals whose supervision terms were ended early ("low risk," "served a minimum amount of time," "in compliance with all of their supervision conditions," and "other"; 1 = yes, 0 = no) and the percentage of cases terminated. Lastly, we asked directors to report whether they planned to release individuals from supervision early in the future (1 = yes, 0 = no).

Directors were asked to report whether COVID-19 specific prevention policies had been implemented (1 = yes, 0 = no). Example items included whether masks were provided for staff and/or individuals on supervision and whether mask use was required. An open-ended response item was included to allow directors to write in other prevention strategies implemented.

Containment strategies

Directors were asked to report whether they had implemented a number of containment strategies, including use of a screening tool to identify people with possible exposure to COVID-19 or at a higher risk of COVID-19 infection, and sharing information and guidance about COVID-19 prevention (1 = yes, 0 = no). An open-ended response item allowed respondents to provide any other containment strategies implemented.

Response strategies

Directors were asked to report whether they engaged in response strategies such as whether they "created medical care plans for individuals on supervision," "provided training for staff on how to respond to possible COVID-19 infections," and whether policies were implemented to support staff who tested positive (e.g., paid sick leave) (1 = yes, 0 = no). Directors were given the opportunity to write in additional response strategies.

Impact of COVID-19

To understand the impact of COVID-19 on staffing, we asked whether and what percent of officers were furloughed or laid off, and whether these reductions in workforce were expected in the future. We asked directors whether there were any positive COVID-19 cases identified among clients or staff in their office. Those who reported positive cases were asked to estimate the number of positives detected and to describe the agency response to the detection of positive tests.

Director perceptions

Lastly, directors were asked two open-ended questions regarding their perceptions of the impact of COVID-19 on their agency. First, we asked directors to report the most beneficial strategy their agency has implemented to support effective operations during the COVID-19 pandemic. Second, we asked directors the most pressing issue facing community corrections' agencies in the current climate.

Analytic plan

All survey data were exported to Qualtrics and uploaded to SPSS version 26 for analysis. Because the focus of this study is to examine the landscape of community corrections during the COVID-19 pandemic, a series of descriptive analyses were conducted. Given the focus of this study is exploratory in nature, inferential analyses were not conducted.

Results

Prevention strategies

Of the 213 agencies participating in the survey to-date, 59.1% reported they were supervising individuals face-to-face in the office, while 46% reported supervising individuals face-to-face in the field, representing 179 unique agencies. Only 15.9% of agencies reported they were not seeing any individuals, in any capacity, face-to-face (see Table 2). Of those meetings in the office, 42.9% reported they met somewhere other than usual office space such as the lobby or a classroom where there was more space to social distance. Of those meetings in the field, 72.4% reported officers met with individuals outside of their homes, 26.5% reported they met somewhere else, such as a community park or place of employment, while 8.2% reported no change in how they conducted field visits.

Of the 179 agencies who reported some face-to-face contact (office or field), 25.7% reported they met with all individuals on their caseload as they normally would. However, 51.9% reported they met with high-risk individuals, 26.9% moderate risk, and

Table 2. Face-to-face contact strategies (N = 213).

	% (*n*)
In office	59.1% (126)
In office, somewhere other than usual office space	42.9% (54)
In office, no change	39.7% (50)
In office, designated place (e.g., lobby, classroom)	32.5% (41)
Outside office, parking lot, curbside	19.8% (25)
In office, behind barrier/plexiglass	11.9% (15)
In field	46.0% (98)
In field, outside home	72.4% (71)
In field, park, place of employment	11.1% (14)
In field, no change	8.2% (8)
No face-to-face meetings occurring	15.9% (34)

8.6% with low-risk individuals. Additionally, 37.9% of directors reported they saw individuals who needed to be drug tested while 45.2% of agencies saw new clients (see Figure 1). In agencies where officers saw all individuals face-to-face as they would have prior to COVID-19 (n = 46), about 48% reported these meetings occurred at the same frequency while 46% reported they occurred less frequently than before COVID-19. Directors reported seeing individuals with mental health (41.8%) and substance use (61.4%) issues less frequently due to COVID-19. The only group seen at the same frequency was individuals convicted of sex offenses (63.1%) (see Figure 2).

Use of technology

The most commonly used technology to continue active supervision of individuals during the COVID-19 pandemic was telephone calls (95.8%). A large percentage of agencies

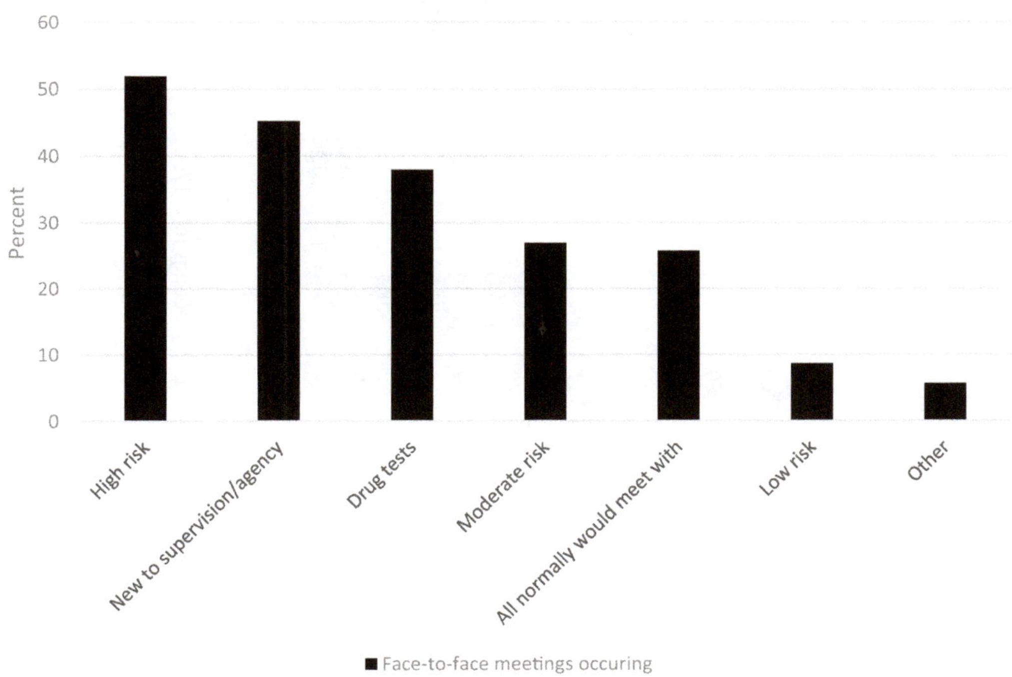

Figure 1. Number of agencies using face-to-face meetings by client type (n = 179).

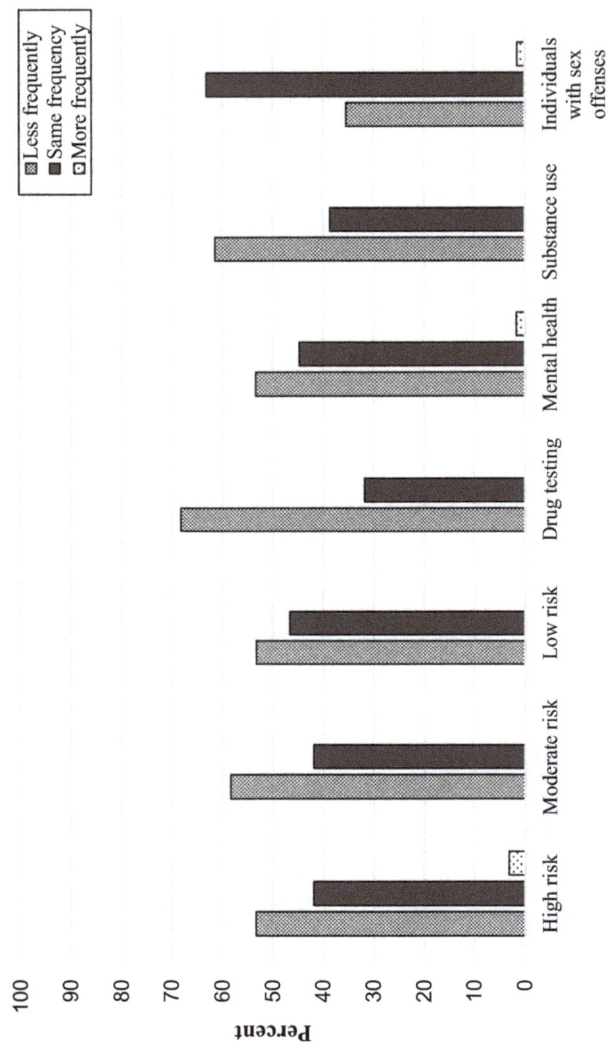

Figure 2. Frequency of face-to-face meetings (n = 179).

reported their officers were also using texting (92%), e-mail (91.1%), and video conferencing (90.6%) to supervise their caseloads (see Figure 3). Approximately 12% of directors reported the use of other technology, including smartphone applications, website reporting, kiosks, electronic monitoring, and social media. Of all strategies, 81% reported that video conferencing was a new technology implemented in response to COVID-19

The majority of directors reported individuals were using telehealth services for mental health (82.6%) and substance use (83.6%). Approximately 35% of agencies reported telehealth for mental health services was a new option, while 41% of agencies reported telehealth for substance use services was newly implemented. Of those implementing telehealth, approximately 48% of directors reported increased use for mental health and 53% increased use for substance use during the COVID-19 pandemic (see Figure 3).

Responses to behavior

For all supervision and case management supervision strategies inquired about, the largest increase in use was reported for electronic monitoring/GPS (25%) (see Table 3). Directors reported decreased use of drug testing (88.7%), community service requirements (77.2%), revocations (76%), and technical violations (75%). Directors reported their office processed fewer violations for all noncompliance, except for commission of a new crime (52%) and possession of a firearm (41%), which agencies were more likely to use violations at the same frequency as prior to COVID-19.

Agency policies

At the time of data collection, approximately 62% of agencies reported they were collecting supervision fees but were not issuing violations for late fees while 14% reported issuing violations for late fees. Only 2.5% of agencies suspended the collection of supervision fees during the pandemic. Roughly 22% of agencies reported they made alterations in their collection process, such as permitting online, mail-in, or phone payments.

Approximately 24% of agencies reported they had terminated supervision terms early because of COVID-19 (see Table 4). The majority reported these individuals were those in full compliance with all conditions of probation (91.7%), while other characteristics used to guide termination decisions included whether they were low risk (68.8%) or served between 50% and 75% of their time (41.7%). Approximately 66% of all agencies reported they were not planning to terminate supervision terms in the future, while 30% reported this was a possibility.

Most agencies reported they received fewer new clients referred for supervision (71.6%), while 31% of agencies reported receiving increased referrals since the start of the COVID-19 pandemic. Of those who experienced a decline, directors reported anywhere from a 1% reduction in caseload to a 100% reduction, representing no new cases referred. In agencies that experienced an increase, the reported range was from 1% to 40% increase (see Table 4).

Provision of PPE

Approximately 83% of agencies provided face masks for staff, while 56% provided masks for individuals on supervision. Approximately 72% required staff to wear a face mask while working, while 65% required individuals on supervision to wear a face mask. When asked to report additional policies implemented, 10% reported conducting temperature screening of all individuals prior to entering the building, 10% reported additional

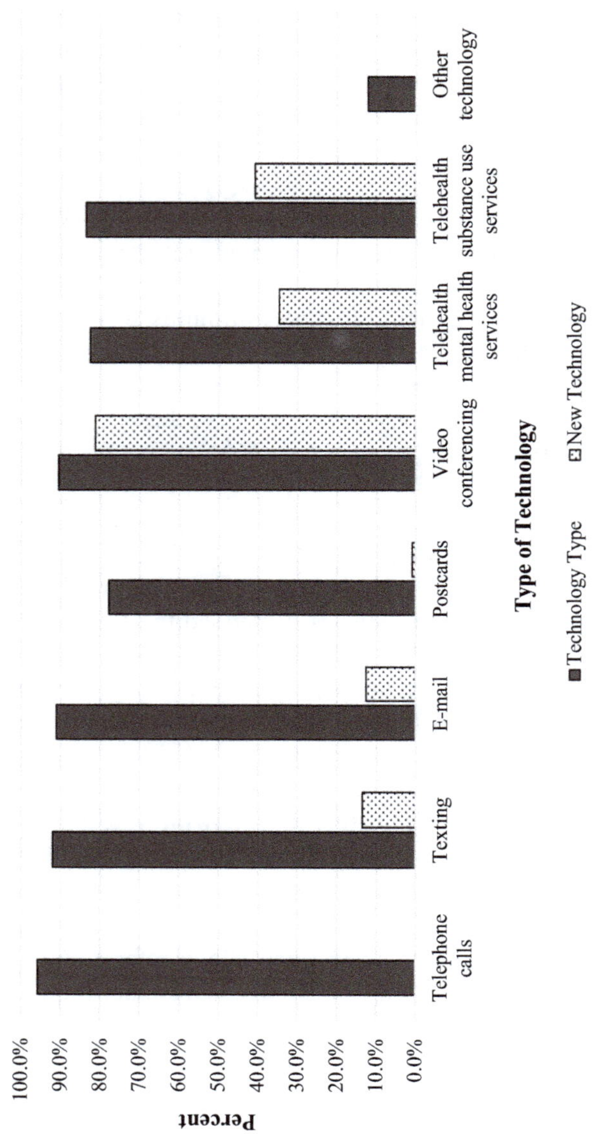

Figure 3. Use of technology to supervise clients (N = 213).

Table 3. Use of supervision strategies and violations compared to pre-COVID-19 (N = 213).

	Less frequently	Same frequency	More frequently
Supervision Strategy Use			
Drug testing	88.7%	10.3%	0.5%
Community service	77.2%	12.9%	3.0%
Revocations	76.1%	16.4%	2.5%
Technical violations	75.1%	18.4%	3.0%
Employment assistance	36.3%	45.3%	10.4%
Substance use treatment	28.1%	62.1%	5.9%
Housing assistance	26.4%	48.3%	7.5%
Risk assessments	23.2%	68.5%	4.4%
Curfews	22.3%	44.6%	11.9%
Mental health treatment	22.2%	64.5%	8.9%
EM/GPS	20.8%	38.6%	24.9%
Help accessing medical care	20.0%	49.3%	5.0%
Use of Violations			
Failed drug/alcohol test	69.4%	14.5%	9.7%
Failed community service	61.9%	12.5%	12.5%
Failed to appear to meeting with office	59.5%	22.1%	11.1%
Failed to maintain employment	53.9%	17.9%	22.9%
Failure to appear for court	53.0%	25.9%	8.6%
Pay supervision fees	51.9%	18.9%	21.6%
Attend treatment program	50.5%	22.2%	15.5%
Associate with prohibited individuals/places	50.5%	29.8%	11.0%
Pay fines/restitution	49.2%	21.7%	20.6%
New crime	25.5%	52.0%	4.4%
Possession of firearm	25.0%	41.7%	4.4%

Table 4. Supervision terminations and change of client referrals.

Early termination of supervision (*n* = 203)	% (*n*)
Yes	23.5% (48)
No	64.7% (132)
Not sure	11.8% (24)
Terminations by client status (*n* = 48)	% (*n*)
In compliance with all conditions	91.7% (44)
Low risk	68.8% (33)
Served minimum time (range from 50%-75%)	41.7% (20)
Other characteristics (e.g., payment of fees, significant progress in treatment)	16.7% (8)
Agency plans to terminate supervision terms in the future (N = 213)	% (*n*)
Yes	4.2% (9)
Maybe	29.7 (60)
No	65.8% (133)
New Client Referrals (*n* =204)	% (*n*)
Decrease in new clients	71.6% (146)
Increase in new clients	8.8% (18)
Estimated percent decline in number of clients (*n* = 146)	% (*n*)
1–20% decline	19.2% (28)
21–40% decline	23.4% (34)
41–60% decline	17.1% (25)
61–80% decline	17.1% (25)
81–100% decline	11.0% (16)
Estimated percent increase in number of clients (*n* = 18)	% (*n*)
1–10% increase	38.9% (7)
11–20% increase	33.3% (6)
21–30% increase	11.1% (2)
31–40% increase	5.6% (1)
Don't know	5.6% (1)

sanitization of office space, 9% enforced social distancing, and 7% installed plexiglass barriers (see Table 5).

Table 5. Reported prevention, containment, and response strategies implemented (N = 213).

Prevention	% (*n*)
Provide face masks to officers	83.1% (177)
Require officers wear a face mask	71.8% (153)
Require individuals on supervise wear a face mask	64.8% (138)
Provide face masks to individuals on supervision	55.9% (119)
Other strategies:	53.1% (113)
Temperature checks before entering building	10.3% (22)
Additional sanitization of building/agency cars	9.8% (21)
All contact 6 ft or greater, including enforcement in lobby/waiting room	9.3% (20)
Plexiglass barriers, sneeze guards, glass barriers, desk guards	6.6% (14)
In planning phase, nothing implemented yet	0.01% (3)
Containment	% (*n*)
Sharing of information and guidance with staff	73.7% (157)
Sharing of information and guidance with individuals on supervision	58.2% (124)
Use of screening tool to identify possible exposure	52.1% (111)
Use of screening tool to identify people at a higher risk of infection	26.8% (57)
Response	% (*n*)
Paid sick leave	62.0% (132)
Provide training for staff for responding to COVID-19	34.7% (74)
Plan for staffing/agency operations if significant portion unable to work	33.8% (72)
Create medical care plans for individuals on supervision	10.3% (22)
Have not implemented anything yet	26.8% (57)

Containment strategies

Approximately 52% of agencies reported implementing a screening tool to identify individuals who may have been exposed to COVID-19. Another 27% reported implementing a screening tool to identify individuals who are at a higher risk of COVID-19 infection. Roughly 74% of directors shared guidance about prevention with their staff, while 58% shared guidance with individuals on supervision. Other less common strategies reported included requiring clients to sign a form stating they do not have COVID-19 and/or do not currently have symptoms, requiring staff to report symptoms each day before coming to work, posting a sign with common symptoms on the front door, and requiring staff to log all contacts (see Table 5).

Response strategies

Ten percent of directors reported creating medical care plans with guidance on accessing emergency care, a transportation plan, and medical insurance. Less than half of participating agencies reported providing training to their staff on procedures to respond to COVID-19 (34.7%). However, 62% of directors implemented a paid sick leave policy while 33.8% reported having a plan for staffing substitutions and/or agency operations if staff were to fall ill. Approximately 27% of agencies had not yet implemented any policies to support staff who became ill with COVID-19 (see Table 5).

Impact of COVID-19

Approximately 38% of offices reported at least one confirmed case of COVID-19 among individuals on supervision, while 15% reported at least one confirmed case among officers. In these offices, the majority reported fewer than 10 positive cases (60% among clients and 88% among staff). In offices where a client tested positive, 32% placed the individual on

Table 6. Policies implemented in response to identification of positive COVID-19 cases in office.

Response	Clients (n = 64)	Staff (n = 24)
Remote supervision for individual until cleared	31.7% (20)	- -
Cleaning service/increased cleaning	20.6% (13)	70.8% (17)
Remote work for staff/skeleton crew in office	19.0% (12)	- -
Contact tracing	6.3% (4)	45.8% (11)
Closed office temporarily	6.3% (4)	20.8% (5)
Encouraged medical attention	6.3% (4)	- -
Test PO, quarantine until negative	6.3% (4)	58.3% (14)

remote supervision until either they tested negative or 14 days had passed (see Table 6). In those offices where a staff member tested positive, 71% increased cleaning protocols and/or hired a cleaning service, 46% conducted contact tracing, 38% required the officer to quarantine until they tested negative, 21% required any other staff who came into contact with the individual to quarantine until they tested negative, and 21% closed the office temporarily.

Director perceptions

Directors were asked to report the single most beneficial policy implemented in their agency in response to COVID-19 to-date. Of the 171 directors who responded, the most reported beneficial policy was the use of remote supervision and technology to continue supervising individuals (46.8%). The next most frequent responses were mask requirements/use of PPE (10.5%), rotating schedules/skeleton crews (7.6%), and requiring an appointment (5.8%).

Directors were also asked to report the most pressing issue for community corrections' agencies currently. The most common issue reported was the inability to hold individuals on supervision accountable (29%). This challenge stemmed from several issues. First, directors noted they had a limited ability to use incarceration as a sanction. Either the jail would not take individuals for probation violations or judges would not sentence individuals to be incarcerated. Second, directors noted there was a backlog of cases in the court system, which equated to a delay in responding to probation violations filed with the court. Third, directors reported courts were not issuing warrants for arrest for probation violations. As a result, directors noted they were struggling to determine both which violations were worth their time to file, and how to respond to noncompliance when issuing a violation was not possible. The second most common issue directors reported was the limited ability to conduct drug tests (14.6%). In these cases, directors noted they suspected increased levels of drug use but could not conduct drug tests as frequently as usual due to remote work, safety concerns, limited resources/staffing to process tests, or closure of labs. Approximately 13% of directors reported that the inability to meet face-to-face was a challenge, often due to the perceived inability to stay current with the individual and provide an adequate level of supervision. And, close to 10% noted budget strains were the most pressing issue. Some agency budgets largely depend on supervision fees, which clients were struggling to pay, and/or decreased referrals to probation equated to decreased collection of fees and not enough demand for officers.

Discussion

The goal of this study was to examine the policies and procedures community corrections' agencies have put into place in response to COVID-19. The current pandemic challenges correctional decision-makers on how to manage large correctional populations, enforce compliance, and provide and/or link to appropriate treatments while supporting public health measures to prevent virus transmission among staff, clients, and the community. Although this effort is descriptive, it provides a preliminary exploration of the primary changes to traditional supervision as well as ongoing challenges. This information is meant to serve as a starting point for developing guidelines for community corrections' agencies both as the pandemic progresses and for future public health emergencies.

The largest, and perhaps most obvious, change reported across community corrections' agencies was the decrease in face-to-face supervision practices. Less than three-quarters of agencies surveyed reported they were still meeting with individuals in the office, and of those who were, agencies largely prioritized individuals assessed as higher risk followed by those who were new clients. And, agencies instructed officers who conducted field visits to do so either outside the individual's home or in another outdoor location (e.g., community park, place of employment) rather than enter the home as they normally would. In place of this face-to-face contact, agencies reported a large increase in the use of technology (e.g., telephone calls, video conferencing, e-mail, and texting) to supervise caseloads. For the majority of agencies, the use of video conferencing was an entirely new technology. While not surprising, given much of the country has shifted to remote work, this is a significant shift for community corrections' agencies.

There is little previous research on the use of technology as a replacement for face-to-face supervision meetings, but when it has been implemented, these technologies have focused on the use of kiosks (Barnes et al., 2010, 2012; Belshaw, 2011; Ogden & Horrocks, 2000; Wilson et al., 2007) and telephone supervision systems (Viglione & Taxman, 2018). Randomized controlled trials found no significant differences in reoffending, arrest, and incarceration rates between individuals supervised by kiosks and those on traditional supervision (Barnes et al., 2010, 2012). However, the use of these technologies was reserved for only individuals assessed as low risk. And even then, officers were hesitant to rely on the technology as the main supervision modality. An evaluation of telephone supervision found officers either refused placement of low-risk individuals on telephone supervision altogether or avoided designating an individual as low risk to prevent them from being placed on the telephone supervision caseload (Viglione & Taxman, 2018). The COVID-19 pandemic has forced agencies to not only implement technology but to implement technology for most of their caseloads, regardless of the risk level. Directors reported this adaptation was the single most beneficial change made in response to COVID-19. The use of technology allowed agencies to prioritize the health and safety of their staff and clients and has removed some traditional barriers for individuals on supervision, including transportation and flexibility to meet with their officers around their work schedules. Despite these reported benefits, there is scant empirical evidence regarding the implementation and effectiveness of teleconferencing for community supervision. However, meta-analytic evidence examining the use of telehealth with criminal justice populations for substance use services finds virtual services were as effective as in-person services (Batastini et al., 2016). While this evidence points to the utility of technology, a critical path forward for future research is to examine the implementation of technologies to supervise individuals and provide support and a range of services.

Despite the reported benefit of technology to continue supervision efforts, directors reported the biggest challenge currently facing the field of community supervision was the inability to hold individuals accountable. This was due to court systems being entirely shut down or were operating with a backlog, inability to obtain arrest warrants, limited processing of violations, and reduced use of jails for probation violations. This left many directors feeling as though they must prioritize only the most serious violations (e.g., new offense or firearm possession) and that they have limited alternatives to keep individuals in compliance. Given the nature of the pandemic and the attention on reducing crowding within jails and prisons, this challenge is one community corrections' agencies may face for the foreseeable future.

A growing body of evidence suggests the use of jail and incarceration as a sanction may not be the strongest strategy to respond to noncompliance (Boman et al., 2019; De Wree et al., 2009; Gil, 2010; Morash et al., 2019; Wodahl et al., 2015). For example, Boman et al. (2019) found no difference between the use of jail-based and community-based sanctions in response to drug use violations, while enhanced treatment sanctions improved the likelihood that an individual would successfully complete intensive supervision probation. Morash et al. (2019) found punitive responses (e.g., jail time, extension of supervision term, increased drug testing) to non-drug-related violations were related to increased violations, while treatment responses (e.g., encouragement, required, or increased drug treatment) were related to decreased recidivism. Additional research found no difference in effectiveness between jail-based sanctions and alternatives (e.g., written assignments, treatment requirements, community service) in promoting compliance and decreased recidivism (De Wree et al., 2009; Gil, 2010; Wodahl et al., 2015). This research supports the use of alternative, community-based responses to noncompliance and suggests support for strengthening systems of graduated sanctions, which aim to provide incremental responses to noncompliance while reserving formal violations for the most serious behaviors (Burke, 1997; Taxman et al., 1999). Examples of incremental responses include those aligned with a rehabilitation goal (e.g., drug court, treatment) or punitive goals (e.g., increased reporting requirements, electronic monitoring, increased drug testing) (Burke, 1997). However, the pandemic presents challenges to many of these options due to limited resources (e.g., limited availability of treatment, inability to drug test). This suggests the need for individual agencies to create a schedule of responses feasible in their jurisdiction as well as creativity in developing alternatives to violations.

The inability to drug test individuals on supervision was also reported as a major challenge during the pandemic. Directors reported significant concern that individuals were likely relapsing and/or using substances at an increased rate during the pandemic and that they were unable to detect this increase in use. Changes in drug testing resulted from either the complete shut down of community supervision offices where drug tests were conducted, the use of skeleton crews which resulted in not enough staff in office at one time to drug test the population at the normal rate, and the shutdown and/or backlog in labs who conduct and/or process drug testing. Additionally, directors reported concerns over the safety of conducting drug tests during the pandemic. Several directors reported they had switched to the use of mouth swabs for drug testing, the use of patch testing for alcohol use, or had actually added a window to their bathrooms so officers could supervise drug tests from a different room. This challenge presents a direct need for community supervision agencies to partner with public health experts, as drug testing does involve risks that are directly relevant in the COVID-19 pandemic. For example, research on COVID-19 finds that viral RNA may be present in urine, but little evidence that this viral RNA is infectious (Nomoto et al., 2020). However, infectious viral RNA is known to be found in saliva (To et al., 2020), which suggests the use of mouth swabs may be riskier than traditional urine screens. However, officer supervision of a urine screen in an enclosed space without proper ventilation (e.g., a bathroom) is also risky for COVID-19 transmission (Morawska et al., 2020). And, with either strategy, appropriate PPE would be required to reduce risks of transmission, which requires the acquisition of resources that have been difficult across the country. Safer alternatives may include bathroom window observation of drug screens or perhaps when proper PPE is available, the use of curbside mouth swab testing. However, creating alternatives to procedures such as drug testing requires careful consideration of the medical and infectious disease research on COVID-19 and should be done in consultation with experts to best protect the safety of staff and clients. Continued shut-downs, lack of resources/staff, and backlogs in labs are likely to persist, which will require the development of protocols that are safe and feasible for community supervision agencies to implement.

Lastly, financial and budget concerns are likely to challenge community supervision agencies for the foreseeable future. While many directors reported current budget crises already, others reported the expectation of financial crises to come. With the inability to collect supervision fees and reduction in the numbers of individuals on supervision, directors have been (anticipate) forced to lay off staff. This is particularly troubling as directors report expectations that their budgets will be drastically reduced for years to come, yet the reduction in caseloads is not expected to last indefinitely. Thus, it is likely that community corrections' agencies may see a surge in cases (e.g., once court backlogs have resolved), yet they will have drastically reduced budgets and workload. This anticipated challenge may be partially addressed through the continued use of technology to supervise clients; however, researchers and practitioners should prioritize developing protocols and guidelines for community supervision agencies to navigate the consequences of the pandemic.

Limitations

The goal of the current study was to provide a descriptive and preliminary analysis of the ways in which community supervision agencies have adapted and responded to the COVID-19 pandemic. Given the nonrandom sample, it is possible that the findings presented here do not generalize to community supervision agencies across the country. However, we were able to report on data from a significant portion of the country and across a number of different settings (e.g., region, populations served). And, this study serves to build knowledge around the contextual factors that may be currently impacting community supervision agencies in the United States as a means to build the foundation for further examining the impact of COVID-19 on practice and outcomes. The data presented in this manuscript represent data from the first month of data collection only. The next steps of this study include an additional month of data collection in wave 1 followed by two additional waves of data collection to examine how responses to COVID-19 and the challenges presented to community supervision agencies change over the course of the pandemic.

Conclusions

The pandemic has drastically altered the nature of community supervision across the United States. Approximately 4 months into the pandemic, community supervision agencies have had to shift to a technological approach to supervising caseloads and grapple with initial challenges of accountability, drug testing, and budget strains. This analysis aimed to shed light on these issues to spark conversation and action to develop strategies that will assist community supervision agencies during these challenging times. Immediate work is needed to support directors and probation staff in addressing noncompliance using alternatives to violations and jail-based sanctions and the monitoring and detection of substance use as well as develop and advance technologies to support supervision efforts during the ongoing pandemic and beyond. This ongoing project sets a foundation for additional inquiry in understanding how agencies response to COVID-19 will shape the future of community corrections.

At a broader level, we are at a critical juncture to consider how the landscape of community corrections might be permanently altered to better define key goals and priorities, and cost-effective methods for achieving these goals. Previous research suggests probation, although designed as an alternative to incarceration, serves as a "net widener" (Phelps, 2013). The imposition of many conditions and punishment for noncompliance with those conditions can result in revocation and incarceration (Doherty, 2016; Klingele, 2013), a system that can feed both mass imprisonment and mass probation (Phelps, 2020). Correctional agency resources were often limited prior to the COVID-19 pandemic, with evidence from the current study suggesting these budgets may become even further strained. Coupled with the current health risks associated with many traditional supervision processes, steps toward reform seems necessary now more than ever. Research on effective correctional practices has emphasized the need to intervene with higher-risk individuals, citing the negative consequences that result from over-supervising those who are a low risk to reoffend (Hanley, 2006; Lowenkamp & Latessa, 2002). And, Phelps (2020) discusses a number of key reforms to move away from a system of mass probation to a system that can provide meaningful supports to individuals on supervision, including a reduction in the use of community supervision, a reduction in the number of probation conditions, especially blanket conditions applied to entire populations, and more liberal use of early terminations. Findings from the current study suggest agencies have been forced to implement some of these measures, suggesting a need for ongoing research to examine the long-term impacts of these changes. Additionally, Phelps (2020) calls for improved guidelines and tools for responding to probation violations, a need that is supported by the findings of the current study. Given the hardships and complexities posed by COVID-19, implementation and evaluation of these reforms could move the field away from the wide use of community supervision to a more targeted approach designed to provide quality, individualized services and support for those with the greatest needs. And, in the context of COVID-19, these steps could assist agencies by reducing the number of individuals they must manage and adapt services for during times of crises, reducing risks for staff, individuals on supervision, and their families and communities.

Note

1. The states represented in the sample are as follows: Northeast: Connecticut, Massachusetts, New Jersey, New York, Pennsylvania, Vermont; Midwest: Illinois, Indiana, Iowa, Missouri, Kansas, Michigan, Nebraska, Ohio; West: Arizona, California, Colorado, Hawaii, Idaho, Montana, Nevada, New Mexico, Oregon, Utah, Washington; South: Alabama, Arkansas, Florida, Georgia, Louisiana, Maryland, South Carolina, Texas, Virginia.

Disclosure statement

No potential conflict of interest was reported by the author(s).

Funding

This study was funded by a grant from the National Science Foundation [grant number 2030344]. The authors gratefully acknowledge the contributions of community corrections agency staff to share their experiences during an extraordinarily difficult time.

References

Ahlin, E. M., Antunes, M. J. L., & Tubman-Carbone, H. (2013). A review of probation home visits: What do we know? *Federal Probation*, *77*(3), 32–37. https://heinonline.org/HOL/Page?handle=hein.journals/fedpro77&div=34&g_sent=1&casa_token=0ouk_J4c23AAAAAA:3eELir3C02gF1P_CzG9f7RrQgh1B24dHqQfCwHEOciH3H0uFfuddXKvuF2v8JUh5j4H1SgzBeg&collection=journals

Ahmed, F., Ahmed, N., Pissarides, C., & Stiglitz, J. (2020). Why inequality could spread COVID-19. *The Lancet*, *5*(12), E240. https://doi.org/10.1016/S2468-2667(20)30085-2

Andrews, D. A., & Bonta, J. (2010). Rehabilitating criminal justice policy and practice. *Psychology, Public Policy and Law*, *16*(1), 39–55. https://doi.org/10.1037/a0018362

Barnes, G. C., Ahlman, L., Gill, C., Sherman, L. W., Kurtz, E., & Malvestuto, R. (2010). Low-intensity community supervision for low-risk offenders: A randomized, controlled trial. *Journal of Experimental Criminology*, *6*(2), 159–189. https://doi.org/10.1007/s11292-010-9094-4

Barnes, G. C., Hyatt, J. M., Ahlman, L. C., & Kent, D. T. (2012). The effects of low-intensity supervision for lower-risk probationers: Updated results from a randomized controlled trial. *Journal of Crime & Justice*, *35*(2), 200–220. https://doi.org/10.1080/0735648X.2012.679874

Batastini, A. B., King, C. M., Morgan, R. D., & McDaniel, B. (2016). Telepsychological services with criminal justice and substance abuse clients: A systematic review and meta-analysis. *Psychological Services*, *13*(1), 20–30. https://doi.org/10.1037/ser0000042

Belshaw, S. H. (2011). Supervising probationers on the information superhighway: Towards an understanding of minimum supervision level probationers in a large Texas county. *International Journal of Punishment and Sentencing*, *7*(3), 98–106. https://heinonline.org/HOL/Page?handle=hein.journals/punisen7&div=15&g_sent=1&casa_token=z5GwGP33VuMAAAAA:-k1PaCVucAfV-OcKH16S2fX8OvI9FGRCw4t-WBojMK7Q49Z1YvgRb4aWr67s6-1zffYpIgjudQ&collection=journals

Boman, J. H., IV, Mowen, T. J., Wodahl, E. J., Lee Miller, B., & Miller, J. M. (2019). Responding to substance-use-related probation and parole violations: Are enhanced treatment sanctions preferable to jail sanctions? *Criminal Justice Studies*, *32*(4), 356–370. https://doi.org/10.1080/1478601X.2019.1664506

Burke, P. (1997). *Policy-driven responses to probation and parole violations*. National Institute of Corrections.

Campedelli, G. M., Aziani, A., & Favarin, S. (2020). Exploring the effect of 2019-nCoV containment policies on crime: The case of Los Angeles. *arXiv Preprint arXiv, 2003*, 11021. https://doi.org/10.31219/osf.io/gcpq8

Clark, C. B., McCullumsmith, C. B., Waesche, M. C., Islam, M. A., Francis, R., & Cropsey, K. L. (2013). HIV-risk characteristics in community corrections. *Journal of Addiction Medicine, 7*(1), 45–51. https://doi.org/10.1097/ADM.0b013e3182781806

De Wree, E., Ruyver, B. D., & Pauwels, L. (2009). Criminal justice responses to drug offences: Recidivism following the application of alternative sanctions in Belgium. *Drugs: Education, Prevention and Policy, 16*(6), 550–560. https://doi.org/10.3109/09687630802133632

Dillman, D. A. (2000). *Mail and web-based survey: The tailored design method.* Wiley.

Doherty, F. (2016). Obey all laws and be good: Probation and the meaning of recidivism. *Georgetown Law Journal, 104*(2), 291–354. https://heinonline.org/HOL/Page?handle=hein.journals/glj104&div=13&g_sent=1&casa_token=&collection=journals

Dong, E., Du, H., & Gardner, L. (2020). An interactive web-based dashboard to track COVID-19 in real time. *Lancet Infectious Diseases, 20*(5), 533–534. https://doi.org/10.1016/S1473-3099(20)30120-1

Executives Transforming Probation and Parole [EXiT]. (2020, March 12). *Statement from community supervision executives on the importance of using best practices during the COVID-19 crisis.* https://www.exitprobationparole.org/Covid19statement.

Fearn, N. E., Vaughn, M. G., Nelson, E. J., Salas-Wright, C. P., DeLisi, M., & Qian, Z. (2016). Trends and correlates of substance use disorders among probationers and parolees in the United States 2002–2014. *Drug and Alcohol Dependence, 167*, 128–139. https://doi.org/10.1016/j.drugalcdep.2016.08.003

Gil, C. (2010). *The effect of sanction severity on criminal conduct: A randomized low intensity probation experiment* [Doctoral dissertation]. University of Pennsylvania.

Ginsburg-Kempany, K., & Kaiser, K. A. (2017). Incorporating procedural justice and legitimacy into the RNR model to improve risk-need assessment. In F. S. Taxman (Ed.), *Handbook on risk and need assessment: Theory and practice* (pp. 269–291). Routledge.

Hanley, D. (2006). Appropriate services: Examining the case classification principle. *Journal of Offender Rehabilitation, 42*(4), 1–22. https://doi.org/10.1300/J076v42n04_01

Igielnik, R. (2020, May 15). *Majority of Americans who lost a job or wages due to COVID-19 concerned states will reopen too quickly.* Pew Research Center. https://www.pewresearch.org/fact-tank/2020/05/15/majority-of-americans-who-lost-a-job-or-wages-due-to-covid-19-concerned-states-will-reopen-too-quickly/

Kaeble, D., & Cowhig, M. (2018). *Correctional populations in the United States, 2016.* Bureau of Justice Statistics (BJS), US Department of Justice, and Office of Justice Programs.

Kaeble, D., & Alpher, M. (2020). *Probation and Parole in the United States, 2017–2018.* Bureau of Justice Statistics (BJS), US Department of Justice, and Office of Justice Programs. https://www.bjs.gov/content/pub/pdf/ppus1718.pdf

Klingele, C. (2013). Rethinking the use of community supervision. *Journal of Criminal Law and Criminology, 103*(4), 1015–1070. https://doi.org/10.2139/ssrn.2232078

Lowenkamp, C. T., & Latessa, E. J. (2002). *Evaluation of Ohio's community based correctional facilities and halfway house programs* (Technical report). University of Cincinnati.

Morash, M., Kashy, D. A., Smith, S. W., & Cobbina, J. E. (2019). Technical violations, treatment and punishment responses, and recidivism of women on probation and parole. *Criminal Justice Policy Review, 30*(5), 788–810. https://doi.org/10.1177/0887403417723425

Morawska, L., Tang, J. W., Bahnfleth, W., Bluyssen, P. M., Boerstra, A., Buonanno, G., … Wierzbicka, A. (2020). How can airborne transmission of COVID-19 indoors be minimised? *Environment International, 142*, 105832. https://doi.org/10.1016/j.envint.2020.105832.

Nomoto, H., Ishikane, M., Katagiri, D., Kinoshita, N., Nagashima, M., Sadamasu, K., … Ohmagari, N. (2020). Cautious handling of urine from moderate to severe COVID-19 patients. *American Journal of Infection Control, 48*(8). https://doi.org/http://doi.10.1016/j.ajic.2020.05.034.

Ogden, T. G., & Horrocks, C. (2000). Pagers, digital audio, and kiosk: Officer assistants. *Federal Probation, 65*(2), 35–44.

Petersilia, J. (1997). Probation in the United States. *Crime and Justice*, *22*, 149–200. https://doi.org/10.1086/449262

Phelps, M. (2013). The paradox of probation: Community supervision in the age of mass incarceration. *Law & Policy*, *35*(1–2), 51–80. https://doi.org/10.1111/lapo.12002

Phelps, M. (2020). Mass probation from micro to macro: Tracing the expansion and consequences of community supervision. *Annual Review of Criminology*, *3*(1), 261–279. https://doi.org/10.1146/annurev-criminol-011419-041352

Prison Policy Initiative. (2020, August 18). *Responses to the COVID-19 Pandemic*. https://www.prisonpolicy.org/virus/virusresponse.html

Schwartzapfel, B. (2020, April 3). *Probation and parole officers are rethinking their rules as coronavirus spreads*. The Marshall Project. https://www.themarshallproject.org/2020/04/03/probation-and-parole-officers-are-rethinking-their-rules-as-coronavirus-spreads

Sharma, D., Li, W., Lavoie, D., & Lauer, C. (2020, June 16). *Prison populations drop by 100,000 during the pandemic*. The Marshall Project. https://www.themarshallproject.org/2020/07/16/prison-populations-drop-by-100-000-during-pandemic

Snow, J., & Mann, M. (2013). *Qualtrics survey software: Handbook for research professionals*. Qualtrics Labs, Inc.

Sumner, A., Hoy, C., & Ortiz-Juarez, E. (2020). *Estimates of the impact of COVID-19 on global poverty. UNU-WIDER, April*, 800-9. United Nations University World Institute for Development Economics Research.

Taxman, F. S., Soule, D., & Gelb, A. (1999). Graduated sanctions: Stepping into accountable systems and offenders. *The Prison Journal*, *79*(2), 182–204. https://doi.org/10.1177/0032885599079002004

The Marshall Project. (2020, August 14). *A state-by-state look at coronavirus in prisons*. https://www.themarshallproject.org/2020/05/01/a-state-by-state-look-at-coronavirus-in-prisons

To, K. K. W., Tsang, O. T. Y., Leung, W. S., Tam, A. R., Wu, T. C., Lung, D. C., . . . Lau, D. P. L. (2020). Temporal profiles of viral load in posterior oropharyngeal saliva samples and serum antibody responses during infection by SARS-CoV-2: An observational cohort study. *The Lancet Infectious Diseases*, *20*(5), 565–574. https://doi.org/10.1016/S1473-3099(20)30196-1

Vaughn, M. G., DeLisi, M., Beaver, K. M., Perron, B. E., & Abdon, A. (2012). Toward a criminal justice epidemiology: Behavioral and physical health of probationers and parolees in the United States. *Journal of Criminal Justice*, *40*(3), 165–173. https://doi.org/10.1016/j.jcrimjus.2012.03.001

Vera Institute of Justice. (2020a, May 14). *New research shows nationwide failure to release people from prison to prevent spread of COVID-19*. Vera Institute of Justice. https://www.vera.org/newsroom/new-research-shows-nationwide-failure-to-release-people-from-prison-to-prevent-spread-of-covid–19

Vera Institute of Justice. (2020b, March 18). *Guidance for preventative and responsive measures to coronavirus for parole, probation, and clemency*. Vera Institute of Justice. https://www.vera.org/downloads/publications/coronavirus-guidance-parole-probation-clemency.pdf

Viglione, J., & Taxman, F. S. (2018). Low risk offenders under probation supervision: Risk management and the risk-needs-responsivity framework. *Criminal Justice and Behavior*, *45*(12), 1809–1831. https://doi.org/10.1177/0093854818790299

Wilson, J. A., Naro, W., & Austin, J. F. (2007). *Innovations in probation: Assessing New York City's automated reporting system*. JFA Associates.

Wodahl, E. J., Boman, J. H., IV, & Garland, B. E. (2015). Responding to probation and parole violations: Are jail sanctions more effective than community-based graduated sanctions? *Journal of Criminal Justice*, *43*(3), 242–250. https://doi.org/10.1016/j.jcrimjus.2015.04.010

The Response to the COVID19 Crisis by the Pennsylvania Department of Corrections

John E. Wetzel and Janeen M. Davis

ABSTRACT
The article is an overview of mitigation efforts and outcomes from a six month timeframe of managing COVID19 at the PA Department of Corrections.

In March 2020, the PA Department of Corrections experienced its first of three outbreaks to date, at three separate facilities. During this unprecedented time, we have been able to pivot, creating protocols with customization based upon the facility needs and physical structure. These protocols have been utilized at each affected facility, with the ability to effectively: limit the spread of infection (i.e., increased sanitation, social distancing/cohorting/facility "zoning"/ population reduction) ease and calm fears with education (i.e. prevention and recognition of symptomology), encourage and support staff and inmates with increased open communication (i.e. town hall meetings and fireside chats), manage/control daily facility activities/movement with innovative data gathering strategies (i.e., sewage and surveillance testing, "mapping" of county/facility hotspots). Today we are more sophisticated in our reviews and analyses resulting in a streamlined and quick decision making process with experiential confidence. Our COVID19 positive rate is approximately 1% lower, and the COVID19 mortality rate 6.1% lower than that of the community rate in Pennsylvania.

Nationally, this is the most prolific pandemic America has experienced in modern times, and it's safe to say that there was not a corrections system in the world prepared for this type of incident. A week into September, there are at least 125,000 incarcerated individuals in American prisons who have tested positive for COVID19 according to the Marshall Project. Sadly, the same publication report. Sadly, the same publication reports over 1,000 deaths in prisons of individuals with COVID19. Additionally, over 27,000 staff members have tested positive and regretfully there's been at least 75 deaths among corrections professionals. Clearly, systems were not prepared for this unforeseen event. (Project, The Marshall, 2020)

While it's true that every corrections system had a "pandemic plan ", which has generally been very successful against influenza (as a result of education, vaccination, and early identification/isolation/quarantine with onset of symptomology), it proved woefully insufficient to manage COVID19, and therefore, I share some numbing reasons why. First, no virus (to include influenza) that we've confronted has been this contagious. Secondly, we have never before had to deal with a contagious virus that is transmittable by people without symptoms. Thirdly, this often invisible, highly contagious virus occurred in America at a time where the political environment has created a situation where people don't believe data and science but rather news from the echo chamber most associated with their beliefs. These three factors created a situation that has become a literal nightmare for almost every corrections system.

Unlike many challenges corrections officials face, COVID19 is an outside/in threat. In other words, as COVID19 invaded America and began to spread across our country – the potential for transmission resided with individuals who routinely, often daily, entered our prisons/jails from the community. This lead to the implementation of several critical steps. Most systems stopped visits from the public very early on. Implementation of staff screenings (for everyone entering the facilities), included daily temperatures, and a questionnaire that assisted in identifying symptomology and contact with those individuals that were positive for the virus. Masking had also quickly become an expected practice. Increased sanitation protocols were mandated with access to cleaning products and hand sanitizer/ soap in an effort to prevent virus spread.

Nevertheless, given the challenging nature of this virus, it literally became a "pressure test" for systems. Similar to turning on the garden hose at the first sign of spring, invisible cracks leak while under pressure and systems experienced problems that likely lead to increased rates of spread from existing shortcomings in part due to new and unparalleled pressure points.

Staffing

Staffing prisons in the COVID19 era is one of the most challenging areas of management. Even with aggressive recruiting strategies; preconceived misconceptions of the correctional environment, personal fear, or other opportunities of interest within the community and/or private sector, affected Pennsylvania; therefore, like many other systems, went into COVID19 with vacancy rates of 20% or more. In addition to mitigation strategies that attempt to keep the virus from entering our facilities, such as staff failing a pre-entry COVID19 screening (preventing them from entering the institution), personal or family illness, and/or a loss of interest in job commitment based on fatigue or "burn out", has quickly become a universal issue.

Crowding

The number of inmates per square foot is emerging as one of the key factors in the amount of virus spread in a facility. Social distancing in a crowded prison is not possible. This is why many systems have reduced their populations. Even a system like ours, in Pennsylvania, that went into COVID19 below operational capacity (97%), found out quickly that operational capacity with social distancing requires further reductions. This is most relevant in dormitory housing settings. Operational capacity reduction is estimated at about 20% to ensure social distancing while the reduction in dorms averaged 50%.

Health care infrastructure

Providing community level health care in prisons has been historically challenging. Given the sheer number of inmates, the health acuity in a population likely to suffer from addictions, and the overrepresentation of mentally ill individuals, health care resources are frequently taxed under normal conditions. Due to the implementation of mitigation strategies (i.e. screening protocols, isolation, quarantine, COVID19 testing, "zoning"/delivery of medical services and/or medication administration, etc.) medical providers and nurses have had to adapt to a change in the way services are delivered and the length of time it takes to complete daily required assignments. An increase in staffing hours may be required to complete the duties as outlined in COVID19 established protocols, which at times may lead to exhaustion or staff burn out. Often, community staffing resources (i.e. nursing agencies, health care vendors) are not able to assist with requests/demands, as their staff have been allocated to the private sector or other county/state/federal agencies (i.e. long-term care). Medical equipment (i.e. thermometers, oxygen cylinders/concentrators, etc.) may also be difficult to obtain, as resources are strained in areas with increased COVID19 cases.

Essential components of a COVID19 management plan

First and foremost, systems must have a robust screening protocol that includes questions about both symptoms and contact with COVID19 positive individuals. Caution as to how shifts revolve through the facility to ensure social distancing is another key area. Ensuring that mask wearing is enforced for both staff and inmates, and easy access to hand sanitizer/ soap is also required.

Cohorting is a practice where managers decide the number of inmates that can be out of their cells at one time. Initially, many systems quarantined entire facilities, keeping inmates in their cells/dorms up to 22 hours per day. However, as this virus has progressed and knowledge gained, the need to increase out of cell time has necessitated the deploying of multiple inmates simultaneously or cohorting. Cohorting works in concert with the critical contact tracing infrastructure that is required. When a positive case is discovered, facilities must track contacts that specific individual has had, going back five days from onset of symptoms or the positive test date for those who are determined to be asymptomatic positives. Cohorts reduce the risk of spread by reducing the number of people who would be considered contacts.

Identification of vulnerable inmates

As defined by, and based on CDC guidelines, the Pennsylvania DOC utilized its Electronic Health Record (EHR) to ascertain "vulnerable" inmates. Information based on inmate medical diagnosis, age, body mass index, and lifestyle choices (i.e. smoking) was identified, and facility specific lists were created. These lists assist nurses when completing a more comprehensive COVID19 medical screen, to aid medical providers while ordering treatment plans for those affected by the virus, and to identify appropriate housing accommodations. Inmates that have been identified as "vulnerable" should be housed in cells, and not in dormitory settings if at all possible.

Isolation and testing

In order to mitigate the spread of infection within facilities, isolation and quarantine practices were implemented. Inmates that present with symptoms are removed from their cohort, placed in isolation and COVID19 tested. Based on test results, a COVID19 positive, asymptomatic inmate will be isolated for 14 days. A COVID19 positive, symptomatic inmate, will be discharged from protocol when they are medically stable, and upon the resolution of symptoms, as defined by the CDC. Cohorts that have been compromised by a COVID19 positive source, or have been identified as having a close contact through contact tracing, will be placed on enhanced quarantine protocols (temperature checks, observation/assessment for Influenza Like Illness "ILI", and pulse oximeters for inmates identified as "vulnerable"). These protocols will occur twice daily, for 14 days, from the day the "source" was removed from the cohort. Parole violators received from the street will also be placed on enhanced quarantine for 21 days after reception. Cohort enhanced quarantine protocols will be lifted on their respective dates, as long as no other person becomes symptomatic, or tests COVID19 positive. Quarantine protocols (temperature checks, and observation/assessment for ILI once daily) are implemented for all correctional (county, state, federal) receptions/transfers, or trips returning from the community (medical appointments, court appointments, etc.) for 14 days, as long as no person becomes symptomatic, or tests COVID19 positive within the cohort.

Lab based PCR testing is required for all inmate transfers and/or releases, inmates that present with symptoms, or PV receptions from the street. If an inmate refuses testing, the inmate will be treated as a presumptive COVID19 positive source, and will be isolated for 14 days (asymptomatic), or when medically cleared (symptomatic) with a resolution of symptoms as defined by the CDC. Abbott Rapid test machines have been implemented in all facilities and are approved for use for reprieves, emergent dental procedures, immediate releases, and at the request of the Department's Chief of Medical Services and/or a community medical provider for treatments or procedures. Rapid, COVID19 positive test results are recognized; however, a rapid COVID19 negative test result requires a lab based PCR test to confirm its validity. Lab based PCR testing is also available for correctional staff that fail pre-entry screening, have been identified as a close contact through contact tracing, or voluntarily request testing. Common tests for COVID-19 may produce "false negatives" up to 30%; therefore, Pennsylvania chose not to mass test its inmate population. However, when staff call-offs increase due to COVID related symptoms, or if there is a noted increase in inmate COVID positive test results in an individual facility, the department has utilized Surveillance Testing. Surveillance testing is a representative, random sample of the population that allows us to make inferences about the level of infection spread within the inmate population, to identify asymptomatic cases, and to assist in making formulated decisions on appropriate interventions and response as it relates to inmate receptions/transfers, activities, and movement within the facility.

Like anything in the public sector, inspections or quality assurance needs to be in place. In our example, we have a team of trained individuals that do unannounced checks at our facilities and rate compliance to mitigation protocols such as mask wearing, social distancing and sanitation.

An emerging tool some systems are exploring is sewage testing to trace amounts of COVID19. We have explored this testing technology for approximately a month at four facilities. It did, in fact, detect COVID19 in the sewage discharge at one test facility which had more than 10 cases with no detection noted at the remaining test facilities.

A population reduction mechanism needs to be in place to allow systems to create space. Both space to allow individuals adequate out of cell time with social distancing, as well as, space to isolate/quarantine individuals.

PA outbreaks

In the past six months, we have experienced three outbreaks at three separate facilities. Based on the knowledge gained with each outbreak, and due to the uniqueness of each facility, we had to adapt, and modify our approach on how to contain and treat COVID19. In sequence, our outbreaks first began at SCI-Phoenix on March 27, 2020 through May, 15' 2020, resulting in fifty positive cases and five deaths. While in the midst of SCI-Phoenix's outbreak, SCI-Huntingdon became the next facility affected. On April 17, 2020 through July 17' 2020, SCI-Huntingdon's outbreak resulted in 195 positive cases and five deaths. Currently, we have an outbreak at SCI-Mercer which began on August 26, 2020 and is still ongoing (September 22, 2020) with a total of 44 positive cases and 0 deaths. Overall, we have tested 14,523 incarcerated individuals; 13,351 have tested negative, 434 have tested positive, another 738 results are still pending, and 11 deaths have resulted as COVID19 related. As previously noted, our COVID19 positive and COVID19 mortality rates are lower than that of the community rate in Pennsylvania.

SCI-Phoenix

As stated above, SCI-Phoenix received its first positive case on March 27, 2020. In response to this notification, we quarantined our entire correctional system. The facility located in Montgomery County, PA, a collar county of Philadelphia and the epicenter of the PA COVID19 outbreak, recorded the first COVID19 positive case in PA on March 13, 2020. The outbreak at SCI-Phoenix was limited to three housing units; therefore, our primary mechanism of controlling the potential spread of infection was pervasive "enhanced quarantine" (only one cell was permitted out of cell time at any given moment). SCI-Phoenix is our newest prison, and is equipped with air conditioning, new cells with Plexiglas enclosed doors, and no dorm space/housing; therefore, the physical design alone positively contributed in our ability to restrict the spread of infection. We requested and completed random COVID19 testing for inmates on the affected housing units to ascertain spread. Our last symptomatic inmate tested positive on May 15, 2020, signaling the end to this outbreak. In all, SCI-Phoenix resulted in 50 positive cases, in a facility with a population of approximately 2500 inmates. We learned from this outbreak that in our newer facilities we have the capability to quarantine on the housing unit by cell and control the spread of infection. However, in retrospect, a more targeted approach would have been equally effective than placing the entire facility on quarantine.

SCI-Huntingdon

Our second outbreak began on April 17, 2020 and lasted until July 17, 2020. SCI-Huntingdon was opened in 1889, and is a classic Auburn style tiered facility with approximately 1900 inmates. This facility has a combination of barred cell doors, three to four tiered housing units, and some dorm style housing, all of which contributed to the spread of infection. The facility also lacks an infirmary; therefore, in the midst of growing COVID19 cases, we were required to turn the gym, and two storage areas, into "field hospital" type infirmaries. As a result of contact tracing, we were able to ascertain, that COVID19 was introduced into the facility by a COVID19 symptomatic kitchen staff member. In a cascading event, this positive staff member infected other kitchen staff and inmate kitchen workers, who, in turn, spread the infection throughout the facility. The food distribution network quickly became a virus distribution network, and likely accounts for the spread of infection to 195 individuals. In the midst of the outbreak, we had also recognized the need for space to properly isolate and quarantine those infected, or potentially exposed; therefore, we transferred 80 soon to be released inmates to a self-contained outside housing unit at another facility. (It's important to note that we tested these individuals prior to transfer and found that nearly half were asymptomatic positives. Those who were COVID19 positive were isolated for 14 days as a cohort, and then transferred. It was critical that all of the cohorted positive inmates were transferred to their own housing units, as not to spread the virus to another facility.) The outbreak at SCI-Huntingdon really highlighted the importance for the necessity of space to both quarantine/isolate, and the need for "recovery units". Recovery units are for people who have completed their isolation period, but remain quarantined in a separate area for another three – ten days prior to returning to a general population unit. Established recovery units provide another layer in erring on the side of caution (ensuring that symptomatic inmates are completely free from symptoms and/or do not experience a relapse of symptoms) and assist in calming the fears of other non-affected inmates. During this outbreak, we developed our surveillance testing approach that has since become an important tool in our response protocols. This outbreak occurred in a small, rural county; therefore, we contributed to maxing out the community's medical infrastructure. We discovered that we needed to be proactive in working with the community's medical infrastructure early on in an outbreak, so that not only the facility, but the community as a whole, could be properly isolated, and treated during this critical time. Finally, the knowledge obtained as it relates to the nexus between food service and the spread of the virus, shaped our approach in immediately removing inmates from food service work detail when we start to identify and/or receive symptomatic positive cases.

SCI-Mercer

We are currently into our fourth week of our third noted outbreak, which began on August 26, 2020, at SCI-Mercer. This facility has a population of approximately 1500 inmates, and we have received 44 COVID19 positive cases to date (it should be noted that three days have passed without a new positive case resulting). When the facility received its first symptomatic positive, we initiated a 72 hour lock down. During those 72 hours, staff worked aggressively to disinfect/decontaminate the entire facility, including all cells and common areas. In order to enhance and monitor the prevalence of COVID19 within the facility, we initiated sewage testing for COVID19 during our second week into the outbreak. The initial sewage test results detected COVID19, then indicated an increase in levels upon later/further testing, and at the end of the third week revealed decreasing levels. We are in the process of placing sewage testing equipment/machines at every facility as a proactive measure/early warning system.

In a system with 24 facilities, limiting our outbreaks to three facilities is a likely testament to our proactive mitigation strategies. However, once the virus enters, it is very clear that food service is an area that requires special attention and assertive protocols. We are also proactively screening all vulnerable inmates, at any facility with symptomatic positives, twice daily with temperature checks, observation for ILI, and pulse oximeter testing, which likely contributes to our low death rate compared to the PA community at large.

In summary, COVID19 has been a challenge for correctional systems across America. It has exacerbated preexisting system weaknesses while creating and identifying several other areas to be fortified. Proactive and aggressive measures that focus on prevention, rapid response, as well as a population reduction strategy to both gain space and limit resource exhaustion will be required moving forward. The actions to address staff and population fatigue are in concert with the pragmatic work to support their wellness and family connections along with appreciation for the tireless efforts and patience of everyone involved. Staff acknowledgment, while providing a safe environment for the population, will only aid in the esprit de corps vital for managing this virus with the greatest amount of success possible. Courageous decision making coupled with science, data, experience and a margin of error will pivot the outcome to one which is far more manageable and embolden the existing foundations of our systems.

A Case Study of the Westchester County New York's Jail Response to COVID-19: Controlling COVID while Balancing Service Needs for the Incarcerated-A National Model for Jails

Kimberly Collica-Cox and Louis Molina

ABSTRACT

Controlling COVID rates, which initially soared within New York State, proved to be more challenging for correctional institutions, which were tasked with trying to protect a captive population. This article profiles the Westchester County Department of Correction (WCDOC), a county jail located 20 miles north of Manhattan; it is the second-largest jail in New York State. By employing a multitude of modalities, the WCDOC was able to lower their COVID-19 rates significantly, while simultaneously providing medical, mental health, drug treatment, and court-related services. By leveraging the use of technology and employing innovative policies for prisoners and staff, the WCDOC can serve as a model for other correctional institutions.

Introduction

As rates of COVID-19 infection appeared to decline in many areas, rates in correctional institutions across the United States continued to rise; inconsistent policies and a deficit in testing made it difficult to ascertain accurate infection rates for the incarcerated (Williams et al., 2020). At the peak of infection in New York State (NYS) (late March and early April of 2020), approximately 800 people died daily of Coronavirus-related illness (Higgins-Dunn, 2020). On March 7, 2020, NYS Governor Andrew M. Cuomo signed Executive Order No 202 declaring a disaster emergency in NYS (New York State [NYS], 2020), which was followed nine days later by a declaration of emergency in Westchester County by County Executive George Latimer (Westchester Government, 2020). High rates in the general population posed significant problems for correctional institutions, where social distancing was difficult and the closed quarters of the correctional environment served as an incubator for the virus (Prison Policy Initiative, 2020).

The rates in NYS' correctional facilities began to mirror rising rates in the general community. Since the beginning of July 2020, there were 541 reported cases of Coronavirus among NYS prisoners, with 16 related deaths (Park & Meagher, 2020). Even though there was a focus on prisoner health, prisoners' health was only one area of concern. With the health of staff and prisoners inextricably linked (each poses a risk to the other), effective policies to limit rates of COVID-19 infection must address both populations simultaneously and effectively. In NYS, there were 1,299 reported cases of the Coronavirus among state prison workers, with five related deaths (Park & Meagher, 2020). Since staff can infect prisoners or vice versa, correctional institutions have a difficult task to manage. Correctional administrators must try to minimize Coronavirus transmission, which occurs when a non-infected person is in close contact with an infected person's respiratory secretions (i.e., through coughing, sneezing, talking or singing) (World Health Organization [WHO], 2020), while still providing care, custody, control, and essential services to a population that suffers from high rates of drug addiction and mental illness (Bronson & Berzofsky, 2017).

Much of the discourse, particularly media attention, surrounding Coronavirus and the incarcerated has focused on state facilities, with little attention paid to jails. Jail administrators have one of the most challenging tasks regarding the control of Coronavirus. Their population is relatively transient and incarceration stays are much shorter when compared to those serving state prison time (25 days compared to 2.6 years) (Zeng, 2018). The risk of infection being brought into the jail via a new admission (or into the community via a new release) is significantly higher when compared to the state prison system, which receives its prisoners from jail facilities. The Westchester County Department of Correction (WCDOC), the second-largest jail in NYS (approximately 20 minutes north of Manhattan), was able to bring its infection rate to zero. Through the implementation of technology and the creation of strategic policy (which pertained to both staff and prisoners), WCDOC was able to maintain the safety of its staff and prisoners, while simultaneously maintaining essential services (i.e., mental health treatment, court appearances, etc.). This article will discuss the various strategies utilized by the WCDOC, which can serve as a model for other correctional institutions that want to minimize the risk of transmission but still provide a pre-pandemic level of service.

The WCDOC

The WCDOC is a county jail located in Valhalla, NY, within the County of Westchester, a large suburb of New York City. Their mission is to serve "the public by providing an efficient, secure and humane means of detaining individuals with criminal matters pending in Westchester County" (Westchester County department of Correction [WCDOC], 2020). The WCDOC consists of a Jail Division, which houses individuals 18 years and older (including males accused of a crime or awaiting sentencing and females accused of a crime, awaiting sentencing or sentenced to terms of a year or less) and a Penitentiary Division, which houses males sentenced to terms of one year or less. This jail facility holds detainees, sentenced offenders and federal detainees, with varying levels of security (i.e., unclassified, low, medium, high and maximum). With the ability to hold a capacity of 1,821 inmates, WCDOC has a current population of approximately 500 prisoners (490 at the time this article was written); almost 30 were women. In total, WCDOC has approximately 877 staff, which includes 836 law enforcement staff (officers, sergeants, etc.), who have contact with prisoners. The Department is accredited by the American Correctional Association (ACA) and operates within local, state and federal guidelines. It was the first jail in NYS to receive PREA (Prison Rape Elimination Act) accreditation and its medical operations were accredited by the National Commission on Correctional Health Care

(NCCHC). WCDOC follows the policies and guidelines mandated by New York's State Commission of Correction (SCOC) (Collica-Cox, 2018).

Pre-COVID

Even though no one was adequately prepared to address the COVID-19 outbreak when the World Health Organization designated it as a public health emergency of international concern on January 30, 2020 (WHO, 2020), there were two factors which assisted the WCDOC in their initial efforts. First, the WCDOC had a longstanding pandemic plan policy, communicable disease policy and a universal precaution policy, which meet and exceed standards set by the SCOC, ACA and NCCHC. The Department's strong foundation of detection, prevention and response to flu and other influenza type viruses was helpful in preparing for this process.

Second, NYS passed a bail reform law, considered one of the most "progressive" bail reforms in the nation, which went into effect January 1, 2020, and eliminated bail for most misdemeanors and nonviolent felonies, drastically reducing jail populations throughout the state (Lartey, 2020). Although the law was modified in April 2020 to expand judicial discretion for determining bail for certain crimes (15 new eligible bail categories were added), the core of the original law remained (Coltin, 2020; Merkl, 2020). As a result, new admissions were low, which made it possible for the WCDOC to discontinue dormitory-style housing. The majority of prisoners moved to single cells, which housed a private toilet and sink. Single showers were cleaned after each use. The only exception was for those prisoners who assisted in food preparation and worked in the kitchen. These residents were housed in quad-style housing units but were separated by distances of greater than twenty feet. They were medically monitored multiple times throughout the day.

Early release & providing unrestrained access to the courts

To enhance efforts to moderate the spread of COVID-19 and further reduce the jail population, the Westchester County District Attorney's Office partnered with the Legal Aid Society of Westchester to review the case files of prisoners who might be eligible for early release (Westchester County New York Office of the District Attorney, 2020). In total, 65 prisoners were released early. Thirty-three prisoners were released early with conditions placed upon their release, while 32 of the releasees, who were initially remanded on a probation violation, were released back to the supervision of probation (Lungariello & Eberhart, 2020). All releasees, who were primarily low-level offenders, had release dates of June 26, 2020 or earlier and were serving one year or less (Lungariello & Eberhart, 2020). The long-term detainees, who were scheduled to take a plea but were unable to do so because of court closures, would have remained in jail longer then their sentence warranted if this action was not taken by the County District Attorney and the Legal Aid Society. To date, none of the releasees have been remanded back to the WCDOC; however, it is unknown if any were arrested (but not remanded) at any point since their release.

Although the WCDOC does not play a deciding role in whether a prisoner is released, they were able to help facilitate court processes by maintaining scheduled court visits via their video platform technology and by assigning six correctional officers fulltime to sustain the court volume. Many prisoners across the country and throughout the state were denied their right to a "speedy resolution" and unable to access justice because of correctional facilities' inability to provide access to the courts during in-person court closures (Weichselbaum, 2020); the WCDOC's willingness to utilize video platform technology (i.e. Skype, WebEx, etc.) allowed them to maintain all of the prisoners' court dates. In cases where prisoners were applying for early release based on an underlying medical condition, WCDOC expediated the forms that were needed by attorneys, such as HIPPA (Health Insurance Portability and Accountability Act) forms and electronic medical records (EMRs), even with reduced staff. During the jail's lockdown to visitors, defense attorneys could continue to confer with their clients using their video technology system. Technology, which many correctional institutions lack due to security concerns (Jewkes & Johnston, 2009), was a tremendous benefit during this pandemic.

Quarantining, testing & partnership

Over 100 prisoners were tested by the WCDOC during the peak of the Coronavirus outbreak, which was more than 20% of their population. This seemed in line with testing overall in NYS, where approximately 25% of residents have been tested (4,673,195 tests for 19 million people) (Jin, 2020). This number may be lower as such data only accounts for the number of tests administered, rather than the number of people tested; it cannot account for repeat testers (i.e., essential workers with repeated exposure). Testing is important because it not only identifies those who may be infected, but it can initiate the process of contact tracing to stop the further spread of infection (Centers For Disease Control and Prevention [CDC], 2020a). Testing determines housing placements, staffing, and delivery of care/ services to the prisoners.

Correctional institutions may have the capacity to conduct higher levels of testing if they partner with an outside medical organization. WCDOC partnered with the Westchester County Department of Health (WCDOH) and their Department's medical provider, Wellpath, to develop a testing process for both staff and residents. WCDOH provided COVID-19 testing kits to WCDOC, which were not commercially available at the time and Wellpath agreed to administer the tests and have them sent for processing. The testing of prisoners allowed WCDOC to safely house those who were symptomatic. Based on several exhibited symptoms at the beginning of the pandemic, all prisoners were placed on a 14-day quarantine. Other prisoners, who may have been in the vicinity of a symptomatic prisoner, were placed under a precautionary quarantine, which enabled WCDOC to monitor them until their test results returned. WCDOC was also able to designate housing for those who completed their 14-day quarantine and remained asymptomatic for three days (i.e., no fever and improved respiratory symptoms such as cough or shortness of breath) or 10 days since symptoms first appeared (as per CDC guidelines). To reduce risk at the state level, all scheduled transfers from the jail to state prisons at the beginning of the pandemic were suspended. Presently, all WCDOC prisoners scheduled to be sentenced by the court to serve incarceration terms exceeding more than one year with the New York State Department of Corrections and Community Supervision (NYSDOCCS) will quarantine for 14 days prior. This assists in minimizing any outbreaks during transfer from one facility to another but still allows for the movement of prisoners. In July 2020, the WCDOC received one new admission who tested positive for COVID-19; due to WCDOC's testing and isolation protocols, infection was detected immediately, while this individual was still being held in initial quarantine (required of all new admissions). This individual remained isolated from the general population for the contagion period, fully recovered, and posed no threat to others. No other staff or prisoner contracted COVID-19 and the WCDOC's COVID-19 rate returned to zero.

To minimize infections being brought from the community to the jail, all non-essential staff (including volunteers and contractors), worked remotely. Uniform staff were essential and since they resided in different communities throughout NYS, they had varying levels of exposure. This necessitated a specific testing protocol for staff. Westchester County implemented various policies to ensure that staff members who were experiencing symptoms did not feel compelled to come to work. Once staff members experienced symptoms, they were tested and remained quarantined at their residence until their test results returned. If they tested negative, they could return to work but until the process was concluded, they were often home for a period of at least five days. If the test results were positive, staff quarantined 14 to 20 days. To encourage staff to report symptoms, a "COVID-sick" policy was implemented; staff were not required to use their sick time for quarantining and if they were previously approved for leave under the Family Medical Leave Act (FMLA), they were not required to use their FMLA hours. Staff were also allowed to take COVID sick leave, without impacting their accrued sick or FLMA hours, if they had a family member with an underlying medical condition or if they were responsible for minor children and were unable to secure childcare during NYS' stay-at-home order. During WCDOC's peak, approximately 150 officers were out of work on a COVID-related issue; these absences (approximately 18% of their security workforce) created countless operational challenges. In total, over 300 employees were tested, accounting for 34% of their staff. Testing prisoners and staff who were symptomatic resulted in the Department experiencing its peak number of cases quite sooner than the rest of NYS. Prisoners and staff both peaked in the number of persons experiencing symptoms and testing positive during the week of March 29, 2020 (See Charts 1 and 2), while the rest of NYS reached its COVID-19 peak on or about April 16, 2020 (Tampone, 2020).

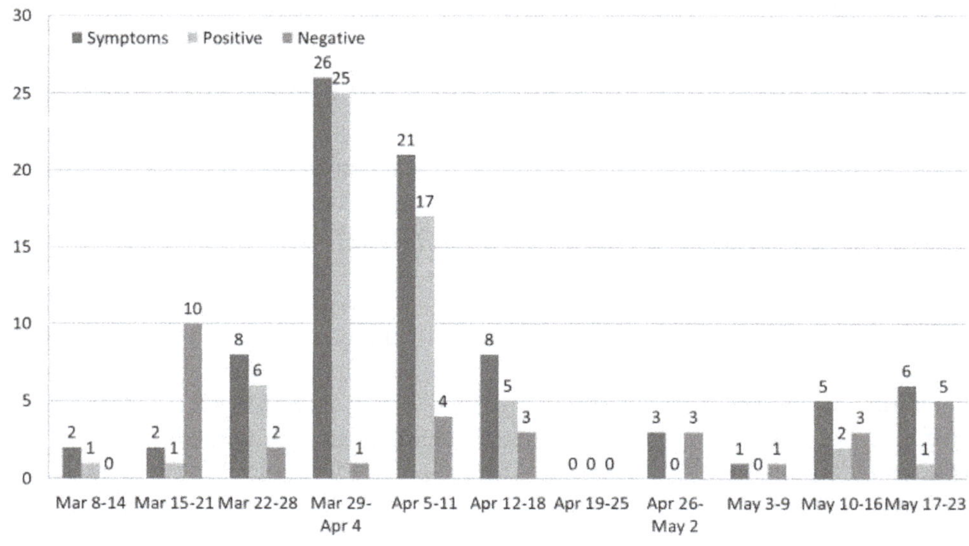

Chart 1. Prisoner symptoms and COVID-19 testing results.

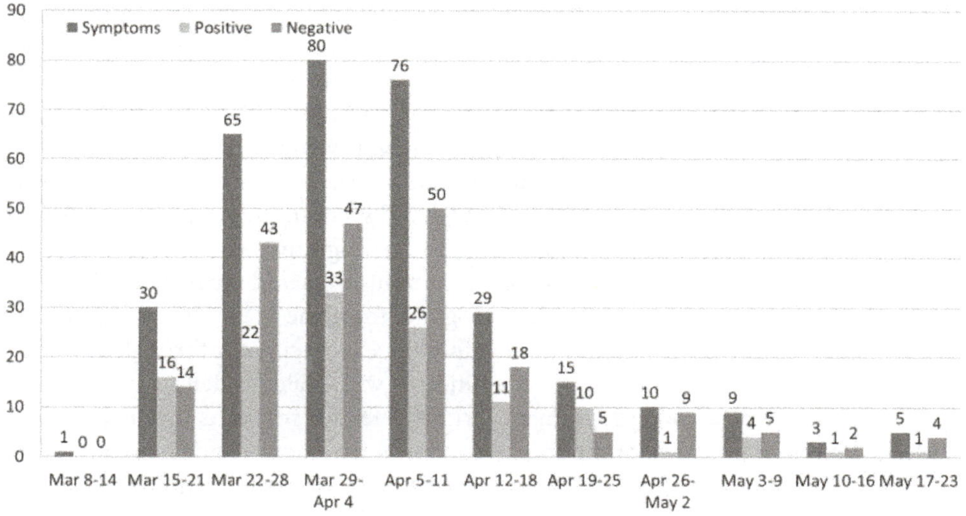

Chart 2. Staff symptoms and COVID-19 testing results.

Cleaning & personal protective equipment (PPE)

While testing was critical to operational planning, more needed to be done to ensure the safety of prisoners and staff. WCDOC engaged in a vigorous cleaning routine. Housing blocks and other areas were sanitized multiple times daily. Correctional Officers performed cleaning and other custodial duties to continuously maintain a sanitized environment throughout the day. Staff and prisoners were encouraged to maintain consistent handwashing and to use hand sanitizing stations placed throughout the facility. Hand sanitizer is still considered contraband in 20 states and in all federal facilities (i.e. security concerns that prisoners might ingest it or utilize it as an accelerant), even though the CDC asked facilities to consider easing restrictions for the benefit of public health initiatives (CDC, 2020b; Tolan, 2020). The WCDOC maintained a strategic inventory of PPE supplies, which included masks that were provided to all staff and prisoners and changed weekly (or more frequently if needed) to lessen community spread. Staff and prisoners were required to wear masks at all times; all prisoners had to wear masks whenever leaving their cells.

Technology & maintaining essential services

The WCDOC has a wide variety of programming which was initially affected by the shutdown. Although medical and mental health staff, deemed essential, were still onsite, many other programs, particularly those under the leadership of contractors and volunteers, were suspended. Many of these programs, albeit not all of them, were able to continue their work through WCDOC's video visitation system. The WCDOC leveraged their existing video visitation technology to ensure that prisoners stayed connected to ongoing academic studies. Students enrolled in college programming with Pace University met with their professor via video visits and those completing their high school/GED course of study through BOCES (Board of Cooperative Educational Services), were able to maintain the same contact with their teachers. With the assistance of a program sergeant, assignments could be distributed and collected. Unfortunately, this was not the case for most correctional institutions – programs were suspended indefinitely, leaving prisoners little to do while quarantined (increasing stress and despondency) and interrupting programming that was geared toward achieving rehabilitative and reintegrative outcomes (Lewis, 2020).

This same technology platform also allowed those receiving treatment for substance abuse to continue receiving support from WCDOC's community-based partner, Saint John's Riverside Hospital. Participants engaged in cognitive behavioral intervention (CBI), via interactive journaling, with another community-based partner, Hudson Valley Community Services, a program funded by a grant from the NYS Division of Criminal Justice Services; prisoners stayed connected with their CBI Facilitator through video visitation. Lastly, Family Services of Westchester connected with male residents who participated in their Navigating Fatherhood program and with the female residents who participated in the EMERGE program (i.e. Educating Mothers to Embrace Reentry and Gain Employment) via video visitation. In-person programming was able to resume at the WCDOC in July 2020. Programs opened slowly and in stages to minimize and monitor potential health risks. In-person programming will continue to be monitored closely.

Technology & maintaining family connections

Family visitation was negatively impacted by the Coronavirus pandemic. To prevent the spread of illness, most facilities, nationwide, suspended all visitation (Kindy et al., 2020). The same held true for the WCDOC – all visits were suspended in March 2020. Normally, family connections are difficult to preserve while one is incarcerated (i.e., difficulty with travel, cost of collect calls, etc.) (New York State Division of Criminal Justice Services, 2013) but the COVID-19 crisis made this process even more challenging. Family connections are important in impacting recidivism; family/marital stability is one of the "central eight" risk factors that correctional-based programs are urged to target (Andrews et al., 2006, 2012). Family relationships affect criminal behavior, with strong family relationships precluding future crime (Collica-Cox & Furst, 2020). Without visitation, families would need to rely upon telephone calls or video visitation, which is not affordable for every family, especially with 1.6 million New Yorkers filing claims for initial unemployment insurance during the onset of the Coronavirus (Marroquin, 2020). Hence, the WCDOC purchased telephone cards, which were issued to residents at no cost, so they could maintain communication and receive updates from their outside support systems. Free calling cards and reduced pricing for video visitation increased family contact with the number of monthly calls rising from 1,700 pre-pandemic to 4,000 during the pandemic. In fact, this process allowed more prisoners the opportunity to stay in contact with family than ever before. Non-contact visitation was able to resume at the WCDOC in September 2020. If COVID-19 rates in the community remain low, contact visiting may return, but this is a process that will occur gradually to minimize and evaluate the potential risk.

Conclusion

The Prison Policy Initiative developed recommendations for how the criminal justice system could slow the spread of COVID-19 (Wagner & Widra, 2020). These recommendations included: reducing the number of prisoners in county jails and state/federal prisons, lessening unnecessary personal 1:1 contact, providing for health care that is humane for both staff and prisoners, and affording methods for family to remain in contact with incarcerated loved ones at no charge. The WCDOC met and exceeded these guidelines. Policies that were enacted during this pandemic can result in long-term changes, which far exceed the longevity of this virus. Consider the expanded use of video technology, which if implemented in more facilities, could expand programming options for correctional institutions. Such technology could also defer costs and increase public safety when prisoners attend court appearances remotely. In addition, family who may have not been able to visit an incarcerated loved one or afford the costs of phone calls, are able to maintain consistent contact through calling cards. If strong family relationships can help to mitigate rates of recidivism (Collica-Cox & Furst, 2020), the costs of these cards are economically beneficial.

Policies implemented by the WCDOC prior to the pandemic, such as communicable disease procedures and bail reform, helped place WCDOC in a good position to manage the complexities of COVID-19. NYS was the epicenter of COVID-19 in the United States (beginning in the City of New Rochelle in Westchester County) at the start of the pandemic (McKinley, 2020), posing numerous challenges for correctional institutions, particularly jails. By helping to facilitate court visits and necessary paperwork for early release consideration, prisoners were given unbridled access to the courts. The use of quarantining, testing, cleaning and mandated use of PPE helped to limit exposure. WCDOC assigned officers to manage the court volume and they assigned personnel to the County Emergency Operations Center to ensure the leadership team had the most up-to-date information regarding the pandemic; this also helped them learn about possible resources which could enhance Departmental operations. WCDOC utilized technology to maintain programming, drug treatment, CBI services and family reunification. The sick policy for staff was modified allowing staff to minimize exposure to others while allowing staff to care for themselves and their families.

The American Civil Liberties Union (ACLU) issued a failing grade for most states' responses to mitigating coronavirus among the incarcerated (Widra & Hayre, 2020), including New York State (NYS). NYS' failing grade was based partly on data from the NYSDOCCS' website (which due to staff shortages may not have been updated regularly), as well as outside agencies that were attempting to collect data during this difficult period. The NYSDOCCS is a state system that reports on state facilities; county jails (there are 58 jails covering 62 counties in NYS) are not reported on their website. Grades were based upon several factors, such as distribution of ample PPE for staff and the incarcerated; reduction of the incarcerated population; a Governor-issued mandate hastening the release of vulnerable prisoners and/or those toward the end of their sentence; and publicly available COVID-19 data. The WCDOC, although not graded independently, did not fail to meet these criteria. As mentioned above, PPE was issued to staff and residents weekly (or more if needed). The NYS State Governor did not issue a mandate regarding Coronavirus and the incarcerated, yet, Westchester County devised a local response to the pandemic when the Westchester County District Attorney's Office partnered with the Legal Aid Society of Westchester to review the case files of prisoners who might be eligible for early release; the WCDOC helped to facilitate these cases quickly and efficiently through their video platform technology. Since January, bail reform coupled with releases during the Coronavirus pandemic allowed WCDOC to reduce its jail population by almost 50% (approximately 1,000 incarcerated to 500 incarcerated). Last, data were released to local news sources and subsequently published, yet, readily available data on the WCDOC website might provide more accessibility for the public. Overall, based on the criteria established by the ACLU, the WCDOC can serve as a model for other correctional institutions, including those in NYS.

To help mitigate the spread of COVID-19, advocates were calling for the early release of the incarcerated. However, these individuals were being released during a pandemic, when there were staff shortages, office closings, limited services (i.e., mental health, substance abuse, housing, etc.), and few resources (Carissimo, 2020; King, 2020). Staff employed with nonprofit agencies, who commonly service the formerly incarcerated, were working remotely. If the formerly incarcerated had difficulty gaining access to technology, they had difficulty obtaining services. Services can be difficult to assess under normal circumstances, but the Coronavirus pandemic made it even more challenging (Westervelt, 2020). Case managers or discharge planners, who normally worked with the incarcerated prior to their release, were also working remotely, which can make it difficult to connect those awaiting release with outside services (Carissimo, 2020). The release process, which is often overwhelmed (i.e., not enough services for the newly released), was inundated with cases during a time that few services could be offered (Carissimo, 2020). Clearly, community-based treatment is an area in need of remediation and increased funding is required to provide these necessary services more efficaciously, especially during a pandemic; otherwise, those who are released early are likely to return (McCarthy et al., 2020). Moreover, those who specifically suffer from opioid addiction have a high probability of overdose following their release; internationally, drug overdoses are the primary cause of death for the newly released (Joudrey et al., 2019). These overdoses occurred pre-pandemic but such rates will continue to increase if community-based treatment/services for the addicted is less accessible as a result of the pandemic (American Medical Association [AMA], 2020; Longley, 2020).

The WCDOC, like many other correctional institutions, found themselves in one of the most challenging times that impacted staff and prisoners and the extended families of both. WCDOC maintained unit cohesion and synergy with their strategic partners, establishing a multitude of best practices and other operational strategies that could be replicated in other jails and prisons throughout the country. WCDOC can serve as a model for other correctional institutions, especially if a second wave of COVID-19 is predicted (Ferre-Sadurni & Schweber, 2020). Future researchers should determine if these methods are as effective as in-person modalities and whether such procedures, when implemented in other correctional institutions, have the same outcomes (i.e., a zero COVID-19 rate).

Acknowledgments

A special thanks to all of the essential workers at the WCDOC for their hard work and dedication during these extremely challenging times.

Disclosure statement

No potential conflict of interest was reported by the author(s).

ORCID

Kimberly Collica-Cox http://orcid.org/0000-0002-6598-8000

References

AMA (American Medical Association). (2020). *Issue brief: Reports of increases in opioid-related overdose and other concerns during COVID pandemic*. https://www.ama-assn.org/system/files/2020-08/issue-brief-increases-in-opioid-related-overdose.pdf b

Andrews, D. A., Bonta, J., & Wormith, J. S. (2006). The recent past and near future of risk and/or need assessment. *Crime and Delinquency*, *52*(1), 7–27. https://doi.org/10.1177/0011128705281756

Andrews, D. A., Guzzo, L., Raynor, P., Rowe, R. C., Rettinger, L. J., Brews, A., & Wormith, J. S. (2012). Are the major risk/need factors predictive of both female and male reoffending? A test with the eight domains of the level of service/case management inventory. *International Journal of Offender Therapy and Comparative Criminology*, *56*(1), 113–133. https://doi.org/10.1177/0306624X10395716

Bronson, J., & Berzofsky, M. (2017, June). *Indicators of mental health problems reported by prisoners and jail inmates, 2011-2012* (NCJ 250612). Bureau of Justice Statistics. https://www.bjs.gov/content/pub/pdf/imhprpji1112.pdf

Carissimo, J. (2020, April 29). Leaving rikers Island and coming home to a pandemic. *CBS News*. https://www.cbsnews.com/news/rikers-island-coronavirus-pandemic-new-york-city-covid-19/

CDC (Centers For Disease Control and Prevention). (2020a). *Coronavirus disease 2019*. https://www.cdc.gov/coronavirus/2019-ncov/php/open-america/contact-tracing-resources.html

CDC (Centers For Disease Control and Prevention). (2020b). *Interim guidance on management of Coronavirus disease 2019 (COVID-19) in correctional and detention facilities*. https://www.cdc.gov/coronavirus/2019-ncov/community/correction-detention/guidance-correctional-detention.html

Collica-Cox, K. (2018). Impossible until it's done: PREA accreditation in Westchester County. *American Jails*, *31*(6), 8–14.

Collica-Cox, K., & Furst, G. (2020). Prisoner parenting: Parenting from a federal jail. *The Journal of Correctional Health Care*, *26*(2), 138–150. https://doi.org/10.1177/1078345820916475

Coltin, J. (2020, April 4). How New York changed its bail law. *City & State New York*. https://www.cityandstateny.com/articles/policy/criminal-justice/how-new-york-changed-its-bail-law.html

Ferre-Sadurni, L., & Schweber, N. (2020, July 14). New York confronts second-wave risk: Visitors from Florida and Texas. *New York Times*. https://www.nytimes.com/2020/07/14/nyregion/coronavirus-ny-travel-cuomo.html

Higgins-Dunn, N. (2020, May 22). New daily coronavirus cases in New York are now lower than at the beginning of the outbreak, Gov. Cuomo says. *CNBC News*. https://www.cnbc.com/2020/05/22/new-daily-coronavirus-cases-in-new-york-are-now-lower-than-at-the-beginning-of-the-outbreak-gov-cuomo-says.html

Jewkes, Y., & Johnston, H. (2009). 'Cavemen in an era of speed-of-light technology': Historical and contemporary perspectives on communication within prisons. *The Howard Journal of Criminal Justice*, *48*(2), 132–143. https://doi.org/10.1111/j.1468-2311.2009.00559.x

Jin, B. (2020). *Live tracker: How many coronavirus cases have been reported in each U.S. state?* Politico. https://www.politico.com/interactives/2020/coronavirus-testing-by-state-chart-of-new-cases/

Joudrey, P. J., Khan, M. R., Wang, E. A., Scheidell, J. D., Edelman, E. J., McInnes, D. K., & Fox, A. D. (2019). A conceptual model for understanding post-release opioid-related overdose risk. *Addiction Science & Clinical Practice*, *14*(7). https://doi.org/10.1186/s13722-019-0145-5

Kindy, K., Berman, M., & Tate, J. (2020, March 17). Jails and prisons suspend visitation to keep coronavirus from spreading. *The Washington Post*. https://www.washingtonpost.com/national/jails-and-prisons-suspend-visitation-to-keep-coronavirus-from-spreading/2020/03/16/0cae4adc-6789-11ea-abef-020f086a3fab_story.html

King, D. H. (2020, May 11). *Pandemic leads to early prisoner release, but finding housing for them remains difficult*. Shelterforce. https://shelterforce.org/2020/05/11/pandemic-leads-to-early-prisoner-release-but-finding-housing-for-them-remains-difficult/

Lartey, J. (2020, April 23). *New York rolled back bail reform. What will the rest of the country do?* The Marshall project. https://www.themarshallproject.org/2020/04/23/in-new-york-s-bail-reform-backlash-a-cautionary-tale-for-other-states

Lewis, N. (2020). *Can college programs in prison survive COVID-19?* The Marshall Project. https://www.themarshallproject.org/2020/05/04/can-college-programs-in-prison-survive-covid-19

Longley, J. (2020). *As overdoses spike during coronavirus, treating addiction in prisons and jails is a matter of life and death*. ACLU. https://www.aclu.org/news/prisoners-rights/as-overdoses-spike-during-coronavirus-treating-addiction-in-prisons-and-jails-is-a-matter-of-life-and-death/

Lungariello, M., & Eberhart, C. J. (2020). 65 people released form Westchester County Jail over COVID-19 fears: DA. *Lohud*. https://www.lohud.com/story/news/coronavirus/2020/04/10/coronavirus-westchester-county-jail-department-of-correction-district-attorney/5134407002/

Marroquin, M. (2020). COVID-19: Unemployment in NYS by the numbers. *Lohud*. https://www.lohud.com/story/money/2020/05/04/covid-19-unemployment-new-york-state-numbers/3064195001/

McCarthy, C., Weissmann, R., & Fitz-Gibbon, J. (2020, April 19). Dozens of NYC inmates back in jail after coronavirus release. *The New York Post*. https://nypost.com/2020/04/19/dozens-of-nyc-inmates-back-in-jail-after-coronavirus-release/

McKinley, J. (2020, March 22). New York City region is now an epicenter of the Coronavirus pandemic. *New York Times*. https://www.nytimes.com/2020/03/22/nyregion/Coronavirus-new-York-epicenter.html

Merkl, T. A. (2020). *New York's latest bail law changes explained*. Brennan Center For Justice. https://www.brennancenter.org/our-work/analysis-opinion/new-yorks-latest-bail-law-changes-explained#:~:text=New%20York's%20new%20bail%20reform,other%20conditions%20of%20pretrial%20release

New York State Division of Criminal Justice Services. (2013). *Children of incarcerated parents in New York State. A data analysis*. https://www.criminaljustice.ny.gov/pio/2013-children-with-inarcerated-parents-report.pdf

NYS (New York State). (2020). *Information on novel Coronavirus*. New York State Government. https://www.governor.ny.gov/news/no-202-declaring-disaster-emergency-state-new-york

Park, K., & Meagher, T. (2020, July 10). *A state-by-sate look at corona virus in prison*. The Marshall Project. https://www.themarshallproject.org/2020/05/01/a-state-by-state-look-at-coronavirus-in-prisons

Prison Policy Initiative. (2020, July 8). *Responses to the Covid-19 pandemic*. https://www.prisonpolicy.org/virus/virusresponse.html

Tampone, K. (2020). *Coronavirus in NY: Deaths at low since April peak as new cases continue to slow*. Syracuse.com. https://www.syracuse.com/coronavirus/2020/06/coronavirus-in-ny-deaths-at-low-since-april-peak-as-new-cases-continue-to-slow.html

Tolan, C. (2020, May, 5). *Hand sanitizer is still considered contraband in some prisons around the country*. CNN. https://www.cnn.com/2020/05/05/us/coronavirus-prison-hand-sanitizer-contraband-invs/index.html

Wagner, P., & Widra, E. (2020). *Five ways the criminal justice system could slow the pandemic*. Prison Policy Initiative. https://www.prisonpolicy.org/blog/2020/03/27/slowpandemic/

WCDOC (Westchester County department of Correction). (2020). Westchester County Government. https://correction.westchestergov.com/

Weichselbaum, S. (2020, May 1). *Can't make bail, sit in jail even longer thanks to coronavirus*. The Marshall Project. https://www.themarshallproject.org/2020/05/01/can-t-make-bail-sit-in-jail-even-longer-thanks-to-coronavirus

Westchester County New York Office of the District Attorney. (2020). *65 inmates released from county jail on COVID-19 concerns*. https://www.westchesterda.net/april-2020/6517-65-inmates-released-from-county-jail-on-covid-19-concers

Westchester Government. (2020). *County executive George Latimer declares 'state of emergency' in response to COVID-19 pandemic*. Westchester County Government. https://www.westchestergov.com/home/all-press-releases/8320-county-executive-george-latimer-declares-state-of-emergency-in-response-to-covid-19-pandemic

Westervelt, E. (2020). *Advocates: Inmates released early due to pandemic need help to safely shelter*. NPR WNYC. https://www.npr.org/2020/04/09/830394249/advocates-inmates-released-early-due-to-pandemic-need-help-to-safely-shelter

WHO (World Health Organization). (2020, July 9). *Transmission of SARS-CoV-2: Implications for infection prevention precautions*. https://www.who.int/news-room/commentaries/detail/transmission-of-sars-cov-2-implications-for-infection-prevention-precautions

Widra, E., & Haye, D. (2020). *Failing grades. States" responses to COVID-19 in jails and prisons*. ACLU. https://www.aclu.org/sites/default/files/field_document/failing_grades_states_responses_to_covid-19_in_jails_prisons.pdf

Williams, T., Seline, L., & Griesbach, R. (2020, June 30). Coronavirus cases rise sharply in prisons even as they plateau nationwide. *New York Times*. https://www.nytimes.com/2020/06/16/us/coronavirus-inmates-prisons-jails.html

Zeng, Z. (2018). *Jail inmates in 2016* (NCJ 251210). Bureau of Justice Statistics. https://www.bjs.gov/content/pub/pdf/ji16.pdf

British Columbia Provincial Corrections' Response to the COVID-19 Pandemic: A Case Study of Correctional Policy and Practice

Danielle J. Murdoch

ABSTRACT

Health and justice officials across North America have described correctional institutions as petri dishes for the transmission of COVID-19. Individuals in custody commonly have health profiles that are more compromised than those of the general population. Institutional infrastructure issues and custody counts that create barriers to protocols, including physical distancing measures, that health authorities recommend to limit the spread of the virus compound these profiles. Many correctional authorities have struggled to implement strategies to mitigate infection rates among custodial populations. This paper examines the strategies employed by one provincial correctional authority in Canada that has to date successfully prevented the spread of COVID-19 in custody centers by adopting a health-informed approach to the crisis rather than a traditional justice-informed response. The findings highlight practices that can inform the responses of other jurisdictions as the pandemic continues and identify areas of future research on the effects of COVID-19 on incarcerated persons, correctional and health-care staff, and communities.

Introduction

Health and justice officials across North America have described correctional institutions as petri dishes for the transmission of COVID-19 (see e.g., Paynter, 2020). Correctional authorities have struggled to implement strategies to mitigate infection rates within custodial populations (Franco-Paredes et al., 2020; Marcum, 2020; Oladeru et al., 2020; Ouellet & Loiero, 2020; Saloner et al., 2020). A preliminary analysis of COVID-19 infection rates among incarcerated populations in Canada conducted in July 2020 found that infection rates were up to five times higher in provincial custodial institutions and nine times higher in federal correctional institutions than infection rates in the community (Ouellet & Loiero, 2020). A study of infection rates among prisoners across the US that used data collected between March 31, 2020 and June 6, 2020 found infection rates were 5.5 times higher in federal and state prisons than infection rates in the community with the research team acknowledging disparities in infection rates are likely greater (Saloner et al., 2020, pp. 602–603).

Individuals in custody typically have diverse, complex, and coexisting physical and mental health needs that include high rates of mental disorders, substance use disorders, communicable diseases (e.g., Tuberculosis, HIV, and hepatitis C), and chronic health conditions (e.g., hypertension, diabetes, asthma; Fazel & Baillargeon, 2010; Kinner & Young, 2018; Kouyoumdjian et al., 2016; McLeod & Martin, 2018). These health profiles are more compromised than those of the general population and in combination with institutional dynamics and infrastructure design, it means that incarcerated populations are likely more vulnerable to COVID-19 outbreaks (World Health Organization [WHO], 2020).

The following discussion examines how one provincial correctional service has been largely successful in preventing the introduction and transmission of COVID-19 among individuals in custody and staff in correctional centers and into the community. The discussion offers a number of recommendations that might assist other correctional authorities in Canada and internationally to respond to the ongoing pandemic and it could inform their responses to other highly communicable viruses as well. The discussion concludes by identifying areas of research that provide evidence-based materials to correctional authorities who may be confronted with similar crises in the future and that can inform correctional policy and practice beyond the pandemic.

While some observers (e.g., Vose et al., 2020) have held that preventing the transmission of the virus in correctional institutions is "impossible," this case study demonstrates that correctional policies and practices can be effective in addressing some of the challenges posed by COVID-19. At the time of writing (mid-August 2020), the British Columbia (BC) correctional service had reported just one case of an infected incarcerated individual and one case of an infected staff member, both of whom recovered from the illness (BC Corrections, 2020a). In July 2020, Ouellet and Loiero (2020) reported that Provincial Health Services Authority's Correctional Health Services was testing individuals in BC provincial custody at a rate of 392 per 1,000 with an infection rate among individuals in custody of 0.7 per 1,000 (Ouellet & Loiero, 2020).[1] The provincial experience is in sharp contrast to that of the federal Correctional Service of Canada in BC where one correctional facility had an outbreak of a total of 120 positive tests among prisoners, resulting in one death (Correctional Service Canada, 2020; testing rate of 222 per 1,000 individuals in custody and an infection rate of 60.68 per 1,000 across federal institutions in BC (Ouellet & Loiero, 2020).[2]

Institutional corrections and COVID-19

As noted, individuals in custody typically have diverse, complex, and co-occurring physical and mental health needs (Fazel & Baillargeon, 2010; Kinner & Young, 2018; Kouyoumdjian et al., 2016; McLeod & Martin, 2018). Compounding the complex health needs among incarcerated populations is institutional infrastructure issues (e.g., shared or poor ventilation systems, small shared spaces), safety and security concerns, inadequate health-care resources, and custody counts that create barriers to protocols, including practicing good hygiene and physical distancing, that health authorities recommend to limit the spread of COVID-19.

Maintaining good hygiene can be difficult for incarcerated populations due to requirements in some jurisdictions that they purchase soap using their own funds and institutional restrictions on providing custodial populations with access to hand sanitizer with a minimum 60% alcohol content for use when soap and water are not available due to concerns prisoners will ingest the sanitizer to become inebriated (Eisen & Weiss-Wolf,

2020; Oladeru et al., 2020; Prisoners' Legal Services, 2020). Maintaining clean surfaces in correctional centers can also be challenging, which is problematic due to the need to disinfect surfaces to reduce the spread of COVID-19. The virus can "survive for prolonged periods on materials that are highly prevalent in custodial settings including nonporous and metallic surfaces" (Franco-Paredes et al., 2020, p. 2).

The WHO (2020) recommends physical distancing – at least one-meter distance from one another – and self-isolation to limit the spread of COVID-19. These recommendations can be impossible to follow in correctional institutions characterized by high levels of human contact and interactions because of overcrowding and other institutional dynamics with some scholars describing "social distancing [as] the antithesis of incarceration" (Franco-Paredes et al., 2020, p. 3).

Failing to provide appropriate health-care services and implement effective strategies to mitigate infection rates among custodial populations during the global pandemic puts incarcerated persons, a majority of whom are marginalized and vulnerable, at risk, as well as correctional and health-care personnel and the community. First, the types of health conditions prominent among incarcerated populations place these individuals at risk of serious illness and complications resulting from COVID-19. For example, populations living with HIV (those not receiving treatment and those with a lower CD4 count), Tuberculosis, and chronic health conditions (e.g., diabetes, lung disease) have been identified as those more likely to develop serious illness and complications from contracting the virus (BC Centre for Disease Control, 2020a, para. 1). The health profiles of incarcerated populations mean these individuals are "among the most likely to contract the virus and among the least likely to overcome the illness and regain full health" (Vose et al., 2020, p. 769).

Second, extant literature highlights how "infections of the prison soon become the infections of the wider community" (International Centre for Prison Studies [ICPS], 2004, p. 24). Institutional outbreaks, including COVID-19 infection rates, have the potential to create community outbreaks due to the number of individuals who enter and leave custody centers on a daily basis (e.g., correctional and health-care personnel, visitors, and clients) and due to the short periods of time individuals are held in custody (ICPS, 2004; McLeod & Martin, 2018; Oladeru et al., 2020). To illustrate the latter point, in 2017/2018 in Canada (the most recent year for which data are available), 51% of remanded adults (those awaiting trial or sentencing) were held for 1 week or less and 59% of males and 68% of females were sentenced to custody for 1 month or less (Malakieh, 2019). As the WHO (2020) argues "efforts to control COVID-19 in the community are likely to fail if strong infection prevention and control measures, adequate testing, treatment and care are not carried out in prisons and other places of detention as well" (p. 1).

Adult custody in Canada

Adult correctional services in Canada are administered by the federal, provincial, and territorial governments. The federal Correctional Service of Canada operates correctional facilities for individuals sentenced to 2 years or more of imprisonment and supervises federal offenders released into the community (e.g., on parole). Provincial and territorial correctional services operate custody centers for individuals sentenced to 2 years less a day, persons awaiting trial or who have been found guilty and are awaiting sentencing (often referred to as "remand"), and also provide supervision for offenders serving community sentences (e.g., probation), and, in some provinces, offenders released on parole (Griffiths & Murdoch, 2018; Malakieh, 2019).

On any given day in 2017/2018, approximately 39,000 adults were in custody in Canada (Malakieh, 2019). The majority (24,657) of adults in custody were under the supervision of provincial and territorial correctional services with the remand population outnumbering the sentenced population by approximately 50% per day (14,812 and 9,543, respectively), a trend that has held constant since 2004/05 (Malakieh, 2019).

A notable feature of provincial and federal correctional systems in Canada is the overrepresentation of Indigenous persons, which is a consequence of a variety of factors, including the ongoing effects of colonialism (Chartrand, 2019; Palmater, 2018). In 2017/2018, Indigenous people represented 29% of admissions to federal custody and 30% of admissions to provincial and territorial custody while comprising only 4% of the general Canadian adult population (Malakieh, 2019).

The high rates of incarceration of Indigenous people places them at a disproportionate risk of contracting COVID-19. COVID-19 outbreaks in prisons in Canada are likely to disproportionately affect Indigenous people and their communities upon their release: individuals and communities who already disproportionately experience adverse health outcomes due to colonialism in Canada (see e.g., National Collaborating Centre for Aboriginal Health, 2013).

In BC, the provincial corrections Adult Custody Division has over 1600 full-time personnel and operates 10 correctional facilities to provide custody for individuals who are sentenced to 2 years less a day of imprisonment, awaiting trial or sentencing (i.e., remand), or pending an immigration review (BC Corrections, 2017; Malakieh, 2019). Prior to BC declaring a provincial state of emergency in March 2020 in response to the coronavirus, the Adult Custody Division was supervising 2,200 individuals in custody and admitting and discharging approximately 50 people per day (BC Corrections, 2020a). Since the start of the pandemic, the Division reported a nearly 32% decrease in their institutional correctional population from pre-COVID levels: as of June 2020, the service was responsible for supervising approximately 1,500 individuals in custody and admitting and discharging roughly 20 individuals per day (BC Corrections, 2020a). Similar to other jurisdictions across Canada, Indigenous people are overrepresented in the province's correctional populations. Data from 2016/2017 indicate that Indigenous people, who comprised just 5% of the adult population in BC, represented 29% of individuals in provincial custody (BC Corrections, 2017).

Correctional authorities in Canada are required to provide individuals in custody with health-care services although the administration of these services varies by jurisdiction (Kouyoumdjian et al., 2016). Since late 2017, individuals in custody in all 10 of BC Corrections' custody centers receive health care from Correctional Health Services: a division within the BC Mental Health & Substances Use Services portfolio of the Provincial Health Services Authority. BC was the third province in Canada to situate health-care responsibilities within the portfolio of the ministry responsible for health services rather than the ministry responsible for justice (McLeod & Martin, 2018). Correctional Health Services team members conduct physical and mental health assessments upon an individual's admission to custody and provide diverse services, such as "medical and nursing care, mental health and substance use treatment programs and services, … and health-related discharge planning to help clients transition successfully to community-based care" (BC Mental Health & Substances Use Services, 2020, para. 4).

Overcrowding in correctional centers has been an ongoing challenge for the Adult Custody Division in BC. In 2010, the Division's average occupancy rate was 176% across all of their institutions, "one of the highest rates of double-bunking among Canadian provinces" (Office of the Auditor General of BC, 2015, p. 5). Concerns with overcrowding and several other issues surrounding the administration of institutional corrections culminated in an investigation of the Division by the provincial Auditor General in 2015. In its final report, the Auditor General found that the Adult Custody Division had failed to "demonstrate that it has the right amount or type of facilities needed to provide safe, secure custody" (Office of the Auditor General of BC, 2015, p. 6). The Auditor-General also criticized the division's failure to ensure effective core programs for sentenced individuals in custody. Further, the Auditor General (Office of the Auditor General of BC, 2015) criticized the Division for failing to adhere to all of its legislated requirements and policy expectations pertaining to the accommodation of individuals in custody, including separating non-sentenced from sentenced individuals, and those that concern providing sentenced individuals in custody with timely access to correctional programming to address their risk of re-offending (p. 6).

A follow-up audit completed in 2019 examined the division's progress in addressing the eight recommendations set forth in the 2015 report. This investigation found that the division had partially acted upon two of the report's eight recommendations, made full/substantial progress toward three others, and had not acted on the remaining three (Office of the Auditor General of BC, 2019).

The division had partially implemented the Auditor General's (2015) recommendation to "implement a complete performance management framework of goals, objectives, strategies, performance measures and targets to achieve safe and secure custody, and reduce criminal behaviour . . . including defining appropriate occupancy levels" (p. 7). The division had also only partially implemented the Auditor General's (2015) recommendation to regularly examine trends "in safety and security within and across their correctional centres" (p. 7) to learn how institutional and operational features contribute to incidents, such as inmate-on-staff assaults. The Auditor General (2019) outlined opportunities for improvement for the division to address these partially implemented recommendations, including the service defining how occupancy levels and targets affect "safe, secure custody and behavioural change" (p. 11) and using data to examine trends in safety and security to reduce the likelihood of future incidents.

Since the 2015 audit, the Adult Custody Division had made full/substantial progress toward three of the report's recommendations. The division had taken the initiative to use forecasting data to determine their long-term facility and programming needs and to make decisions about the use of facility resources and programming informed by the attributes of the persons in custody. The division had also taken the initiative to assess the effectiveness of some of their correctional programs and use that data to enhance the programs (Office of the Auditor General of BC, 2019).

The division had not taken any action toward three of the report's recommendations. They had not created a structure to "monitor and continuously improve the classification and case management" (Office of the Auditor General of BC, 2015, p. 7) process across correctional centers. No progress was made toward examining the consequences "of housing sentenced and remanded clients together" (Office of the Auditor General of BC, 2015, p. 7) or changing their practices to meet the policy set out in the *Correction Act Regulation* (2005). Last, the division had not taken action to examine the case management process to "identify and address barriers to offenders getting timely access to the programs they need to reduce criminal behaviour" (Office of the Auditor General of BC, 2015, p. 7) and to develop an evidence-based risk/needs assessment tool to match offenders with required programming.

The progress audit demonstrated that the Adult Custody Division was in the process of completing the required reforms when the pandemic hit. Despite the outstanding unaddressed issues, the division took quick action to mitigate the potential impact of the virus by adopting a health-informed response to COVID-19 rather than employing a traditional justice-informed approach to the crisis.

A health-informed response to the COVID-19 pandemic

As of mid-August 2020, the various strategies employed by provincial correctional authorities in BC have been successful in preventing the spread of COVID-19 in custody centers.[3] Their response to the global pandemic is informed by the Provincial Health Officer's recommendations to minimize transmission of COVID-19 and reflects the Service's ongoing collaboration with various government partners, including the Provincial Health Services Authority, Occupational Health and Safety, and WorkSafe BC, among others. The response of correctional authorities is premised on a number of components:

Ongoing education about COVID-19 for individuals in custody and correctional staff

The correctional service provides ongoing education about COVID-19 for individuals in custody and correctional staff. In collaboration with the Provincial Health Services Authority's Correctional Health Services, the Division offers information sessions and provides handouts to staff and individuals in custody so they remain informed about COVID-19, its transmission, and how to minimize exposure through their behavior, including frequent hand washing and sanitation (E. Gunnarson, personal communication, August 5, 2020).

Screening and testing

The correctional service screens everyone who enters the custody facilities, including staff, contractors, legal counsel, and individuals being admitted to custody (BC Corrections, 2020a). Staff and contractors are screened at the start of their shifts at the entry to each correctional center. A questionnaire is administered to assess whether these individuals present symptoms of COVID-19 and whether they have traveled outside of Canada in the past 14 days. Those who have traveled outside of Canada and/or who are experiencing symptoms of the virus cannot enter the facility. Legal counsel is also subject to this screening process should they have a face-to-face meeting with a client in a custody center (BC Corrections, 2020a).

A Correctional Health Services nurse administers a questionnaire and conducts a temperature check on all individuals who are admitted to custody. Asymptomatic individuals go to an induction unit for 14 days (see below); a medically directed isolation protocol is followed for individuals who are symptomatic. Suspected or confirmed cases of COVID-19, and those individuals who have had close contact with people who are suspected of or confirmed to have contracted the virus, are tested and monitored by Provincial Health Services Authority health-care personnel. This monitoring occurs in a regular living unit that allows the individual to be confined separately from others, or in an alternative unit (BC Corrections, 2020a; E. Gunnarson, personal communication, August 5, 2020).

Institutional policy dictates individuals living on a regular living unit who present symptoms of the virus will be immediately isolated and monitored by Provincial Health Services Authority health-care personnel. Should medical staff determine that an individual must be tested for COVID-19, results are obtained within 24 hours to facilitate contact tracing. The correctional service has also limited movement of staff and individuals in custody within and between their correctional centers. When circumstances require moves, individuals in custody are tested for the virus prior to their transfer (BC Corrections, 2020a).

Induction units

As a preventative measure, induction units have been created that subject new admissions to custody who are asymptomatic to a 14-day assessment period to address any healthcare-related matters before they are integrated into the custodial population. This 14-day isolation period complies with global health guidelines for quarantine after possible exposure to COVID-19 as symptoms can take up to 14 days to appear (WHO, 2020).

Induction units can be any unit within the correctional centers, have single-cell bunking to facilitate physical distancing, and health-care staff conduct frequent health-care checks. Individuals in induction units are assigned to cohorts comprised of individuals who were admitted on the same day. The cohorts receive more limited programming than in a regular living unit although they are offered free phone access and as much time as possible outside of their cells, including access to amenities (e.g., canteen, exercise). The policy also provides that individuals who are being assessed in the induction units and who are "contact concerns" must be provided with "alone time" out of their cells (BC Corrections, 2020a). Time out of one's cell and amenity use depend on the number of cohorts in each induction unit, meaning that individuals in induction units might not receive as much time out of their cells as they would in a regular living unit (BC Corrections, 2020a).

Since individuals risk contracting COVID-19 when they leave the custody center to attend court in person, they are placed in an induction unit for another 14-day assessment when they return to the facility (BC Corrections, 2020a). For this reason, the correctional service encourages individuals in custody, their legal counsel, and their justice partners to use video court wherever possible to minimize the likelihood individuals in custody will be exposed to COVID-19 and to avoid another 14-day induction period upon their return from court (BC Corrections, 2020a).

Individuals required to attend trial over multiple days are placed in separate confinement, most often in the health-care unit, to monitor their health status on an ongoing basis. When their trial is over, they are placed in an induction unit for 14 days before being transferred to a regular living unit in a custody center. Separate confinement cells are the same size as regular cells, individuals maintain access to free telephone calls, and they are single-bunked; however, they receive less time out of their cells (BC Corrections, 2020a).

As of mid-June, 2020, the correctional service noted no clients had attended a lengthy in-person trial (BC Corrections, 2020a). The correctional service acknowledged that experiencing separate confinement could be very challenging for individuals with multi-day or multi-week trials and that the service needed to develop appropriate strategies to provide individuals in separate confinement with meaningful opportunities to have time out of their cells, particularly on weekends when they did not attend court, to prevent the negative effects of separate confinement (BC Corrections, 2020a).

The correctional service described the induction units as "the single most effective tool for keeping the virus from entering and spreading in centres" (BC Corrections, 2020a, at 19:11). The Service anticipates they will operate induction units until such time as a vaccination is found or a new strategy is developed to prevent the spread of COVID-19 (BC Corrections, 2020a).

Changes to visitation practices

The correctional service has restricted in-person visits "unless there are urgent, exceptional circumstances" (BC Corrections, 2020a, at 21:56) due to concerns about visitors exposing staff and individuals in custody to the virus. When these restrictions were imposed at the beginning of the pandemic, the service simultaneously eliminated the costs of local and long-distance telephone calls and individuals in custody have an unlimited number of calls to increase their ability to maintain contact with their loved ones (BC Corrections, 2020a). Communication with loved ones through phone calls and video visits offers incarcerated populations social support that may minimize the pains of imprisonment, increase their adherence to institutional policies and practices, and promote their reintegration back into society (Duwe & McNeeley, 2020; Hewson et al., 2020; Murdoch & King, 2020).

BC Corrections also reduced and/or suspended volunteer programming and contracted services for non-essential program delivery. Legal counsel are encouraged to use video or telephone means to connect with their clients although BC Corrections provides a room with a built-in glass partition should an in-person meeting be required (BC Corrections, 2020a).

Cleaning, sanitizing, and staff use of personal protective equipment

Since the pandemic started, BC Corrections intensified their cleaning and disinfecting procedures, including increasing the frequency of contracted cleaning services and the cleaning of high-contact surface points. Induction and living units are sanitized multiple times throughout the day. People who enter the custody centers are subject to mandatory handwashing and cleaning protocols (BC Corrections, 2020a).

In April 2020, at the recommendation of their health-care partners, the correctional service changed their policy to require staff use personal protective equipment (PPE) when they cannot maintain 2-m distance from their clients. The Service has different types of masks to minimize the risk of transmission of COVID-19 to individuals in custody (BC Corrections, 2020a).

Physical distancing

The correctional service encourages their staff and individuals in custody to maintain 2-m distance from one another. To that end, they have added lines on the floor in the custody centers to provide visual guidance to their clients during mealtimes and individuals in custody are allowed to have their meals in their cells if they choose to do so. Individuals in custody are also encouraged to maintain physical distance during unit activities and programming (BC Corrections, 2020a). Staff members are also required to remain

2-m distant from their clients when possible, and when they cannot do so, they must wear PPE. The Service has determined that individuals in custody do not require masks, as they have completed a 14-day induction period (BC Corrections, 2020a).

Improving the response of BC corrections to the COVID-19 pandemic

While BC Corrections has been largely successful in preventing the introduction of COVID-19 into custody centers and preventing the transmission of the virus to individuals in custody, personnel, and their communities, the service could improve their response by increasing their use of temporary absences. As per s. 22(1)(a-b) of the *Correction Act* (2004), the service can release individuals from custody on temporary absences for medical, educational, humanitarian, rehabilitation, or reintegration-related reasons. The Assistant Deputy Minister of BC Corrections publicly acknowledged:

> Many of the individuals who come into custody have compromised health to begin with, and so really, are at much higher risk to contract the virus and the consequences as we know of the virus. So really, our focus is really on keeping the virus out of the centres and doing everything that we need to, to keep them safe. (BC Corrections, 2020a, at 44:10)

To that end, the Service could be more proactive in using temporary absences in line with existing regulations in their *Adult Custody Policy* (Adult Custody Division: Corrections Branch, 2005). Specifically: s.5.2.9 allows for a humanitarian absence for compassionate reasons and s. 5.2.11 for communicable disease absence. The application of these sections of the *Adult Custody Policy* (Adult Custody Division: Corrections Branch, 2005) would allow BC Corrections to release more individuals from custody – a population that they themselves acknowledge is vulnerable of contracting and getting seriously ill from COVID-19 – but it would require BC Corrections to focus on both public safety and the health of the individuals in custody rather than solely on public safety.

As a temporary measure implemented since the beginning of the pandemic, BC Corrections has been conducting proactive assessments of both individuals with less than 60 days remaining of their intermittent sentences (a sentence of 90 days or less wherein the convicted individual usually serves their time on weekends in a provincial correctional center; Government of BC, 2020) and nonviolent-sentenced offenders. The assessment focuses on a variety of risk-focused factors, including public and victim safety, criminal history, sentence length, and offense type, and support in the community (BC Corrections, 2020a). Between the middle of March and the beginning of June, only 80 individuals were released on temporary absences: 50 who were serving intermittent sentences (with less than 60 days remaining) and 30 who were serving sentences (BC Corrections, 2020a). Thus, the Service's use of temporary absences has had a minimal effect on their custodial count (BC Corrections, 2020a). Expanding their use of temporary absences to consider both public safety and the health of individuals in custody rather than focusing solely on public safety is one way the correctional service can work toward maintaining their reduced custodial counts.

Discussion

Population management strategies made possible with reduced custodial counts are fundamental to protecting medically vulnerable and elderly prisoners, staff, and the communities to which these individuals return (Franco-Paredes et al., 2020; Vose et al., 2020; WHO, 2020). Custodial populations fluctuate due to external factors such as changes in crime rates and decision-making practices at earlier points of the criminal justice system (Office of the Auditor General of BC, 2015). Of specific relevance to BC Corrections' post-COVID-reduced custodial count – from 2,200 to 1,500 – is that regular operations of the provincial and supreme courts were suspended in BC shortly after the province declared a state of emergency in response to the pandemic (Supreme Court of British Columbia, 2020; The Provincial Court of British Columbia, 2020).[4] These changes led to decreased court activity in the province, which have likely contributed to the correctional service admitting fewer individuals to custody at the same time that existing clients were completing their sentences (BC Corrections, 2020a). BC Corrections (2020a) also describes judges' increased use of bail and decreased use of remand after the pandemic started as key contributors to their reduced custody counts. Judges across Canada are considering COVID-19 in their bail and sentencing decisions, including releasing individuals accused of nonviolent offenses on bail when they have presented reasonable release plans even though under normal circumstances they would likely have been subject to pretrial detention (The Factum, 2020).

Maintaining the reduced custodial count is vital to the ongoing success of BC Corrections' response to the pandemic. First, BC Corrections (2020a) acknowledged that the pre-COVID population count of 2,200 individuals in custody meant many were double-bunked. Two adults, two bunks, a toilet, and occasionally a desk, in a cell roughly the size of a standard parking spot means double-bunked individuals in custody cannot possibly maintain appropriate physical distance – defined by BC's Provincial Health Officer as a distance of 2-m– from each other (BC Centre for Disease Control, 2020b; BC Corrections, 2020a). Thus, reduced custody counts since the start of the pandemic – a decrease of nearly 32% – have allowed the service to single-bunk many of the individuals in their custody, which given the need for physical distancing to reduce the transmission of COVID-19, has been a critical piece of their strategy of responding to the pandemic (BC Corrections, 2020a).

Second, BC Corrections' ongoing ability to operate induction units, providing single-bunking and offering individuals in custody an appropriate amount of meaningful time outside of their cells, is also connected to custodial counts. In June 2020, a time with decreased court activity in the province and a time that was characterized by judges' increased use of bail and decreased use of remand, the correctional service reported approximately 16% (n = 240) of their custodial population was being assessed in induction units. The service's two remand centers were busiest, operating two or three induction units at any given time with an average of 50 to 60 people in each unit (BC Corrections, 2020a, at 62:40). Increases in the custodial count are likely to negatively affect the operation of induction units and those being assessed within them.

Interestingly, at a time when COVID-19 restrictions and changes to regular routines and activities have increased tensions in prisons worldwide (see e.g., Perkel, 2020; Scott, 2020), conflicts *appear* to be decreasing in BC Corrections' custody centers where inmate-on-inmate and inmate-on-staff assaults and use of force incidents have decreased from pre-COVID numbers (BC Corrections, 2020a). Senior management attribute reductions in assaults and use of force incidents to their decreased use of double-bunking and having fewer people on each living unit, changes made possible by reduced population counts (BC Corrections, 2020a). Pre-COVID numbers (August 2018) demonstrate that six of BC Corrections' 10 adult correctional centers were relying on double-bunking due to unit closures largely attributed to staff shortages: the percentage of individuals in custody double-bunked ranged from 17% at Prince George Regional Correctional Center to 66% at Vancouver Island Regional Correctional Center (Office of the Auditor General of BC, 2019). Of concern in the months ahead, as long as a vaccination or viable treatment for the virus are not available, is the correctional service's previous estimate that 35% of their custodial population would be double-bunked by 2022/2023 (Office of the Auditor General of BC, 2015).

Increased custodial counts will not only challenge the Service's ability to continue utilizing their current response to COVID-19 (BC Corrections, 2020a), but also, such increases could potentially result in a return to pre-COVID numbers of inmate-on-inmate, inmate-on-staff, and use of force incidents. Extant literature identifies a plethora of negative effects for incarcerated populations living in, and personnel working within, overcrowded institutions, such as increasing tension and conflict between prisoners and between prisoners and staff, impeding rehabilitative, recreational, vocational, and educational programming, and contributing to an increase in illness, such as the spread of infectious and communicable diseases (Simpson et al., 2019), self-harm, and suicide among prisoners (Haney, 2006; Office of the Auditor General of BC, 2015; Pitts et al., 2014; Sharkey, 2010).

Lessons learned: recommendations for other jurisdictions to consider implementing in response to the pandemic

Many of the strategies developed and implemented by provincial correctional authorities in BC in response to the pandemic follow guidance from the WHO (2020) to prevent the "introduction of the infectious agent into prisons or other places of detention, [limit] the spread within the prison, and [reduce] the possibility of spread from the prison to the outside community" (p. 2). Best practices learned from the success of BC Corrections to date and for correctional authorities in other jurisdictions to consider adapting include those described in earlier paragraphs: providing ongoing education about COVID-19 for individuals in custody and correctional staff, screening and testing everyone who enters custody centers, creating and operating induction units, limiting visitors' access to centers while ensuring other modalities of communication are widely available (i.e., video visitation, unlimited free local and long-distance calling), enhancing sanitization and cleaning practices, and providing staff with PPE when physical distance cannot be maintained.

Other jurisdictions must carefully consider the appropriateness of implementing the strategies that have worked for BC Corrections in terms of their own service's client characteristics, institutional custody counts, and institutional infrastructure, among other factors, such as infection rates in the wider community. Best practices that emerged from this case study of BC Corrections' response to the pandemic, supported by extant literature, are described below.

Adapt a health-informed rather than justice-informed response to COVID-19

BC Corrections has experienced success in keeping COVID-19 out of custody centers by opting for a health-informed rather than a justice-informed approach that has been characterized by close collaboration and coordination between justice and health agencies, an approach recommended by the WHO (2020). Correctional Health Services are independent from BC Corrections in their provision of health-care services for individuals in BC provincial custody facilities and BC Corrections has worked closely with – and followed – the Provincial Health Services Authority's and Provincial Health Officer's recommendations to mitigate the spread of the virus (BC Corrections, 2020a).

Examples of BC Corrections' health-informed approach include screening and testing everyone who enters custody, operating induction units for asymptomatic individuals and isolation for suspected and confirmed individuals, and providing staff with PPE when physical distance cannot be maintained. BC Corrections also has a procedure that allows for contact tracing, which Clarke et al. (2020) argue is a key component of controlling transmission of COVID-19 in correctional institutions. Another primary component of responding to the pandemic through a health-informed approach is ensuring that correctional authorities do not simply default to solitary confinement as the primary solution to minimize transmission of the virus.

Do not default to solitary confinement as the primary solution to minimize transmission of COVID-19

BC Corrections has utilized diverse strategies informed by public health recommendations: strategies that move beyond solitary confinement to mitigate the risk of COVID-19 entering and spreading within custody. Considering alternatives to solitary confinement is vital in light of existing research evidence of the various negative mental and physical health effects on incarcerated persons subject to separate confinement including anxiety, psychosis, perceptual distortions, heart palpitations, worsening of preexisting medical conditions, depression, hopelessness, and higher overall mortality within 5-years post-release (see e.g., Reiter et al., 2020; Shalev, 2008; West Coast Prison Justice Society, 2016; Wildeman & Andersen, 2020).

Further, some correctional services have abolished solitary confinement, and as such, they should be implementing alternative strategies to ensure adherence to policy and legal precedent. Violating the human rights of prisoners and contravening existing regulations is not excused by the existence of a global pandemic (Prisoners' Legal Services, 2020; WHO, 2020). Correctional authorities should maintain opportunities for incarcerated populations to access their community supports, meaningfully engage with other prisoners, and access amenities and outdoor activities to support their mental and physical health during the pandemic (Prisoners' Legal Services, 2020).

Develop a multi-pronged approach to decarceration

Decarceration promotes the health of individuals diverted and released from custody by keeping them out of prisons, "epicentres for infectious diseases" (Kinner et al., 2020, p. E188), and in some jurisdictions, allows them to access higher quality health-care resources in the community than they could access in custody (Henry, 2020).

Decarceration allows both those who *remain* incarcerated (e.g., individuals with higher risk profiles) and staff greater ability to practice social distancing, access existing health-care resources, and quarantine when necessary while also providing opportunities for enhanced cleaning procedures (Henry, 2020; Oladeru et al., 2020; Vose et al., 2020).

BC Corrections' ability to implement diverse strategies (e.g., induction units) and to practice physical distancing, including single-bunking, in response to COVID-19 has been largely influenced by external factors. Judicial decision-making can play an important role by reducing custody populations by judges relying more on bail than remand for those who come before the courts. When appropriate, judges should consider imposing community sentences – such as home confinement – for individuals convicted of nonviolent offenses and those with low-risk profiles and caring responsibilities (WHO, 2020). At earlier stages of the criminal justice system, police officers should be encouraged to issue citations and divert low-level offenders who do not pose a risk to public safety (Henry, 2020) and prosecutors can exercise their discretion in what charges to lay and whether to lay any charges at all.

Correctional authorities and the ministries responsible for their portfolios also have an obligation to examine how they can release individuals from custody, such as by using temporary absences, without increasing the risk to the community. Correctional authorities should prioritize their use of temporary absences for those most at-risk of becoming seriously ill from the virus: elderly individuals and those with chronic conditions (Simpson & Butler, 2020). Correctional authorities should also offer temporary absences to those with imminent release dates and low-risk profiles as determined by the risk-need-responsivity model of offender management. Correctional authorities can use validated assessment instruments that identify the risks and needs of offenders to target the release of individuals into the community in a manner that promotes both the health of incarcerated populations and the safety of the communities to which they reenter (Vose et al., 2020).

Correctional and paroling authorities should also examine how to alter their decision-making practices for those who have violated the conditions of their release by examining whether those incarcerated for violations of the conditions of their release can be safely re-released into their communities. Additionally, community corrections officers should carefully consider whether breaches of conditions warrant a revocation to custody (Wurcel et al., 2020).

Provide incarcerated populations with ongoing information about COVID-19 and the institution's response and provide them with free access to the items they need to prevent transmission of the virus

Correctional authorities should provide custodial populations with information about the institution's response to COVID-19 as this might alleviate their anxiety about contracting the virus (Pyrooz et al., 2020). Additionally, correctional authorities should reassure individuals in custody that they will have opportunities to maintain connections with their loved ones to support their psychological and emotional well-being during the pandemic (WHO, 2020).

Health guidelines demonstrate the importance of frequent hand washing, sanitizing, and cleaning of high contact points (WHO, 2020). Incarcerated populations should have free access to soap, sanitizer, and cleaning supplies to maintain their personal hygiene and cleanliness of their living spaces and common areas (Wurcel et al., 2020). They should also have access to masks given high levels of human interactions that characterize imprisonment (Wurcel et al., 2020). Correctional authorities that charge incarcerated populations co-pay fees to see doctors to access medication and testing should eliminate these fees during the pandemic to encourage their populations to access medical treatment, which promotes institutional and public health (Prison Policy Initiative, 2020; Wurcel et al., 2020).

Maintain ongoing contact with existing oversight agencies

Engaging in ongoing communication with existing oversight agencies is a key component of the strategy to mitigate COVID-19 transmission in prison. Oversight agencies are uniquely situated to identify problematic practices that do not promote the rule of law in prison and human rights for prisoners and that may in fact put incarcerated populations, personnel, and communities at risk.

Coordinate support for incarcerated populations upon their release into the community

Now more than ever, prison health *is* community health (McLeod & Martin, 2018). As such, efforts must be made to ensure released individuals have support as they return to their communities. This support requires coordination across health, not-for-profit, and justice providers (Simpson & Butler, 2020) and includes providing individuals returning to their communities with knowledge of the most current COVID-19-related information about transmission and prevention measures, suitable housing arrangements, transportation to their residence, continuity of care (e.g, for opioid agonist treatment), and masks to protect their community. These efforts will likely prove challenging due to increased unemployment rates and additional barriers (e.g., fewer resources) to the delivery of services that support prisoner reentry (Abraham et al., 2020).

Future research

The preceding discussion examined the strategies employed by one provincial correctional authority in Canada that, as of mid-August 2020, have successfully prevented the spread of COVID-19 in custody centers. Lessons from this experience can serve as the focus for future research: findings from these future studies can inform correctional policy and practice.

The research literature suggests that correctional services that have integrated public and prison health services report many improvements: importantly, medical staff can act independently of the correctional authority and "put the needs of the patient before institutional requirements" (ICPS, 2004, p. 24), promote strategies that enhance public health, and coordinate more effective responses to health-care issues that arise, including infections (ICPS, 2004).

Health-care services in BC provincial correctional centers are administered by an independent health provider, Correctional Health Services. Future comparative research should be undertaken to examine how the independent health-care services and health-informed approach utilized by BC Corrections in their response to

COVID-19 differs from the approaches implemented by other jurisdictions in Canada that followed more of a justice-informed response without independent health-care providers. How do outcomes differ in light of the existing research that identifies the benefits of integrated public and prison health services? Outcomes to examine include infection rates, mortality rates, inmate-on-inmate and inmate-on-staff assaults, staff use of force incidents, perceptions and experiences of incarcerated populations and personnel and their families, and recidivism rates. What lessons can be learned for the provision of health-care services to incarcerated populations both during pandemic and "normal" times?

BC Corrections (2020a) reported that reduced custody counts allowed for their enhanced use of single-bunking, which they believe has contributed to decreased inmate-on-inmate and inmate-on-staff assaults, as well as fewer incidents of staff use of force. Additional analyses are required to determine whether these changes are actually significant and not simply a reflection of reduced daily custodial counts. Future research should also explore whether reduced custody counts that allowed for extensive use of single-bunking contributed to decreases in these negative correctional measures, or whether BC Corrections' use of induction units fostered a more positive prison subculture than their regular intake and assessment process. There are possible lessons for population management that BC Corrections could adapt from this research; for example, if induction units are indeed contributing to a more positive prison subculture than the service may wish to continue using these units moving forward under "normal" circumstances to promote the safety and security of individuals in custody, staff, and institutions.

People concerned with public safety may argue that BC Corrections' success in mitigating infection rates in their correctional centers calls into question decision-making practices that allowed for the early release of thousands of incarcerated persons to save their lives and counteract institutional outbreaks. For example, in late March, the California Department of Corrections and Rehabilitation paroled 3,500 individuals early, and in July, they announced that as many as 8,000 others – those with approaching release dates and those deemed to be medically vulnerable – could be released by the end of August 2020 (Prison Policy Initiative, 2020). Future research should thus examine trends in crime rates pre-, during, and post-pandemic to evaluate how policies and practices triggered by the pandemic contributed to crime rates and thus, whether the continued use of incarceration for nonviolent offenders and reliance on pretrial detention (i.e., remand) are warranted to promote public safety.

In BC, this research should examine trends in crime rates pre-, during, and post-pandemic to evaluate the effects of BC Corrections' (minimal) use of temporary absences to release offenders into the community early and judicial decision-making to release individuals on bail rather than remand them to custody. Remand custody populations have outnumbered sentenced custody populations in Canada for approximately 15 years (Malakieh, 2019), and BC Corrections has experienced challenges separating remand from sentenced individuals even though they acknowledge separation is good correctional practice as outlined in the *Correction Act Regulation* (2005, Office of the Auditor General of BC, 2019). Examining whether judges can reduce their use of remand and increase their use of bail without sacrificing public safety is an important avenue of future research. Research should also investigate how COVID-19 release strategies and reentry programming – where they exist – compare to pre-

COVID release and reentry programming to determine if traditional strategies could be enhanced (Abraham et al., 2020).

Indigenous people are vastly overrepresented in correctional populations in Canada due to the intergenerational consequences of colonialism in this country (Chartrand, 2019; Palmater, 2018). Given this overrepresentation, it is important to invite Indigenous communities to engage in research to examine the negative consequences of COVID-19 resulting from the incarceration of their people during these unprecedented times. One goal of this research should be to identify opportunities to support nation-specific initiatives designed to meet the unique needs of each nation to counteract any negative effects resulting from the pandemic and to develop policies and practices to decrease the overrepresentation of Indigenous people in correctional populations in the years ahead.

Moving forward, an identified need to learn more about BC Corrections' response to the pandemic from the perspective of those most heavily affected by their approach remains: individuals in custody and those working on the frontlines. The narrative to date has largely been dominated by the Service's voice, limiting what we know about their response and the experiences of a vulnerable and marginalized population (individuals in custody) and their families, and frontline staff. What are the consequences of their response to the pandemic for prisoners and personnel (both correctional and health-care) and their family members? As noted by the WHO (2020), health-care workers' families and communities may avoid them due to fear of contracting the virus and stigma about the work they complete in custody. Future research should examine this stigma for correctional and health-care personnel alike. Further, research should examine how personnel and individuals in custody perceive their own risks and the institutional responses put in place (see e.g., Pyrooz et al., 2020). How do individuals in custody, who have limited autonomy in correctional environments, cope with the stressors associated with the virus and BC Corrections' response? What recommendations might prisoners and personnel offer to inform BC Corrections' – and other jurisdictions' – response to the pandemic in the months ahead? What recommendations might they offer to inform population management practices in post-pandemic times?

Conclusion

Addressing COVID-19 within correctional centers is a key aspect of the global response to the virus as such facilities are "epicentres for infectious diseases" (Kinner et al., 2020, p. E188). Keeping COVID-19 out of correctional institutions to protect vulnerable individuals in custody who often have poor health profiles and have been identified as vulnerable to COVID-19 infection (WHO, 2020), correctional personnel, and the public, is a shared responsibility. BC Corrections has implemented various strategies (e.g., screening and testing, induction units) to minimize the risk of COVID-19 entering their custody centers, but their success to date has largely been dictated by external factors. As noted, BC Corrections' predominant use of single-bunking and induction units is contingent on low provincial custody counts (BC Corrections, 2020a). In the months ahead, crime rates, police decision-making, increased court activity, judicial decision-making, community infection rates, and other factors will fundamentally determine whether BC Corrections can continue to utilize the strategies they have implemented to address the pandemic and that have to date been so effective in preventing major outbreaks of COVID-19 in custody centers while other correctional authorities have failed to do so (see Franco-Paredes et al., 2020; Marcum, 2020; Oladeru et al., 2020; Ouellet & Loiero, 2020; Saloner et al., 2020).

Notes

1. It is possible this testing rate includes multiple tests of the same person. Further, the rates were calculated using a one-day snapshot of the inmate population from May through July 01 2020 (Ouellet & Loiero, 2020).
2. It is possible this testing rate includes multiple tests of the same person. Further, the rates were calculated using a one-day snapshot of the inmate population from May through July 01 2020 (Ouellet & Loiero, 2020). As of August 7 2020, with a testing rate of 46,782 per 1,000,000, there have been only 3,934 total cases and 195 confirmed deaths in BC, which has a population of approximately five million (BC Centre for Disease Control, 2020c; BC Stats, 2020).
3. To learn more about how BC Corrections has responded to COVID-19 in the community setting, see: BC Corrections (2020a) and (2020b).
4. For further information about these suspensions, see: Supreme Court of British Columbia (2020) and The Provincial Court of British Columbia (2020).

Acknowledgments

The author would like to thank Drs Sheri Fabian and Curt Taylor Griffiths for their feedback on earlier drafts of this manuscript. The author would also like to thank Erin Gunnarson, Director, Policy and Programs, Strategic Operations Division, of BC Corrections for providing feedback about the Adult Custody Division's response to the pandemic. Any errors are my own.

Disclosure statement

No potential conflict of interest was reported by the author(s).

ORCID

Danielle J. Murdoch http://orcid.org/0000-0001-9358-3265

References

Abraham, L. A., Brown, T. C., & Thomas, S. A. (2020). How COVID-19's disruption of the U.S. correctional system provides an opportunity for decarceration. *American Journal of Criminal Justice*, *45*(4), 780–792. https://doi.org/10.1007/s12103-020-09537-1

Adult Custody Division: Corrections Branch. (2005). *Adult custody policy*. Ministry of Justice. http://docs.openinfo.gov.bc.ca/d26445513a_response_package_jag-2013-00337.pdf

BC Centre for Disease Control. (2020a). *Priority populations*. Provincial Health Services Authority. http://www.bccdc.ca/health-info/diseases-conditions/covid-19/priority-populations

BC Centre for Disease Control. (2020b). *Physical distancing*. Provincial Health Services Authority. http://www.bccdc.ca/health-info/diseases-conditions/covid-19/prevention-risks/physical-distancing

BC Centre for Disease Control. (2020c, August 7). *BC COVID-19 data: COVID-19 dashboard*. Provincial Health Services Authority. Retrieved August 9 2020, from http://www.bccdc.ca/health-info/diseases-conditions/covid-19/data?bcgovtm=20200506_GCPE_AM_COVID_9_NOTIFICATION_BCGOV_BCGOV_EN_BC__NOTIFICATION

BC Corrections. (2017). *A profile of BC corrections: Reduce reoffending, protect communities*. Ministry of Public Safety and Solicitor General. https://www2.gov.bc.ca/assets/gov/law-crime-and-justice/criminal-justice/corrections/reports-publications/bc-corrections-profile.pdf

BC Corrections. (2020a). *BC corrections' response to COVID-19*. The Canadian Bar Association: British Columbia Branch. Retrieved July 17 2020, from https://www.cbabc.org/Publications-and-Resources/COVID-19-Resource-Hub/PD-Programming/BC-Corrections-Response-to-COVID-19

BC Corrections. (2020b). *COVID 19 information for judicial sector*. Government of British Columbia. Retrieved July 17 2020, from https://www2.gov.bc.ca/gov/content/justice/criminal-justice/corrections/covid-19-judicial

BC Mental Health & Substances Use Services. (2020). *Correctional health services*. Provincial Health Services Authority. http://www.bcmhsus.ca/our-services/health-services-for-people-in-custody/correctional-health-services

BC Stats. (2020, June 30). *Issue 20-123: Quarterly population highlights*. Province of British Columbia. https://www2.gov.bc.ca/gov/content/data/statistics/infoline/infoline-2020/20-123-quarterly-population-highlights

Chartrand, V. (2019). Unsettled times: Indigenous incarceration and the links between colonialism and the penitentiary in Canada. *Canadian Journal of Criminology and Criminal Justice*, *61*(3), 67–89. https://doi.org/10.3138/cjccj.2018-0029

Clarke, M., Devlin, J., Conroy, E., Kelly, E., & Sturup-Toft, S. (2020). Establishing prison-led contact tracing to prevent outbreaks of COVID-19 in prisons in Ireland. *Journal of Public Health*, *42*(3), 1–6. https://doi.org/10.1093/pubmed/fdaa092

Correction Act. (2004). *[SBC 2004] Chapter 46*. Retrieved from BC Laws website: https://www.bclaws.ca/civix/document/id/complete/statreg/04046_01#section22

Correction Act Regulation. (2005). *B.C. Reg. 58/2005*. Retrieved from BC Laws website: https://www.bclaws.ca/civix/document/id/complete/statreg/10_58_2005

Correctional Service Canada. (2020, August 7). *Inmate COVID-19 testing in federal correctional institutions August 6, 2020*. Government of Canada. Retrieved August 08 2020, from https://www.csc-scc.gc.ca/001/006/001006-1014-en.shtml

Duwe, G., & McNeeley, S. (2020). Just as good as the real thing? The effects of prison video visitation on recidivism. *Crime & Delinquency* (online first), 001112872094316. https://doi.org/10.1177/0011128720943168

Eisen, L. B., & Weiss-Wolf, J. (2020, April 10). *No soap. Broken sinks. We will all pay for coronavirus ravaging prisons*. Brennan Center for Justice. https://www.brennancenter.org/our-work/analysis-opinion/no-soap-broken-sinks-we-will-all-pay-coronavirus-ravaging-prisons

Fazel, S., & Baillargeon, J. (2010). The health of prisoners. *The Lancet*, *377*(9769), 956–965. https://doi.org/10.1016/S0140-6736(10)61053-7

Franco-Paredes, C., Jankousky, K., Schultz, J., Bernfeld, J., Cullen, K., Quan, N. G., Kon, S., Hotez, P., Henao-Martínez, A. F., Krsak, M., & Kamhawi, S. (2020). COVID-19 in jails and prisons: A neglected infection in a marginalized population. *PLOS Neglected Tropical Diseases*, *14*(6), e0008409. https://doi.org/10.1371/journal.pntd.0008409

Government of British Columbia. (2020). *Custody sentences*. https://www2.gov.bc.ca/gov/content/justice/criminal-justice/bcs-criminal-justice-system/if-you-are-convicted-of-a-crime/understanding-your-sentence/custody-sentences

Griffiths, C. T., & Murdoch, D. J. (2018). *Canadian corrections* (5th ed.). Nelson Education Ltd.

Haney, C. (2006). The wages of prison overcrowding: Harmful psychological consequences and dysfunctional correctional reactions. *Washington University Journal of Law & Policy*, *22*, 265–294. https://openscholarship.wustl.edu/cgi/viewcontent.cgi?article=1360&context=law_journal_law_policy

Henry, B. F. (2020). Social distancing and incarceration: Policy and management strategies to reduce COVID-19 transmission and promote health equity through decarceration. *Health Education & Behavior, 47*(4), 536–539. https://doi.org/10.1177/1090198120927318

Hewson, T., Shepherd, A., Hard, J., & Shaw, J. (2020). Effects of the COVID-19 pandemic on the mental health of prisoners. *The Lancet, 7*(7), 568–570. https://doi.org/10.1016/S2215-0366(20)30241-8

International Centre for Prison Studies. (2004, April 2). *Prison health and public health: The integration of prison health services: Report from a conference.* https://www.prisonstudies.org/sites/default/files/resources/downloads/prison_health_4.pdf

Kinner, S. A., & Young, J. T. (2018). Understanding and improving the health of people who experience incarceration: An overview and synthesis. *Epidemiologic Reviews, 40*(1), 4–11. https://doi.org/10.1093/epirev/mxx018

Kinner, S. A., Young, J. T., Snow, K., Southalan, L., Lopez-Acuña, D., Ferreira-Borges, C., & O'Moore, E. (2020). Prisons and custodial settings are part of a comprehensive response to COVID-19. *The Lancet, 5*(4), E188–E189. https://doi.org/10.1016/.S2468-2667(20)30058-X

Kouyoumdjian, F., Schuler, A., Matheson, F. I., & Hwang, S. W. (2016). Health status of prisoners in Canada: Narrative review. *Canadian Family Physician, 62*(3), 215–222. https://pubmed.ncbi.nlm.nih.gov/27427562/

Malakieh, J. (2019). *Adult and youth correctional statistics in Canada, 2017/2018.* Statistics Canada website: https://www150.statcan.gc.ca/n1/pub/85-002-x/2019001/article/00010-eng.htm

Marcum, C. D. (2020). American corrections system response to COVID-19: An examination of the procedures and policies used in spring 2020. *American Journal of Criminal Justice, 45*(4), 759–768. https://doi.org/10.1007/s12103-020-09535-3

McLeod, K. E., & Martin, R. E. (2018). Health in correctional facilities is health in our communities. *CMAJ, 190*(10), E274–E275. https://doi.org/10.1503/cmaj.171357

Murdoch, D. J., & King, L. L. (2020). 'Not feeling like a caged animal:' Prisoner perceptions of a remote video visitation system. *Journal of Crime and Justice, 43*(2). https://doi.org/10.1080/0735648X.2019.1653216.

National Collaborating Centre for Aboriginal Health. (2013). *Setting the context: An overview of aboriginal health in Canada.* https://www.ccnsa-nccah.ca/docs/context/FS-OverviewAbororiginalHealth-EN.pdf

Office of the Auditor General of British Columbia. (2015). *An audit of the adult custody division's correctional facilities and programs.* https://www.bcauditor.com/sites/default/files/publications/2015/special/report/AGBC%20Corrections%20report%20FINAL.pdf

Office of the Auditor General of British Columbia. (2019). *Progress audit: Correctional facilities and programs: An independent audit report.* https://www.bcauditor.com/sites/default/files/publications/reports/OAGBC_Adult-Custody-Division_RPT.pdf

Oladeru, O. T., Tran, N.-T., Al-Rousan, T., Williams, B., & Zaller, N. (2020). A call to protect patients, correctional staff and healthcare professionals in jails and prisons during the COVID-19 pandemic. *Health and Justice, 8*(1), 1–3. https://doi.org/10.1186/s40352-020-00119-1

Ouellet, V., & Loiero, J. (2020, July 17). COVID-19 taking toll in prisons, with high infection rates, CBC News analysis shows. *CBC News.* https://www.cbc.ca/news/canada/prisons-jails-inmates-covid-19-1.5652470

Palmater, P. (2018). Confronting racism and over-incarceration of Indigenous peoples in Canada. *Journal of Community Corrections, 27*(2), 5–20. https://www.civicresearchinstitute.com/online/article_abstract.php?pid=9&aid=8530&iid=1304

Paynter, M. (2020, March 3). Martha Paynter: Prisons as petri dishes for coronavirus. *The Chronicle Herald.* https://www.thechronicleherald.ca/opinion/local-perspectives/martha-paynter-prisons-petri-dishes-for-coronavirus-418686/

Perkel, C. (2020, April, 23). Federal prison tensions rise amid COVID lockdowns; activists want releases. *National Post.* https://nationalpost.com/pmn/news-pmn/canada-news-pmn/federal-prison-tensions-rise-amid-covid-lockdowns-activists-want-releases

Pitts, J., Griffin, H., & Johnson, W. (2014). Contemporary prison overcrowding: Short- term fixes to a perpetual problem. *Contemporary Justice Review*, *17*(1), 124–139. https://doi.org//10.1080/10282580.2014.883844

Prison Policy Initiative. (2020, July 29). *Responses to the COVID-19 pandemic*. Retrieved August 1 2020, from https://www.prisonpolicy.org/virus/virusresponse.html#state

Prisoners' Legal Services. (2020, March 20). *Re: Call to reduce incarceration during COVID-19 pandemic*. https://prisonjustice.org/wp-content/uploads/2020/04/20200319-Call-to-Reduce-Incarceration-During-COVID-19-Pandemic.pdf

Pyrooz, D. C., Labrecque, R. M., Tostlebe, J. J., & Useem, B. (2020). Views on COVID-19 from inside prison: Perspectives of high-security prisoners. *Justice Evaluation Journal* (online first), 1–13. https://doi.org/10.1080/24751979.2020.1777578

Reiter, K., Ventura, J., Lovell, D., Augustine, D., Barragan, M., Blair, T., Chesnut, K., Dashtgard, P., Gonzalez, G., Pifer, N., & Strong, J. (2020). Psychological distress in solitary confinement: Symptoms, severity, and prevalence in the United States, 2017-2018. *American Journal of Public Health*, *110*(S1), S56–S62. https://doi.org/10.2105/AJPH.2019.305375

Saloner, B., Parish, K., Ward, J. A., DiLaura, G., & Dolovich, S. (2020). COVID-19 cases and deaths in federal and state prisons. *JAMA*, *324*(6), 602. https://doi.org/10.1001/jama.2020.12528

Scott, B. J. (2020). Special section article: A pandemic in prisons. *Social Anthropology*, *28*(2), 352–353. https://doi.org/10.1111/1469-8676.12857

Shalev, S. (2008, October). *A sourcebook on solitary confinement*. Mannheim Centre for Criminology. http://solitaryconfinement.org/uploads/sourcebook_web.pdf

Sharkey, L. (2010). Does overcrowding in prisons exacerbate the risk of suicide among women prisoners? *The Howard Journal of Criminal Justice*, *49*(2), 111–124. https://doi.org/10.1111/j.1468-2311.2009.00602.x

Simpson, P. L., & Butler, T. G. (2020). COVID-19, prison crowding, and release policies. *BMJ*, *369*. https://doi.org/10.1136/bmj.m1551

Simpson, P. L., Simpson, M., Adily, A., Grant, L., & Butler, T. (2019). Prison cell spatial density and infectious and communicable diseases: A systematic review. *BMP Open*, *9*(7), 1–10. https://doi.org/10.1136/bmjopen-2018-026806

Supreme Court of British Columbia. (2020). *Notice to the profession, the public and the media regarding criminal proceedings*. https://www.policevictimservices.bc.ca/wp-content/uploads/2020/03/Supension-of-Criminal-Proceedings-with-appendices-Supreme-Court-of-BC.pdf

The Factum. (2020). *How COVID-19 is affecting bail and sentencing decisions*. MyLawBC. http://factum.mylawbc.com/posts/2020/5/1/how-covid-19-is-affecting-bail-and-sentencing-decisions

The Provincial Court of British Columbia. (2020, March 19). *Notice to the profession and public: COVID-19: Suspension of regular court operations*. https://www.policevictimservices.bc.ca/wp-content/uploads/2020/03/Suspension-of-Provincial-Court-Operations-COVID-19.pdf

Vose, B., Cullen, F. T., & Lee, H. (2020). Targeted release in the COVID-19 correctional crisis: Using the RNR model to save lives. *American Journal of Criminal Justice*, *45*(4), 769–779. https://doi.org/10.1007/s12103-020-09539-z

West Coast Prison Justice Society. (2016, November). *Solitary: A case for abolition*. https://prisonjustice.org/wp-content/uploads/2018/11/solitary-confinement-report.pdf

Wildeman, C., & Andersen, L. H. (2020). Solitary confinement placement and post- release mortality risk among formerly incarcerated individuals: A population-based study. *The Lancet*, *5*(2), E107–E113. https://doi.org/10.1016/S2468-2667(19)30271-3

World Health Organization. (2020, March 15). *Preparedness, prevention and control of COVID-19 in prisons and other places of detention: Interim guidance*. https://www.euro.who.int/__data/assets/pdf_file/0019/434026/Preparedness-prevention-and-control-of-COVID-19-in-prisons.pdf?ua=1

Wurcel, A. G., Dauria, E., Zaller, N., Nijhawan, A., Beckwith, C., Nowotny, K., & Brinkley-Rubinstein, L. (2020). Spotlight on jails: COVID-19 mitigation policies needed now. *Clinical Infectious Diseases*, *71*(15), 891–892. https://doi.org/10.1093/cid/ciaa346

Management of COVID-19 for Persons with Mental Illness in Secure Units: A Rapid International Review to Inform Practice in Québec

Ashley J. Lemieux, Audrey-Anne Dumais Michaud, Jean Damasse, Julie-Katia Morin-Major, To Nhu Nguyen, Alain Lesage, and Anne G. Crocker

ABSTRACT

Most countries have implemented guidelines and policies in response to COVID-19 that have had a direct impact on institutionalized or incarcerated persons with mental health problems. Although these strategies are essential to protect these vulnerable persons from the pandemic, they can also have significant consequences on recovery, well-being, as well as rights and freedoms. Accordingly, we conducted a rapid review to identify strategies, challenges and recommendations for dealing with the COVID-19 outbreak in secure settings for persons with mental illness. While most available publications are not empirical in nature, this knowledge synthesis can nevertheless guide managers of psychiatric and forensic psychiatric institutions, and correctional facilities in dealing with the COVID-19 pandemic.

Introduction

As COVID-19 spreads around the world, more and more countries are implementing guidelines and policies in order to flatten the infection curve and avoid overtaxing health-care systems. For example, social distancing and confinement measures have been applied in the general population, and several countries have had to reassign medical and psycho-social staff to COVID-19 screening, management, and treatment services in order to avoid the worst-case transmission scenarios.

These government measures and guidelines have a direct impact on institutionalized or incarcerated persons with mental health problems. Specialized mental health resources have been reassigned to short-term hospital services and long-term care facilities, and social distancing measures have limited visitors' access to mental health institutions. In addition, institutionalized or incarcerated persons with mental health problems have seen decreases in their access to practitioners and non-essential services, which has led to reduced care (Hewson et al., 2020; Moreno et al., 2020). Although these strategies are essential to protect these vulnerable persons from the pandemic, they can also have significant consequences on their recovery and well-being. Indeed, persons with mental illness in closed settings are particularly susceptible to such consequences, as they were experiencing some form of confinement *prior* to the pandemic.

Local context in Canada and Québec

The first official cases of COVID-19 in Canada appeared on January 23, 2020; by the end of August 2020, Canada will have had a total of 125 969 cases and 9 090 deaths (Government of Canada, 2020). Long-term care facilities were hard hit: this is where the majority of outbreaks and deaths occurred (Flood et al., 2020). However, there have been outbreaks reported in correctional settings, as well as psychiatric institutions across the country. Correctional services in Canada have reported 360 cases and two deaths as of August 25, 2020, one of which occurred in a correctional facility in the province of Québec (Correctional Service Canada, 2020). The perceived mismanagement of the COVID-19 pandemic in federal correctional facilities sparked a class action lawsuit on behalf of all federal inmates in the province, alleging that appropriate dispositions were not taken to contain contagion and that inmates who presented symptoms were discredited and diminished (Iftene, 2020).

Within Canada, the province with the highest COVID-19 death rate is Québec, with a total of 61 945 cases and 5 747 deaths for a population of 8.485 million (Gouvernement du Québec 2020); this represents a death rate of 677.31 per one million population, making it the third-deadliest place in the world (Statista, 2020). Montréal with a population of 2 million, bore the brunt of the pandemic in the province of Québec and reported 29 714 cases and 3 465 deaths as of August 26, 2020.

Montréal is home to the *Institut national de psychiatrie légale Philippe-Pinel* (INPLPP), Québec's only high secure forensic psychiatric institution and Canada's largest, with its 15 20-bed units. Because of its particular expertise in forensic mental health, the INPLPP has a provincial mandate to exercise an advisory role with government agencies dealing with issues at the intersection of mental health and justice involvement, including offenders with mental illness within the criminal justice system. Montreal is also home to the Montreal Mental Health University Institute (IUSMM),[1] a 389-bed institution, which includes a low-medium secure forensic psychiatry unit of 18 patients.

As of August 26, 2020, the INPLPP reported two positive COVID-19 cases among patients upon admission over the course of the pandemic, while the IUSMM forensic psychiatry unit recorded none. The successful management of this health crisis by these institutions is in part due to the rapid mobilization of management and staff in implementing changes based on the best available information.

Supporting clinical leadership through health technology assessment

On March 13, 2020, the Government of Québec declared a public health emergency for the entire province of Quebec, due to the COVID-19 pandemic. This triggered an immediate mobilization by the INPLPP, through the creation of a COVID-19 crisis management unit and of a special inter-council COVID-19 committee. The crisis unit is composed of INPLPP managers, and meets daily to plan rapid and effective responses to pandemic-related issues. The inter-council committee is composed of the heads of the various clinical councils and provides recommendations for the INPLPP's executive committee and COVID crisis unit.

The INPLPP's safety, justice, and mental health technology assessment unit[2] was invited to participate in the inter-council committee to orient recommendations and decision-making based on available evidence. The IUSMM put a similar crisis response structure in place. In response to questions raised by the crisis units and the inter-council committee, the INPLPP's heath technology assessment unit collaborated with the IUSMM's mental health technology assessment unit[3] to support their clinical leadership in the management of the pandemic by conducing a rapid review.

Aim

It is essential to examine the potential impact of changes in practice of various kinds (legislative, organizational, clinical, ethical) on institutionalized or incarcerated persons with mental health problems. Doing so will allow managers and clinicians to respond to the health issues raised by the COVID-19 pandemic and take appropriate action. Accordingly, a rapid review was conducted to answer the following question: *What strategies have been implemented in response to the COVID-19 outbreak in clinical and legal environments (general-psychiatry services, forensic-psychiatry services, correctional services) in which persons with mental health problems are confined?* This review also addresses a logical corollary of this question, namely: *Given the potential impact of these strategies in these environments, should they be maintained after the pandemic?*

Methods

Search strategy

A rapid review of the gray and scientific literature on clinical and legal environments (general and forensic psychiatric services, correctional services housing persons with mental health problems) was carried out between May 10 and May 16, 2020. From this date on, a literature watch was set up to identify any relevant papers, up until August 18, 2020. Moreover, an additional search was conducted in Google Scholar on August 18, 2020. To be included in the review, the publications had to be in French or English, and published from December 2019 (when Chinese health authorities identified the first cases of COVID-19 in Wuhan, China) onwards. Two librarians searched the Medline, Pubmed, PsycInfo, CINAHL, EMBASE, EBM Reviews, and HeinOnline bibliographic databases, as well as Internet sites of some international organizations active in health technology assessment (HTA), some national and international health organizations, and Google Scholar. The primary keywords used included terms related to psychiatry (e.g., psychiatric, mental disorder, mental illness), correctional activities (correctional, offender), and forensic psychiatry (e.g., forensic); these were then combined with keywords related to COVID-19 (e.g., coronavirus, SARSCoV-2).

Selection of documents

The initial reference search yielded 679 publications. Of these, 561 were in the seven reference databases, 110 were found using Google Scholar, and 8 were found through manual searches of the references of previously identified publications and scientific journal newsletters. Elimination of duplicates (n = 216) resulted in 463 publications, of which 368 were not retained; this reduced the number of eligible publications to 95. These 95 publications were read, and after applying inclusion and exclusion criteria, 49 were included into the review. An additional 137 papers were identified through information watch (17) and Google Scholar (120) after the original search was conducted; of these, 20 were identified as relevant. This review is therefore based on 69 publications. The flow chart for the Preferred Reporting Items for Systematic Reviews and Meta-Analysis (PRISMA) model can be found in Figure 1. For the complete list of references, please contact the authors.

For the first 49 publications, the documents were independently selected by two professionals trained in HTA (AJ, JD, and JM). Inter-rater reliability was assessed using a 25% sample of the publications retained after the first selection stage and 20% of the publications retained after the second. In the case of divergent evaluations, a third professional cast the deciding vote. Because of the explosion in the number of publications since May 26, 2020, the following 20 papers were selected based on inclusion criteria as well as relevance. Specifically, because a majority of publications in the first iteration pertained to psychiatric institutions, the second iteration favored publications focusing on correctional and forensic institutions.

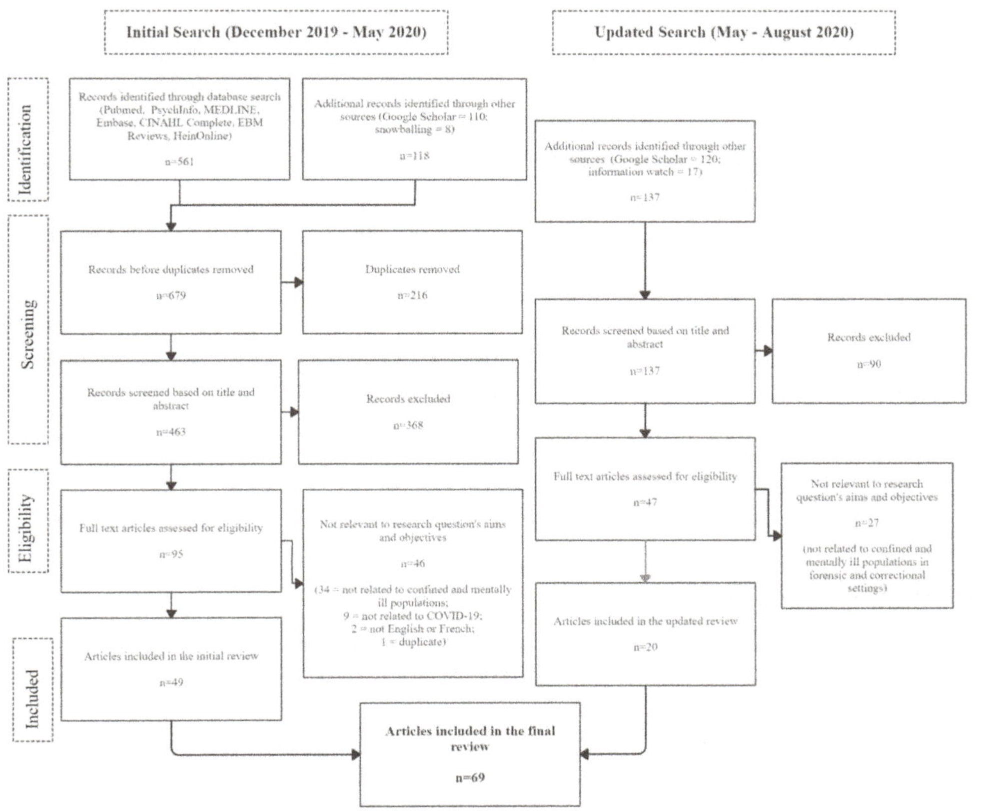

Figure 1. PRISMA flow chart (Moher et al., 2015).

Data extraction, coding, analysis, and synthesis

The three HTA professionals developed an extraction form, and extracted data from the publications after an analysis of inter-rater reliability using a 20% sample of the documents retained for analysis. For the first 49 publications, information extracted pertained to: 1) description of the measures implemented (and, if described or measured, their impact); 2) primary clinical, practical, or ethical issues; and 3) recommendations for changes in practice (the data extraction form is available upon request). The data was then coded by the three HTA professionals and grouped into thematic categories. For the subsequent 20 publications, only new information was extracted (AJ and AD) into the relevant themes and one additional theme was identified. The quality of the studies was not evaluated. The results are presented below in narrative form.

Summary of results

The 69 publications reviewed were all published in 2020 in, most commonly, the United States (14 publications), China (13), Italy (8), the United Kingdom (6), France (5), Germany (3), and Ireland (3). Singapore, Brazil, Canada, Spain, and Australia contributed two publications each, and India, Israel, Poland, New Zealand, South Korea, Scandinavia, and Switzerland contributed one each.

These publications were primarily (n = 50) opinion pieces by experts (editorials, letters to the editor, position papers and other correspondences). There were also four rapid literature reviews, seven narrative (i.e. non-systematic) literature reviews, and eight empirical studies (three surveys and five descriptive/case studies). Reference documents (laws, standards, guidelines, etc.) were also consulted for context (for a list of complementary resources, please consult the original rapid response guide linked in the Acknowledgments or contact the authors).

The rest of this section presents a synthesis of information collected from the literature reviewed. The authors of the publications primarily discuss issues related to the management of the pandemic in psychiatric environments, and present recommendations based on their own experience with COVID-19 or on previous studies. Nine main themes are discussed: 1) increased vulnerability of confined persons with mental health problems; 2) composition and management of mental health teams; 3) release from prison, and return to the community; 4) management of transmission and physical spaces on secure units; 5) sanitary issues; 6) continuity, suspension, or reduction of services; 7) remote technologies; 8) patient rights; and 9) longer-term effects of the pandemic.

Increased vulnerability of patients

Persons with mental health problems are more vulnerable to COVID-19: both morbidity and mortality are greater in this population, in large part because of multiple physical comorbidities as well as lifestyle factors, such as sedentary lifestyle and smoking (C. Brown et al., 2020; Kozloff et al., 2020). Special attention should be paid to the interaction between COVID-19 and psychiatric medication (Chevance et al., 2020; Cranshaw & Harikumar, 2020). This is especially important to consider when using sedation to ensure compliance with measures of isolation in their rooms, as it may aggravate respiratory symptoms

(Chevance et al., 2020). Another issue identified in correctional settings is the increased risk of withdrawal symptoms in response to reduced access to illicit psychoactive substances as a result of restricted access to the community (Fovet et al., 2020).

Living environment

Transmission of COVID-19 is greater in secure units, such as forensic and psychiatric hospitals, remand centers, and prisons (De Girolamo et al., 2020; Liebrenz et al., 2020) as social distancing is challenging due to population density (Kothari et al., 2020; Kozloff et al., 2020). Moreover, in order to prevent suicide or unauthorized leaves, windows are often locked, which leads to poor ventilation, itself a risk factor for transmission (Kozloff et al., 2020). Correctional environments, already underfunded and overcrowded prior to the pandemic, struggle as austerity measures amplify preexisting challenges (Kothari et al., 2020).

Clinical issues

Some patients need constant reminders of social distancing rules due to illness-related cognitive problems or disorganized behavior (Chevance et al., 2020; Kozloff et al., 2020). Concomitant substance use affects some persons' judgment, and ability to comply with these rules (Kozloff et al., 2020). Some patients suffering from psychosis are less motivated to comply with rules regarding social distancing and infection control (E. Brown et al., 2020; Rajkumar, 2020). Agitated patients may spit on staff or other patients, which increases the risk of transmission (C. Brown et al., 2020). The circumstances of the pandemic may also lead to atypical psychiatric presentations that may complexify treatment and compliance (Türközer & Öngür, 2020). Moreover, rising tension, distress and anger in the face of an ever-increasing number of restrictions coupled with fear of falling ill, have led to acts of rebellion such as hunger strikes, protests and riots in prisons, along with escapes, deaths and injuries (Caputo et al., 2020; De Carvalho et al., 2020).

Relapse

The impact of COVID-management measures on psychiatric relapses must be emphasized. Relapses may be triggered by increased stress secondary to confinement or pandemic-related discharge and early return to the community (Garriga et al., 2020), as well as by exposure to constant negative media coverage and worries about friends and family in the community with whom the patient or inmate has lost contact (Fovet et al., 2020). In additions, individuals with mental illness and those who are already confined in prisons or in psychiatric facilities are at increased risk of developing a pandemic acute stress disorder (Heitzman, 2020). Because suicide and self-harm rates are generally high in correctional settings, globally, especially for those who are on remand, some authors are concerned that increased isolation may increase this risk (Hewson et al., 2020).

Staff composition and personnel management in mental health

The management of the COVID-19 pandemic has led to significant changes to the organization of care, and especially to staff composition and personnel management in clinical settings. In the current context, it may prove useful to create an inter-profession task force, which includes representatives of all clinical and non-clinical departments, that meet on a daily basis to oversee the operational aspects of interventions and procedures (L. Li, 2020). Transparent communications within the institution as well as with the public can be facilitated though intranet, podcasts, and institutional websites (Kreuzer et al., 2020). Increased collaboration between professionals and community agencies has had some positive impacts, as stated by Hewson et al. (2020), in the United Kingdom: clinicians have been advocating for whole prisons and communities, which has generated a sense of belonging for inmates within their communities and a greater camaraderie between staff and inmates.

Healthcare professionals must not only take on new roles and responsibilities but also rapidly adapt to work environments characterized by tense relationships and uncertainty about COVID-19 transmission (Muirhead, 2020). Several authors recommend that the management of front-line staff (psychiatrists, psychologists, social workers, etc.) be based on six principles: 1) implementation of a staff-management plan (canceling and rescheduling holidays, financial compensation); 2) equitable treatment of staff, and attention to their well-being; 3) training and appropriate supervision of staff; 4) psychological support for teams facing challenging situations daily; 5) good communication and strong collaboration between professionals and teams; and 6) validation of the work and skills of those most at risk (Kothari et al., 2020; Ornell et al., 2020; Poremski et al., 2020). To reinforce affiliation and allow debriefing after each work shift, an employee-manager buddy system can be established (Kothari et al., 2020). Discussing practical changes in team briefings through examples across disciplines may help support staff behavioral changes (Boland & Dratcu, 2020).

Teams of healthcare professionals should be reduced in size, in order to create standby replacement teams that can incorporate providers in non-clinical administrative roles. This would permit the staff most at risk of infection (workers who are older, pregnant, or in fragile health) to avoid undue exposure and allow work teams to have rest periods (L. Li, 2020). A survey can be used to identify staff with specific needs, such as those with health risks or those with children to care for during lock down (Kreuzer et al., 2020).

It is clear from the literature that there is a need for training programs on COVID-19 risk and prevention strategies, in order to equip professionals to deliver appropriate care that minimizes the risk of infection, and rapidly identify the signs and symptoms of the infection (C. Brown et al., 2020; Druss, 2020). Guidelines on the evaluation of symptoms, patient transfers to intensive care units, and the functional links between services should be produced and disseminated (Thome et al., 2020). It is recommended that posters and e-mail be used to regularly communicate up-to-date information, as there seems to exist a knowledge gap about the pandemic among staff (Kothari et al., 2020; Zhu et al., 2020).

Conditional discharge and community release

The increased criminalization of some social groups (ethnic minorities, homeless persons, persons with substance-use problems, persons with mental health problems) is reported to increase transmission of COVID-19 in correctional settings (Akiyama et al., 2020). Moreover, repeated transitions to and from their living environment and prison (i.e. "the revolving doors of justice") increase the transmission of COVID-19 in both the community and correctional settings.

In response to this problem, Akiyama et al. (2020) have formulated recommendations for this population, most notably: 1) release from prison of persons with the lowest risk of recidivism, of older inmates, and of persons with health problems; 2) provisional suspension of arrests and court proceedings for minor offenses; 3) isolation of persons who are, or are suspected of being, COVID-positive; 4) preparation of protocols for the transfer and hospitalization of inmates with severe cases of COVID-19; and 5) identification of infected and recovered staff who may have acquired greater immunity and could therefore be assigned to duties related to the hygiene and care of COVID-positive inmates.

To prevent transmission of the virus in prisons, the Bazelon Center for Mental Health (Washington DC, United States) recommends the immediate release of inmates with mental health problems, and the exclusion from prisons of any arrested person with a mental health problem (Canady, 2020a). In the United Kingdom, new legislation had been proposed to modify the admission and diversion conditions for legally detained persons with mental health problems, and strongly incites Mental Health Trusts to transfer these persons to, and treat them in, the community (C. Brown et al., 2020). On the other hand, although public health authorities in England have also recommended early release of correctional detainees, this has only been carried out partially, and has been ineffective in reducing prison deaths due to COVID-19 (Kothari et al., 2020). In Italy, a government decree was introduced on March 17 which gave approximately 4 000 prisoners the possibility of home detention, with electronic bracelets for those with less than 18 months left to serve (Caputo et al., 2020). However, releasing individuals from prison into precarious living situations or into the streets, in a context where many emergency resources have reduced their services, may in fact increase the “revolving doors of justice” phenomenon (Fovet et al., 2020).

The diversion of COVID-negative patients from psychiatric hospitals to psychiatric services in the community must be planned (Choi et al., 2020), though sometimes, relocation of hospitalized patients to community-based services occurred very rapidly, without any transition period (Muirhead, 2020). Rapid discharge poses ethical and clinical challenges with regards to the evaluation of risk of transmission as well as the suitability and availability of community services (Moreno et al., 2020).

In the United Kingdom, patients who tested positive for COVID-19 were prioritized for discharge if they were medically well and responded positively to psychiatric treatment (Boland & Dratcu, 2020). In France, patients who could be quarantined (14 days), had a stable psychiatric state, and were able to comply with confinement requirements were released early from psychiatric hospitals in order to free up psychiatric beds for pandemic patients (Chevance et al., 2020). In Italy however, psychiatric hospitalizations lasted longer in March 2020 than in March 2019 in some regions, because of difficulties ensuring that patients could return to a safe home environment (Clerici et al., 2020).

Management of transmission and physical spaces in secure units

Admissions

Many hospitals have suspended admissions (D’Agostino et al., 2020) or tightened admission criteria (Muirhead, 2020; Xiang et al., 2020). Prior to admission, all patients and detainees should be screened for COVID-19 symptoms, including a history of travel to high-risk regions, and a history of contacts with persons confirmed to be COVID-positive or exhibiting COVID-like symptoms (D'Agostino et al., 2020; Starace & Ferrara, 2020). Isolation of new admissions was standard practice in mental health (Starace & Ferrara, 2020) and correctional settings (Burton et al., in press).

Detection of positive cases and "cohorting"

Vigilance for COVID-19 symptoms should be constant and dynamic, in order to prevent outbreaks on units (D'Agostino et al., 2020). Individuals with severe mental illness often presented with atypical symptoms and were unable to correctly and rapidly identify their own symptoms (Ji et al., 2020). It has also been reported that inmates in correctional facilities were reluctant to report symptoms, out of fear that they would be subjected to additional isolation precisely when they were feeling particularly vulnerable and alone (Kothari et al., 2020). When a COVID-positive case is identified, all individuals on the unit should be tested for COVID-19, and a protocol should be in place for their transfer to a designated COVID care unit should their health deteriorate.

Several authors have reported the creation of distinct units ("patient cohorting"): 1) Hot zones, in which COVID-positive patients or inmates receive appropriate treatment; 2) Warm zones, which house suspected/symptomatic COVID cases for 14 days while they await the results of screening tests; and 3) Cold zones, which house COVID-negative individuals (Arango, 2020; L. Li, 2020). In addition, distinct corridors may be created within these units for staff and patients, in order to limit the risk of transmission (Chevance et al., 2020). If necessary, patients or inmates suspected of being or known to be COVID-positive may be separated from the general population and isolated in designated individual rooms for 14 days (Akiyama et al., 2020; L. Li, 2020). Dedicated isolation units should include seclusion rooms for behavioral disturbances with dedicated personnel and full use of personal protective equipement (A. I. F. Simpson et al., 2020).

Symptomatic patients in isolation should also be monitored closely should they exhibit suicidal or violent behaviors (L. Li, 2020). The decision to transfer a patient to a designated hospital should be based on the patient's level of risk and needs, determined through a procedure established by the local government (Zhu et al., 2020). In their narrative review of the impact of the pandemic on psychiatric care, Bojdani et al. (2020) underline several challenges faced by institutions when dealing with contagion. One of the difficulties in dealing with COVID-positive patients is the inability to predict the course of a patient's infection. Psychiatric and correctional facilities seldom have access to emergency material, supplies and expertise for physical interventions, such as intubation, if a patient were to rapidly develop complications. Strategies to effectively and rapidly transfer patients and inmates to appropriately resourced medical units are essential.

Hygiene, sanitation, and protection

Personal protective equipment

The implementation of enhanced hygiene measures and of personal protective equipment (PPE, e.g., masks, face coverings, protective suits) faces many obstacles, especially with regards to supply, safety, training, and use. First, both psychiatric and correctional institutions have difficulty obtaining adequate supplies due in part to the fact that they lie outside traditional supply chains and maintain little PPE on the premises (Enos, 2020; Kothari et al., 2020). It is also important to consider the inherent hazard of some situations in secure units: masks may be used as ligatures (Enos, 2020), and alcohol-based hand sanitizers may be prohibited in units, due to the risk of patients or inmates consuming them. Their use may therefore require additional monitoring by staff (Burton et al., in press).

All staff should wear masks and be trained in the use of PPE, in order to reduce the risks of infection (Enos, 2020; Percudani et al., 2020). When the supply of PPE is limited, the equipment should be reserved for interactions with patients with fever and respiratory symptoms (L. Li, 2020). Changing rooms should be set up to allow staff to don surgical masks and disposable suits before entering units with COVID-positive patients (Chevance et al., 2020; Percudani et al., 2020). However, staff must be mindful that masks might inadvertently appear threatening to patients experiencing emotional distress and paranoid thoughts (The Lancet Psychiatry, 2020). Moreover, to foster empowerment, patients should be offered the choice of wearing or not wearing a mask, so that they can feel that they have some control over their situation (Canady, 2020b). If a patient is incapable of wearing a mask due to their psychiatric symptoms or safety considerations, those near them should wear a mask or face covering, in order to reduce the risk of transmission (Enos, 2020).

Enhanced hygiene measure

In the current context, it is essential to increase the availability of alcohol-based hand sanitizer and to educate not only patients, but also staff, about hand hygiene, how to cough safely and how to dispose of tissues (A. I. F. Simpson et al., 2020). Some authors recommend using highly visible posters that provide information on COVID-19, the virus' means of transmission, and the different safety protocols applicable to staff and patients (Canady, 2020a). Surfaces (e.g., doors, shared computers, identity cards, metal or plastic surfaces that facilitate virus transmission) and frequently used locations (e.g., dining rooms) should be disinfected (L. Li, 2020). Additional measures should be put in place in hot zones, such as regular disinfection of all equipment (e.g., keys, telephones), assigning specific equipment to each patient or, when this is not possible, disinfecting it between each patient interaction (Chevance et al., 2020). Food and equipment of any kind should be inspected and disinfected by staff before their distribution (C. Li et al., 2020). Increased ventilation can be achieved by keeping windows open whenever safe to do so, in all clinical and non-clinical rooms in the ward (Boland & Dratcu, 2020).

Continuity, reduction, or suspension of services

Restriction of admissions

Several authors reported difficulties in maintaining services to persons with mental health problems due in part to restricted admissions policies (Arango, 2020; Choi et al., 2020) and closure of community-based clinical and psychosocial services (L. Li, 2020). In addition, the admission of new patients takes longer, which contributes to overtaxing psychiatric emergency services. Zuffranieri and Zanalda (2020), in Italy, report that court orders were temporarily put on hold for admission to rehabilitative psychiatric health facilities for offenders who are mentally incapacitated and considered to be highly dangerous to society; admission were limited to individuals who were already in prison as well as those who were difficult to control in the community during lockdown.

Suspension of group activities

Several authors have recommended the reduction, if not complete suspension, of group activities and activities held in common rooms, as well as the restriction of the number of participants in groups, especially those involving older patients with multiple comorbidities (L. Li, 2020; Tomlin, 2020). However, limiting group activities could lead to greater loneliness in already isolated patients, and exacerbate psychiatric symptoms (Xiang et al., 2020). Group activities where social distancing can be applied, such as gardening, should be expanded and maintained (Boland & Dratcu, 2020). In forensic psychiatric residential facilities in Italy, group activities were reorganized with the help of patients, by limiting the number of participants, by enforcing physical distancing and the use of surgical masks, and by choosing to do the activities in large well-ventilated spaces, or outdoors (Zuffranieri & Zanalda, 2020). Boland and Dratcu (2020) report offering occupational therapy activities and educational sessions on COVID-19 on a one-on-one basis as opposed to group settings. While transforming group activities into individual session may be resources-intensive, the reduction of the number of inpatients through community release and restricted admissions will allow institutions to increase resources for those remaining (Kreuzer et al., 2020).

Individual activities and interventions

Poremski et al. (2020) state that the decision to reduce individual activities should take into account the risk posed by the activity, patient needs, and existing alternative services. Cullen et al. (2020) fear that reducing services will lead to a deterioration of patients' mental and physical states, and recommend increasing care during this period of crisis. Tomlin (2020) recommends that forensic mental health environments plan how often patients go outdoors and enjoy exercise periods, to ensure that they receive the minimum time outdoors recommended by the United Nations' Nelson Mandela Rules (at least one hour of outdoor physical activity per day, weather permitting). Kothari et al. (2020) recommend that prisoners in cells receive entertaining material such as jigsaw puzzles and playing cards, as well as personal-development material such as guides to yoga or physical fitness. A variety of levels should be available, with activities for beginners and experts. They also report that detainees greatly appreciate these basic interventions.

Reduction of mental health services in prisons

Many therapeutic and recreational activities have been suspended in prisons while time in cells has increased, with reports stating some prisoners are isolated up to 23 hours a day (Hewson et al., 2020). Liebrenz et al. (2020) emphasize that mental health problems are disproportionately frequent among incarcerated persons. Even under normal conditions, psychiatric care in prison environments is inadequate – during a crisis, the psychiatric and psychological needs are that much greater, due to increased feelings of fear and uncertainty, and the undesirable effects of isolation measures. Ensuring the continuity of psychiatric and psychological services during the COVID-19 pandemic is paramount. To this end, Kothari et al. (2020) recommend regional coordination of psychiatric and correctional services, as well as liaison with courts and probation officers to screen for mental health problems and ensure adequate follow-up. They also emphasize the need to triage persons with serious mental health problems, by identifying risk factors – such as preexisting mental health problems, the risk of harm to self or others, violent or aggressive behavior, and refusal to eat – and to consider the recommendations of professionals with prior knowledge of the detainee. These individuals should be prioritized for care (Kothari et al., 2020). Furthermore, professionals who provide psychosocial care should be regularly informed of the evolution of symptoms (Liebrenz et al., 2020). In order to ensure that follow-up is congruent with the constantly evolving situation, new practices should be regularly reevaluated and redeveloped, and all changes should be clearly explained to staff and detainees (Kothari et al., 2020). Spaces may even need to be reorganized in order to allow for the respect of social distancing measures (Fovet et al., 2020).

Suspension of legal proceedings

Treatment orders and involuntary admissions take longer to process when court proceedings are suspended or limited, and this may exacerbate existing psychiatric problems (L. Li, 2020). Suspension of court hearings and jury trials have increased time spend in remand centers. In their commentary, Hewson et al. (2020) highlight that time spent in remand is often difficult for prisoners, as it is characterized by uncertainty and anxiety about possible legal outcomes. This is compounded by the distress and insecurity brought on by the ongoing pandemic. They suggest that additional assistance be offered by court-liaison services in order to reduce delays in court processing and offer much-needed support.

Remote technologies

Technology as the interface for patient-family meetings

Several countries have promoted the use of remote technologies to ensure hospitalized patients remain in contact with their families. In the absence of in-person visits, videoconferencing (when available) and telephones have become the principal means of contact between these groups (Garriga et al., 2020). In Madrid, one psychiatric unit prohibited in-person visits, but families could turn to a psychiatric-liaison department, which provided videoconferencing technology for virtual visits to patients (Arango, 2020). In addition to videoconferencing with patients' close relatives and friends, some hospitals used remote technology to provide psychological support to grieving families (De Girolamo et al., 2020). In the United States, the National Association of State Mental Health Program Directors (2020) recommends patients stay in touch with their loved ones, which can be done via videoconferencing (Muirhead, 2020), FaceTime, or Skype (Canady, 2020a). In addition, the National Alliance on Mental Illness (2020) published a guide that explains, among other things, how to contact an incarcerated close relative or friend with a mental health problem.

Remote interventions

In response to the COVID-19 pandemic, some public authorities rapidly turned to remote delivery of patient services, with the justice environment being no exception. In Ireland, the experience has been positive (Kennedy et al., 2020): the use of video court appearances has resulted in meetings adhering more closely to the agenda, triage being more rigorous and effective, and detainees being more likely to appear. Regarding telemedicine, some care units, such as those of the Irish National Forensic Mental Health Service and the Irish Prison Service, offer videoconferencing interventions. Kennedy et al. (2020) believe that video court appearances and telemedicine accelerate some elements of the judicial process and propose that they be continued after the COVID-19 crisis. Although virtual contacts may be used in secure rooms or cells for interventions or mental state checks, they may present some challenges in shared spaces, such as prison cells and double-occupancy rooms, where they compromise confidentiality and may increase stigmatization and feelings of shame (Kothari et al., 2020). Hewson et al. (2020) recommend that other communication methods should be encouraged: writing letters, increased access to telephone landlines, and use of the prison voicemail service.

Prior to the COVID-19 pandemic, communication technologies dedicated to intervention were not always available or used for this purpose in psychiatric settings (Shalev & Shapiro, 2020). A survey conducted by S. A. Simpson et al. (2020) in March 2020 – in which 101 psychiatrists in 29 US states were asked to assess the quality of, and access to, mental health services – reveals that even today, these technologies are not always used when available. Psychiatrists reported being more likely to use telemedicine technologies for outpatients than for inpatients, whose health status increases their susceptibility to COVID-19 infection (S. A. Simpson et al., 2020). The current situation may reflect the apprehension some health professionals have in the use of these technologies as alternatives to in-person meetings with clients. Nevertheless, this apprehension is continually diminishing as the value of these communication technologies in hospital environments is recognized; as a result, uptake of the technologies is growing.

The recourse to remote technologies, be they videoconferencing or telephone consultations between professionals and patients (Arango, 2020), or FaceTime or Skype discussions between staff, requires staff training in the technology in question (Canady, 2020a). Moreover, remote technologies should be used not only for consultations but also for the management of medication and communications with patients' close relatives and friends (De Girolamo et al., 2020). In fact, the value of these technologies is increasingly recognized, and remote consultations with patients are becoming widespread in the face of social distancing measures applicable to patients and healthcare personnel (S. Li & Zhang, 2020; Muirhead, 2020). Furthermore, the use of computers, cellular telephones, and tablets for virtual team meetings is increasingly common, and is consistent with recommendations by institutional authorities to find alternatives to in-person meetings (Shalev & Shapiro, 2020; Shao & Fei, 2020). However, if telepsychiatry becomes the new norm (Türközer & Öngür, 2020), it is unclear whether telehealth services will be reimbursed differently from face-to-face services, which will probably increase inequalities in fractured health-care systems (Moreno et al., 2020).

Patient rights: from loss to empowerment

Loss of rights and confinement

Preventive isolation measures have forced many psychiatric-care and residential-treatment care settings to confine patients who were normally free to come and go. This has been reported in Italy (De Girolamo et al., 2020; Starace & Ferrara, 2020), Scotland (C. Brown et al., 2020), New Zealand (Muirhead, 2020), and China (Zhu et al., 2020), and is also true generally in forensic psychiatry environments (Tomlin, 2020). However, the loss of rights and freedoms is a fundamental concern when implementing isolation measures with populations that are already confined. One of the issues raised for some patients is their difficulty observing guidelines for in-room isolation without resorting to sedation which could aggravate respiratory symptoms (Chevance et al., 2020). Zuffranieri and Zanalda (2020) pointed out the psychological impact of isolation for all people, but more attention should be given to patients who are already limited in their freedom. In fact, isolation measures within the prison context results in a superposition of confinements, which De Carvalho et al. (2020) call "overisolation".

Video court appearances and tele-assessment: not as good an idea as it seems?

Kelly (2020) reports that COVID-motivated temporary legislative changes in the Republic of Ireland affect the assessment, treatment, and judicial process of persons with mental health problems. The most noteworthy changes concern assessment procedure (both remote and in-person evaluations are now allowed), composition of the members of the tribunal assessing mental health problems (the tribunal can now be composed of only one person rather than three), and procedures of the tribunal (both video and in-person appearances are now allowed). C. Brown et al. (2020) reported similar temporary legislative changes in the United Kingdom.

Although these provisional changes to the law were proposed in response to the heightened need for psychiatrists dispatched to other sectors, Kelly (2020) notes that they may have significant impact on patient rights. Specifically, video appearances may raise additional barriers to access for patients with literacy or cognitive difficulties, placing a further burden on the patient's legal representative, who must ensure that their client comprehends and participates in the proceedings. Also, the mental health tribunal's reduced size and wider powers may compromise the fairness and equity of hearings. As such, the authors recommend that such changes be avoided in future mental health legislation. Moreover, Farrell and Hann (2020) mentioned that the measures to contain the spread of COVID-19 should always be carried out in strict accordance with human rights standards.

Loss of rights and isolation

The proposed provisional changes in the United Kingdom were also meant to facilitate the isolation and detention of persons with mental health problems, in the interest of preventing transmission (C. Brown et al., 2020). Isolation and deprivation of liberties is a crucial issue in secure units, in light of increased vulnerability factors and possible inability to provide informed consent (due to cognitive impairment and psychiatric symptoms). These measures must therefore be applied with caution, as they constitute a significant infringement on individual rights (C. Brown et al., 2020). Moreover, involuntary hospitalization in response to an inability to follow sanitary guidelines may exacerbate the mental health state which led to this inability to begin with (Gold et al., 2020). Conversely, one may be tempted to use involuntary confinement as a means to reduce the risk of transmission to the patients or others, even when the behavior is not directly related to psychiatric symptomatology (for example, individuals who refuse to quarantine in order to purchase illicit substances). This would represent an abuse of the commitment law (Gold et al., 2020).

In order to avoid COVID-19 transmission in the community or in institutions, protocols that ensure the observation of isolation guidelines, as well as the respect of patient rights, must be put in place. Isolation should only be implemented after measures more respectful of individual liberties (e.g., discharge, parole and patient cohorting) have failed. In C. Brown et al.'s (2020) view, existing laws regarding the confinement of psychiatric patients who are, or are suspected of being, COVID-positive are deficient. Moreover, the use of isolation to prevent COVID-19 transmission is a security and contamination risk-management issue, not a mental health treatment issue. The legal apparatus surrounding isolation must reflect this, and public-health acts must be adapted to reflect the situation of persons with mental health problems. The authors recommend that, in light of this legal gray zone, governments issue clear and concrete guidelines regarding COVID-19 isolation measures for individuals with severe mental illness, and that the power to implement isolation measures under public-health acts be delegated to care providers. In the absence of formal recommendations, each health institution should develop clear COVID-19 isolation policies which are the least restrictive of individual liberties.

Favoring empowerment and trauma-informed approaches

In Mental Health Weekly paper, Canady (2020a) pointed out that measures in place in hospitals and prisons may trigger painful memories of trauma. In response, the National Association of State Mental Health Program Directors (2020) shared peer-led recommendations emphasizing safety, empowerment, transparency, collaboration, peer support, and cultural sensitivity. Empowerment may also be reinforced by the continuous communication of decisions, based on reliable sources, which affect patients and inmates – if the stream of communications does not overload them or staff. In the same vein, regularly and adequately informing inmates or patients of the current situation and of the reasons for the measures taken to protect their health is essential (L. Li, 2020; Zhu et al., 2020). To ensure decision-making transparency, patients and inmates should therefore be informed of changes in procedures and of measures underway in their environment (Canady, 2020a). To this end, they must be able to have discussions with staff and obtain accurate and relevant information about the pandemic that they can easily understand (De Carvalho et al., 2020; Hewson et al., 2020). Tomlin (2020) reviewed the literature on the effects of restrictive measures on the perceived freedom of patients in forensic-psychiatry environments, and concluded that these measures are perceived as punitive, provoke fear, and deny the dignity of patients. Patients subjected to these measures feel diminished, bored, frustrated, and dehumanized. Echoing Canady (2020a), Tomlin (2020) states that measures that patients perceive to be fair, less restrictive, and contextually appropriate are also perceived as more legitimate, and are thus more likely to be respected.

The post COVID world: dealing with lasting effects and changes

A new theme that emerged with the updated literature review was a preoccupation with the lasting effects of the pandemic, in terms of mental health impacts as well as service delivery.

On mental health

In their paper on pandemic acute stress disorder, which is defined as a "prolonged anxiety reaction and inability to break away from permanent trauma", Heitzman (2020) describes the diagnostic criteria, which includes obsessive symptoms, mood disorder symptoms, dissociative symptoms, avoidance symptoms, and as well as symptoms of hyperactivity. The author states that individuals with preexisting mental illness, as well as those who are deprived of liberty, such as those who are incarcerated, are more vulnerable to developing this disorder. As such, the author proposes strategies, which include providing organizational security (procedures, standards and guidelines to direct decision-making, management, and responsibility); informative security (limit information to proven and reliable sources); and medical security (discussions on how to manage and control symptoms of mental illness and strategies to reduce their impact). They also suggest undertaking educational and informational work with families and supporting health professionals (Heitzman, 2020). Strategies to mitigate the lasting effects on mental health could include community monitoring and mental health screening of vulnerable groups using digital technologies to identify the specific needs of each geographic area (Moreno et al., 2020).

On the economy

It is no surprise that after months of restrictive measures, most nations are now faced with an economic crisis in addition to a global pandemic. Individuals in secure settings are not immune to the long-term effects of this pandemic on the economy. Economic recessions have been found to increase rates of mental health disorders, homelessness, suicide, substance use, all of which are already highly prevalent in populations with mental illness in secure settings (Türközer & Öngür, 2020). Mental health services are already struggling to meet higher demands, and the long-term effects of the pandemic and economic crises are likely to add additional strain. As such, mental health, addiction, housings, and social services must prepare to meet these new challenges.

On practice

Many measures have been rapidly put into place in the past several months to quickly respond to a pandemic that took everyone by surprise. Now that these structures are in place, it is critical to thoroughly consider their impact by defining indicators and outcomes (Moreno et al., 2020). These indicators should include outcomes related to COVID-19 monitoring and treatment (testing, cases, intensive-care cases, mortality, vaccination, etc.), and service use (use of face-to-face, video or phone contact with different mental health providers, availability and uptake of COVID-19 information, rates of prescription medication, rates of psychiatric hospitalization, discharge, loss to follow-up, etc.).

In line with decreased populations in secure settings to minimize infection, efforts will have to be made to increase access and maintain community supports for people with severe mental illness through home-based treatment and monitoring (Moreno et al., 2020). This will imply, on one hand, increased resources to ensure that community services have the capacity to guarantee sufficient services and, on the other, changes in practice for all stakeholders to move away from institutionalizing offending patients and toward increased residential support (Zuffranieri & Zanalda, 2020).

Moreno et al. (2020)'s review of mental health practice changes in the face of COVID-19 underlines the new roles that can be taken by service users. Faced with limited resources, services can increase peer worker involvement in service delivery. Moreover, changes in practice should be spearheaded by service users, as they have been pivotal in the development of recovery-oriented approaches across the globe. It is essential that the current need for rapid decision-making is not used as a pretext to evacuate service users and should instead be used as an opportunity for the co-creation of new protocols and practice.

On research

This pandemic has had a considerable impact on research in forensic mental health: most activities with participants have been suspended to minimize infection risk and researchers and their teams have been affected like most professionals by stay at-home orders. Research funding has been massively turned toward COVID-related initiatives. Clinical research resources have been dedicated to patient care, while basic research has been reoriented to support laboratory testing (Kreuzer et al., 2020). While confinement measures have been slowly easing in the general population, this likely will not be the case immediately in secure settings, given their additional vulnerability factors. This may demand that researchers adapt their protocols to this new reality, for example, through the use of digital technologies (Türközer & Öngür, 2020). This may, however, pose an additional challenge to recruitment, especially in secure settings where the use of digital technologies is often monitored and restricted. Moreover, existing tools may need to be adapted and validated for use in digital settings. Finally, the pandemic, and its effect on physical health, mental health and disruptive behaviors will represent a significant confounder for research in forensic mental health which will have to be accounted for in non-pandemic research (Türközer & Öngür, 2020). While this may not have an immediate impact on the individuals who are confined in correctional or mental health settings, we can expect that long-term changes might influence how we conduct research in these environments for practitioners, researchers, and service users.

Discussion

The objective of this rapid response guide was to identify strategies that have been developed in response to the COVID-19 pandemic and applied in clinical, forensic, and correctional environments housing legally detained persons with mental health problems. More specifically, the intent was to characterize the impact of these measures, in order to identify the best practices to promote, now and going forward. The literature reports transformations around the world, primarily in psychiatric environments, but also in correctional and forensic-psychiatry environments. The publications reviewed describe real-world situations, identify issues relevant to patient and detainee management, and issue recommendations.

Seven major conclusions can be drawn from this literature review. First, persons confined in psychiatric or correctional environments are more vulnerable to COVID-19, due to their multiple physical and psychiatric comorbidities, and to the characteristics of the environments themselves. It is therefore necessary to take these factors into account when planning patient management strategies during this health emergency, when vulnerability factors are accentuated. Although certain group activities should be suspended to minimize the risk of transmission, patients/detainees will probably require additional individual interventions.

Second, frequent, and transparent communication between management, treatment teams, and patients/detainees is essential to ensure effective and acceptable changes in the organization of services in response to the pandemic. Involving patients/detainees in communication activities and changes gives them a feeling of control that helps reduce the negative impacts of disruptions and may enhance compliance.

Third, changes in care trajectories due to early release or to restricted admission policies must be compensated for by intensive community services and ongoing follow-up. While services move from institutions to communities, it will be essential to broaden the scope of interventions to include those with higher needs in terms of mental health and therapeutic security. This may include favoring options such as mental health probation or forensic assertive community teams (ACT), and should comprise sufficient community services so as to not encourage the revolving door phenomenon (Cuddeback et al., 2020).

Fourth, contagion-control measures that are least restrictive of individual liberties should be favored. When in-room or in-cell isolation is necessary, it should be compensated for by more extensive psychosocial services.

Fifth, managers of these institutions must ensure supplies are adequate, staff is trained, PPE is used, and equipment to support enhanced hygiene measures is available. Clear protocols that are proportionate to the risk of transmission must be implemented, and staff and patients/detainees should be informed of them.

Sixth, the use of remote technologies (videoconferencing, computers, tablets, telephones, etc.) appears to be a valuable strategy for maintaining contacts between patients and their families, between patients and their treatment teams (telemedicine), and between professionals (for professional discussions and team meetings). It also appears to be useful for maintaining the continuity of essential judicial activities (video court appearances, tele-assessment). Although these technologies appear promising in facilitating access and continuity of care, effective and efficient, it is necessary to consider their impacts on confidentiality, their suitability for persons with literacy or cognitive deficits, and the subjective experience of patients/detainees, who may feel that they are not understood as well as during in-person interactions.

Finally, this reorganization of services should be seized as an opportunity to further involve service users in the planning, development, and delivery of care, as well as an occasion to evolve toward more trauma-informed and recovery-oriented approaches.

It is important to bear in mind that although there are specific issues to be considered when planning service delivery to forensic psychiatric patients – such as the risk of violence and the higher prevalence of functional deficits (Beach et al., 2013; Nijdam-Jones et al., 2017) – the scientific literature reviewed only identified a small number of publications which related specifically to the forensic mental health context. The gray literature reviewed somewhat fills this gap by noting the importance of the factors mentioned in this review, but also by pointing out the need to take into account the following factors upon admission, detention, or hospitalization: 1) transfer and follow-up procedures; 2) the patient/detainee's legal status; 3) the patient/detainee's individual risk factors (e.g., family violence, sexual violence, pedophilia); and 4) the use of isolation and restraint measures when behavioral problems arise (Association des jeunes psychiatres et des jeunes addictologues, 2020; Royal College of Psychiatrists, 2020).

Another noteworthy point is the scarcity of literature specifically focusing on persons who have mental health problems and are in correctional settings. This literature review has demonstrated that mental health problems are an additional challenge to be taken into account in the management of persons in detention, but did not undertake an in-depth analysis of the specific situation in correctional environments, which pose specific challenges, such as inadequate psychosocial care and relatively heterogeneous populations (Mulvey & Schubert, 2017).

Health technology assessment in support of rapid changes

Locally, this review produced a rapid response guide that was essential in guiding decision makers in the implementation of practices in uncertain times. It was the product of the collaboration of two leading mental health institutions in the province. During the course of the process, communication was maintained between researchers and managers of the crises teams so as to ensure that daily decisions were made with the best available knowledge. This likely contributed to low infection rate throughout.

The rapid turn around resulted in response guides being produced in both official languages (French and English), a brief, five-minute capsule on social media which conveyed complex information in an accessible manner to practitioners, service users, and family members alike, as well as an online webinar which was widely viewed by practitioners and managers in the fields of psychiatry, forensic mental health, corrections and social services across the province. The rapid response guide is also being used in the development of an implementation plan for a potential second COVID-19 wave. This project is a successful example of how health technology assessment can be rapidly put into practice to inform decision-making in times of crises.

Limitations of the rapid review

This rapid review has some limitations that should be taken into consideration when interpreting the results presented. The first limitation pertains to the type of literature reviewed: given the novelty of the COVID-19 pandemic, it was decided not to limit the review to reports of empirical studies. In fact, the publications reviewed are mostly opinion pieces by experts (editorials, letters to the editor, other correspondence).

The review period corresponds to the period that saw a rapid outbreak of COVID-19 around the world. The content of the publications analyzed reflects the urgency of the situation in psychiatric and correctional environments in many countries. Most of the publications report recommendations, issued by practitioners and local authorities, which modify professional practice and the organization of services offered to persons with serious mental health problems and who are confined in one of these environments. Although these recommendations are based on clinical knowledge or previous research, it should be noted that they are not systematically based on empirical knowledge of the impact of COVID-19 or of the measures implemented.

The second limitation pertains to the timeframe of the review relative to the sheer quantity of information that has been produced in response to the pandemic. The period covered by our initial search strategy spanned approximately six months (December 2019 to May 2020). When we sought to re-run the same strategy to update our review in August, we were faced with more than three times the amount of literature for half the period. We therefore chose to restrict our search strategy to one database. Though we had reached a certain level of thematic saturation, it is likely that we missed pertinent papers published between May and August 2020. Moreover, by the time this is published, many more papers will have been published. In the short time we conducted this review, the nature of publications has also evolved: more papers of an empirical or descriptive nature are being published as time progresses. The next step in responding to our framework question would therefore be to revisit our research when enough time has elapsed to allow empirical research to have been conducted in this area. This second review could contrast the COVID-related recommendations reported here with the results of empirical studies and develop guidelines for future health emergencies of this kind. Finally, given the need for a rapid response, methodological quality was not evaluated in this review. Readers should therefore be cautious in their interpretation of the results and recommendations reported.

Conclusion

This rapid review was intended to identify best practices for persons who have serious mental health problems and are confined in secure units during the COVID-19 pandemic. Although the literature review and the conclusions thereafter are based primarily on opinion pieces rather than empirical studies, this review will nevertheless help managers of psychiatric services in forensic-psychiatry and correctional environments make decisions related to the management of the COVID-19 pandemic. It should also stimulate reflection on the best way to ensure the safe management of patients and detainees that minimizes undesirable effects on recovery from mental illness.

Notes

1. Institut universitaire en santé mentale de Montréal.
2. Unité d'évaluation des technologies et modes d'intervention en santé mentale, justice et sécurité.
3. Unité d'évaluation des technologies et modes d'intervention en santé mentale.

Acknowledgments

This rapid review was produced by the *Institut national de psychiatrie légale Philippe-Pinel*'s *Unité d'évaluation des technologies et modes d'intervention en santé mentale, justice, sécurité* (UETMI-SMJS; https://pinel.qc.ca/unite-devaluation-des-technologies-et-modes-dintervention/), in collaboration with the *Centre intégré universitaire en santé et services sociaux (CIUSSS) de l'Est-de-l'Île-de-Montréal*'s *Unité d'évaluation des technologies et des modes d'intervention en santé mentale - Institut universitaire en santé mentale de Montréal* (UETMISM-IUSMM; https://ciusss-estmtl.gouv.qc.ca/ressources/documentation/qualite-des-services). A first iteration of this rapid review, prior to peer review, is available on each institution's website.

Disclosure statement

No potential conflict of interest was reported by the author(s).

ORCID

Ashley J. Lemieux http://orcid.org/0000-0001-8630-2752
Alain Lesage http://orcid.org/0000-0002-4226-4683
Anne G. Crocker http://orcid.org/0000-0003-0571-8890

References

Akiyama, M. J., Spaulding, A. C., & Rich, J. D. (2020). Flattening the curve for incarcerated populations—Covid-19 in jails and prisons. *New England Journal of Medicine*, *382*(22), 2075–2077. https://www.nejm.org/doi/full/10.1056/NEJMp2005687

Arango, C. (2020). Lessons learned from the coronavirus health crisis in Madrid, Spain: How COVID-19 has changed our lives in the last 2 weeks. *Biological Psychiatry*, *88*(7), e33–e34. files/16839/abstract.html

Association des jeunes psychiatres et des jeunes addictologues. (2020). *Recommandations en psychiatrie légale - épidémie Covid-19* [Recommendations in Forensic Psychiatry – Covid-19 Epidemic].

Retrieved March 2020, from https://www.ajpja.fr/uploads/file/5e853089ec30b_EUhPsvPWAAE6au1.jpeg

Beach, C., Dykema, L.-R., Appelbaum, P. S., Deng, L., Leckman-Westin, E., Manuel, J. I., McReynolds, L., & Finnerty, M. T. (2013). Forensic and nonforensic clients in assertive community treatment: A longitudinal study. *Psychiatric Services, 64*(5), 437–444. https://doi.org/10.1176/appi.ps.201200170

Bojdani, E., Rajagopalan, A., Chen, A., Gearin, P., Olcott, W., Shankar, V., Solomon, H., Naqvi, N. Z., Batty, N., Festin, F. E. D., Tahera, D., Chang, G., DeLisi, L. E., & Cloutier, A. (2020). COVID-19 pandemic: Impact on psychiatric care in the United States, a review. *Psychiatry Research, 289*, 113069. https://doi.org/10.1016/j.psychres.2020.113069

Boland, X., & Dratcu, L. (2020). COVID-19 and acute inpatient psychiatry: The shape of things to come. *International Journal of Psychiatry in Clinical Practice*, 1–3. https://doi.org/10.1080/13651501.2020.1801755

Brown, C., Keene, A. R., Hooper, C. R., & O'Brien, A. (2020). Isolation of patients in psychiatric hospitals in the context of the COVID-19 pandemic: An ethical, legal, and practical challenge. *International Journal of Law and Psychiatry, 71*, 101572. https://doi.org/10.1016/j.ijlp.2020.101572

Brown, E., Gray, R., Lo Monaco, S., O'Donoghue, B., Nelson, B., Thompson, A., ... McGorry, P. (2020). The potential impact of COVID-19 on psychosis: A rapid review of contemporary epidemic and pandemic research. *Schizophrenia Research*. https://doi.org/10.1016/j.schres.2020.05.005

Burton, P. R. S., Morris, N. P., & Hirschtritt, M. E. (in press). Mental health services in a U.S. prison during the COVID-19 pandemic. *Psychiatric Services*. Prepublication. https://doi.org/10.1176/appi.ps.202000476

Canady, V. A. (2020a). Bazelon center urges reduction of jail population with MI. *Mental Health Weekly, 30*(15), 7. https://doi.org/10.1002/mhw.32318

Canady, V. A. (2020b). NASMHPD issues guidance to maintain hospital patients' health in crisis. *Mental Health Weekly, 30*(18), 1–3. https://doi.org/10.1002/mhw.32343

Caputo, F., Gratteri, S., Sacco, M. A., Scalise, C., Cacciatore, G., Bonetta, F., ... Cordasco, F. (2020). Covid-19 emergency in prison: Current management and forensic perspectives. *Medico-Legal Journal*, 0025817220923693. https://doi.org/10.1177/0025817220923693

Chevance, A., Gourion, D., Hoertel, N., Llorca, P. M., Thomas, P., Bocher, R., ... Gaillard, R. (2020). Ensuring mental health care during the SARS-CoV-2 epidemic in France: A narrative review. *Encephale, 46*(3), 193–201. https://doi.org/10.1016/j.encep.2020.03.001

Choi, K. R., Heilemann, M. V., Fauer, A., & Mead, M. (2020). A second pandemic: Mental health spillover from the novel coronavirus (COVID-19). *Journal of the American Psychiatric Nurses Association*, 1078390320919803. https://doi.org/10.1177/1078390320919803

Clerici, M., Durbano, F., Spinogatti, F., Vita, A., de Girolamo, G., & Micciolo, R. (2020). Psychiatric hospitalization rates in Italy before and during COVID-19: Did they change? An analysis of register data. *Irish Journal of Psychological Medicine, 26*(4), 1–8. https://doi.org/10.1017/ipm.2020.29

Correctional Service Canada. (2020). *Inmate COVID-19 testing in federal correctional institutions August 26 2020*. Retrieved August 29, 2020, from https://www.csc-scc.gc.ca/001/006/001006-1014-en.shtml

Cranshaw, T., & Harikumar, T. (2020). COVID-19 infection may cause clozapine intoxication: Case report and discussion. *Schizophrenia Bulletin, 46*(4), 751. https://doi.org/10.1093/schbul/sbaa070

Cuddeback, G. S. S., Jennie, M., & Wu, J. C. (2020). A comprehensive literature review of forensic assertive community treatment (fact): Directions for practice, policy and research. *International Journal of Mental Health, 49*(2), 106–127. No-Specified. https://doi.org/10.1080/00207411.2020.1717054

Cullen, W., Gulati, G., & Kelly, B. D. (2020). Mental health in the Covid-19 pandemic. *QJM: An International Journal of Medicine, 113*(5), 311–312. files/16949/PMC7184387.htmlfiles/16951/5813733.html

D'Agostino, A., Demartini, B., Cavallotti, S., & Gambini, O. (2020). Mental health services in Italy during the COVID-19 outbreak. *The Lancet Psychiatry*, *7*(5), 385–387. https://doi.org/10.1016/s2215-0366(20)30133-4

de Carvalho, S. G., Santos, I. M., & Dos Santos, A. B. S. (2020). *The pandemic in prison: Interventions and overisolation*. https://doi.org/10.1590/SciELOPreprints.570

de Girolamo, G., Cerveri, G., Clerici, M., Monzani, E., Spinogatti, F., Starace, F., ... Vita, A. (2020). Mental health in the coronavirus disease 2019 emergency-the Italian response. *JAMA Psychiatry*, *77*(9), 974. https://doi.org/10.1001/jamapsychiatry.2020.1276

Druss, B. G. (2020). Addressing the COVID-19 pandemic in populations with serious mental illness. *JAMA Psychiatry*, *77*(9), 891. https://doi.org/10.1001/jamapsychiatry.2020.0894

Enos, G. (2020). Few organizations immune to perils of securing PPE for staff, patients. *Mental Health Weekly*, *30*(19), 1–8. https://doi.org/10.1002/mhw.32355

Farrell, A.-M., & Hann, P. (2020). Mental health and capacity laws in Northern Ireland and the COVID-19 pandemic: Examining powers, procedures and protections under emergency legislation. *International Journal of Law and Psychiatry*, *71*(July–August), 101602. https://doi.org/10.1016/j.ijlp.2020.101602

Flood, C. M., MacDonnell, V., Philpott, J., Thériault, S., & Venkatapuram, S. (2020). Overview of COVID-19: Old and new vulnerabilities. In C. M. Flood, V. MacDonnell, J. Philpott, S. Thériault, & S. Venkatapuram (Eds.), *Vulnerable: The law, policy and ethics of COVID-19* (pp. 1–30). University of Ottawa Press.

Fovet, T., Lancelevée, C., Eck, M., Scouflaire, T., Bécache, E., Dandelot, D., ... Lacambre, M. (2020). Mental health care in French correctional facilities during the Covid-19 pandemic. *L'Encéphale*, *46* (3). https://doi.org/10.1016/j.encep.2020.05.002

Garriga, M., Agasi, I., Fedida, E., Pinzón-Espinosa, J., Vazquez, M., Pacchiarotti, I., & Vieta, E. (2020). The role of mental health home hospitalization care during the COVID-19 pandemic. *Acta Psychiatrica Scandinavica*, *141*(5), 479–480. https://doi.org/10.1111/acps.13173

Gold, A., Strous, R. D., & Appelbaum, P. S. (2020). COVID-19 and involuntary hospitalisation: Navigating the challenge. *The Lancet Psychiatry*, *7*(7), 572–573. https://doi.org/10.1016/S2215-0366(20)30246-7

Government of Canada. (2020). *Coronavirus disease (COVID-19)*. Retrieved August 29, 2020, from https://www.canada.ca/fr/sante-publique/services/maladies/maladie-coronavirus-covid-19.html

Heitzman, J. (2020). Impact of COVID-19 pandemic on mental health. *Psychiatria Polska*, *52*(2), 187–198. https://doi.org/10.12740/PP/120373

Hewson, T., Shepherd, A., Hard, J., & Shaw, J. (2020). Effects of the COVID-19 pandemic on the mental health of prisoners. *The Lancet Psychiatry*, *7*(7), 568–570. https://doi.org/10.1016/S2215-0366(20)30241-8

Iftene, A. (2020). COVID-19 in Canadian prisons: Policies, practices and concerns. In C. M. Flood, V. MacDonnell, J. Philpott, S. Thériault, & S. Venkatapuram (Eds.), *Vulnerable: The law, policy and ethics of COVID-19* (pp. 367–380). University of Ottawa Press.

Ji, H., Li, L., Huang, T., & Zhu, Y. (2020). Nosocomial infections in psychiatric hospitals during the new coronavirus pneumonia outbreak. *The European Journal of Psychiatry*, *34*(3), 177–179. https://doi.org/10.1016/j.ejpsy.2020.04.001

Kelly, B. D. (2020). Emergency mental health legislation in response to the Covid-19 (Coronavirus) pandemic in Ireland: Urgency, necessity and proportionality. *International Journal of Law and Psychiatry*, *70*(May–June), 101564. https://doi.org/10.1016/j.ijlp.2020.101564

Kennedy, H. G., Mohan, D., & Davoren, M. (2020). Forensic psychiatry and Covid-19: Accelerating transformation in forensic psychiatry. *Irish Journal of Psychological Medicine*, 1–26. https://doi.org/10.1017/ipm.2020.58

Kothari, R., Forrester, A., Greenberg, N., Sarkissian, N., & Tracy, D. K. (2020). *COVID-19 and prisons: Providing mental health care for people in prison, minimising moral injury and psychological distress in mental health staff*. SAGE Publications Sage UK.

Kozloff, N., Mulsant, B. H., Stergiopoulos, V., & Voineskos, A. N. (2020). The COVID-19 global pandemic: Implications for people with Schizophrenia and related disorders. *Schizophrenia Bulletin*, *46*(4), 752–757. https://doi.org/10.1093/schbul/sbaa051

Kreuzer, P. M., Baghai, T. C., Rupprecht, R., Wittmann, M., Steffling, D., Ziereis, M., . . . Langguth, B. (2020). SARS-CoV-2 risk management in clinical psychiatry: A few considerations on how to deal with an unrivaled threat. *Frontiers in Psychiatry*, *11*(550), 1–8. https://doi.org/10.3389/fpsyt.2020.00550

Li, C., Zhao, W., He, C., Wu, D., Yue, Y., & Chen, Y. (2020). COVID-19 prevention and control strategies for psychiatric hospitals. *Psychiatry Research*, *289*(July), 112935. https://doi.org/10.1016/j.psychres.2020.112935

Li, L. (2020). Challenges and priorities in responding to COVID-19 in inpatient psychiatry. *Psychiatric Services*, *33*(2), appips202000166. https://doi.org/10.1176/appi.ps.202000166

Li, S., & Zhang, Y. (2020). Mental healthcare for psychiatric inpatients during the COVID-19 epidemic. *General Psychiatry*, *33*(2), e100216. https://doi.org/10.1136/gpsych-2020-100216

Liebrenz, M., Bhugra, D., Buadze, A., & Schleifer, R. (2020). Caring for persons in detention suffering with mental illness during the Covid-19 outbreak. *Forensic Science International: Mind and Law*, *1* (November), 100013. https://doi.org/10.1016/j.fsiml.2020.100013

Moher, D., Shamseer, L., Clarke, M., Ghersi, D., Liberati, A., Petticrew, M., Shekelle, P., & Stewart, L. A.; PRISMA-P Group. (2015). Preferred reporting items for systematic review and meta-analysis protocols (PRISMA-P) 2015 statement. *Systematic Reviews*, *4*(1), 1–9. https://doi.org/10.1186/2046-4053-4-1

Moreno, C., Wykes, T., Galderisi, S., Nordentoft, M., Crossley, N., Jones, N., . . . Arango, C. (2020). How mental health care should change as a consequence of the COVID-19 pandemic. *The Lancet Psychiatry*, *7*(9), 813–824. https://doi.org/10.1016/S2215-0366(20)30307-2

Muirhead, C. (2020). A pandemic within our borders, but what about the impact for our people in acute inpatients? *Journal of Psychiatric and Mental Health Nursing*. https://doi.org/10.1111/jpm.12650

Mulvey, E. P., & Schubert, C. A. (2017). Mentally ill individuals in jails and prisons. *Crime and Justice*, *71*(1), 231–277. https://doi.org/10.1086/688461

National Alliance on Mental Illness. (2020). *COVID-19*. Resource and Information Guide. https://www.nami.org/Support-Education/NAMI-HelpLine/COVID-19-Information-and-Resources

National Association of State Mental Health Program Directors. (2020). *Peer-led recommendations for supporting individuals receiving care in state psychiatric facilities during the COVID-19 crisis*. Retrieved in March 2020, from https://www.nasmhpd.org/content/peer-led-recommendations-supporting-individuals-receiving-care-state-psychiatric-facilities

Nijdam-Jones, A., Nicholls, T. L., Crocker, A. G., Roy, L., & Somers, J. M. (2017). History of forensic mental health service use among homeless adults with mental illness. *International Journal of Forensic Mental Health*, *16*(1), 69–82. https://doi.org/10.1080/14999013.2016.1255281

Ornell, F., Schuch, J. B., Sordi, A. O., & Kessler, F. H. P. (2020). "Pandemic fear" and COVID-19: Mental health burden and strategies. *Brazilian Journal of Psychiatry(AHEAD)*, *42*(3), 232–235. files/16878/scielo.html

Percudani, M., Corradin, M., Moreno, M., Indelicato, A., & Vita, A. (2020). Mental health services in Lombardy during COVID-19 outbreak. *Psychiatry Research*, *288*(June), 1–3. https://doi.org/10.1016/j.psychres.2020.112980

Poremski, D., Subner, S., Lam, G., Kin, F., Dev, R., Mok, Y. M., . . . Fung, D. S. S. (2020). Effective infection prevention and control strategies in a large accredited psychiatric facility in Singapore. *Infection Control and Hospital Epidemiology*, *41*(10), 1238–1240. https://doi.org/http://dx.doi.10.1017/ice.2020.163

Gouvernement du Québec. (2020). *Situation du coronavirus (COVID-19) au Québec*. Retrieved August 29, 2020 from https://www.quebec.ca/sante/problemes-de-sante/a-z/coronavirus-2019/situation-coronavirus-quebec/

Rajkumar, R. P. (2020). COVID-19 and mental health: A review of the existing literature. *Asian Journal of Psychiatry*, *52*(August), 102066. https://doi.org/10.1016/j.ajp.2020.102066

Royal College of Psychiatrists. (2020). *COVID-19: Secure hospital and criminal justice settings*. Retrieved in June 2020, from https://www.rcpsych.ac.uk/about-us/responding-to-covid-19/responding-to-covid-19-guidance-for-clinicians/community-and-inpatient-services/secure-hospital-and-criminal-justice-settings

Shalev, D., & Shapiro, P. A. (2020). Epidemic psychiatry: The opportunities and challenges of COVID-19. *General Hospital Psychiatry, 64*(May–June), 68–71. https://doi.org/10.1016/j.genhosppsych.2020.03.009

Shao, Y., & Fei, J. M. (2020). Psychiatry hospital management facing COVID-19: From medical staff to patients. *Brain, Behavior, and Immunity, 88*(August), 947. https://doi.org/10.1016/j.bbi.2020.04.018

Simpson, A. I. F., Chatterjee, S., Darby, P., Jones, R. M., Maheandiran, M., Penney, S. R., . . . Wilkie, T. (2020). Management of COVID-19 response in a secure forensic mental health setting. *The Canadian Journal of Psychiatry*, 65(10), 695–700. https://doi.org/10.1177/0706743720935648

Simpson, S. A., Dumas, A., McDowell, A. K., & Westmoreland, P. (2020). Novel coronavirus and related public health interventions are negatively impacting mental health services. *Psychosomatics, 61*(5), 568–571. https://doi.org/10.1016/j.psym.2020.04.004

Starace, F., & Ferrara, M. (2020). COVID-19 disease emergency operational instructions for mental health departments issued by the Italian society of epidemiological psychiatry. *Epidemiology and Psychiatric Sciences, 29*(e116), 1–4. https://doi.org/10.1017/s2045796020000372

Statista. (2020). *COVID-19 deaths worldwide per on million population as of August 27, 2020 by country*. Retrieved on August 27, 2020, from https://www.statista.com/statistics/1104709/coronavirus-deaths-worldwide-per-million-inhabitants/

The Lancet Psychiatry. (2020). Mental health and COVID-19: Change the conversation. *The Lancet Psychiatry, 7*(6), 463. https://doi.org/10.1016/S2215-0366(20)30194-2

Thome, J., Coogan, A., Fischer, M., Tucha, O., & Faltraco, F. (2020). Challenges for mental health services during the 2020 Covid-19 outbreak in Germany. *Psychiatry and Clinical Neurosciences, 74* (7), 407. https://doi.org/10.1111/pcn.13019

Tomlin, J. (2020). What does social distancing mean for patients in forensic mental health settings? *Forensic Science International: Mind and Law, 1*, 1–2. https://doi.org/10.1016/j.fsiml.2020.100018

Türközer, H. B., & Öngür, D. (2020). A projection for psychiatry in the post-COVID-19 era: Potential trends, challenges, and directions. *Molecular Psychiatry, 25*(October), 2214–2219. https://doi.org/10.1038/s41380-020-0841-2

Xiang, Y. T., Zhao, Y. J., Liu, Z. H., Li, X. H., Zhao, N., Cheung, T., & Ng, C. H. (2020). The COVID-19 outbreak and psychiatric hospitals in China: Managing challenges through mental health service reform. *International Journal of Biological Sciences, 16*(10), 1741–1744. https://doi.org/10.7150/ijbs.45072

Zhu, Y., Chen, L., Ji, H., Xi, M., Fang, Y., & Li, Y. (2020). The risk and prevention of novel coronavirus pneumonia infections among inpatients in psychiatric hospitals. *Neuroscience Bulletin, 36*(3), 299–302. https://doi.org/10.1007/s12264-020-00476-9

Zuffranieri, M., & Zanalda, E. (2020). The forensic psychiatry in the time of coronavirus: The Italian security residences put to the test in a public health emergency. *Psychiatry and Clinical Neurosciences, 74*(9), 507–508. https://doi.org/10.1111/pcn.13100

Oceania Regional Overview and Reports from Australia and New Zealand

An Examination of COVID-19 Outbreaks in Prisons and Jails in Oceania

Sabrina S. Rapisarda and James M. Byrne

ABSTRACT

This article highlights the unique nature of the Oceanic region and its impact on the extent of COVID-19 outbreaks in the Oceanic region, both within correctional and community settings. Mitigation strategies implemented in Australia, New Zealand, Papa New Guinea, and Fiji are identified, and the reasons for the differences we identified in how governments in this region defined the problem, and developed mitigation strategies, are explored.

Introduction and overview

The Oceanic region includes islandic countries such as Australia, New Zealand, Papa New Guinea, French Polynesia, Fiji, Solomon Islands, Samoa, and more. Compared to other regions of the world, these countries exist in relative isolation. In theory, it is much easier to blockade and restrict the arrival of a disease such as COVID-19, so long as border crossing is limited and importations are monitored early on. Consequently, the outbreak of COVID-19 in the Oceanic region has been much smaller than other regions of the world (Worldometer, 2020). Once penetrating the border of island communities, however, these benefits may transform into foes. Isolation, particularly in the case of Oceania's smaller islands, often equates to more barriers in providing and accessing medical care (Buhre, 2020). It also means that certain items may be more challenging to secure or to rely on due to scarcities or price fluctuations of imported goods (Buhre, 2020). Thus, while still holding the lowest cumulative prevalence of COVID-19 cases among all continental regions, Oceania has, nevertheless, experienced outbreaks across its islands (Worldometer, 2020). Just under 28,000 cases and 600 COVID-19 related deaths region-wide have been confirmed to date, according to the John Hopkins Coronavirus Resource Center (Coronavirus Resource Center, 2020).[1]

Despite the relatively low rates of COVID-19 across Oceania, due to the vulnerability of prison populations, prison and jail inmates in this region have the potential to be disproportionately impacted by the virus. Once the virus enters the prisons, transmission can be more rapid than within the broader community due to living in close quarters, overcrowding, inadequate sanitation materials and procedures, and reduced access to health services while in prison (Kinner et al., 2020). Additionally, individual-level factors including drug use, pre-existing health conditions, and more can further exacerbate this population's susceptibility.

Communicable diseases, in general, are much more difficult to contain within prisons than other community-based settings. Demonstration of such a trend includes the already high prevalence rates of Hepatitis C infections in Australian prisons, which currently comprises 30% of the prison population (The Kirby Institute, 2020). Given that Australia also has the largest prison system in the Oceanic region (World Prison Brief, 2020) and that its prisons are presently struggling with the spread of other communicable diseases such as Hepatitis C, the prison population is highly susceptible to the spread of COVID-19. To date, of the nearly 28,000 positive COVID-19 cases present in Oceania,[2] over 25,300 have been detected in Australia among prisons and the community at large, which is approximately 90% of Oceania's cumulative total count (Coronavirus Resource Center, 2020).

The Australian prison system and COVID-19 outbreaks

Australia currently houses over 44,000 inmates, which equates to an incarceration rate of approximately 174 inmates per 100,000 individuals (World Prison Brief, 2020).[3] Overall, Australia ranks 43rd in the top 50 largest prison systems globally and is the only country in the Oceanic region that is represented in the top 50 (World Prison Brief, 2020; see Figure 1). This is unsurprising, considering that Australia has the largest landmass size and population (N = 25 million) among all countries in the Oceanic region (Australian Population [LIVE], 2020).

Despite that Aboriginal Australians comprise only 3.3% of Australia's total population, they are 11.6 times more likely to be incarcerated than non-Aboriginal Australians

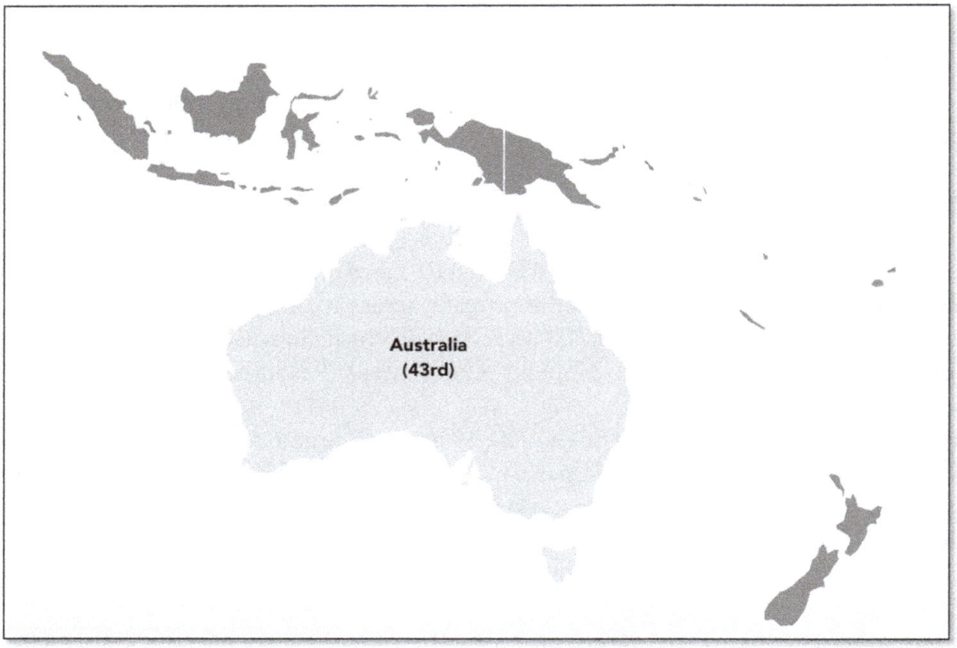

Figure 1. Oceania's largest prison system. *Australia is ranked 43rd in the world's top 50 largest prison systems (World Prison Brief, 2020).

(Australian Bureau of Statistics, 2020). In December of 2019, the rate of incarceration among Aboriginal Australians was 2,536 per 100,000 individuals, while non-Aboriginal Australians were imprisoned at a rate of 218 per 100,000 (Australian Bureau of Statistics, 2020). Therefore, general concerns have been raised regarding the disproportionate number of Aboriginal inmates (many of which have pre-existing health issues) represented within Australian correctional populations. More specifically, attention has been drawn to the potentially detrimental effect of disproportionate representation on Aboriginal inmates, such that they are at higher-risk of contracting COVID-19, among an already vulnerable population (Waight, 2020).

Through March and June of 2020, Australia reported zero cases among inmates nationwide (Wahlquist, 2020). However, there were reported cases among prison staff, which triggered scares among inmate populations. For example, in late April, though ultimately testing negative for COVID-19, 20 inmates were quarantined for 14 days after a prison staff worker in Brisbane tested positive (Layt & Lynch, 2020). Nevertheless, governments in South Australia, Queensland, and Western Australia took precautionary measures and prepared to manage the threat. By late March, correctional facilities in New South Wales and Queensland temporarily suspended all prison visits and equipped inmates with the tools necessary (e.g., computer tablets) to conduct video calls in lieu of in-person visitations (Doneman, 2020; Wahlquist, 2020). By March, if not having already instituted visitation bans, regions had – at minimum – adopted policies that highly discouraged members of the community with suspected infections or exposure to the virus from entering custodial settings (Wahlquist, 2020). Correctional staff members were also subjected to screening (e.g., temperatures were taken to detect fevers) prior to entering correctional facilities (Doneman, 2020).

New South Wales was the first Australian state to introduce legislation, ratified on March 25th, that would enable certain inmates to be released in order to relieve overcrowding among its prison population (Searle, 2020). Serving a similar purpose, eligible remand inmates in Queensland were encouraged to apply to the courts to be granted parole, bail, or even discharge (Doneman, 2020). Prisons throughout Australia had reported decreases in incarceration rates between February and June (Gleeson, 2020). New South Wales's Bureau of Crime Statistics and Research reported releasing 1,508 inmates between the months of March and May, while Corrections Victoria released data that its prisons experienced a 13% population decrease between February and June (Gleeson, 2020). Lawyers and advocates have conveyed that the pandemic has helped illuminate preexisting flaws within Australia's prison system, such as the sheer number of inmates that are incarcerated due to minor charges. Conversely, the pandemic has also demonstrated that decreasing the prison population is feasible and has the potential to be informed by current circumstances in the long term (Gleeson, 2020).

On July 17, 2020, coronavirus entered Melbourne's Metropolitan Remand Center, when an inmate tested positive after being swabbed upon arrival (Chapman, 2020). According to a Department of Justice and Community Safety spokesperson, the inmate underwent a 14-day protective quarantine period in an isolated part of the prison to contain the virus (Chapman, 2020). On July 21st, 2020, six Victorian prisons were placed on lockdown after a guard at Ravenhall Correctional Center tested positive for the virus (Visontay & Wahlquist, 2020). Simultaneously, Victoria reported 374 new cases in the community to add to roughly 2,700 already-active cases and 3 COVID-19-related deaths in a 24-hour period (Visontay & Wahlquist, 2020). At the Malmsbury Youth Justice Facility, an incoming youth offender tested positive in late July, which prompted a lockdown.

More recently, on August 8th, 2020, Brisbane Youth Detention Center in Queensland went on lockdown when a positive case was identified among a 77-year-old prison supervisor (Kleyn, 2020). Nearly 130 inmates and over 500 staff members underwent testing. While no cases have been reported among the youth, through tracing, at least 6 more reported cases were connected to the prison supervisor (Rendall, 2020). In late August, a prison staff worker in Queensland tested positive, spurring the lockdown of 12 Queensland correctional facilities (Daoud & Barnsley, 2020). The Victorian attorney general confirmed in late August that a combined total of at least 50 inmates and prison staff had tested positive in Victoria since the start of the pandemic, 23 of which were adult inmates, 6 of which were prison staff workers, 19 were juvenile inmates, and 5 were juveniles being supervised in the community (Kolovos, 2020).

COVID-19 outbreaks in New Zealand

Relative to other countries in the world, New Zealand has demonstrated great success in preventing and containing COVID-19 in its prisons and the broader community. Not only has the government successfully achieved more than 100 days without a reported case of the virus, there has also yet to be a single reported case among inmates within correctional facilities and only two positive cases among prison staff (Block, 2020; Godin, 2020). The government has approached its prison population with the same tenacity as it has the community. Mitigation strategies were executed swiftly and effectively, which can be largely attributed to public buy-in and support of measures in place, such as a nationwide lockdown (Shepherd, 2020). Among its prison population, various mitigation strategies have been implemented, including widespread dissemination of information regarding COVID-19 and the importance of taking health and safety precautions among inmates and staff (Adair, 2020), the use of personal protective equipment and the implementation of health screenings for prison staff (Boshier, 2020), a 14-day isolation period for newly admitted inmates (RNZ, 2020), and suspension of visitation in the initial stages of the pandemic (RNZ, 2020).

COVID-19 outbreaks in other countries in Oceania

Other countries in Oceania such as Papa New Guinea (N = 424) and Fiji (N = 28) have reported very few total COVID-19 cases as of late August (Coronavirus Resource Center, 2020), and no cases among inmates to our knowledge. Regardless, vigilant and preventative measures within prison settings have been taken. In Papa New Guinea, a small number of low-risk offenders[4] were released to reduce overcrowding (Graue, 2020), while Fiji closed its doors to all visitors, supplementing with remote conferencing (United Nations in the Pacific, in press).

Concluding comments

Our review has highlighted an important point: even islandic countries are susceptible to COVID-19, both in the community and prison systems alike. However, the prevalence rates are lower in this region than the rest of the world, at least as of this point in time (September, 2020). Unfortunately, this may not last. The reported rates of COVID-19 in both the community and in prisons do appear to be on the rise, despite some fairly aggressive mitigation strategies employed in Australia and New Zealand.[5]

Notes

1. As of August 27, 2020.
2. As of August 27, 2020.
3. This number is based on data reported in March of 2020.
4. Low-risk is in reference to the nature of the crime for which the inmates were incarcerated.
5. See the country-specific reports for both countries included in this volume.

Disclosure statement

No potential conflict of interest was reported by the author(s).

References

4512.0 - Corrective services, Australia, March quarter 2020: Key statistics. (2020, July 25). Australian Bureau of Statistics. https://www.abs.gov.au/ausstats/abs@.nsf/mf/4512.0

Adair, J. (2020). *Latest COVID-19 update from Chief Inspector.* Office of the Inspectorate. https://inspectorate.corrections.govt.nz/news/news_items/latest_covid-19_update_from_chief_inspector

Australia Population (LIVE). (2020, August). *Worldometer.* https://www.worldometers.info/world-population/australia-population/

Block, G. (2020, May 8). *Rise in spitting attacks on corrections officers during coronavirus pandemic.* Stuff. https://www.stuff.co.nz/national/health/coronavirus/300008110/rise-in-spitting-attacks-on-corrections-officers-during-coronavirus-pandemic

Boshier, P. (2020, June). *OPCAT COVID-19 report: Report on inspections of prisons under the Crimes of Torture Act 1989.* Office of the Ombudsman. https://www.ombudsman.parliament.nz/sites/default/files/2020-06/Report_on_inspections_of_prisons_under_the_Crimes_of_Torture_Act_1989_062020.pdf

Buhre, M. L. (2020, May 7). *Many Pacific islands are untouched by COVID-19. Its arrival could be disastrous.* PBS. https://www.pbs.org/newshour/world/many-pacific-islands-are-untouched-by-covid-19-its-arrival-could-be-disastrous

Chapman, A. (2020, July 17). *Coronavirus enters Melbourne prison system for first time, results in demands for some inmates' release.* 7 News. https://7news.com.au/lifestyle/health-wellbeing/coronavirus-enters-victorian-prison-system-for-first-time-results-in-demands-for-some-inmates-release-c-1174015

Coronavirus Resource Center. (2020, August 24). *COVID-19 dashboard by the center for systems science and engineering (CSSE) at Johns Hopkins University (JHU).* John Hopkins University & Medicine. https://coronavirus.jhu.edu/map.html

Daoud, E., & Barnsley, W. (2020, August 27). Queensland prisons in lockdown after officer tests positive to coronavirus. *7 News.* https://7news.com.au/lifestyle/health-wellbeing/queensland-prisons-in-lockdown-after-officer-tests-positive-to-coronavirus-c-1269395

Doneman, P. (2020, April 13). *Coronavirus Australia: Queensland prisons taking drastic measures to prevent COVID-19 outbreaks.* 7 News. https://7news.com.au/lifestyle/health-wellbeing/coronavirus-australia-queensland-prisons-taking-drastic-measures-to-prevent-covid-19-outbreaks-c-973426

Gleeson, H. (2020, August 8). *Coronavirus triggers drop in prisoner numbers and an opportunity to reinvent the criminal justice system, lawyers say*. ABC News. https://www.abc.net.au/news/2020-08-09/remarkable-declines-prisoner-numbers-coronavirus-pandemic/12533218

Godin, M. (2020, August 14). *Can New Zealand contain its new coronavirus outbreak?* Time. https://time.com/5879177/new-zealand-coronavirus-cases/?utm_source=newsletter

Graue, C. (2020, April 30). *Small number of low-risk prisoners to be released in PNG as part of COVID-19 plans*. Pacific Beat. https://www.abc.net.au/radio-australia/programs/pacificbeat/png-prisons-covid/12199870

Kinner, S. A., Young, J. T., Snow, K., Southalan, L., Lopez-Acuna, D., Ferreira-Borges, C., & O'Moore, E. (2020, March 17). Prisons and custodial settings are part of a comprehensive response to COVID-19. *The Lancet*, *5*(4), E188–E189. https://doi.org/10.1016/S2468-2667(20)30058-X

Kleyn, B. (2020, August 20). *Young inmates locked in cells as authorities brace for a potential coronavirus outbreak at the Brisbane youth detention centre*. ABC News. https://www.abc.net.au/news/2020-08-21/coronavirus-queensland-wacol-youth-detention-centre-in-lockdown/12564750

Kolovos, B. (2020, August 26). *50 Vic inmates, staff contract COVID-19*. The Islander. https://www.theislanderonline.com.au/story/6896123/50-vic-inmates-staff-contract-covid-19/?cs=7

Layt, S., & Lynch, L. (2020). *More than 20 inmates quarantined in maximum security Brisbane prison*. Brisbane Times. https://www.brisbanetimes.com.au/national/queensland/more-than-20-inmates-quarantined-in-maximum-security-brisbane-prison-20200423-p54mp7.html

Rendall, J. (2020, August 22). *Here's what we know so far about Queensland's coronavirus outbreak in the Brisbane youth detention centre*. ABC News. https://www.abc.net.au/news/2020-08-22/coronavirus-queensland-youth-detention-outbreak-wacol-explained/12582764

RNZ. (2020, April 6). *Covid 19 coronavirus: Prisoners in cells up to 23 hours a day*. New Zealand Herald. https://www.rnz.co.nz/news/in-depth/413538/covid-19-prisoners-in-cells-up-to-23-hours-a-day-guards

Searle, J. (2020, March 24). *Explainer: How will the emergency release of NSW prisoners due to Coronavirus work?* The Conversation. https://theconversation.com/explainer-how-will-the-emergency-release-of-nsw-prisoners-due-to-coronavirus-work-134523

Shepherd, M. (2020, August 10). *How geography helped New Zealand Beat Coronavirus*. Forbes. https://www.forbes.com/sites/marshallshepherd/2020/08/10/how-geography- helped-new-zealand-beat-coronavirus/

Surveillance and treatment of prisoners with Hepatitis C (SToP-C). (2020, August 28). The Kirby Institute. https://kirby.unsw.edu.au/project/stop-c

United Nations in the Pacific. (in press). *Reunited virtually with families in prisons*. United Nations: COVID-19 Response. https://www.un.org/en/coronavirus/reunited-virtually-families-prisons

Visontay, E., & Wahlquist, C. (2020, July 21). *Six Victorian prisons in lockdown after worker tests positive – As it happened*. The Guardian. https://www.theguardian.com/australia-news/live/2020/jul/21/coronavirus-australia-live-update-jobkeeper-nsw-hotspots-victoria-masks-jobseeker-daniel-andrews-gladys-berejiklian-latest-news

Wahlquist, C. (2020, March 19). *Australia's overcrowded prisons could struggle to control coronavirus, expert says*. The Guardian. https://www.theguardian.com/australia-news/2020/mar/19/australias-overcrowded-prisons-could-struggle-to-control-coronavirus-expert-says

Waight, N. (2020, July 30). *Hundreds have died in US prisons from Covid-19. Will Australia act before it's too late?* The Guardian. https://www.theguardian.com/commentisfree/2020/jul/30/thousands-have-died-in-us-prisons-from-covid-19-will-australia-act-before-its-too-late

World Prison Brief. (2020, August). *World prison brief data*. Institute for Crime & Justice Policy Research (ICPR). https://www.prisonstudies.org/world-prison-brief-data

Worldometer. (2020). *COVID-19 coronavirus pandemic*. https://www.worldometers.info/coronavirus/

COVID-19 and Corrections in Australia: A Summary Review of the Available Data and Literature

Jason L. Payne and Natalia Hanley

ABSTRACT

In March 2020, COVID-19 was declared a global pandemic and at the time of writing, there were more than 13 million known cases and more than 500,000 deaths. Not since the Spanish Flu of 1918 has the world needed to respond to the potential threat of a communicable disease with such a high rate of infection and fatality. Using publicly available data, media sources, and literature, this paper maps Australian corrective services' responses to COVID-19. We find evidence of a concerted effort to reduce prison population numbers, as well as to recalibrate corrections practice in an effort to meet new social-distancing rules and regulations. Our analysis is motivated by the knowledge that prior to COVID-19, Australia had a rising prison population, a disproportionate growth in female and remand populations, and significant Indigenous overrepresentation. In this paper, we explore whether the immediate benefits of COVID-19 have helped or hindered efforts to address these wider concerns.

Introduction

On January 30 2020, the World Health Organization (WHO) declared the novel coronavirus disease 2019 (COVID-19) as a public health emergency of international concern. Caused by an outbreak of severe acute respiratory syndrome coronavirus-2 (SARS-CoV-2), COVID-19 was later declared a global pandemic and has required governments around the world to implement a wide range of proactive and reactive measures to limit its spread. SARS-CoV-2 is genetically similar to the coronaviruses responsible for previous pandemic outbreaks (SARS-CoV and MERS-CoV). What makes it different, however, is that while it is less lethal, it appears to have a higher rate of transmission, a longer period of incubation and a shorter interval between symptom onset and maximum infectivity (Peterson et al., 2020). What this ultimately means is that SARS-CoV-2 presents a distinct and heightened risk of transmission in contexts where appropriate physical and social distancing cannot be enforced or maintained.

In the criminal justice context, this has important implications for the administration of justice and the management of corrective services. The health and wellbeing of incarcerated populations and custodial staff have been of particular concern in Australia (see Walhquist, 2020) and there has been much anxiety about how best to protect the health and human rights of the nation's prisoners. Prisoners, by virtue of their incarceration, cannot willfully elect to socially distance and can be subject to mandatory prison lockdowns that significantly restrict access to activities outside the confines of their prison cell. In the community corrections context, there are concerns about how best to enforce community-based orders when social-distancing regulations prohibit the gathering or congregation of small groups, or which restrict access to those communities and other treatment programs that form part of the conditions of an offender's community order. These concerns are shared by many countries around the globe (Kinner et al., 2020), although it is the objective of this paper to document the unique Australian experience of COVID-19 and its impact on the policy debate in corrective services.

COVID-19 in Australia

At the time of writing, Australia had recorded 26,912 confirmed infections of SARS-CoV-2 and 851 deaths (Department of Health, 2020). The first recorded infection was discovered on January 25, and the highest number of new daily cases during the first "wave" was 458 (see Figure 1). Since then, efforts to suppress community transmission had been generally effective until late June when case numbers began to increase. The most recent "second-wave" of infection has been almost exclusively felt in the south-eastern state of Victoria.

The Australian policy response to the impending threat of COVID-19 has been widely acknowledged by the international community as swift and effective (Duckett & Stobary, 2020). Nationwide, containment measures were coordinated by the federal government through a newly established National Cabinet (see Bonyhady & Duke, 2020), although individual states and territories had the autonomy to choose which restrictions to implement, and the timeline upon which to implement them. On 1 February, foreign nationals from China were banned and Australian citizens returning from China were required to self-quarantine for 14 days. Travel bans were later imposed on arrivals from Iran, South Korea, and Italy and a general travel ban for all arrivals was introduced on March 20. In late February, the Australian Prime Minister activated the *Australian Health Sector Emergency Response Plan* and created a new National Cabinet on March 13 – the first such national cabinet since World War II (Bonyhady & Duke, 2020).

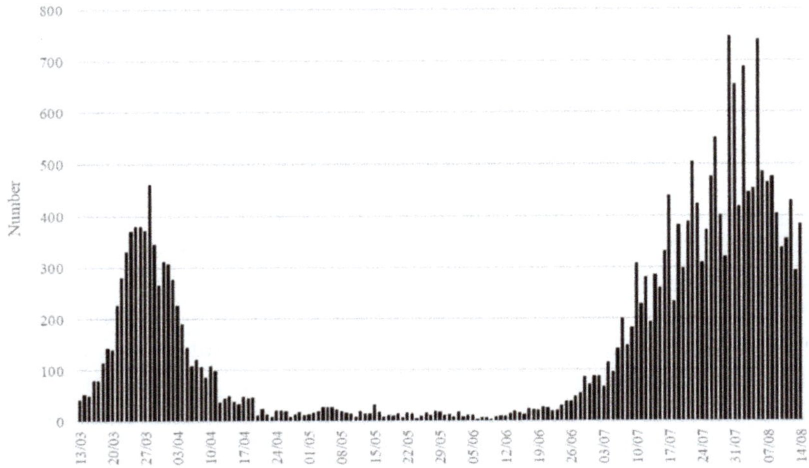

Figure 1. Daily cases of COVID-19 in Australia (March 13 – August 14, 2020). Source: www.covid19data.com.au

The first of the key social-distancing restrictions came into effect on March 15 with the cancellation and restriction of gatherings of more than 500 people. At the time, this excluded schools, universities, and public transport sites. On March 30, stricter rules were imposed, limiting indoor and outdoor gatherings to a maximum of two people (Morrison, 2020). Public spaces, such as parks, community halls, and gyms, were closed and the government issued strong advice for people to stay at home unless necessary. Implementation of these nationally agreed principles was then undertaken at the state level, with some additions and variations including the closure of schools and interstate borders and the restriction of interstate travel.

In early May, as suppression efforts appeared to be successful in curbing transmission, social-distancing restrictions were slowly relaxed in most states and territories (Harris, 2020). That was until late June when transmission rates began to increase again in Victoria. As a response, the Victorian government announced the immediate and temporary lock-down of nine high-rise public housing buildings and strict restrictions on resident and nonresident movement in 10 postcode areas, including the Melbourne Metropolitan area. Not long after, interstate travel was closed to residents and recent travelers from Victoria, extending to residents and recent travelers from certain emerging hotspots in New South Wales (see, for example, the Queensland Border restrictions Direction No.11 (Queensland Government, 2020)).

Prisons in Australia before COVID-19

As of June 2019, there were 43,028 prisoners in Australia (Australian Bureau of Statistics, 2019). The national imprisonment rate is 219 prisoners per 100,000 of the adult population. Australia's largest prison is the newly opened Clarence Correctional Center in New South Wales. It has a capacity to contain 1,700 prisoners and 600 operational staff and it reflects a longer-term shift in Australia toward the building so-called "mega-prisons". Others include the 2017-built Ravenhall prison in Victoria which already a planned extension beyond its current capacity of 1,300 prisoners. Casuarina prison in Western Australia is also scheduled for expansion from its current capacity of 1,033 to 1,782 in the next 3 years. In all, nine facilities across Australia are considered "private prisons," operated by private corporations under contractual arrangements with the relevant state and territory governments. Although Australia has relatively few prison facilities, the proportion of Australian prisoners incarcerated in private facilities is reported as being among the highest in the world (Andrew, Baker & Roberts 2016).

Unlike the United States, imprisonment in Australia has been increasing steadily over the last 10 years – a trend that has been shared by all states and territories. In New South Wales, the largest Australian jurisdiction by population, imprisonment rates have grown as much as 36% in the last 7 years (Bureau of Crime Statistics and Research, 2020) and these trends have been underpinned by a disproportionate increase in the rate of unsentenced imprisonment (i.e. remand and pre-trial custody) and the imprisonment of female and Indigenous Australians (Australian Bureau of Statistics, 2019).

Despite the building of new and expansion of old facilities to accommodate this growth, prison over-crowding has been common in Australia (Mackay, 2015). COVID-19 and the threat of a highly infectious communicable disease has brought the design and architecture of prisons into sharp relief. Prisoners live in close proximity to each other, and commonly share cells or units. However, even in prisons that are able to retain single-cell occupancy despite population increases, facilities such as bathrooms, dining, and recreational spaces are shared and large numbers of people use these spaces each day.

Notwithstanding the rapid expansion of prisons in Australia making custodial facilities more vulnerable to the spread of infectious diseases, Australian prisoners are also disproportionately more likely to experience adverse health outcomes. Prisoners are overwhelmingly drawn from groups that have a greater incidence and co-occurrence of various health issues and emerging data links some of these conditions with the most severe incidences of COVID-19. For example, 22% of prison entrants reported that they had been told they had asthma at some point in their lives. The community rate of asthma is 11%. The rate of tobacco smoking is 4–5 times higher in the prison population compared to the general community population, with 75% of Australian prison entrants reporting that they currently smoke (Australian Institute of Health and Welfare, 2019). There is some evidence that both asthma and smoking may be associated with severe instances of COVID-19 (Centers for Disease Control and Prevention, 2020). While the rates of diabetes in the Australian population are comparable to the community incidence of diabetes (6% and 5%, respectively) diabetes is four times more prevalent in the Aboriginal and Torres Strait Islander population (Australian Institute of Health and Welfare, 2019) a group enormously over-represented in Australian prisons (Australian Bureau of Statistics, 2020). Type 2 diabetes in particular has been identified as increasing the risk of more severe COVID-19 symptoms (Centers for Disease Control and Prevention, 2020). The Australian Institute of Health and Welfare's (AIHW) Health of Australia's Prisoners report does not disaggregate the proportional occurrence of each type of diabetes, but overall it is likely that type 2 diabetes is more common in the Aboriginal and Torres Strait Islander prisoner population.

Taken together, these data highlight that the architecture, use, and high population in prison facilities, coupled with some prisoners' increased vulnerability to more severe instances of COVID-19 presents a potential public health crisis in Australia. The recognition of the significant consequences of COVID-19 infection in the prison estate resulted in the unusual move to implement a national response to shut all Australian prison facilities to social and, in some cases, professional visitors followed by a series of adapted and new practices to reduce the risk. Criminal justice is a state and territory responsibility and there are varied examples of jurisdictions implementing differential practices as a result including, for example, "three strikes" legislation in Western Australia (Hinds, 2005) and the "dual track" system in Victoria for young adult offenders (Victorian Government, 2020). However, COVID-19 appears to offer a unique case study in converging policy and practice across Australia. Analysis of publicly available information about corrective services responses around Australia highlights three inter-related themes; visitation and contact, health provisions, and service delivery modes. Each theme is explored below following an overview of the broad events that have shaped policy in this area.

Prisons in Australia during COVID-19

Major events shaping policy

During the first wave of the COVID-19 pandemic in Australia, there were no confirmed cases of SARS-CoV-2 in any custodial or correctional center. The screening of inmates, visitors, and staff was widely implemented early in the pandemic (ABC News, 2020a) and in at least one jurisdiction (the Australian Capital Territory) all prison visits were suspended until further notice (ABC News, 2020b). Special medical facilities were set up in some prisons as corrective services agencies were on high alert after three justice health workers in New South Wales tested positive in late May (Clun, 2020)

The first recorded case of COVID-19 in custody was reported on July 17 when a remand prisoner in Victoria tested positive during routine testing. At the time, prisons in Victoria had implemented new procedures, mandating the testing and 14-day quarantine of all new custodial receptions (Corrections Victoria, 2020). It was during this routine testing that the positive result was detected, but not before the remandee had been in close contact with a number of other prisoners and prison staff. Responding to the risk of local transmission, the Victorian government placed six prison centers into lockdown. Later that month, a custodial officer in Victoria tested positive (Russell, 2020).

While Australian prisons have experienced only a small number of transmission events, the early experience of COVID-19 in countries such as Italy and the United States provided a foreground for early preparation and policy debate. Watching from afar, the Australian professional and academic community were particularly exercised by the rapid rate of transmission in some U.S.-based custodial centers and so on March 20 an open letter to Australian Governments was published calling for action to prevent the spread of COVID-19 in prisons (Bartels, Anthony & Fletcher, 2020). This was the first of three open letters that have been published since the start of the pandemic (Personal Communication). All three called for the release of prisoners from custody.

Visitation and contact

Following the National Cabinet meeting in March 2020, all jurisdictions in Australia ceased in-person social visitation within prisons. At the time of writing, visitation had recommenced in several jurisdictions including, for example, the Northern Territory, Tasmania and Western Australia. Social visitation recommenced and was temporarily suspended again in South Australia in August 2020 due to heightened infection risk in the community. Visitation is a core pillar of prisoners' rights because of the varied and well-documented benefits associated with regular contact with family and friends. These benefits include promoting positive mental health, maintaining family connections, and reduced recidivism (Duwe & Clark, 2011; McLeod & Bonsu, 2018). The benefits extend beyond prisoners. For children with a parent in prison, visitation offers some protection from the negative impacts of parental incarceration (Schubert et al., 2016).

When social visitation ceased at the end of March all Australian jurisdictions identified alternative solutions to maintain some visitation contact.[1] Most commonly, video-calling was implemented or extended using programs such as zoom and skype and, in some jurisdictions, such as Tasmania, tablet devices were provided to people in prison to facilitate video-visits. However, only Victoria mentioned the provision of technical support to community visitors to assist with the use of this new visitation mode. The picture is unclear in the Northern Territory[2] as the most recently available information states that Corrective Services are considering other modes of communication, including video-calls, where available, and that there will be "increased access" to telephone and video calls. This careful rhetoric is ambiguous about the extent to which visitation is continuing, and in what forms. This is particularly concerning given that "non-essential" service visits have been suspended in the Northern Territory, including visits by non-government organizations and volunteers.

The extent of take-up in alternative social visitation such as video-calling, and the level of effectiveness, access, and satisfaction with the technology is unknown. Where social visitation has, or will soon resume, the number of visitors and/or duration of the visit has been limited, visitors are subject to enhanced health screening, and physical distancing is in place, even in jurisdictions that have exempted prisons from distancing rules, such as Tasmania. For example, in South Australia visitors will be excluded if they present as 'unwell', in the Northern Territory visits are limited to one hour with a smaller number of people, gradually scaled up to larger groups of visitors, and in Tasmania only two visitors are allowed, including children. For example, in South Australia visitors will be excluded if they present as "unwell" and in the Northern Territory visits are limited to 1 hour, with a smaller number of people, gradually scaled up to larger groups of visitors. Meanwhile New South Wales has restricted the consumption of food during visits and physical touching. Video-calling has continued in most jurisdictions to alleviate these restricted face to face visits. The use of video-calling for professional visits is more variable. In the Australian Capital Territory, professional visits continued in person, but were discouraged, whereas in the Northern Territory professional visits were suspended.

Traditional modes of contact have remained, with some variations to increase prisoners' access. Increased phone call allowances, such as an additional weekly AUD$20 credit in the Australian Capital Territory also featured in most jurisdictions. This was further supported by new access to voicemail and e-mail communication. Most jurisdictions noted that letter-writing was encouraged. More broadly there was a "business as usual" thread in several jurisdictions where physical exercise, cultural activities, and existing modes of recreation were highlighted as providing essential structure to the day. While these practices are not new, or even varied, their significance from the perspective of prison management strategy is noteworthy, particularly given that there has been "disturbances" in several Australian prisons attributed to prisoners' frustrations about the lack of social visitation (ABC News, 2020c).

Health provisions

While the use of video-calling represents an adapted strategy for maintaining an existing provision within prisons, there have also been entirely new practices that have emerged in response to the COVID-19 risk. Most obviously, health screening and hygiene practices have been implemented in all jurisdictions, although the form that it takes is somewhat variable from hand washing and physical distancing to dedicated accommodation for people in quarantine. For example, the Australian Capital Territory is one of the jurisdictions to use a COVID-19 screening questionnaire. While most jurisdictions have implemented temperature checking, the temperature thresholds differ. In Tasmania the temperature threshold for concern is 37.3 degrees Celsius compared to 37.5 in New South Wales and 38 in Queensland. In New South Wales the temperature threshold for concern is 37.5□ compared to 38 in Queensland. Examples of hygiene measures include hand sanitation, physical distancing, directions not to hug or shake hands, and more frequent cleaning of facilities. Information provided by Western Australia Correctional Services has a significant emphasis on hygiene measures and included the provision that staff are required to use PPE where a person is suspected of having COVID-19, though the form of PPE was not specified. Mask-wearing does not appear to be a common practice as masks are only mentioned by South Australia Correctional Services, most likely for the reasons that South Australia set out about screening and security concerns.

A corollary of the attention on hygiene is the increased provision of information to prisoners and staff about effective hygiene practices and physical distancing. Only the Northern Territory referred specifically to the provision of health information in "plain English and in Aboriginal languages about what coronavirus is and what is being done to protect prisoners from potential infection." (Northern Territory Government, 2020). Queensland Corrective Services noted that information about what to do if symptoms develop post-release was provided to eligible prisoners. Transition into the community was, overall, rarely mentioned.

There was considerable variation in the response to identified COVID-19 cases in the prison population. Corrections Victoria referred to quarantine reception units for new receptions to ensure that testing could be undertaken before a prisoner was in contact with the prison population. The Tasmanian Prison Service has also implemented a 14-day quarantine period for all receptions. In Queensland, the mandatory 14-day quarantine provision has been abandoned and now, as in the ACT, only people displaying symptoms will be quarantined until test results are available. New South Wales had established a field hospital prepared to treat prisoners with COVID-19. In Queensland, prisoners with COVID-19 would be transferred into a community hospital setting. In Western Australia "each facility has its own operational plan in place to ensure that they are prepared to receive a prisoner or detainee who has, or is suspected of having, COVID-19. Anyone who presents with symptoms can be isolated from the mainstream population and be cared for appropriately by staff and health care professionals." (Western Australia Government, 2020) This approach reflects other jurisdictions in that new receptions are screened, isolation measures are in place, and prisoners remain in a prison rather than a community health setting. The information for Western Australia also raises the possibility of varied practices within-jurisdiction as COVID-19 response plans appear to have been developed at a facility rather than service level. The extent to which this is the case elsewhere is unknown.

Finally, as earlier mentioned nine of Australia's custodial facilities are operated by private enterprise under contract with the relevant state or territory government. These nine private prisons are among some of the largest in Australia, meaning that a sizable proportion of Australian prisoners is incarcerated in privately run facilities. To what extent the facility-level response to COVID-19 has differed between private and state-run prisons is not yet clear and questions remain about the level of influence and control that state governments might have in mandating specific infection control and management protocols. An early account of the situation by the Australian Center for Corporate Responsibility (ACCR) noted that while custodial center service provision contracts might provide a framework for state-mandated COVID-19 requirements, what happens at the ground-level is still a matter for the private contractor (Australian Centre for Corporate Responsibility [ACCR], 2020). The Workers' Union representing staff at one of Australia's largest private custodial service providers, Serco, have made public their concerns that facilities have not provided sufficient personal protective equipment, have not engaged full-time health professionals, and have not supported staff with sufficient personal leave provisions should they develop COVID-19 related symptoms and require home isolation (Australian Centre for Corporate Responsibility [ACCR], 2020). This will be an important area to monitor in Australia as private facilities have not been spared of the need to implement new policies and practices. In Victoria, for example, the main COVID-19 related incident so far – afflicting at least one remanded inmate and at least two staff – occurred at the privately run Ravenhall Remand Center (Mills, 2020).

Service delivery modes

A key area of adapted practices concern offender programs both within and outside of the prison setting. Here there is considerable variation in practice, and less clarity about service revisions, with most jurisdictions adapting programs to reduce infection risk. In the Northern Territory offense-based treatment programs have continued with smaller group sizes and physical distancing. However, at least some prisoner education programs have been temporarily suspended in face-to-face delivery mode. In the Northern Territory, some areas are subject to biosecurity restrictions which have directed Corrective Service options for some program delivery in the community including the Family Violence and Elders Visiting Programs. In the Australian Capital Territory, like Western Australia, community programs have continued except for in proscribed circumstances such as following a direction to isolate by a medical professional. For programs that have continued there are enhanced safety measures such as physical distancing. In South Australia, like Queensland, several programs have resumed including rehabilitation programs in the Aboriginal Services unit and substance testing. A number of jurisdictions have noted that some programs have been moved to an online delivery mode, such as AOD programs, though the rationale for which programs, their effectiveness online, and participation rates is not known.

Overall, corrective services in all Australian jurisdictions have taken substantial steps to manage the risk of COVID-19. Based on publicly available information, which is variable in volume and detail across the jurisdictions, there are two clear strategies that have been pursued to date. First, suspension of social and some professional visitation and the provision of alternative communication approaches including video-visitation. Second, significantly enhanced hygiene practices, COVID-19 screening and procedures for managing staff and prisoners who display symptoms or test positive. Changes to the provision of programs, activities, and requirements in Community Corrective Services have also occurred but the information about Community Corrective Services is comparatively less well documented. Presumably, the attention on the prison as opposed to community setting reflects the greater responsibility of Corrective Services to prisoners due to their confinement.

That said, some states and territories have released a broad set of Community Corrections policy and practice guidelines. In Victoria, for example, Community Corrections have clearly acknowledged a shift to physically distanced supervision protocols which has significantly limited in-person meetings and physical visitations. As an alternative, digital video technology is being progressively rolled out where remote supervision is deemed appropriate (Corrections Victoria, 2020). The use of electronic monitoring (EM) in Victoria will continue, although there is no indication that EM capacities have been increased to meet the higher demand for community supervision alternatives to imprisonment. Unpaid community work has been temporarily suspended while other program attendance (such as drug and alcohol treatment programming) continues in Victoria so long as social and physical distancing can be maintained (Corrections Victoria, 2020). In

Queensland, a four-stage response protocol was developed for community corrections which outlines the service and practice requirements needed at different levels of COVID-19 risk (Queensland Corrective Services, 2020). The protocol can be applied at varying levels to different geographical regions and community corrections offices ranging from Stage 1, which requires basic social and physical distancing, to Stage 4, which prevents staff and all other members of the public from accessing a specific community corrections office or site. At the time of writing, most Queensland Community Corrections offices in the south of the state were at Stage 2 restrictions. This means that programs and services can continue under an approved COVID-19 management plan, although non-essential face-to-face meetings have been limited (Queensland Corrective Services, 2020).

Prisoner trends

The impact of COVID-19 on incarceration rates in Australia is difficult to ascertain, largely because few Australian States and territories regularly release information about their custodial population. Annual national and jurisdictional data collection is conducted by the Australian Bureau of Statistics (ABS) and reported in its *Corrections in Australia* (Australian Bureau of Statistics, 2020) and *Prisoners in Australia* (Australian Bureau of Statistics, 2019) series. The national reports containing data for the period between April and June 2020 have not yet been released, however, at the state-level, some jurisdictions do provide interim quarterly or monthly reports. For example, the New South Wales Bureau of Crime Statistics and Research (BOCSAR) reports quarterly on New South Wales prison and custodial data and their Quarter 2, 2020 (May–June) was recently released. In Victoria and Queensland, the second and third largest states by population, monthly custodial and community corrections data are made publicly available through their respective Open Government Data Portals.

The available data suggest that since the onset of the pandemic in Australia, prison population numbers have declined. In New South Wales, Australia's most populated jurisdiction, the prison population in February 2020 was at an all-time-high of 13,974. By May 2020, that number had dropped to 12,588 (down by 10%) and it remained relatively consistent in June (Figure 2). In Victoria, there were 8,142 prisoners in custody at the end of February 2020 and the 12-month average for 2019 was 8,126. By the end of June 2020, this number had fallen to 7,151 prisoners – the lowest for that state since early-2018 representing a 12% decline since February 2020. Never in the history of the available data series have the New South Wales or Victorian prison populations declined so considerably in such a short period of time.

In Queensland, the available series of monthly data is much shorter, providing only a 12 month snapshot in the period prior to the onset of the pandemic (Figure 3). Still, we note that the custodial population in May 2020 (8,756) was the lowest recorded in the available series and represents a more than 5% decline from its peak in March 2020 (9,226). Of course, the recent decline in prisoner numbers in Queensland follows a substantial increase throughout the first three months of 2020 and some readers might describe this as a "return to trend" rather than a direct response to COVID-19. In our view, however, a reduction of the magnitude witnessed between March and May is unlikely to occur in a custodial population without some meaningful change in policy or practice.

Two mechanisms are likely to have contributed to the decline in prison numbers – an increase in the rate of prison discharge and a decrease in the rate of new prison receptions.

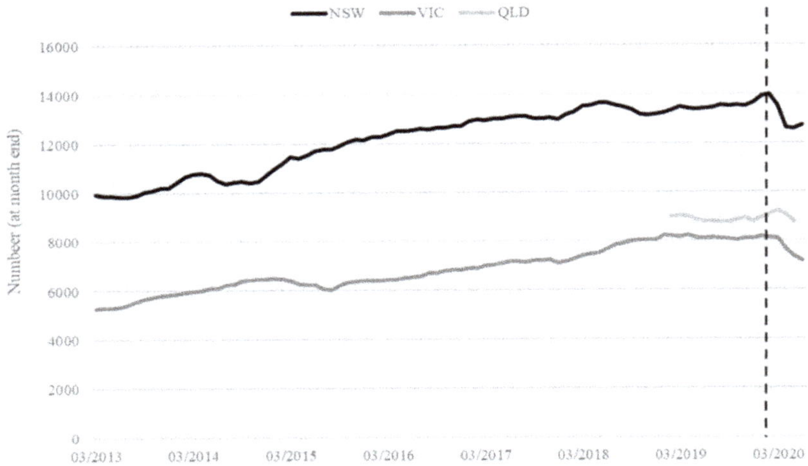

Figure 2. Custodial Prisoner Numbers. Vertical line denotes February 2020. Source: New South Wales Bureau of Crime Statistics; Corrections Victoria; Queensland Government Open Data Portal

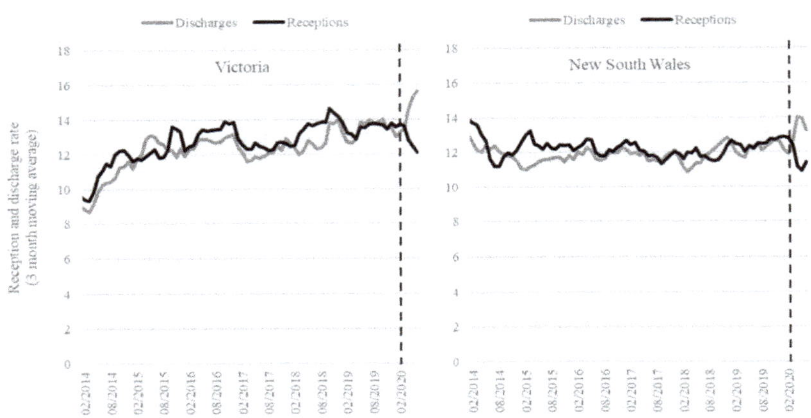

Figure 3. Prison discharge and reception rates, Victoria and New South Wales. Monthly discharge rates are calculated as the number of prisoners discharged in 1 month, divided by the number of prisoners in custody at the end of the previous month. Reception rates are calculated as the number of new receptions divided by the number of prisoners in custody at the end of the same month. Source: New South Wales Bureau of Crime Statistics; Corrections Victoria

Only in New South Wales and Victoria are these data currently available (Figure 3). Using an estimate of the three-monthly moving average (to smooth an otherwise volatile series), Figure 3 shows that both the prison reception and discharge rates in New South Wales and Victoria changed considerably from March 2020 onwards. Discharge rates are the highest they have been in recent history and the rate of new-receptions is also lower than average. Rarely has the discharge rate exceeded the reception rate in either state, and never before has the magnitude of the difference been so large. Put simply, the prison population in New South Wales and Victoria rapidly declined because more prisoners (than average) have been released, and fewer prisoners (than average) have been received into custody.

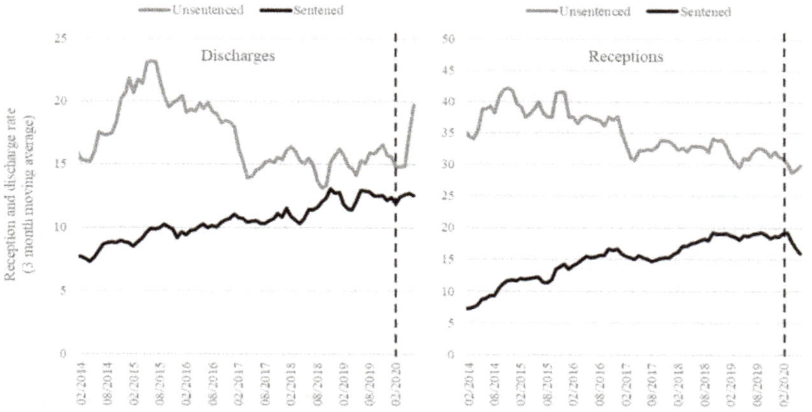

Figure 4. Sentenced and unsentenced prisoner discharge and reception rates, Victoria. Monthly discharge rates are calculated as the number of prisoners discharged in one month, divided by the number of prisoners in custody at the end of the previous month. Reception rates are calculated as the number of new receptions divided by the number of prisoners in custody at the end of the same month. Source: Corrections Victoria

Finally, discharge rates only increased above trend for unsentenced prisoners (Figure 4) while reception rates declined only for sentenced prisoners. In other words, the overall change in the prison population was the result of releasing a larger than average number of unsentenced prisoners, and receiving a smaller than average number of new prisoners on sentence from the courts. The latter is likely the result of some purposeful policy to release prisoners on bail, where appropriate, while the former is likely a result of the slowdown in court processing that occurred while stay-at-home orders were in place and non-essential business activities were temporarily suspended (Wells, 2020). Only in New South Wales has there been an official announcement of a change in policy, with the Commissioner of Corrective Services New South Wales announcing the intention to "conditionally release some low risk and vulnerable inmates from prison, if this is necessary for the safety and effectiveness of our prisons" (New South Wales Government Department of Communities and Justice, 2020). To date, no prisoners have "officially" been released to mitigate COVID-19 risk, but the prisoner trends suggest that these provisions are being informally enacted in all jurisdictions.

Alternatives to imprisonment

The sudden apparent changes in custodial numbers across Australia raise important questions about alternatives to imprisonment. On this topic, however, the publicly available information has been comparatively sparse. For example, it is not clear whether there has been a commensurate increase in the use of alternatives such as home detention or electronic monitoring. In part, this is explained by the fact that a significant proportion of the change in prison numbers has come from a change in the incarceration of pre-trial offenders. The creative use of strict bail conditions has likely been sufficient to manage the unusually high number of offenders who are being released back into the community.

Prisons in Australia after COVID-19

It is too early in the cycle of the COVID-19 pandemic to predict how Australian prisons, prisoners, and prison staff will fare. So far, we have successfully avoided a significant custodial transmission event, but whether COVID-19 will eventually breach the walls is anyone's guess. What matters from here is whether Australian corrective services have sufficiently safeguarded against the ever-present risk and whether any of the reactive COVID-19-related policy and practice changes will have longer term impacts (either positive or negative) on custodial populations and imprisonment trends.

Importantly, as a once-in-a-generation public health crisis of international reach, COVID-19 also offers new opportunities to both reimagine and reinvent corrective services practice. For the first time in a long time, significant effort has been invested into ways of keeping people out of prison and better connecting those who are in prison with family and services beyond the prison walls. This new (and hopefully not temporary) policy orientation offers fertile ground for reform.

Impact on key priority issues and trends

As noted earlier, Australia has seen a continued growth in the use of imprisonment, with imprisonment rates higher now than at any other time in recent history. In addition to this, the overrepresentation of Indigenous Australians remains a significant national problem and the subject of considerable international concern and condemnation (United Nations Human Rights Office of the High Commissioner, 2017). Australia has also seen a disproportionate increase in the rate of female imprisonment, which a sharp incline between 2011 and 2018 (Australian Bureau of Statistics, 2018), and an increase in the imprisonment of unsentenced (pre-trial) offenders since 2010 (Australian Bureau of Statistics, 2019). Each of these issues has been hotly debated across both academic and policy settings and there are emerging concerns that COVID-19 might exacerbate these trends or halt existing efforts to reverse them.

Perhaps the first observation to make here is that the greatest decline in prison numbers has occurred within the unsentenced prison population. This is a consistent trend across the three most populated states (New South Wales, Queensland, and Victoria) and it is a positive indication that police, courts and corrective services agencies have begun to reevaluate the use of pre-trial incarceration. In a pandemic, the costs and consequences of denying bail are conceivably very different. Remanded offenders enter custodial institutions from the community and they are the most likely source of new transmission within a prison setting. For the relevant gatekeepers making the decision to grant or deny bail, the risk of introducing COVID-19 into a custodial environment must now be weighed against the risk of (re)offending. In all, we see this as a positive step toward a wider re-evaluation of the principles underpinning the use of remand and pre-trial custody in Australia. However, it remains to be seen whether these changes can be formalized into a consistent approach that mutes the growth of unsentenced imprisonment well beyond the end of the pandemic.

For the issue of Indigenous over-representation, the early data are mixed and require ongoing monitoring. In Queensland, for example, the number of incarcerated Indigenous offenders has decreased by just 1% since February 2020 and this compares to an overall decline of 5% for their non-Indigenous peers (Figure 5). Even where prison populations

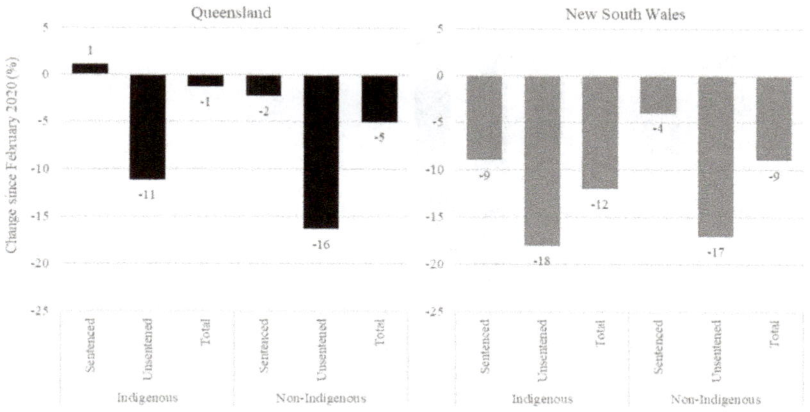

Figure 5. Change in prison population as at May 2020, by Indigenous status, Queensland and New South Wales. Change is calculated as the percentage difference between the prisoner number in February and June 2020. Source: New South Wales Bureau of Crime Statistics; Queensland Government Open Data Portal

have declined the most – i.e unsentenced imprisonment – the decline since February has not been as large for Indigenous prisoners in Queensland (−11% vs. −16%) and this suggests that over-representation in that state could worsen throughout the pandemic. In New South Wales, the data paint a more positive picture where the decline in both sentenced and unsentenced imprisonment has been disproportionally greater for Indigenous prisoners than for their non-Indigenous peers. The number of sentenced Indigenous prisoners in New South Wales declined by 9% (cf –4%) and the number of unsentenced Indigenous prisoners declined by 18% (cf −17%).

Of course, we are reminded that Indigenous Australians are incarcerated at a rate 15 times higher than non-Indigenous Australians and any disproportionate benefit during COVID-19 is but a small fraction of what is needed to redress this most pressing issue. Still, it is positive to see that in Australia's largest jurisdiction the recent decline in prison numbers has disproportionally favored Indigenous prisoners.

By gender, data from Victoria and New South Wales indicate that female prisoner populations have declined more rapidly during the pandemic than male prisoner numbers (Figure 6). In Victoria, the female prison population declined by 23% between February and June 2020 (cf. −11% for men) and the decline was larger for women in both the sentenced and unsentenced categories (Figure 6). In New South Wales, female imprisonment numbers were down by 17% over the same time period (cf –9% for men).

Although in the short term it seems that COVID-19 has not exacerbated Indigenous over-representation, nor further hastened the growth in female or unsentenced imprisonment, what happens in Australia over the longer term should be monitored carefully. A consequence of the dramatic decline in prison numbers since the start of the pandemic is that previously occupied prison beds are now empty. These beds, and possibly more in coming months, will likely remain empty until the pandemic passes. But, once it has, and once the risks of transmission are muted, there is a real possibility that this underutilized capacity is quickly re-used if current policies are

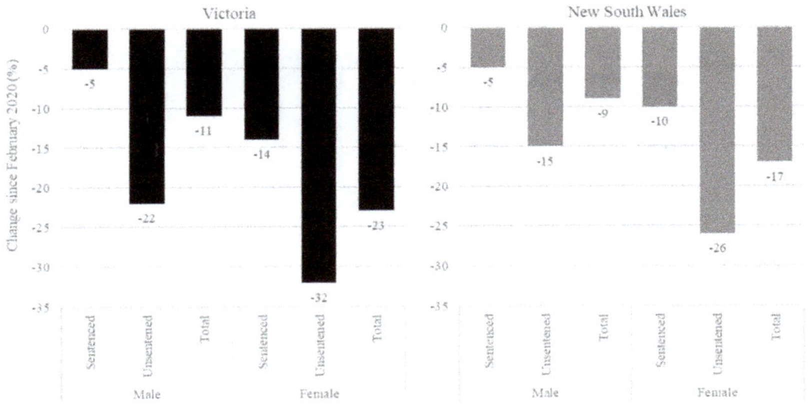

Figure 6. Change in prison population as at June 2020, by gender, Victoria and New South Wales. Change is calculated as the percentage difference between the prisoner number February and June 2020. Source: New South Wales Bureau of Crime Statistics; Corrections Victoria

not examined, evaluated and, where appropriate, embedded into an ongoing practice. This is not likely to be a unique problem for Australia, but we must be extra vigilant to ensure that any "return to trend" does not come at the cost of those populations who are most vulnerable and at risk of incarceration.

Technology and reform

In addition to the decline in prison populations, COVID-19 has also necessitated the rapid evolution of policy, practice, and services offered within the prison. As highlighted earlier, significant effort was made to accommodate the use of tele- and video-conferencing alternatives to in-person social visitation. Although it is important for in-person visitation to resume as soon as practicable and safe, the wide-spread trial and expansion of digital communication facilities within prisons should offer flexible opportunities to connect prisoners with their family and other services. This is particularly promising in the area of program and service delivery, where the rapid investment in new digital and online facilities during the pandemic may be appropriated as a means to overcome a number of long-standing oft-cited barriers to education, program, and service delivery. For example, the availability and accessibility of prison programs have been documented as a barrier to rehabilitation, particularly in remote or regional facilities (Australian Law Reform Commission, 2018). Similarly, resourcing constraints often limit the availability of education and rehabilitation programs to sentenced prisoners, and even then, only those prisoners with sufficient time in custody to wait for the next available vacancy (Australian Law Reform Commission, 2018). Finally, post-release planning and through-care programs are regularly criticized for insufficiently connecting prisoners to community-based services and supports with enough time to solidify positive working relationships and develop truly individualized transition plans (Council of Australian Governments, 2016). While each of these issues may not be completely solved by the use of tele- and video-conferencing facilities, their rapid expansion and widespread implementation during COVID-19 have paved the way for new and innovative approaches that have previously been too costly or too difficult to trial and implement.

Discussion and conclusion

The global pandemic of 2020 represents a once-in-a-generation health crisis that has demanded a rapid reevaluation and reconfiguration of a range of government and community services. Few sectors have been spared and the Australian corrective services system is no exception. Since the onset of the pandemic, it appears that efforts have been made to reduce the number of people in prison mostly by limiting the reception of new unsentenced prisoners (opting instead for a wider use of bail) and releasing sentenced prisoners to community supervised parole. Of the available data for Australia's three most populated states (New South Wales, Victoria and Queensland), the decline in the prison population has been universal, ranging from between 5% in Queensland (to May) and 10percent in New South Wales (to June). Never in the history of the available data for Victoria and New South Wales has there been such a large month-on-month decline in the prison population.

In conjunction with there being fewer prison receptions and more prison discharges than usual, Australian corrective services agencies have taken steps to mitigate the risk of COVID-19 transmission within the custodial setting. For example, special quarantine principles have been adopted for newly received pre-trial prisoners in several jurisdictions, and new health and social-distancing practices have been widely implemented across the country. Social visitation has been temporarily suspended and digital tele- and video-conferencing alternatives have been rapidly implemented or expanded. In some respects, much like the pandemic itself, the pace of policy and practice change in the first half of 2020 has been unprecedented.

Australia is by no means unique in its experience of COVID-19, nor is it unique in the way in which corrective services have responded. Nevertheless, Australian corrective services entered the pandemic with a bleak outlook; where incarceration rates have been persistently increasing over the last 20 years, where per-head of population Australia's Indigenous and First Nations peoples are incarcerated at one of the highest rates of any minority population in the world (Anthony, 2017) and where the increase in female incarceration has been accelerating faster than for their male peers, and especially in the case of Indigenous women (Phelan et al., 2019). Whether COVID-19 will positively affect or exacerbate these disparities makes Australia a country to watch as the pandemic continues. For now, the data is showing some positive signs with equal or better outcomes for Indigenous people and women in prison. There remains a cause for careful monitoring given that the data are emerging, partial, and indicate that the prison population reduction gains are not being evenly felt by Indigenous people in all jurisdictions.

Finally, we believe that COVID-19 presents a once-in-a-generation opportunity to reevaluate and reimagine Australian corrective services policy and practice. Recommendations and decisions once considered too risky or too politically unpalatable have now been given new life as health and viral transmission risks are weighed against recidivism and community safety concerns. For the first time in a long time, there is an opportunity to revitalize arguments for keeping non-serious and low-risk offenders out of prison – it is better for the community as a whole if the transmission of COVID-19 within custody can be prevented. We are hopeful that while the pandemic is likely to be temporary, the efforts taken to reduce incarceration and improve services for prisoners in custody are not short-lived.

Notes

1. This section summarizes information gathered from each of the State and Territory websites. A list of web links and sources is provided in the reference list.
2. Overall, the Northern Territory had the least publicly available information about Corrective Services responses to COVID-19 and the information that was available was difficult to navigate.

Disclosure statement

No potential conflict of interest was reported by the author(s).

References

ABC News. (2020a, March 13). *Sydney news: Coronavirus closes Katoomba High School, prisons begin screening.* https://www.abc.net.au/news/2020-03-13/sydney-morning-briefing-friday-march-13/12051582

ABC News. (2020b, March 21). *Canberra coronavirus cases increase as Health Minister halts prison visits.* https://www.abc.net.au/news/2020-03-21/canberra-records-new-cases-of-covid-19-prison-visits-stopped/12077734

ABC News. (2020c, April 15). *Coronavirus lockdown measures lead to more disturbances in New South Wales prisons.* https://www.abc.net.au/news/2020-04-15/coronavirus-restrictions-ignite-tensions-in-NewSouth Wales-prison-system/12150076

Andrew, J., Baker, M., & Roberts, P. (2016). *Prison privatisation in Australia: The state of the nation.* Sydney Universoty Business School, Sydney. https://www.sydney.edu.au/content/dam/corporate/documents/business-school/research/accounting/Prison_Privatisation_in_Australia-_The_State_of_the_Nation_June_2016.pdf

Anthony, T. (2017, June 6). FactCheck Q&A: Are Indigenous Australians the most incarcerated people on Earth? *The Conversation.* https://theconversation.com/factcheck-qanda-are-indigenous-australians-the-most-incarcerated-people-on-earth-78528

Australian Bureau of Statistics. (2018). *Prisoners in Australia, 2018* (Cat. no 4517.0). https://www.abs.gov.au/ausstats/abs@.nsf/Lookup/by%20Subject/4517.0~2018~Main%20Features~Sex~7

Australian Bureau of Statistics. (2019). *Prisoners in Australia, 2019* (Cat. no 4517.0). https://www.abs.gov.au/AUSSTATS/abs@.nsf/Lookup/4517.0Main+Features12019?OpenDocument

Australian Bureau of Statistics. (2020). *Corrective services, Australia, March Quarter 2020* (Cat. no 4512.0). Retrieved July 28, 2020, from https://www.abs.gov.au/ausstats/abs@.nsf/mf/4512.0

Australian Centre for Corporate Responsibility [ACCR]. (2020). *Private prisons, immigration detention and COVID-19* (ACCR Briefing Note). https://www.accr.org.au/news/private-prisons-immigration-detention-and-covid-19/

Australian Institute of Health and Welfare. (2019). *The health of Australia's prisoners 2018* (Cat. no. PHE 246). AIHW.

Australian Law Reform Commission. (2018). *Key gaps. Pathways to justice–inquiry into the incarceration rate of Aboriginal and Torres Strait Islander peoples* (ALRC Report 133). https://www.alrc.gov.au/publication/pathways-to-justice-inquiry-into-the-incarceration-rate-of-aboriginal-and-torres-strait-islander-peoples-alrc-report-133/9-prison-programs-and-parole/key-gaps/

Bartels, L., Anthony, T., & Fletcher, K. (2020). *Open letter to Australian governments on the impact of COVID-19 on the criminal justice system* (pp. 2).

Bonyhady, N., & Duke, J. (2020, March 13). Leaders in unprecedented 'national cabinet' to tackle coronavirus. *The Sydney Morning Herald.* https://www.smh.com.au/politics/federal/leaders-in-unprecedented-national-cabinet-to-tackle-coronavirus-20200313-p549wd.html

Bureau of Crime Statistics and Research. (2020). *New South Wales Prison Statistics*. Retrieved July 30, 2020, from https://www.bocsar.NewSouthWales.gov.au/Pages/bocsar_custody_stats/bocsar_custody_stats.aspx

Centers for Disease Control and Prevention. (2020). *People with certain medical conditions*. Retrieved July 30, 2020, from https://www.cdc.gov/coronavirus/2019-ncov/need-extra-precautions/people-with-medical-conditions.html

Clun, R. (2020, May 22). The people keeping COVID-19 out of prison. *Sydney Morning Herald*. https://www.smh.com.au/national/NewSouthWales/the-people-keeping-covid-19-out-of-prison-20200515-p54tg6.html

Corrections Victoria. (2020). *Our response to coronavirus (COVID-19)*. https://www.corrections.vic.gov.au/covid19#update

Council of Australian Governments. (2016). *Prison to Work Report*. Commonwealth of Australia. https://www.coag.gov.au/sites/default/files/reports/prison-to-work-report.pdf

Department of Health. (2020). *Coronavirus (COVID-19) at a glance – 10 August 2020*. https://www.health.gov.au/resources/publications/coronavirus-covid-19-at-a-glance-10-august-2020

Duckett, S., & Stobary, A. (2020, June 11). *Australia's COVID-19 response: The story so far. Grattan Institute*. Grattan Institute. https://grattan.edu.au/news/australias-covid-19-response-the-story-so-far/

Duwe, G., & Clark, V. (2011). Blessed be the social tie that binds: The effects of prison visitation on offender recidivism. *Criminal Justice Policy Review*, *24*(3), 271–296. https://doi.org/10.1177/0887403411429724

Harris, R. (2020, May 21). Australians wary about rushing to lift COVID-19 restrictions, survey finds. *Sydney Morning Herald*. https://www.smh.com.au/politics/federal/australians-wary-about-rushing-to-lift-covid-19-restrictions-survey-finds-20200521-p54v9q.html

Hinds, L. (2005). 'Three strikes and you're out in the west: A study of newspaper coverage of crime control in Western Australia. *Current Issues in Criminal Justice*, *17*(2), 239–253. https://doi.org/10.1080/10345329.2005.12036352

Kinner, S. A., Young, J. T., Snow, K., Southalan, L., Lopez-Acuña, D., Ferreira-Borges, C., & O'Moore, É. (2020). Prisons and custodial settings are part of a comprehensive response to COVID-19. *The Lancet Public Health*, *5*(4), e188–e189. https://doi.org/10.1016/S2468-2667(20)30058-X

Mackay, A. (2015, May/June). Overcrowding in Australian prisons: The Human Rights Implications (2015). *Precedent*, *37*(128). SSRN. https://ssrn.com/abstract=2625347

McLeod, B. A., & Bonsu, J. (2018). The benefits and challenges of visitation practices in correctional settings: Will video visitation assist incarcerated fathers and their children? *Children and Youth Services Review*, *93*(October), 30–35. https://doi.org/10.1016/j.childyouth.2018.07.004

Mills, T. (2020, July 18). Knife-edge': Remand centre prisoner tests positive sparking outbreak fears. *The Age*. https://www.theage.com.au/national/victoria/knife-edge-remand-centre-prisoner-tests-positive-sparking-outbreak-fears-20200717-p55d4r.html

Morrison, S. (2020, March 29). *National cabinet statement* (Press release). Office of the Prime Minister of Australia. https://www.pm.gov.au/media/national-cabinet-statement

New South Wales Government Department of Communities and Justice. (2020). *Corrective services*. https://www.coronavirus.dcj.NewSouthWales.gov.au/services/corrective-services

Northern Territory Government. (2020). *Measures to Protect Prisoners*. https://coronavirus.nt.gov.au/updates/items/2020-04-08-measures-to-protect-prisoners

Peterson, E., Koopmans, M., Go, U., Hamer, D. H., Petrosillo, N., Castelli, F., Storgaard, M., Al Khalili, S., & Simonsen, L. (2020). Comparing SARS-CoV-2 with SARS-CoV and influenza pandemics. *The Lancet Infectious Diseases*, *20*(9), e238–e244. https://doi.org/10.1016/S1473-3099(20)30484-9

Phelan, L., Sotiri, M., & Scott, M. (2019). *Keeping women out of prison coalition. Profile of women in New South Wales. Part A: A snapshot*. https://www.sydneycommunityfoundation.org.au/wp-content/uploads/2020/04/KWOOP-Coalition-Profile-of-women-in-prison-in-NewSouth Wales.-Part-A.-A-snapshot.-Final-9-March-2020.pdf

Queensland Corrective Services. (2020). *COVID-19 (Coronavirus): Information for stakeholders*. https://corrections.qld.gov.au/covid-19-coronavirus-information-for-stakeholders/#How_are_Community_Corrections_managing_offenders_during_COVID19

Queensland Government. (2020). *Border restrictions Direction (No.11) - Direction from Chief Health Officer in accordance with emergency powers arising from the declared public health emergency*. https://www.health.qld.gov.au/system-governance/legislation/cho-public-health-directions-under-expanded-public-health-act-powers/border-restrictions

Russell, L. (2020, July 23). Why prisons in Victoria are locked up and locked down. *The Conversation*. https://theconversation.com/why-prisons-in-victoria-are-locked-up-and-locked-down-143178

Schubert, E. C., Duininck, M., & Shlafer, R. J. (2016). Visiting Mom: A pilot evaluation of a prison-based visiting program serving incarcerated mothers and their minor children. *Journal of Offender Rehabilitation*, *55*(4), 213–234. https://doi.org/10.1080/10509674.2016.1159641

United Nations Human Rights Office of the High Commissioner. (2017). *End of mission statement by the United Nations Special Rapporteur on the rights of indigenous peoples, Victoria Tauli-Corpuz on her visit to Australia*. https://www.ohchr.org/EN/NewsEvents/Pages/DisplayNews.aspx?NewsID=21473&LangID=E

Victorian Government. (2020). *Youth Justice Strategic Plan 2020–2030*. https://www.justice.vic.gov.au/sites/default/files/embridge_cache/emshare/original/public/2020/06/89/79b442d3c/Youth-Justice-Strategic-Plan.pdf

Walhquist, C. (2020, March 19). Australia's overcrowded prisons could struggle to control coronavirus, expert says. *The Guardian Australia*. https://www.theguardian.com/australia-news/2020/mar/19/australias-overcrowded-prisons-could-struggle-to-control-coronavirus-expert-says

Wells, G. (2020, June 14). New South Wales courts set to reopen after coronavirus, with Virtual Court to continue for some matters. *ABC News*. https://www.abc.net.au/news/2020-06-14/NewSouthWales-courts-to-open-to-jury-trials-after-coronavirus-lockdown/12349390

Western Australia Government. (2020). *Corrective Services response to the COVID-19 pandemic*. https://www.wa.gov.au/organisation/department-of-justice/corrective-services-response-the-covid-19-pandemic

Corrective Services Sources

This paper has been written with reference to a large number of digital sources and news updates from each state and territory. A link to each jurisdiction is provided below.

Australian Capital Territory Corrective Services:
https://www.coronavirus.dcj.nsw.gov.au/
Northern Territory Correctional Services:
https://coronavirus.nt.gov.au/
Queensland Corrective Services:
https://corrections.qld.gov.au/
South Australia Department for Correctional Services:
https://www.corrections.sa.gov.au/
Corrections Victoria:
https://www.corrections.vic.gov.au/covid19
Western Australia Corrective Services:
https://www.correctiveservices.wa.gov.au/

"We Must Go Hard and We Must Go Early": How New Zealand Halted Coronavirus in the Community and Corrections

Laura J. Murray and Kimberly R. Kras

ABSTRACT

New Zealand's success at containing the coronavirus, despite a potential reemergence in August, is viewed by the World Health Organization as a model for handling a pandemic. This same success also appears within one of its most vulnerable locales—prisons. While New Zealand's Department of Corrections has not experienced a single COVID-19 case within prison walls, the efforts to contain the virus have also come at costs to incarcerated individuals' rights. This article demonstrates the successful efforts to contain the coronavirus pandemic in New Zealand and how these efforts have been met with both praise and criticism. In particular, we will highlight the ways in which prison officials have quickly responded to the pandemic as well as their ongoing efforts to improve the conditions for those incarcerated.

Introduction

As the rest of the world grapples with the surge of coronavirus, New Zealand has emerged as a success story (O'Grady & Farzan, 2020; World Health Organization, 2020). New Zealand, home to around 5 million residents, holds one of the lowest COVID infection rates at 1,827cases and 25 deaths[1] (Ministry of Health, 2020). Prime Minister Jacinda Ardern's decisive response in implementing effective communications, extensive contact tracing, isolation, increased testing, lockdowns, and swift border closures made it one of the first COVID-free countries in the world (Godin, 2020; www.dw.com, D. W., 2020). While geography has been noted as one advantage New Zealand had on controlling virus transmission (Shepherd, 2020), the citizens of New Zealand also collectively abided by the strict guidelines set by the prime minister, with only 8% of the public opposed to the lock-down measures set forth.

On June 8, 2020, New Zealand declared itself a COVID-free and loosened restriction on citizens (Cave & Solomon, 2020). On August 14, 2020, New Zealand broke its 102-day COVID-free status with an outbreak in Auckland. Quick action by Prime Minister Janice Ardern aimed to curtail this outbreak stating, "It's being dealt with in an urgent but calm and methodical way" (Godin, 2020). When coronavirus first appeared in New Zealand, the government tightened its borders, ordered a lockdown, enforced social distancing, and increased testing to quash the spread of the novel virus. In the face of new cases emerging at the end of the summer, more masks have been provided to the public and a contract tracing app has been implemented to help identify case clusters (Godin, 2020).

One area that remains less understood is how coronavirus has impacted the correctional system. As the correctional systems in many countries work to reduce the conditions promoting the transmission of the virus, New Zealand's response is reflective of its national approach to the pandemic. This article examines how COVID-19 affects the current incarcerated populations in New Zealand and what is being done to balance public safety and prevent the potential hazards to a vulnerable population.

Consistent with movements in other counties, justice reform advocates are demanding that the prison population to be lowered in order to halt the spread of COVID-19 (Boyle, 2020). Despite the fact that there are no existing cases in New Zealand prisons or jails as of this writing, advocates warn that the likelihood of infection is high in these conditions. Sir Kim Workman, a justice reformist, said prisons are a "breeding ground for infectious disease" highlighting dense quarters and preexisting conditions (Boyle, 2020). Sir Workman stated:

> It is a population which is extremely susceptible to infectious disease and would be classified, I think under any criteria, as a vulnerable population. And you have got them all sitting next to one another. The potential for the spread of coronavirus is incredibly high. (Boyle, 2020).

Advocates suggest prioritizing release of the elderly, those with preexisting health conditions, and those waiting in custody pre-trial. However, achieving the early release of selected incarcerated subgroups is easier said than done. According to National Commissioner Rachel Leota, the "corrections' chief executive does not hold the powers to grant early releases, and any decision to change these policy settings would be a matter for the Government to decide" (Boyle, 2020). Because the corrections department does not make release decisions, the courts and parole board do, there is no plan to release prisoners early (Boyle, 2020; Forbes, 2020).

In this article, we outline and discuss the context of the correctional system in New Zealand and highlight the steps toward mitigating COVID-19 outbreaks as well as the remaining challenges in the face of a potential resurgence.

New Zealand corrections

The New Zealand Department of Corrections (Ara Poutama Aotearoa) operates a centralized system of prisons and community supervision. With over 10,000 staff, the prison system operates 18 prisons and 100 community correction offices across the country (Annual Report – Department of Corrections, 2019; Leota, 2020). Despite the increase of private in prisons Oceania (see Byrne et al., 2019), New Zealand hosts only one privately run facility – the Auckland South Correctional Facility, a 960-bed prison, housing minimum to high-security men, and operated by British company Serco (Department of Corrections (DOC), 2020a).

As of June 2020, there were 9,469 individuals in New Zealand prisons (Prison facts and statistics – June 2020, 2020), a rate of 188 incarcerated individuals per 100,000 residents (World Prison Brief, 2020). The majority of this population is male (93.4%), and one-third of those incarcerated are in the 30–39 age group. The most common offense type is violence (40.9%), and 38% of individuals are there on remand (not sentenced) (DOC, 2020b; Prison facts and statistics – June 2020, 2020). Most of the prison population is Minimum (33.3%), Low (22%), or Low Medium (25.4%) security classification.

A larger portion of the convicted population overseen by the Department of Corrections is on community-based supervision. There are approximately 30,000 individuals serving sentences in the community, the majority of whom are male (80%) (Community Statistics, 2020). In 2020, there were 24,878 individuals serving a community sentence, with 6,295 on direct supervision, 4, 632 on intensive supervision, 1, 263 on community detention, 1,419 on home detention, and 10,639 on a community work supervision[2] (Department of Corrections, 2020b). Another 2,580 individuals were being supervised on a term of parole (DOC, 2020b).

As in other correctional systems around the world, the indigenous population and people of color are over-represented. In New Zealand, over half of the prison population is Maori (52.3%), while only making up 15% of the general population (Annual Report – Department of Corrections, 2019; Prison facts and statistics – June 2020, 2020). Individuals classified as European make up 31%, with Pacific, Other, and Unknown categories making of the remaining proportion. Nearly 60% of women incarcerated and 70% of young people incarcerated are Maori (Annual Report – Department of Corrections, 2019). Similar statistics are reported for the community supervision population with 32% European, 46% Maori, 10% Pacific, and Other or Not recorded comprising the remaining categories (DOC, 2020b).

Mechanisms of success in fighting COVID-19

There have been no reported cases among the incarcerated population,[3] and only two positive cases among staff, which were deemed contracted outside of the prison facility (Block, 2020a). There are no reported data on infections among individuals on community-based forms of supervision or staff. There are several reasons for the success of New Zealand corrections in fighting the coronavirus.

First, the swift response of the government as a whole, including corrections, meant that citizens and incarcerated persons were better equipped to implement mitigation strategies, such as hygiene, social distancing, and interaction procedures. The Office of the Inspectorate, who is responsible for prison oversight, resumed prison inspections after initial strategies have been in place. A primary goal of the Office of the Inspectorate is to ensure that prisons are being operated humanely and in accordance with the Nelson Mandela Rules. At the beginning of the lockdown, the Office of the Inspectorate became available seven days a week and doubled its staff to respond to concerns and complaints from within the prison system (Adair, 2020). In a report from May 2020, Chief Inspector Janis Adair noted that both incarcerated individuals and staff had a "shared understanding of the effects of COVID-19 and the importance of taking health and safety precautions" (Adair, 2020). The report also noted that staff were properly wearing PPE and undergoing temperature checks and health screenings (Boshier, 2020).

New prisoners and those who had been transported outside the facility were isolating for 14 days upon entry into institutions (RNZ, 2020). Any new admits to prison facilities underwent temperature checks and health screenings to determine potential exposure (Boshier, 2020), but no testing protocols have been reported. In contrast to many other prison facilities around the world, New Zealand does not have an overcrowding problem at just 93.8% capacity (World Prison Brief, 2020a), instead of maintaining "a small buffer of vacant capacity at all times" to remain flexible in response to fluctuations in the court system (Annual Report – Department of Corrections, 2019, p. 12). In fact, only 38% of prisoners share a cell, as shown in Figure 1 (DOC, 2020b).

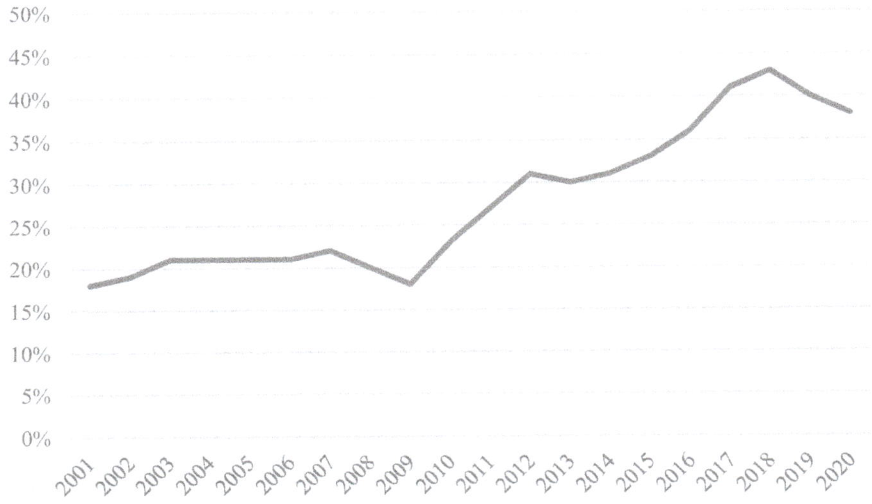

Figure 1. Proportion of New Zealand prisoners cell sharing. *Figure from the New Zealand Department of Corrections, Corrections Volume 2019–2020.*

Nonetheless, at the beginning of the country's lockdown, many facilities were instituting strict lockdown protocols within institutions where individuals were in cells between 20 and 22 hours a day (RNZ, 2020). Staff had implemented cohort "bubbles" to maintain isolation and increased "unlock" times to allow incarcerated individuals minimum daily access outside their cells and were cleaning and disinfecting common areas between each unlock time (Boshier, 2020). However, in one prison setting, the Inspector found inadequate cleaning supplies to accomplish this task, and in two other prison's recreational areas there were no handwashing or hygiene accommodations (Boshier, 2020). In response to this critique, officials noted the arduous and complex task of isolating individuals in different security classifications, especially with the nature and variability of prison architecture, with some prisons having more open floor plans, while others being comprised of many smaller wings with tight quarters (Boshier, 2020). Despite these challenges, during the COVID-19 pandemic, correction workers have been praised by community members and the Department of Corrections for the response to the lockdowns and guidelines in order to protect the health of both their families and incarcerated individuals (Block, 2020).

Outside visitors to correction facilities were also suspended, along with the receipt of any outside materials by family members or friends (RNZ, 2020). In lieu of suspended visits, correction officials provided phone cards; however, there were some reports that the lines to use the phones were long and there were not enough to meet demand (RNZ, 2020). When visits resumed on June 6, some facilities continued to adhere to strict social distancing measures, despite being downgraded to Alert Level 1 which eases some restrictions, and the dismay of inmates' family members[4] (Witton, 2020). Officials indicated each prison was operating differently based on circumstances.

On August 12, 2020, in response to the new community cases in Auckland, the DOC implemented Alert Level 3 protocol in its Auckland facilities while the rest of the country's facilities remained at Alert Level 2 (Leota, 2020). Alert Level 3 limits physical interactions, which includes in-person visits, but the DOC is supporting and encouraging increased communication with family members and friends through telephone and video calls, and letters and e-mails. Approximately 15% of incarcerated New Zealanders are in the Auckland facilities (Prison facts and statistics – June 2020, 2020). All out-of-prison work, such as programming and work activities, are suspended in the Auckland facilities. The DOC is taking a "deliberately cautious approach" and making decisions about restrictions and mitigation strategies on a facility-by-facility basis (Leota, 2020). For example, in Alert Level 2 facilities, regular programming and work will continue but with social distancing protocols in place. As of this writing, Auckland prisons remain at Alert Level 2 while the rest of New Zealand's prisons are at Alert Level 1 (DOC, 2020). To facilitate the proper screening of visitors, institutions have implemented thermal cameras to capture temperature prior to entering a facility, as well as provision of medical-grade masks (DOC, 2020).

The Ombudsman's June 2020 report suggests that prisons were providing access to health care at a normal pace and general practitioners continued to visit facilities or provide care via teleconference (Boshier, 2020). Mental health counseling and drug and alcohol treatment continued in virtual or telephonic sessions (Boshier, 2020). A 2012 Ombudsman's investigation found that prisoner's access to health care was "equivalent to that of the general public" but highlighted areas for improvement including the process of requesting health care, wait times, medicine waste, and access to medically assisted substance use treatment and mental health services (Wakem & McGee, 2020, p. 3). Access to health care in New Zealand's prisons has been improving. In 2019, the Department of Corrections received a 128 USD million dollar increase in funding to attend to mental health and substance use concerns (Cheng, 2020).

The DOC began conducting parole hearings by teleconference, totaling nearly 600 during the lockdown and before resuming in person hearings on July 6 (Scoop, 2020b). Another strategy aligned with the larger governmental response of closing borders involved sentence adjustments for foreign detainees (Gay, 2020). In May, eight individuals had their parole revoked, days after it was granted but before they were released from prison, in an effort to avoid deporting potentially exposed people to other countries (Gay, 2020). While a controversial decision, it was in line with the Alert Level 4 guidelines which grounded flights and international travel.

Community corrections are also responding in like fashion. All in-person visits have been suspended and clients are reporting to their officers by phone. Home visits remain authorized, but must be pertinent to the supervision requirements, and staff and clients must engage in proper social distancing and protective measures, such as masks (Leota, 2020). Although the community correction offices are open, they operate with a reduced staff and no clients are able to report in person.

Continuing challenges

As the pandemic continues to surge around the world, New Zealand remains prepared to confront the challenge country-wide, but ongoing problems preceding the pandemic adversely affect the justice-involved population. A primary concern relates to adequate access to health care. While the Ombudsman's recent report suggests a positive degree of health care provided to incarcerated individuals (Boshier, 2020), other officials have been less optimistic about the Ombudsman's equivalence of in-custody care to that of the public. For instance, Deputy Health and Disability Commissioner Kevin Allan stated,

> A person being held in custody does not have the same choices or ability to access health services as a person living in the community. People in custody do not have direct access to over-the-counter medications or to a GP (General Practioner), and are entirely reliant on prison staff to assess, evaluate, monitor, and treat them appropriately (Scoop, 2020).

Data on prison health care in the midst of COVID-19 remain relatively sparse. Looking into prior reports on health care practices of the past may present a realistic view of things to come. According to a report on access to health care in Christchurch Men's Prison was extremely limited, with a backlog of medical requests from individuals waiting to be seen for various medical issues (RNZ, 2020). Attending to medical concerns during incarceration is necessary, as individuals will reenter society, bringing with them new threats of diseases, such as coronavirus, and untreated illnesses and endangering the community to which they return. As health inequities persist amongst the incarcerated populations, their safe return to communities is a critical social justice issue (Enggist et al., 2019). As well as considering the vulnerabilities presented by individuals returning to communities, the New Zealand DOC had previously established relationships with Housing New Zealand to advance resettlement centers in an attempt to also curb homelessness amongst the population returning to their communities (Annual Report – Department of Corrections, 2019).

Another challenge is related to the number of individuals incarcerated on remand, or pre-sentence. Approximately nearly 40% of the prison population in New Zealand is incarcerated while awaiting trial, as shown in Figure 2 (Stats New Zealand, 2020; World Prison Brief, 2020a). In an interview with Chief Justice Dame Helen Winkelmann, she stated,

> The amount of people in remand in prison is unacceptable. Often, they are not even convicted and are simply awaiting trial, they don't have access to rehabilitation so they can often be sentenced and released immediately. This should be a great concern to all of us as a society (RNZ, 2020a).

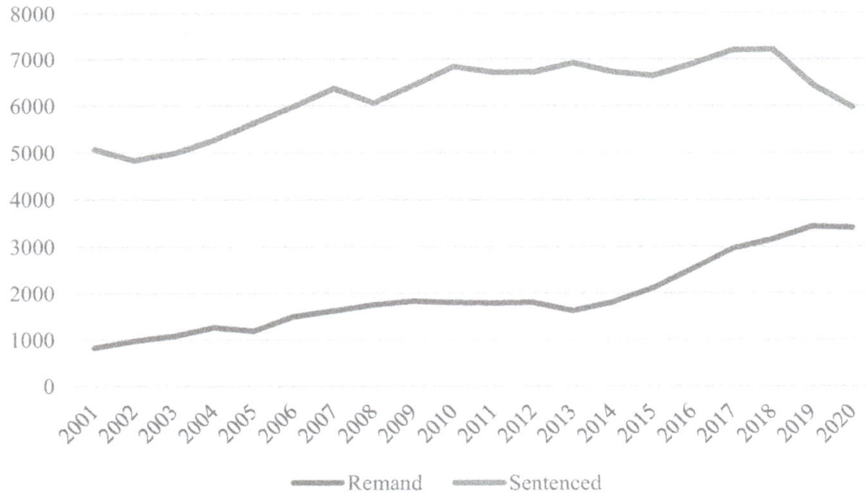

Figure 2. Prisoners in New Zealand: sentenced compared to remand. *Figure from the New Zealand Department of Corrections, Corrections Volume 2019–2020.*

Further, the Chief Justice remarked that one reason for the court backlog is the reliance on "paper trials" and an irrational resistance to digitizing court hearings to establish bail or resolve cases (RNZ, 2020a). And additional category contributing to the incarcerated population are those who are scheduled to be deported. Because the lockdown prohibited entering or exiting the country and the police escort services were postponed, incarcerated individuals scheduled to be deported remain in prison (Wellington District Court Reporter, 2020).

Attending to ethnic disparities among the prison population remains at the forefront who is most susceptible to the coronavirus. Both incarceration and health inequalities are structurally driven challenges exacerbated by a slow response to ameliorate the disparities in sentencing and criminal justice involvement as well as providing adequate access to health care in marginalized communities (Kukutai et al., 2020) Being incarcerated only widens the gap between cultures and leads to further socio-economic disenfranchisement and constrained choice of the returning citizen (Johnsen, 2020; Kukutai et al., 2020).

In particular, the immediate response to limit family visitation in prison facilities serves to avoid possible infection and spread, but is not accompanied by suitable replacement for the family and friend support garnered by visits and other types of contacts. New Zealand prison tensions mount in response to a lack of access to legal advice, rehabilitation, and face to face visits, the prisoners are dependent on the poor and outdated communication infrastructures of the prisons (Block, 2020a). Due to COVID-19 the new restrictions on prison access to outsiders and what appears to be inadequate audio-visual alternatives would disproportionately affect Māori who have less access to modern technology and are adversely affected by economic disparity and poverty (Ministry of Health, 2013). In addition to the lack of outside contact, incarcerated individuals are locked down for as much as 23 hours a day, adding to an already stressed environment (Block, 2020). In an Auckland women's prison, one report suggests incarcerated individuals are remaining in cells for up to 29 hours at a time (Espiner, 2020a).

This concern also stems from what is perceived to be a lack of transparency among correction officials. In an April 2020 report, Chief Ombudsman Peter Boshier indicated he was discouraged by prison officials from coming to facilities (Espiner, 2020b). Boshier reiterated his chief monitoring role in ensuring policies and procedures are followed inside institutions and suggested that the current lockdowns within facilities amounted to solitary confinement and was not a sustainable solution to prevent the spread of coronavirus (Espiner, 2020b).

Advocates are worried about the suspension of prisoner rights during these mandated lockdowns. One of these ways includes not releasing an inmate due to a positive COVID-19 test. While the rationale is to quarantine a potentially infectious person, this decision is at odds with legal rights to release (Espiner, 2020). Similar situations have occurred in pre-trial situations where individuals who have tested positive for COVID-19 are being denied bail. Defense lawyer Douglas Ewen said refusing bail to people suspected of having COVID-19 was not only unlawful but was unsafe, especially given about a third of the country's 10,000 prisoners are double-bunked (Espiner, 2020c).

As in other countries, New Zealand's success in containing the coronavirus is also met with related emerging challenges of being on lockdown. First, economists are preparing New Zealanders for severe economic downturn (Goff, 2020). This form of recession exacerbates economic disparities. For instance, the top 1% of New Zealanders owns 16% of the country's wealth – with the richest 5% owns 38% – while half the population, including beneficiaries and pensioners, earn less than 24,000 USD (Fyers, 2017). Since 2014, polls have consistently shown that New Zealanders rate inequality as the single largest issue facing the country (Inequality.org). The effects of the predicted economic downturn due to COVID-19 combined with the moderate wealth inequality the country already suffers from remains to be seen.

Relatedly, although New Zealand experienced a "chilling effect" on reported crime, police are projecting increases in crime and new class of people involved in criminal behavior: middle-class individuals who have not experienced financial strain and those working in the tourist industry (Ensor, 2020; Ensor & Devlin, 2020). Police speculate these New Zealanders, faced with their new economic circumstances due to reduced commerce and a shut-down tourism industry, will turn to crime to make ends meet (Ensor & Devlin, 2020). Similarly, reports of increased substance use in response to the lockdown have impacted the illegal drug market, which faces challenges meeting demand due to closed borders (Ensor, 2020a). As New Zealand eases its coronavirus containment procedures, it will next face the aftermath of the virus on its citizens.

Conclusion

The swift action of the New Zealand government, including the Department of Corrections, has been credited with the successful suppression of the coronavirus spread. The prioritization of implementing WHO guidelines while doing their best to uphold human rights per the Nelson Mandela Rules serves as an example to others as a model way to address a pandemic, or other contagious disease outbreak, in prisons.

The mitigation efforts of prison officials have largely been tied to isolating individuals and practicing social distancing and hygiene guidance. New Zealand has not announced any plans to release individuals, especially those being held pre-trial, despite the high proportion of unsentenced people. Similarly, correction officials have been challenged by parole, where the board is reluctant to grant release decisions or execute them for public safety reasons. The lack of within-facility population reduction is at odds with current trends in other countries to depopulate as a pandemic prevention measure, as well as to uphold prisoner's rights.

Aside from this critique, New Zealand's leadership had a clear goal not to just contain Coronavirus but to eradicate it from the country all together. An important factor not to be understated is that the citizens of New Zealand trust their government. According to the latest Colmar Brunton poll, 88% of New Zealanders trust their government to make the right choices when it comes to protecting them from the coronavirus (Shaw, 2020). Prime Minister Ardern has been transparent, concise, and clear to the public urging them to shelter in place, saves lives and be kind, and they listened (Shaw, 2020).

This culture of kindness and concern not only extends to the citizenry but seems to appear in the prison culture as well, as correctional and prison staff interact with New Zealand prisoners on a daily basis as frontline workers (Block, 2020). They face the practical challenges of containing the virus within prison walls, while also embodying the caring and concern for human safety and rights necessary for a properly functioning correctional system. While new challenges emerge in the wake of the unknown duration and effect of COVID-19, New Zealand, and its correctional institutions appear to have risen to the task.

Notes

1. As of September 24, 2020.
2. Home detention refers to the entire supervision period occurring at the individual's residence, Community detention refers to electronic monitoring with curfew, and Community work refers to supervision through community service projects (DOC, 2020b).
3. As of September, 24th, 2020. This is with exception of a woman who was imprisoned for refusing medical treatment for a positive COVID test while in the community (Block, 2020b).
4. Alert Level 1: Prepare, the disease is contained; Alert Level 2: Reduce, the disease is contained, but the risk of community transmission remains; Alert Level 3: Restrict, High risk the disease is not contained; Alert Level 4: Lockdown, the disease is not contained (https://covid19.govt.nz/assets/resources/tables/COVID-19-alert-levels-summary.pdf).

Disclosure statement

No potential conflict of interest was reported by the author(s).

ORCID

Laura J. Murray http://orcid.org/0000-0001-6828-5119

References

Adair, J. (2020). *Latest COVID-19 update from chief inspector*. Office of the Inspectorate. https://inspectorate.corrections.govt.nz/news/news_items/latest_covid- 19_update_from_chief_inspector

Annual Report - Department of Corrections. (2019). https://www.corrections.govt.nz/__data/assets/pdf_file/0008/38852/Annual_Report_2018_2019_Web_Version_Final.pdf

Block, G. (2020, May 18). *Coronavirus: The Kiwi corrections officers who helped stop an outbreak of Covid-19*. Stuff. https://www.stuff.co.nz/national/health/coronavirus/300011688/coronavirus-the-kiwi-corrections-officers-who-helped-stop-an-outbreak-of-covid19

Block, G. (2020a, May 8). *Coronavirus: Prison 'timebomb' fears as frustration and boredom build*. https://www.stuff.co.nz/national/300007046/coronavirus-prison-timebomb-fears-as-frustration-and-boredom-build

Block, G. (2020b, March 11). *Coronavirus: Woman jailed for refusing Covid-19 medical examination, tests positive after release from Auckland prison*. Stuff. https://www.stuff.co.nz/national/health/coronavirus/300009845/coronavirus-woman- jailed-for-refusing-covid19-medical-examination-tests-positive-after-release-from- auckland-prison

Boshier, P. (2020, June). *OPCAT COVID-19 report: Report on inspections of prisons under the crimes of torture act 1989*. Office of the Ombudsman.

Boyle, C. (2020, March 26). *Covid 19 coronavirus: Call to lower prison population to combat spread of virus. New Zealand Herald*. https://www.nzherald.co.nz/nz/news/article.cfm?c_id=1&objectid=12319392

Byrne, J., Kras, K. R., & Marmolejo, L. M. (2019). International perspectives on the privatization of corrections. *Criminology & Public Policy*, *18*(2), 477–503. https://doi.org/10.1111/1745-9133.12440

Cave, D., & Solomon, S. (2020, August 13). *New Zealand beat the virus once. Can it do it again? The New York Times*. https://www.nytimes.com/2020/08/13/world/asia/new-zealand-coronavirus-lockdown-elimination.html?campaign_id=9

Cheng, D. (2020). *Covid 19 coronavirus: Virus-positive ... - nzherald.co.nz*. Horrible sense of déjà vu over Government border blunders. https://www.nzherald.co.nz/nz/news/article.cfm?c_id=1&objectid=12331137

Community-based sentence and order facts and statistics - June 2020. (2020, July 29). *Department of corrections*. https://www.corrections.govt.nz/resources/research_and_statistics/community_sentences_and_orders/community_stats_june_2020

Department of Corrections. (2020). https://www.corrections.govt.nz/.
Department of Corrections. (2020a). *Auckland South correctional facility*. https://www.corrections.govt.nz/about_us/getting_in_touch/our_locations/auckland_sout h_corrections_facility
Department of Corrections. (2020b). *Corrections volume 2020*. https://www.corrections.govt.nz/__data/assets/pdf_file/0016/41191/Corrections_Volumes _2020.pdf
Devlin, B. (2020, July 25). *Coronavirus: Police predict the emergence of a new group of criminals post Covid-19*. Retrieved September 07, 2020, from https://www.stuff.co.nz/national/crime/122223019/coronavirus-police-predict-the-emergence-of-a-new-group-of-criminals-post-covid19
Enggist, S., Møller, S., Galea, G., & Udesen, C. (2019). *Prisons and health*. World Health Organization. https://www.euro.who.int/__data/assets/pdf_file/0005/249188/Prisons-and- Health.pdf?ua=1
Ensor, B. (2020, April 23). *Coronavirus: Reported crime is well down but police fear hidden cases - and a post-Covid-19 lockdown surge*. Stuff. https://www.stuff.co.nz/national/crime/121205785/coronavirus-reported-crime-is-well-down-but-police-fear-hidden-cases–and-a-postcovid19-lockdown-surge
Ensor, B. (2020a, May 13). *Coronavirus: Meth prices double in parts of New Zealand during Covid-19 lockdown*. Stuff. https://www.stuff.co.nz/national/crime/121494987/coronavirus-meth-prices-double-in-parts-of-new-zealand-during-covid19-lockdown?rm=a
Ensor, B., & Devlin, C. (2020, July 26). *Coronavirus: Police predict the emergence of a new group of criminals post Covid-19*. Stuff. https://www.stuff.co.nz/national/crime/122223019/coronavirus-police-predict-the-emergence-of-a-new-group-of-criminals-post-covid19
Espiner, G. (2020, April 16). *Recommendations to push back release of virus-risk prisoners condemned*. https://www.rnz.co.nz/news/national/414370/recommendations-to-push- back-release-of-virus-risk-prisoners-condemned
Espiner, G. (2020a, May 1). *Covid-19: Prisoners confined to cells for up to 29 hours, diary shows*. https://www.rnz.co.nz/news/national/415563/covid-19-prisoners-confined-to- cells-for-up-to-29-hours-diary-shows
Espiner, G. (2020b, April 24). *Ombudsman 'discouraged' from accessing prisons amidst Covid- 19 lockdown concerns*. https://www.rnz.co.nz/news/in-depth/415026/ombudsman- discouraged-from -accessing-prisons-amidst-covid-19-lockdown-concerns
Espiner, G. (2020c, April 22). *Concerns prisons will turn into Covid-19 'quarantine facilities'*. https://www.rnz.co.nz/news/in-depth/414834/concerns-prisons-will-turn-into-covid-19- quarantine-facilities
Forbes, M. (2020, March 29). *Coronavirus: No plans to release low-risk prisoners during COVID-19 crisis. News Hub*. https://www.newshub.co.nz/home/new- zealand/2020/03/coronavirus-no-plans-to-release-low-risk-prisoners-during-covid-19- crisis.html
Fyers, A. (2017, January 17). *The truth about inequality in New Zealand*. Stuff. https://www.stuff.co.nz/business/88455171/the-truth-about-inequality-in-new-zealand
Gay, E. (2020, April 11). *Coronavirus: Parole revoked for eight foreign prisoners due to leave New Zealand*. Stuff. https://www.stuff.co.nz/national/crime/120949523/coronavirus- parole-revoked-for-eight-foreign-prisoners-due-to-leave-new-zealand
Godin, M. (2020, August 14). *Can New Zealand contain its new coronavirus outbreak?* Time. https://time.com/5879177/new-zealand-coronavirus-cases/?utm_source=newsletter
Goff, P. (2020, May 28). *Coronavirus: Auckland's greatest challenge is still to come*. Stuff. https://www.stuff.co.nz/national/300023199/coronavirus-aucklands-greatest-challenge-is-still-to-come
Johnsen, M. (2020, April 21). *Government's Māori Covid-19 response all words, no action - response group*. RNZ. https://www.rnz.co.nz/news/te-manu-korihi/414667/government-s-maori-covid-19-response-all-words-no-action-response-group
Kukutai, T., Moewaka Barnes, H., McCreanor, T., & Mcintosh, T. (2020, September 6). *Recession hits Māori and Pasifika harder. They must be part of planning New Zealand's COVID-19 recovery*. The Conversation. https://theconversation.com/recession-hits-maori-and-pasifika-harder-they-must-be-part-of-planning-new-zealands-covid-19-recovery-137763
Leota, R. (2020, August 13). *COVID-19 alert level 2 and 3: Corrections update*. Department of corrections. https://www.corrections.govt.nz/news/2020/update_on_corrections_moving_to_covid- 19_alert_level_4

Ministry of Health. (2013). *Socioeconomic indicators, by gender, Māori and non-Māori, 2013.* https://www.health.govt.nz/our-work/populations/maori-health/tatau-kahukura- maori-health-statistics/nga-awe-o-te-hauora-socioeconomic-determinants- health/socioeconomic-indicators

Ministry of Health New Zealand. (2020). *COVID-19: Current issues.* https://www.health.govt.nz/our-work/diseases-and-conditions/covid-19-novel- coronavirus/covid-19-current-situation/covid-19-current-cases

O'Grady, S., & Farzan, A. N. (2020, September 21). *New Zealand, an early success story, set to ease most restrictions once again as second outbreak slows. Washington Post.* https://www.washingtonpost.com/world/2020/09/21/new-zealand-an-early-success-story- set-ease-most-restrictions-once-again-second-outbreak-slows/

Prison facts and statistics - June 2020. (2020, July 29). *Department of corrections.* https://www.corrections.govt.nz/resources/research_and_statistics/quarterly_prison_statistics/prison_stats_june_2020

RNZ. (2020, April 6). *Covid 19 coronavirus: Prisoners in cells up to 23 hours a day.* New Zealand Herald. https://www.nzherald.co.nz/nz/news/article.cfm?c_id=1&objectid=12322673

RNZ. (2020a, June 17). *NZ's high number of remand prisoners 'unacceptable' - Chief justice.* https://www.rnz.co.nz/news/national/419207/nz-s-high-number-of-remand-prisoners- unacceptable-chief-justice

Scoop. (2020, February 17). *Inadequate medical care of a prison inmate.* https://www.scoop.co.nz/stories/AK2002/S00371/inadequate-medical-care-of-a-prison- inmate.htm

Scoop. (2020b, July 7). *Parole hearings return to prisons.* Scoop. https://www.scoop.co.nz/stories/PO2007/S00075/parole-hearings-return-to-prisons.htm

Shaw, R. (2020, April 14). *Coronavirus: Trust in government is high in New Zealand, but will it last until the election?* Stuff. https://www.stuff.co.nz/national/politics/opinion/120999344/coronavirus-trust-in-government-is-high-in-new-zealand-but-will-it-last-until-the-election

Shepherd, M. (2020, August 10). *How geography helped New Zealand beat coronavirus.* Forbes. https://www.forbes.com/sites/marshallshepherd/2020/08/10/how-geography-helped-new-zealand-beat-coronavirus/

Stats New Zealand. (2020). *NZ Stat.* http://nzdotstat.stats.govt.nz/wbos/Index.aspx?_ga=2.234880990.1530601590.1534467838-1884899923.1534467838

Wakem, & McGee (2020). *ombudsmen act 1975 - legislation.govt.nz.* http://www.legislation.govt.nz/act/public/1975/0009/latest/096be8ed819f9dec.pdf

Wellington District Court Reporter. (2020, April 30). *Coronavirus: Deportees are sitting in prison cells after police cancel escort duties.* Stuff. https://www.stuff.co.nz/national/crime/121152913/coronavirus-deportees-are-sitting-in-prison-cells-after-police-cancel-escort-duties

Witton, B. (2020, June 26). *Rimutaka Prison: Inmates still can't hug family and children in 'mind-boggling' rule.* Stuff. https://www.stuff.co.nz/national/health/coronavirus/121923450/rimutaka-prison-inmates-still-cant-hug-family-and-children-in-mindboggling-rule

World Health Organization. (2020). *New Zealand takes early and hard action to tackle COVID-19.* https://www.who.int/westernpacific/news/feature-stories/detail/new-zealand- takes-early-and-hard-action-to-tackle-covid-19

World Prison Brief. (2020). *COVID-19 in prisons – A major public health risk.* COVID-19 in prisons – a major public health risk | https://www.prisonstudies.org/news/covid-19-prisons-–major-public-health-risk.

World Prison Brief. (2020a). *New Zealand.* https://www.prisonstudies.org/country/new-zealand

www.dw.com, D. W. (2020). *Coronavirus: 5 things New Zealand got right: DW: 08. 06.2020.* DW.COM. https://www.dw.com/en/jacinda-ardern-leadership-in-coronavirus-response/a-53733397

Index

Notes: This has the reference of figures as "Italics" and tables as "Bold".

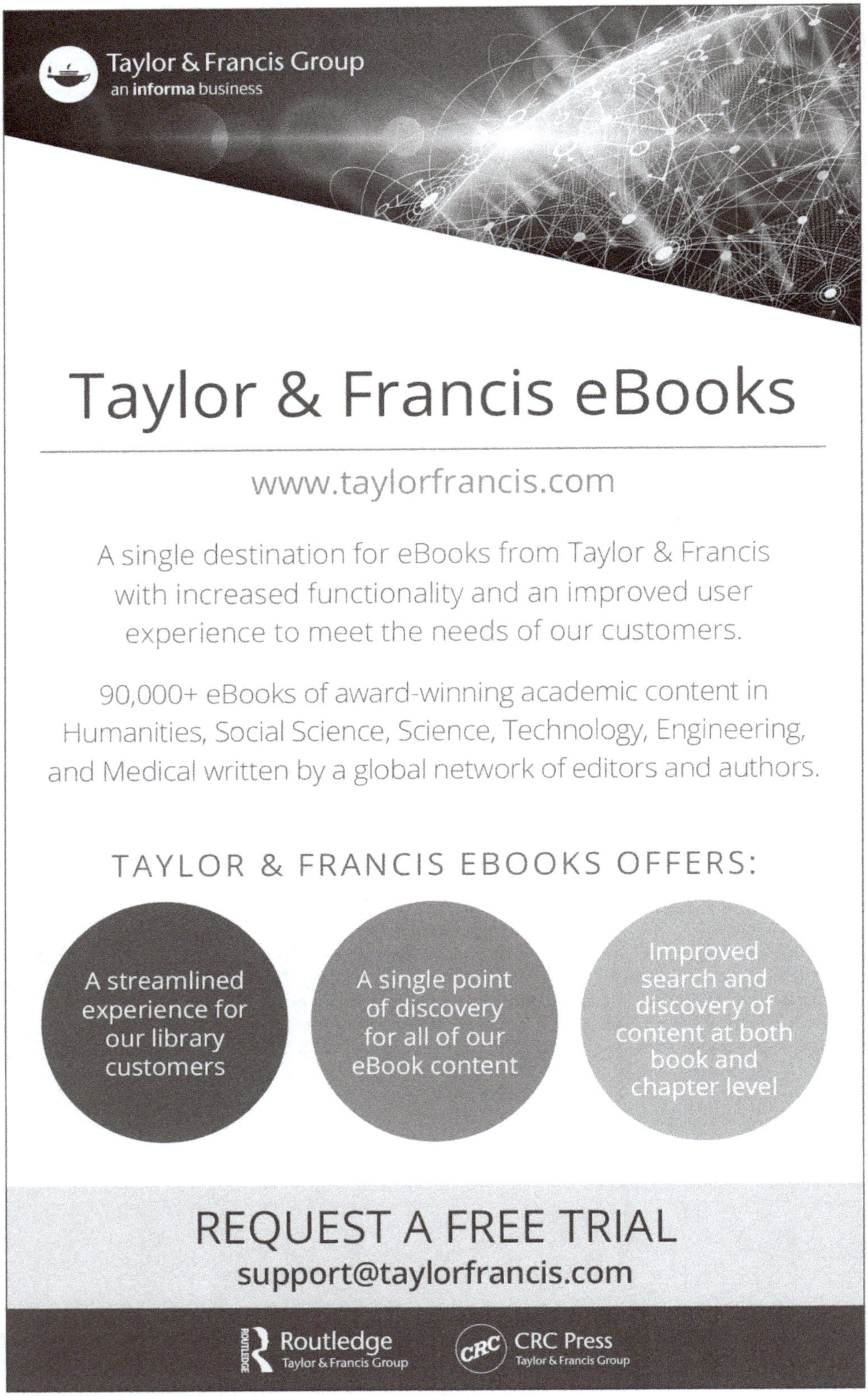
Taylor & Francis Group
an informa business
Taylor & Francis eBooks
www.taylorfrancis.com
A single destination for eBooks from Taylor & Francis with increased functionality and an improved user experience to meet the needs of our customers.
90,000+ eBooks of award-winning academic content in Humanities, Social Science, Science, Technology, Engineering, and Medical written by a global network of editors and authors.
TAYLOR & FRANCIS EBOOKS OFFERS:
A streamlined experience for our library customers
A single point of discovery for all of our eBook content
Improved search and discovery of content at both book and chapter level
REQUEST A FREE TRIAL
support@taylorfrancis.com
Routledge
Taylor & Francis Group
CRC Press
Taylor & Francis Group

Lightning Source UK Ltd.
Milton Keynes UK
UKHW030715270422
402119UK00005B/263

9 781032 014913